Prefix
MTW

0104198

KT-385-014

THE LIBRARY
KENT & SUSSEX HOSPITAL
TUNBRIDGE WELLS
KENT TN1 8AT

PATHOPHYSIOLOGY:
AN ESSENTIAL TEXT FOR THE ALLIED HEALTH PROFESSIONS

vn

15

201ʳ

For Elsevier:

Senior Commissioning Editor: Heidi Harrison
Development Editor: Siobhan Campbell
Project Manager: Joannah Duncan
Designer: George Ajayi
Illustration Manager: Bruce Hogarth
Illustrator: Ethan Danielson

PATHOPHYSIOLOGY:
AN ESSENTIAL TEXT FOR THE ALLIED HEALTH PROFESSIONS

Edited by

Delva Shamley PhD

Senior Lecturer in Physiotherapy and Assistant Director for Research, School of Health and Social Care, Oxford Brookes University, Oxford, UK

Foreword by

Louis Gifford MAppSc BSc FCSP

Private Practitioner, Falmouth Physiotherapy Clinic, Cornwall, UK

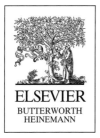

ELSEVIER
BUTTERWORTH
HEINEMANN

Edinburgh London New York Oxford Philadelphia St Louis Sydney Toronto 2005

A 052134

Q2 140

THE LIBRARY
KENT & SUSSEX HOSPITAL
TUNBRIDGE WELLS
KENT TN4 8AT

ELSEVIER
BUTTERWORTH
HEINEMANN

© 2005, Elsevier Limited. All rights reserved.

No part of this publication may be reproduced, stored in a retrieval system, or transmitted in any form or by any means, electronic, mechanical, photocopying, recording or otherwise, without either the prior permission of the publishers or a licence permitting restricted copying in the United Kingdom issued by the Copyright Licensing Agency, 90 Tottenham Court Road, London W1T 4LP. Permissions may be sought directly from Elsevier's Health Sciences Rights Department in Philadelphia, USA: phone: (+1) 215 238 7869, fax: (+1) 215 238 2239, e-mail: healthpermissions@elsevier.com. You may also complete your request on-line via the Elsevier Science homepage (http://www.elsevier.com), by selecting 'Customer Support' and then 'Obtaining Permissions'.

First published 2005

ISBN 0 7506 5234 9

British Library Cataloguing in Publication Data
A catalogue record for this book is available from the British Library

Library of Congress Cataloging in Publication Data
A catalog record for this book is available from the Library of Congress

Notice
Knowledge and best practice in this field are constantly changing. As new research and experience broaden our knowledge, changes in practice, treatment and drug therapy may become necessary or appropriate. Readers are advised to check the most current information provided (i) on procedures featured or (ii) by the manufacturer of each product to be administered, to verify the recommended dose or formula, the method and duration of administration, and contraindications. It is the responsibility of the practitioner, relying on their own experience and knowledge of the patient, to make diagnoses, to determine dosages and the best treatment for each individual patient, and to take all appropriate safety precautions. To the fullest extent of the law, neither the publisher nor the editors assumes any liability for any injury and/or damage.

The Publisher

Working together to grow
libraries in developing countries

www.elsevier.com | www.bookaid.org | www.sabre.org

ELSEVIER   **BOOK AID**
International   Sabre Foundation

ELSEVIER   your source for books,
journals and multimedia
in the health sciences
www.elsevierhealth.com

The
Publisher's
policy is to use
**paper manufactured
from sustainable forests**

Printed in China

Contents

THE LIBRARY
KENT & SUSSEX HOSPITAL
TUNBRIDGE WELLS
KENT TN4 8AT

Foreword

When I trained as a physiotherapist in the early 1980s pathophysiology regularly shifted from being on one hand a necessary evil, and on the other a sometimes fascinating insight into some of the disorders that were treated. Much of the time, the pure pathophysiology studied appeared remote from the practical application of 'physical' therapy to patients on hospital wards and in the departments. I can recall witnessing a great many excellent physiotherapists skilfully guide bed-ridden patients from postoperative misery and fear to confident mastery of movement and healthy laughter – often within minutes. Back then it seemed that the best part of the job, after recording and measuring what the patient had difficulty doing or could not do, was to get people moving, to instil confidence and to give healthy guidance with exercises appropriate to the impairments revealed.

Early in my first year of qualifying I treated a patient who had chronic neck and arm pain. His presentation, along with a great many others like him, had a significant impact on my career and my subsequent thinking and reasoning. He was in his 50s and had been off work for 3 years. He described his pain quite dramatically as 'knives digging into my shoulder blade', 'electric shocks shooting from my shoulder to my hand', 'swelling feelings and throbbing in the hand' and a great deal more. I spent an hour listening and examining him, he could hardly move his neck or his arm without wincing or squirming with pain, I could barely touch him, everything was incredibly hypersensitive. No teacher, no book, no lecture had ever described this or prepared me for it. Then he said, 'You are the first person who has really listened to me and taken an interest in my problem, I've seen doctors, specialists, physios, chiropractors and many others and they've not really listened, they've told me all sorts of different things: spondylosis, wear and tear, locked joints, "inflamed nerves" and more and more frequently it's been "psychological" and stress'. Then he said, 'What do you think causes this, or is it really something in my mind?' I could not answer his question, I hadn't a clue. It made me angry to be put in a situation with a patient like this and to not have any reasonable answers for him, or for me! All I really knew about were 'treatments' like electrotherapy and mobilisations where the prime concerns were target identity and the skills of application, and physical examinations which basically revealed and measured lost function and impairments. So the confused and pain riddled patient got my stuttering response: 'It's most likely coming from your neck', and by avoiding eye contact for a moment or two and getting on with a tentative treatment to his neck, I managed to dodge the question and survive. The answer was nowhere near good enough – he knew it, and I knew it. I also knew that I had either better come up with some better and more useful explanations, or learn a few more phrases that would help me comfortably dodge questions asked!

If I think back and reflect on the core driving force throughout my career as a clinician and teacher/lecturer/writer it has been two-fold: firstly, it has been to simply know and be able to explain the relevant science that can help answer questions like those posed by the patient described with his chronic neck pain. This is still a hugely challenging area that requires more input. For example, if we know that healing of collagenous tissue (see Chapter 1 and a great deal of Section 2) is impressively slow, why is it that acute back or neck pain following some sort of trauma can often recover within a few days? Discs don't suddenly heal up, yet many clinical paradigms over the years have focused on the disc as a 'likely' primary cause. It just does not seem to fit, which brings me to the second of my driving forces: to feel comfortable with the underlying scientific rationale of all management, treatment and rehabilitation approaches that physiotherapists use. If I am doing something with or to a patient I want to be able to answer their simple and reasonable question, 'what does this do?' and other questions like, 'is it safe to start ... bending, lifting, walking, swimming, etc...?'

Approaching 25 years into my career, though still very challenging, it is generally much more possible to rationally and reasonably answer virtually any question a patient may ask about their condition! For example, why pain behaves the way it does, what caused it, what predisposes to it, what helps it recover, how it recovers, the likely time course of recovery of the tissues and their often complicated relationship to pain, what factors might influence recovery; whether it might be safe to start loading and getting function back; why movement is helpful; the types of movement that are helpful; how fear, anxiety, anger, confidence, well-being, positive and negative thinking, optimism, pessimism, acceptance, coping, stress can impact positive or negative physiological processes or behaviours; and a great many more.

For the reasons already given, my own study and my own interest has taken me into the medical sciences related to pain physiology and pathophysiology; neuroplasticity, memory and learning; psychoneuroimmunology; tissue inflammation and healing; stress and endocrinology; circulation and training effects on the cardiovascular and peripheral circulatory systems; bone, cartilage, muscle, tendon and ligament metabolism, healing, training and health; ageing; the detrimental effects of immobilisation; the peripheral nervous system – from understanding transduction and impulse propagation, to its special adaptations to movement and its nutritional requirements. Many congratulations to Delva Shamley and all her contributing colleagues. This impressive book contains a great deal from this list and a great deal more. To me, what is contained here is essential, it's for your confidence, it's for the sake of the future of rational management and treatment approaches, it's for all of our profession's standing and recognition, but above all it's for the patient and it should not be kept a secret or forgotten once we are qualified. My passion is not just to know it and understand it but also to be able to translate it into realistic and meaningful, positive messages and treatments for those who suffer yet who have the capacity to manage better, improve or completely overcome their problem. Read it, study it, think about it, use it and continuously re-refer to it!

Louis Gifford
Chartered Physiotherapist, UK, 2005

Contributors

Karen Barker, MSc, PhD, MCSP
Head of Physiotherapy, Nuffield Orthopaedic Centre NHS Trust, Headington, Oxford OX3 7LD, UK

Susan A. Brooks, PhD
Senior Lecturer in Cell Biology, School of Biological and Molecular Sciences, Oxford Brookes University, Gypsy Lane, Headington, Oxford OX3 0BP, UK

R. Chen
Human Cortical Physiology Section and Human Motor Control Section, Medical Neurology Branch, National Institutes of Neurological Disorders and Stroke, National Institutes of Health Building 10, Room 5N226, 10 Center Drive MSC 1428, Bethesda, MD 20892-1428, USA

L.G. Cohen, MD
Director, Human Cortical Physiology Section, National Institute of Neurological Disorders and Stroke, National Institutes of Health, Building 10, Room 5N226, 10 Center Drive MSC 1428, Bethesda, MD 20892-1428, USA

Richard Craven, BSc (Hons), PhD
Principal Lecturer in Physiology, School of Biological and Molecular Sciences, Oxford Brookes University, Gypsy Lane, Headington, Oxford OX3 0BP, UK

Mary Dyson, PhD, FCSP (Hon), FAIUM (Hon)
Emeritus Reader in Biology of Tissue Repair, GKT School of Biomedical Sciences (KCL), Guy's Campus, London Bridge, London SE1 1UL, UK
(now retired)

Lukas Foggensteiner, BSc, BM, MRCP, PhD
Consultant Nephrologist, Renal Unit, Queen Elizabeth Hospital, Birmingham B15 2TH, UK

M. Hallett, MD
Chief, Human Motor Control Section, Medical Neurology Branch, National Institute of Neurological Disorders and Stroke, National Institutes of Health, Building 10, Room 5N226, 10 Center Drive MSC 1428, Bethesda, MD 20892-1428, USA

Alex Hough, PhD
Respiratory Clinical Specialist Physiotherapist, East Sussex Hospitals NHS Trust, Eastbourne, UK

W. John Kalk, MB, BCh, FRCP (Lond)
Lead Clinician, Diabetes and Endocrinology, Diabetes Centre, Derbyshire Royal Infirmary, London Road, Derby DE1 2QY, UK

Udo Kischka, MD
Consultant Neurologist, Oxford Centre for Enablement, NOC, Windmill Road, Oxford, OX3 7LD, UK and Visiting Professor, University of Hertfordshire, Hatfield, UK

Sue Madden, PhD, BSc (Hons), MCSP
Senior Lecturer Physiotherapy, School of Health and Social Care, Oxford Brookes University, 58 London Road, Headington, Oxford OX7 3PE, UK

Carolyn Mason, Cert Ed EdD, BA (Hons), GradDip Phys, MCSP, SRP
Senior Lecturer, Physiotherapy, School of Health and Social Care, Oxford Brookes University, 58 London Road, Headington, Oxford OX7 3PE, UK

Jacek L. Mostwin, MD, DPhil (Oxon)
Professor of Urology, Johns Hopkins Hospital, Baltimore, Maryland 21287-2411, USA

Mohi Rezvani, BSc, MSc, PhD
Reader in Radiobiology and Director, Research Institute, University of Oxford, Churchill Hospital, Oxford OX3 7LJ, UK

Christine M. Schnitzler, MD, FRCS (Edin)
Professorial Research Fellow, MRC Mineral Metabolism Research Unit, University of the Witwatersrand, Johannesburg, South Africa

Delva Shamley, PhD, MCSP
Senior Lecturer in Physiotherapy and Assistant Director for Research, School of Health and Social Care, Oxford Brookes University, 58 London Road, Headington, Oxford OX7 3PE, UK

Mel Siff, PhD (deceased)

Leif Rune Skymoen MSc (Pharm)
Pharkin AS, Olaf Schous vei 18, N-0572, Oslo, Norway

Sue Syndica-Drummond, BSc (Hons) Physiotherapy
Senior Lecturer, Physiotherapy, School of Health and Social Care, Oxford Brookes University, 58 London Road, Headington, Oxford OX7 3PE, UK

Derek G. Waller, BSc (Hons), DM, MB, BS (Hons), FRCP
Consultant Cardiovascular Physician and Senior Lecturer in Medicine and Clinical Pharmacology, Southampton General Hospital, Mail Point 47, Tremona Road, Southampton SO16 6YD, UK

Angela J. Woodiwiss, BSc, BSc Physiotherapy, MSc, PhD
Associate Professor, School of Physiology, University of the Witwatersrand, Medical School, 7 York Road, Parktown 2193, Johannesburg, Gauteng, South Africa

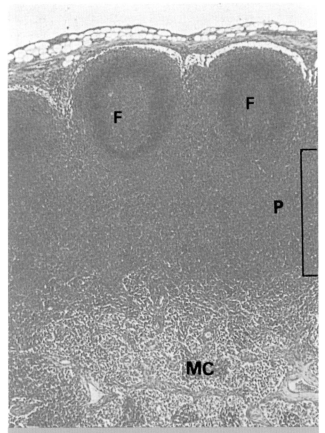

Plate I. Histology of a lymph node. (Reproduced with permission from Young and Heath, 2000).

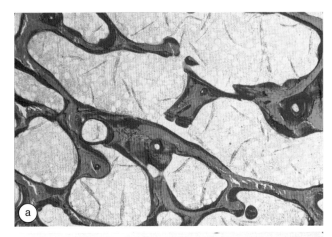

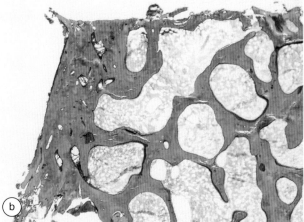

Plate III. Photomicrographs of osteomalacic (a) and normal bone (b). An abnormally large proportion of the osteomalacic bone (a) consists of osteoid, i.e. unmineralized bone matrix (osteoid in red; mineralized bone in green, and bone marrow in lighter colours; Masson–Goldner trichrome stain of undecalcified bone). Although the osteomalacic bone shows fairly well-preserved trabecular connectivity, the bone is weak because its mineralized portion (green), on which structural integrity depends, lacks connectivity.

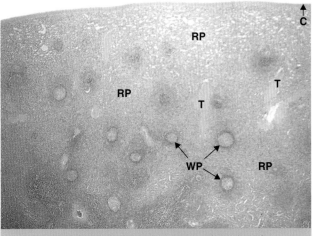

Plate II. Histology of spleen. (Reproduced with permission from Young and Heath, 2000.)

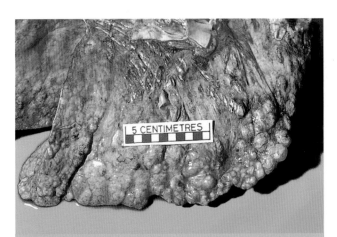

Plate IV. Emphysema. This is severe emphysematous change characterized by large bullae at the pleural surface. (Reproduced with permission from Underwood, 2000.)

AN INTRODUCTION TO DISEASE PROCESSES

Section **1**

Inflammation, Wounds and Wound Healing

Mary Dyson

1

Inflammation is the response of vascularized living tissue to trauma and infection. It is triggered by a wide range of adverse events including incision, excision, tissue necrosis other than apoptosis, excessive heat, cold and pressure, irritant and corrosive chemicals, and most infections, exceptions being Creutzfeldt–Jakob disease and opportunistic infections in AIDS. A tissue-based 'startle' reaction to trauma and infection, it progresses by a series of steps each of which is controlled by molecular signals. Inflammation provides a vigilant and vital involuntary defence against injury and attack by pathogens. The cardinal signs of inflammation are, according to Celsus, a physician of Rome at around AD40, *calor* (heat), *rubor* (redness), *tumor* (swelling) and *dolor* (pain). A fifth cardinal sign *functio laesa* (loss of function) was added much later by Virchow. Today much more is known about inflammation, but still not enough. When subject to precise regulation it initiates wound healing and can be life-saving, but if this regulation is lost it causes morbidity and can be life-threatening. Persistent inflammation arrests wound healing and can damage DNA sufficiently badly to promote neoplastic transformation.

Inflammation is generally localized to living tissue adjacent to the site of injury. Such inflammation is termed *acute* if it rapidly initiates the rest of the healing process, or *chronic* if it does not. Chronic inflammation must be replaced by acute inflammation for healing to occur. The most severe type of inflammation, *whole body inflammation*, has no role in wound healing. It produces multiple organ failure. During it cytokines (non-antibody proteins that act as intercellular mediators) leak into the bloodstream, more free radicals are produced than can be neutralized by free radical scavengers, local ischaemia kills tissues, and leakage of heatshock proteins can lead to irreversible shock and death.

Acute inflammation is the normal response of healthy tissue to injury. It is regulated by cellular activity, which results in the release of growth factors and other cytokines, the latter including interleukins. Recently a neural pathway that reflexively monitors and adjusts the inflammatory response has been identified.

If, as is usual, there has been damage to blood vessels, then oedema and temporary haemostasis involving blood clotting occur. Following this, debris and necrotic tissue are cleared from the wound site and growth factors are released which initiate the proliferative phase of healing. Proliferation, which overlaps with and then follows acute inflammation, results in the formation and growth of either a blastema or granulation tissue. A blastema differentiates into replacement tissues identical to those present at the wound site prior to injury, producing regeneration. In contrast, granulation tissue develops into highly collagenous scar tissue, repairing the wound rapidly but in doing so inhibiting regeneration.

Acute inflammation is self-limiting in time and space. It is not a disease, but an essential part of the healing process. In contrast, chronic inflammation, which is not self-limiting, is a disease which must be resolved and replaced by acute inflammation if wound healing is to proceed successfully.

ACUTE INFLAMMATION

Acute inflammation usually lasts for 3–7 days. It is a vital part of the healing process. It is induced and controlled by prostaglandins and other chemical mediators of inflammation. The information flow involved in its control is illustrated in Figure 1.1.

During acute inflammation oedema and blood clotting usually occur, the injury site is cleared of debris, bacteria are killed by the neutrophils, and pro-inflammatory cytokines and growth factors are secreted. These growth factors are low-molecular-weight polypeptides whose main collective function is to initiate and control the proliferative phase of repair; the macrophage is a key cell in their production.

Acute inflammation is generally subdivided into early and late phases for descriptive convenience. The early phase includes those activities induced by injury that result in haemostasis and produce local oedema, vasodilatation and pain. The late phase consists of the recruitment and activation of inflammatory cells.

Early inflammation

The early part of inflammation is under the control of *inflammatory mediators*. These include:

1. Vasoactive amines such as histamine and serotonin, both derived from mast cells and platelets, which signal changes resulting in immediate oedema.

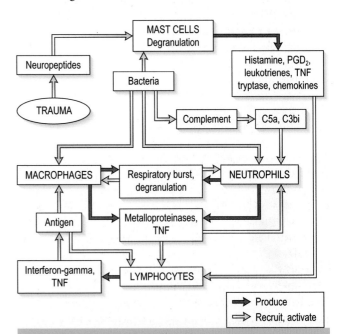

Figure 1.1.   Information flow during acute inflammation, excluding that involved in haemostasis. The different cell types involved recruit and activate other cells, after receiving multiple chemical signals. Collectively they amplify inflammation. (After Nathan, 2002.)

2. Components of the complement system (see Ch. 2):
   - the anaphylatoxins C3a and C5a that bind to mast cells and cause them to liberate histamine
   - the opsonin C3b
   - the membrane-damaging complex C5b-9.
3. The kinin system, a group of proteins that produce bradykinin, which increases vascular permeability, dilates blood vessels and causes pain.
4. Prostaglandins, products of the cyclo-oxygenase pathway of arachidonic acid metabolism. They include:
   - thromboxane A2 (TXA_2), a platelet product that aggregates platelets and constricts blood vessels
   - prostacyclin (PGI_2), from blood vessel walls; it prevents platelet aggregation and dilates blood vessels
   - prostaglandin E (PGE), perhaps the most potent vasodilator.
5. Leukotrienes, products of the lipo-oxygenase pathway of arachidonic acid metabolism. Formerly known as slow-reacting substances (SRSs), they are produced by all the inflammatory cells except lymphocytes and include:
   - leukotriene C4 and its products D4 and E4, which increase vascular permeability
   - leukotriene B4, which is a powerful chemoattractant and makes neutrophils adhere to endothelium.
6. Other pro-inflammatory cytokines, polypeptide mediators released by platelets, mast cells, inflammatory cells and other cells. They include:
   - tumour necrosis factor-alpha (TNF-α); made by macrophages, this amplifies and prolongs the inflammatory response by stimulating the release of inflammatory mediators from other cells
   - interleukin-1 alpha (IL-1α)
   - interleukin-1 beta (IL-1β)
   - interleukin-6 (IL-6).
7. Inorganic inflammatory mediators such as nitric oxide and reactive oxygen species.
8. The clotting system (see below).

In recent years new non-steroidal anti-inflammatory drugs (NSAIDs), some of which are non-selective cyclo-oxygenase (COX) inhibitors whereas others inhibit either COX-1 or COX-2 selectively, have been developed. This has allowed the effects on inflammation and proliferation of these isoforms of COX and their principal products, prostaglandins D_2 and E_2 (PGD_2 and PGE_2), to be explored. In an excised wound model, COX-1 inhibition brings about increased production of TNF-α, which has an adverse effect on healing, with a reduction in re-epithelialization and the loss of granulation tissue. Inflammation can be suppressed by the application of the COX-2 inhibitor celecoxib; this is followed by reduced formation of granulation tissue and less scarring without compromising tensile strength, a clear indication that what happens during inflammation affects subsequent changes in the healing wound.

The totality of the wound healing process is largely regulated by the ordered production of cytokines that control the gene activation responsible for cell migration, proliferation and synthesis. The release of the various cytokines is regulated by changes in the tissue environment.

Haemostasis

If the endothelial lining of any vessel is breached, potentially vital blood clotting and haemostasis follow rapidly. Haemostasis includes blood clotting, which is accompanied by oedema, and followed by the emigration of leucocytes from the microcirculation into the oedematous tissue.

Haemostasis consists of the following major events:

- *Temporary vasoconstriction*. This reduces bleeding by limiting the flow of blood to the injured tissue; it is under neural control.
- *Blood clotting or coagulation*. This takes place by either intrinsic or extrinsic biochemical pathways involving proteinaceous clotting factors. The intrinsic pathway occurs in response to vascular abnormalities in the absence of tissue injury. The extrinsic pathway occurs in the presence of tissue injury. Both converge onto a common pathway, producing a blood clot. This pathway consists of three stages: (1) platelet activation; (2) stabilization of the platelet plug; and (3) red thrombus formation.

1. Platelet activation. This is induced when thrombin binds to specific receptors on the surface of platelets, initiating a signal transduction cascade leading to the release of intracellular Ca^{2+} and the activation of the enzymes phospholipase A_2, protein kinase C (PKC), and myosin light chain kinase (MLCK). Phospholipase A_2 hydrolyses membrane phospholipids, resulting in the liberation of arachidonic acid, which is followed by increased production and release of thromboxane A_2, another platelet activator. One of the many actions of PKC is the phosphorylation of a platelet protein that induces platelet degranulation, and the release of adenosine diphosphate (ADP) and the other contents of the granules. ADP stimulates the activation of more platelets. MLCK phosphorylates the light chain of myosin, which then interacts with actin within the platelets, changing their motility and morphology. The surface of the platelets becomes adhesive, causing them to stick to the collagen exposed when the endothelium ruptures. This is mediated by von Willebrand factor (vWF), a glycoprotein produced by the platelets and stored in their granules. When released, vWF acts as a link between collagen and a specific glycoprotein on the surface of the platelets, which also adhere to each other, forming a loose platelet clump. When the platelets degranulate, they release, in addition to the ADP and vWF described above, serotonin, phospholipids, lipoproteins and other proteins. Surface phospholipids of activated platelets play an important role in the activation of the cascade of biochemical events which results in coagulation. Activated platelets also secrete a plethora of growth factors including:

- platelet-derived growth factor (PDGF)
- epidermal growth factor (EGF)

- heparin-binding epidermal growth factor (HB-EGF)
- insulin-like growth factor-1 (IGF-1)
- transforming growth factor-β (TGF-β).

These growth factors are chemotactic, attracting neutrophils and macrophages to the wound site. They also stimulate cell division and the synthesis of matrix components by fibroblasts.

2. Stabilization of the platelet plug. ADP released from activated platelets modifies the platelet membrane in a manner that allows fibrinogen to link together two platelet surface glycoproteins, termed GPIIb and GPIIIa, resulting in fibrinogen-induced platelet aggregation. Fibrinogen is also converted to fibrin, a fibrous protein that polymerizes within the platelet plug, strengthening it and producing a stable three-dimensional network, the fibrin clot or white thrombus.

3. Red thrombus formation. The fibrin clot traps erythrocytes and other blood cells, producing a red thrombus. This usually stops further bleeding and provides a temporary or provisional matrix through which cells can migrate during late inflammation and the proliferative phase of healing in response to the growth factors retained in the clot.

Oedema formation

Vessels of the microcirculation in the intact tissue adjacent to the injury dilate and flow within them slows down (Fig. 1.2). Chemical mediators of acute inflammation cause the endothelial cells to swell and retract, so that they no longer line the vessels completely. The permeability of the vessels therefore increases. Water, electrolytes and some small proteins including fibrinogen leak out of the vessels into the surrounding tissue matrix forming a fluid exudate containing growth factors (Fig. 1.3).

The process of exudation can continue for over 24 hours. There is an immediate response, either followed by or overlapped by a delayed response. These responses are as follows:

1. An immediate but transient exudation, peaking at 5–10 minutes, and lasting for 30–60 minutes. It involves only

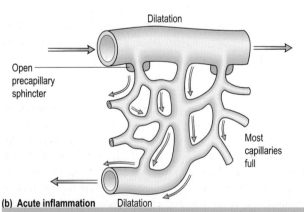

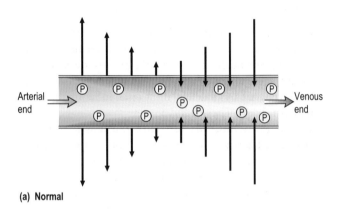

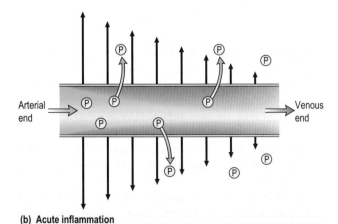

Figure 1.2. Vascular dilatation in acute inflammation. (a) Normally, most of the capillary bed is closed down by precapillary sphincters. (b) In acute inflammation, the sphincters open, causing blood to flow through all capillaries. (Reproduced with permission from Underwood, 2000.)

Figure 1.3. Ultrafiltration of fluid across the small blood vessel wall. (a) Normally, fluid leaving and entering the vessel is in equilibrium. (b) In acute inflammation, there is a net loss of fluid together with plasma protein molecules (P) into the extracellular space, resulting in oedema. (Reproduced with permission from Underwood, 2000.)

the venules, and is mediated by a host of chemical mediators, including prostaglandins, serotonin and histamine.

2. A longer-lasting immediate response that occurs if the injury has killed endothelial cells. It can affect any vessel and persists until ended by either thrombosis or vessel regeneration.
3. A delayed response, in which further exudation typically begins some hours or days after injury. It is preceded by apoptosis of the endothelial cells and the exposure of increased areas of basement membrane to the plasma. Affecting venules and capillaries, it is generally associated with burns.

Oedema is one of the first signs of types of injuries, such as pressure ulcers, that start deep within the tissues. It can be detected non-invasively by ultrasound biomicroscopy before there are visible signs of damage, allowing preventative action to be taken in a timely manner.

Blood flow changes
The following changes occur sequentially:

- Reduction in the volume of blood entering the damaged tissue due to neurally controlled vasoconstriction, causing temporary blanching at the site of injury. Blood coagulates, arresting bleeding.
- The capillaries adjacent to the wound become dilated, producing a dull reddening resembling a flush.
- Arteriolar dilatation, termed *active hyperaemia*, lasting for a few minutes to several hours depending on the severity of the injury, increases the local blood flow up to 10-fold.
- Blood flow then slows as plasma exudes, mainly via venules, increasing the viscosity of the remaining blood. Plasma proteins leak from these vessels, increasing the osmotic pressure of the interstitial fluid; water is drawn out of the vessels by osmosis and oedema (swelling) results. Much of this fluid is returned to the general circulation via the lymphatics. The vessels become increasingly permeable to proteins as their endothelial cells swell and contract in response to mediator release following injury, opening up gaps between the cells and thus exposing more of the basement membrane to the plasma. Polyanions are also lost from the basement membrane. The worse the injury, the larger the proteins that can leak out of the vessels. If fibrinogen escapes, it forms a network of fibrin fibres within the inflamed tissues.
- As fluid leaks out of the venules and other vessels of the microcirculation, the concentration of the blood cells increases. Capillaries can become blocked by erythrocytes, producing red cell stasis. The flow of the increasingly viscous blood becomes slow enough for leucocytes, which are usually swept away from the endothelial lining of the vessels by the fast-flowing plasma, to make contact with the endothelium and adhere to it, a process referred to as *pavementing*. Some of the leucocytes contribute to leakiness by inflicting further damage. Pavementing is followed by leucocyte emigration into the extravascular tissue; emigration is generally described as occurring during late inflammation.

Late inflammation

Late inflammation is characterized by the emigration of leucocytes from the blood vessels into the inflamed tissue. Also known as inflammatory cells, they include neutrophils, monocytes and T-lymphocytes. They are attracted to the wound site by chemoattractants. These include:

1. monocyte chemoattractant protein-1 (MCP-1)
2. interleukin-8 (IL-8)
3. growth-related oncogene alpha (GROα)
4. fragments of collagen, elastin and fibronectin
5. fibrin degradation products
6. platelet-derived growth factor (PDGF)
7. platelet factor 4.

Numbers 1, 2 and 3 of the list above are highly specific, MCP-1 attracting monocytes while IL-8 and GROα attract neutrophils. The others are less specific.

Generally neutrophils are the first cells to enter the inflamed tissue, closely followed by monocytes and lymphocytes. Following entry into the inflamed tissue, the monocytes become activated, forming macrophages. The following processes are involved in leucocyte emigration (Fig. 1.4):

- margination or pavementing
- adhesion to endothelial cells
- diapedesis.

Margination
As a result of the slowing of blood flow, the leucocytes, initially mainly neutrophils, can move from the axial stream of the venules to the peripheral region adjacent to the endothelium. They roll along the endothelium until leucocyte adhesion molecules on their surfaces interact with endothelial adhesion molecules on the endothelial cells.

Adhesion to endothelial cells
Adhesion of leucocytes to endothelial cells occurs when leucocyte L-selectin adhesion molecules on the surface of the leucocytes bind to endothelial adhesion molecules on the endothelial cells. The latter include ELAM-1, which binds neutrophils, and ICAM-1, which binds neutrophils, monocytes and lymphocytes. The stimulation of pain fibres causes the local neutrophils to stop expressing L-selectin adhesion molecules, limiting the acute inflammatory response. It is noteworthy that the leucocytes and endothelial cells of alcoholics, diabetics and patients on long-term glucocorticoid therapy have a reduced ability to express adhesion molecules; this may be one of the reasons they have difficulty coping with bacterial infections, adversely affecting their ability to heal wounds.

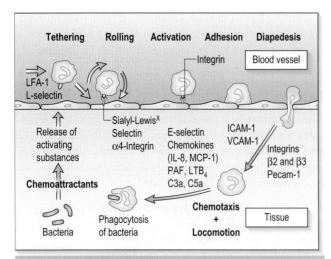

Figure 1.4. Neutrophil migration. Neutrophils arrive at the site of the inflammation, attracted by chemoattractants. They roll along the blood-vessel wall and their progress is halted by L-selectin, on their surface, binding to a carbohydrate structure, e.g. sialyl-Lewis^x, an adhesion molecule. On activation, the L-selectin is replaced by another cell surface adhesion molecule, e.g. integrin which binds to E-selectin. Various other chemokines, e.g. interleukin-8 (IL-8), macrophage chemoattractant factor (MCP), TNF-α and other inflammatory mediators are involved. These inflammatory markers attract the activated neutrophil into the tissue where it phagocytoses and destroys C3b-coated bacteria. The inflammation releases activating substances attracting more neutrophils. LFA, leucocyte function antigen; PAF, platelet-activating factor, LTB$_4$, leukotriene B4; ICAM, intracellular adhesion molecule; VCAM, vascular cell adhesion molecule; PECAM, platelet/endothelial cell adhesion molecule. (Reproduced with permission from Kumar and Clark, 2002.)

Diapedesis

This occurs when the leucocytes that have adhered to the endothelial cells move into the spaces between the retracted or apoptotic endothelial cells, and then cross the basement membrane that the neutrophils weaken by the secretion of proteolytic enzymes. Surviving endothelial cells then repair the damaged basement membrane.

The process of leucocyte emigration is made possible and enhanced by chemical mediators. Some cause chemokinesis (increased locomotion) and others chemotaxis (directional migration) of the leucocytes. Chemotactic agents include:

- bacterial breakdown products
- leukotriene B
- complement components such as C5a
- some lymphokines and monokines
- mast cell-derived eosinophilic factor of anaphylaxis.

They interact with the cell membrane, which in turn triggers changes in the cytoskeleton that affect movement. The migration of the cells into the injured tissue is assisted by their production of proteinases, proteolytic enzymes that clear a route in front of the migrating cells.

Having entered the inflamed tissue, the monocytes develop into macrophages. Neutrophils and macrophages become phagocytic, ingesting and digesting bacteria and other infectious organisms, necrotic tissue and dying cells.

Phagocytosis

Neutrophils are the main phagocytic cells of acute inflammation. Foreign bodies such as bacteria and debris that have entered the body through a wound are first coated by IgG (either subtype 1 or subtype 3) or by C3b. This process of coating with protein is called *opsonization*. Because the neutrophils have receptors for these opsonins on their cell surfaces, the coated particles adhere to these receptors. The cell membrane engulfs each particle, forming a phagosome, which fuses with one or more of the neutrophil's primary lysosomes to form a secondary lysosome. The hydrolytic enzymes stored in the primary lysosomes now digest the particle and its components are recycled by the neutrophils.

Living bacteria that are phagocytosed are killed within the secondary lysosomes either by the H_2O_2-myeloperoxidase system, less effective oxygen-dependent and oxygen-independent systems, or by microbe-killing proteins such as lysozyme and lactoferrin. Sometimes the bacteria kill the neutrophils, in which case the neutrophils break down releasing lysosomal enzymes, H_2O_2, free radicals and other materials that produce local damage. Release of these substances, termed cytotoxic release, can also occur from living neutrophils by regurgitation. A wound can therefore be increased in size by the body's own defence mechanisms; a military analogy would be friendly fire. Usually the neutrophils undergo apoptosis and are engulfed by macrophages. Neutrophil apoptosis regulates their longevity and is integral to the resolution of inflammation. In vitro experiments have shown that it is downregulated by contact with endothelial cells. Monocytes become phagocytic macrophages shortly after emigrating into the inflamed tissue and respond to opsonized particles in a similar fashion.

Diabetes and glucocorticoids interfere with the phagocytic activity of leucocytes; so diabetic patients and those being treated with glucocorticoids are at particular risk of developing infected wounds and even septicaemia.

Pathogen elimination

This is a major function of neutrophils. Bacteria and other foreign materials are either phagocytosed and destroyed within the neutrophils or killed by toxic reactive oxygen species, also known as free radicals, released by the cells. Hypochlorite anions, superoxide anions and hydroxy radicals are examples of these weapons of mass destruction, not only killing pathogens but also damaging the host tissues unless neutralized by free radical scavenger molecules such as superoxide dismutase which healthy cells generate.

Debridement

Wound eschar is debrided by *neutrophils* and *macrophages* by means of phagocytosis and by releasing proteinases. These enzymes consist of the following groups:

1. Serine proteinases:
   - human leucocyte elastase (HLE)
   - cathepsin G
   - protease-3
   - urokinase-type plasminogen activator (uPA).
2. Metalloproteinases:
   - neutrophil collagenase (MMP-8)
   - gelatinase B (MMP-9).
3. Cysteine proteinases.
4. Aspartic proteinases.

These proteinases are normally held in granules within the cells and are released when the cells degranulate in response to membrane changes usually induced by inflammatory mediators. Groups 1 and 2 are of particular importance in debridement. The damage they could do to healthy tissue on their release is limited by proteinase inhibitors.

In acute wounds the proteinase levels usually rise shortly after injury, peaking after a few days, and then falling to pre-wounding levels. A second rise in proteinase levels, unrelated to inflammation, occurs during remodelling.

The number of neutrophils in the blood increases (neutrophilia) in patients with infected wounds because mediators released by other cells increase the production of neutrophils by the bone marrow and also cause their early release. In severe infection neutrophils may be killed faster than they are produced, causing their number in the blood to be reduced (neutropenia). Although the infiltration of neutrophils into wounds protects the body from invading pathogens, the recent studies involving neutrophil depletion suggest that they can inhibit epidermal healing but not dermal healing. Neutrophils killed at the wound site during the battle against infection either become part of the wound eschar or are phagocytosed locally by macrophages.

Macrophages play a crucial role in late inflammation and the subsequent phases of wound healing, acting as a central stimulator (Fig. 1.5) for many of the cell types involved in the process. Like neutrophils, macrophages are derived from stem cells located in the bone marrow. These enter the circulation as monocytes, are attracted to the wound site by chemoattractants and on arrival are activated, becoming macrophages. As the number of neutrophils at the wound site decreases, the number of macrophages increases and they remain after acute inflammation is over, forming a physiologically important component of the granulation tissue that develops during the proliferative phase of wound healing.

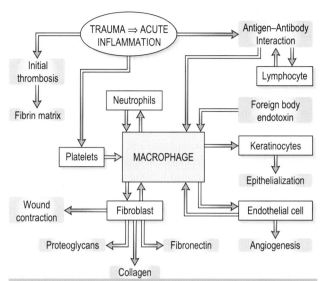

Figure 1.5. The central role of the macrophage in the late inflammatory and subsequent phases of wound healing. (Based on Monaco and Lawrence, 2003.)

Like neutrophils, they respond to cytokines and growth factors in the injured tissue by synthesizing and secreting proteinases, mainly matrix metalloproteinases (MMPs) that digest collagen, fibronectin, laminin, proteoglycans and elastin. Tissue inhibitors of these metalloproteinases (TIMPs), specifically TIMP-1 and TIMP-2, limit tissue breakdown by the MMPs. The enzymatic attack of the MMPs is generally sufficient to separate the eschar without excessive damage to the living tissue deep to it.

Macrophages also secrete the serine proteinase uPA, which converts plasminogen, present in most body fluids, to plasmin, a fibrinolytic protease that breaks down the blood clot at the wound site, allowing granulation tissue to develop in its place. Plasmin may also activate some MMPs and growth factors, including TGF-β.

Macrophages have dual functions:

- wound debridement
- orchestration of the proliferative phase of wound healing by means of a range of signalling molecules that include cytokines and growth factors.

Cytokines and growth factors

Cytokines are polypeptide mediators. Those derived from macrophages are termed monokines and include IL-1 and TNF-α. Those derived from lymphocytes are termed lymphokines. Although many cytokines are pro-inflammatory (e.g. IL-1 and TNF-α), others are anti-inflammatory (e.g. IL-10, interleukin-1 receptor antagonist and TNF-α receptor antagonist which respectively compete with IL-1α and TNF-α for their receptors on the target cells). Growth factors are polypeptides with mitogenic and/or angiogenic activity.

Being cell-derived, they are also cytokines, though not all cytokines are growth factors since many cytokines have functions other than being mitogenic and/or angiogenic. Growth factors and other cytokines can be autocrine (acting on the cell producing them), juxtacrine (acting on an adjacent cell), paracrine (acting on nearby cells) or endocrine (acting on distant cells), the last being rare in wound healing. During early inflammation many cytokines are produced by platelets; later neutrophils and then macrophages and T-lymphocytes become increasingly important in cytokine production (see Ch. 2).

The totality of the wound healing process is largely regulated by the ordered production of cytokines that control the gene activation responsible for cell migration, proliferation and synthesis. The release of the various cytokines is controlled by other cytokines and by changes in the tissue environment or milieu. Tissue hypoxia is described by Monaco and Lawrence (2003) as 'an often underreported signal for cytokine release'. Hypoxia stimulates the releases of TNF-α, TNF-β, vascular endothelial growth factor (VEGF) and IL-8 from macrophages, endothelial cells and fibroblasts.

A vast number of the subset of cytokines termed growth factors have been identified (Table 1.1).

Collectively they, and pro-inflammatory cytokines such as IL-1, play an important role in regulating cellular responses to skin injury with the result that most wounds heal. Their use as a means of facilitating the healing of chronic wounds continues to be investigated. The application of multiple growth factors may produce better results than the application of single factors, the alphabet soup of growth factors being collectively more effective than the individual parts of the recipe. This can be achieved by applying to the wound a dressing incorporating cells such as fibroblasts that produce many of these factors. Another technique is to use physical modalities such as ultrasound to stimulate cells at and adjacent to the wound site to secrete the soup of growth factors.

Cytokine networks, in which different cell types have receptors for the same cytokine, permit a single cytokine to initiate many different actions. The concentration of a cytokine may determine its activity; for example, TGF-β is a macrophage chemoattractant when in the fentomolar range, but cannot stimulate collagen synthesis by fibroblasts until it is in the nanomolar range. Similarly PDGF, which stimulates fibroblast proliferation, is also chemotactic for fibroblasts, but only at a 100-fold greater concentration than that required for stimulating mitogenesis in these cells.

Some cytokines and cytokine isoforms have conflicting actions; for example, TGF-β is a bifunctional regulator of cell growth because some of its isoforms are stimulatory and others inhibitory. The balance determines the activity of the target cells and shifts as healing progresses. Loss of network balance has been implicated in chronic wound healing pathways, though perhaps the problem is lack of shifting of the balance and therefore lack of progression from inflammation to proliferation.

T-Lymphocytes

The recruitment of T-lymphocytes into wounds occurs somewhat later than that of neutrophils and macrophages. Their chemoattractants are thought to include molecules produced later on in the inflammatory process. T-lymphocytes may have a regulatory role in wound healing, being another source of growth factors and other regulatory molecules. Typically, both CD4-positive and CD8-positive T-lymphocytes peak within the wound bed at 5 to 7 days post-injury due to the influence of IL-2 and other immunomodulatory factors. The CD4 lymphocytes in particular are important sources of a host of cytokines including IL-1, IL-2, TNF-α, fibroblast-activating factor, EGF and TGF-β. Among their other functions, these cytokines regulate T-cell proliferation and differentiation in an autocrine fashion. T-lymphocytes effect cell-mediated immunity. Subsets of T-lymphocytes develop into cytotoxic cells that lyse virus-infected cells and cells detected as being foreign.

The removal of T-lymphocytes from the circulation of an injured mammal inhibits the cascade of activities that constitutes healing, indicating that they play a crucial role in the process. In contrast, no role has been assigned to B-lymphocytes.

The inflammatory reflex

A neural pathway reflexively monitors and adjusts the acute inflammatory response. Inflammatory stimuli activate sensory pathways that relay information to the hypothalamus and via this to the autonomic system and to the pituitary gland. Inflammatory input activates an anti-inflammatory response that is rapid and subconscious; it limits local inflammation and prevents the spillover of potentially lethal toxins into the circulation. The nervous system integrates the inflammatory response. It gathers information about the site or sites of injury and pathogenic attack, mobilizes defences and creates a memory of these events to improve our chances of survival.

Table 1.1.   Examples of the subset of cytokines termed growth factors

- Platelet-derived growth factor (PDGF)
- Colony stimulating factor (CSF-1)
- Nerve growth factor (NGF)
- Hepatocyte growth factor (HGF)
- Macrophage-stimulating protein (MSP)
- Fibroblast growth factor
- Transforming growth factor alpha (TGF-α)
- Transforming growth factor beta (TGF-β)
- Progranulin
- Keratinocyte growth factor (KGF)
- Insulin-like growth factor
- Vascular endothelial growth factor (VEGF)

The neural control of acute inflammation has been described as being reflexive, interconnected and controllable. The cholinergic anti-inflammatory pathway has been shown to inhibit the activation of macrophages and the release of cytokines. Stimulation of the vagus nerve, either electrically or pharmacologically, prevents inflammation and cytokine release. One of these cytokines is TNF, which causes the cardinal clinical signs of inflammation. TNF is essential for inflammation, and the ending of inflammation is characterized by a decrease in TNF activity. Endogenous anti-inflammatory pathways involve the action of anti-inflammatory agents such as interleukin-10 (IL-10) and stress hormones such as adrenaline and the glucocorticoids. The activation of pituitary-dependent adrenal responses after endotoxin administration provided early evidence that inflammatory stimuli can activate anti-inflammatory signals in the central nervous system. Inflammation has also been shown to alter neuronal signalling in the hypothalamus.

The nervous and immune systems use a common molecular basis for communication, with cells from each system expressing signalling ligands and receptors for the other. The molecular dovetail between the cholinergic nervous system and the immune system is a nicotinic, α-bungarotoxin-sensitive macrophage acetylcholine receptor. Exposure of macrophages to nicotine or acetylcholine inhibits their production of TNF-α and other cytokines in response to endotoxin, damping down the inflammatory response. The macrophages still produce TNF-α messenger RNA, but do not make TNF-α when acetylcholine activates their cholinergic receptors, indicating that these receptors transduce the signal in an intracellular manner that inhibits cytokine synthesis at a post-transcriptional stage.

The main advantage of neural signalling is its speed. A typical, diffusible inflammatory response takes hours, but neural signalling only milliseconds. Another advantage is that it is short-lived; after a short refractory period the target cells resume their normal function. Inhibition of the immune system is transient, allowing local inflammatory responses to recur if trauma or infection persists. The proper functioning of the immune and neural pathways provides exquisite control of inflammation. Damage to these endogenous pathways converts a protective, self-limiting response into a potentially lethal one.

Possible outcomes of acute inflammation

It is now generally accepted that acute inflammation is an essential component of the process of wound healing. In some ways it can be considered as a necessary evil; it is essential, but it inevitably produces some local damage to the tissue around the wound. Acute inflammation is a battle and the tissue around the wound the battlefield. As in any battle, casualties occur on both sides and some are the result of friendly fire. Acute inflammation normally leads to recovery from infection and healing, but it can become blocked so that it persists, leading to excessive tissue damage by leucocytes (Fig. 1.6). Its progress can be considered in terms of reaching a series of checkpoints, at each of which binary or higher-order molecular signals drive it forwards. What the molecules that mediate acute inflammation do depends on timing and context. They can collectively progress the inflammation or arrest it. It should be appreciated that the non-inflammatory state is not the passive result of an absence of inflammatory mediators. Recent studies indicate that the maintenance of health requires the positive actions of specific gene products that suppress reactions to potentially inflammatory stimuli that do not warrant a full response. Battles may end, but minor skirmishes persist.

The possible outcomes of acute inflammation are as follows:

* *Complete resolution.* The damaged tissue is restored to its original form by regeneration via a blastema. This occurs in the limbs of some poikilothermic animals and in some organs, e.g. the liver, in humans.
* *Tissue repair.* This is the most likely outcome in humans. Growth factors produced during acute inflammation cause granulation tissue to form and this develops into highly collagenous scar tissue. This develops rapidly and allows return to function, albeit abnormal though generally effective function.

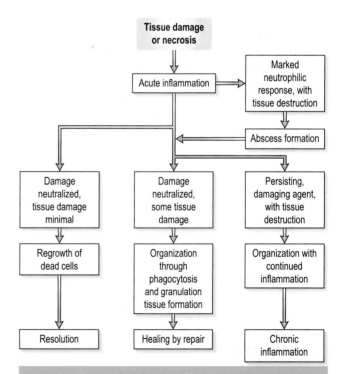

Figure 1.6. Flow diagram of outcomes of acute inflammation. (Reproduced with permission from Stevens and Lowe, 2000.)

- *Abscess formation.* Neutrophils, bacteria, necrotic tissue and debris collected together at loci of infection during acute inflammation can form pus which the body may then wall off by fibrous tissue, forming an abscess. The pus is yellowy-green in colour because of the myeloperoxidase it contains. Proteases in the pus increase its osmotic pressure causing the abscess to take up water and swell. The pressure is painful and is alleviated when the abscess bursts or is lanced.
- *Progress to chronic inflammation.* This happens if the infection or other noxious agent remains or if local pro-inflammatory mediators continue to induce and/or maintain inflammation. Neither regeneration nor repair can occur where there is chronic inflammation.

Prostaglandins, in addition to their pro-inflammatory activities, have recently been shown to be beneficial in the resolution of inflammation. Inhibition of cyclo-oxygenase-2 (COX-2), the predominant prostaglandin endoperoxide synthetase, may attenuate acute inflammation and in doing so delay tissue repair and regeneration. There is prominent expression of COX isozymes in macrophages, endothelial cells, Langerhans cells and keratinocytes in and around an injury, but it is the COX-2 isozyme that affects the healing of that injury.

In normal wound healing, the action of pro-inflammatory cytokines is limited by naturally occurring control systems. For example, IL-1 is regulated by another cytokine, namely IL-1 receptor antagonist, which blocks IL-1 receptors on the target cells. Similarly the activity of TNF-α is regulated by the production of soluble receptors for TNF-α, which compete with it for its receptors on its target cells. In addition to pro-inflammatory cytokines, there are also anti-inflammatory cytokines, e.g. IL-10, that reduce inflammatory activity at the wound site. A shift in the balance between these conflicting agents away from inflammation during the normal response of the body to injury is an important step in allowing healing to progress to completion. It should be appreciated, however, that there is still much to learn about the mechanisms by which acute inflammation is succeeded by the remaining phases of wound healing.

CHRONIC INFLAMMATION

Wounds that fail to heal in the expected time range are generally referred to as chronic. All chronic wounds, regardless of their underlying medical cause (e.g. vascular insufficiency, diabetes, unrelieved pressure), are characterized by unresolved inflammation. Chronic inflammation can be thought of as a two-edged sword:

1. Its pro-inflammatory cytokines forestall the progress of the wound into the proliferative phase of healing.
2. Its proteinases produce erosion of the previously intact tissue at the margins of the wound.

During normal wound healing, pro-inflammatory stimuli are lost within a few days of injury and the acute inflammatory phase, characterized by neutrophil-induced local damage and debridement, is succeeded by the proliferative phase of healing, in which the emphasis shifts to the formation of new tissue. However, if pro-inflammatory signals persist, inflammation becomes chronic as neutrophils continue to enter the wound bed, producing pro-inflammatory cytokines and releasing proteinases that cause local tissue damage, and the wound fails to heal. Anti-inflammatory cytokines such as interleukin-10 are specific gene products that reduce inflammatory action of the wound site, as do soluble TNF receptors. The presence of these agents in chronically inflamed venous ulcers suggests that even here elements of the normal control mechanisms persist. What is necessary is to change the environmental conditions so that the balance shifts towards ending inflammation. Table 1.2 lists many of the causes of persistence of the pro-inflammatory signals.

In 1998, Ashcroft, Horan and Ferguson showed that ageing could be accompanied by increase in neutrophils and decrease in macrophages in the wound bed following injury, shifting the balance towards damage and away from proliferation. This change in cell recruitment profile may be due to age-related changes in cell adhesion molecule (CAM) expression on endothelial cells. The possibility that abnormal CAM expression may be implicated in chronic inflammation is supported by the report that certain CAMs increase markedly in lipodermatosclerotic skin bordering on chronic venous leg ulcers. In acute inflammation, levels of these CAMs are only raised for a few days, limiting the level of inflammatory cell recruitment, but in chronic inflammation these levels remain high, so that inflammatory cell recruitment with its adverse sequelae continues unabated (Fig. 1.7). Some inflammatory cell recruitment is essential for healing, but too much produces increased damage. Topical oestrogen application can reduce neutrophil recruitment and stop chronic inflammation, hastening repair in elderly patients, suggesting that reduced

---

Table 1.2.   Causes of persisting pro-inflammatory signals

- Recurrent physical trauma such as that possible at pressure points
- Uncontrolled bacterial infection, either overt or subclinical
- Contamination of the wound bed by foreign products, e.g. particles of dressings
- Reperfusion injury in tissue cyclically exposed to blood stasis and flow, e.g. during changes in the positioning of the legs of a patient with venous leg ulcers
- Advanced age with its associated physiological changes including adverse alteration in the recruitment of inflammatory cells to the wound bed

---

Several of the above may occur simultaneously.

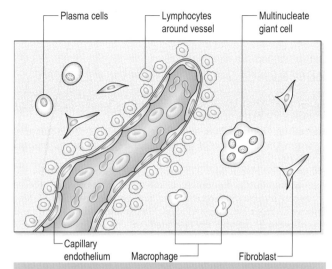

Figure 1.7.   The cells involved in chronic inflammation. Neutrophil polymorphs have disappeared from the site, and mononuclear cells such as lymphocytes and macrophages are prominent. Some specialized lymphocytes called plasma cells are present; these produce immunoglobulins. Some of the macrophages may become multinucleate giant cells. Fibroblasts migrate into the area and lay down collagen. (Reproduced with permission from Underwood, 2000.)

sex hormone production during ageing may adversely affect healing. If so, then this could be a further reason to advocate hormone replacement therapy. The effect of topical testosterone should also be explored.

The neutrophils that persist at the wound site during chronic inflammation continue to produce tissue-digesting proteinases, damaging free radicals and pro-inflammatory cytokines that promote further recruitment of neutrophils, thus completing the vicious circle (Fig. 1.8). Chronic wounds appear to contain excessive amounts of the matrix metalloproteinase MMP-8, also termed neutrophil collagenase, which is produced exclusively by neutrophils and damages the dermis by digesting collagen fibrils. Elevated levels of several other MMPs, including MMP-2 (gelatinase A) and MMP-9 (gelatinase B), the latter invariably associated with neutrophils, have also been reported in chronic wounds, providing further evidence that these wounds are chronically inflamed.

Several serine proteinases are also elevated in chronic wounds, including leucocyte elastase and urokinase-type plasminogen activator. Wound fluid from chronic venous ulcers has been shown to contain about 40 times the elastase activity of wound fluid from acute wounds. Elastase activity may be elevated because of the degradation of its inhibitor, α1-proteinase inhibitor, by other proteinase enzymes present

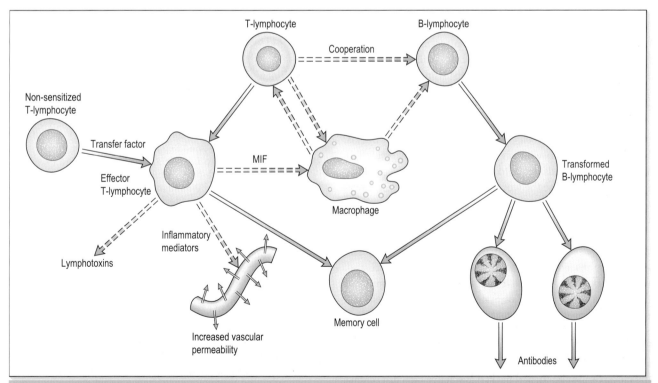

Figure 1.8.   Cellular cooperation in chronic inflammation. Solid arrows show pathways of cellular differentiation. Dotted arrows show intercellular communication. MIF, migration inhibition factors. (Reproduced with permission from Underwood, 2000.)

in the chronic wound fluid. Elastase degrades elastin and fibrononectin, the latter being an important component of the provisional matrix provided by coagulation. Chronic wounds have a shortage of plasminogen activation inhibitor-1, normally produced by endothelial cells and fibroblasts; this leads to abnormally high levels of plasmin, another serine proteinase that degrades the provisional matrix. Since this matrix is the substrate through which cells migrate into the wound bed during late inflammation and proliferation, damage to it has an adverse effect on healing.

It should be appreciated that the proteinases, though damaging if excessive, are necessary for normal wound healing where their action separates necrotic tissue from healthy tissue, debriding the wound. In such conditions the intact tissues are shielded from them by inhibitors or antiproteinases. Chronic wounds have reduced levels of these protective materials, exacerbating their problems. Neutrophils are likely to be active in destruction of this shield since neutrophil elastase and neutrophil collagenase (MMP-8) degrade shield components including proteinase inhibitor TIMP-1.

It is hoped that as knowledge of the proteinase imbalances that occur in chronic inflammation are better understood, therapeutic techniques to deal with them will develop. Therapies aimed at limiting proteolytic activity in chronic wounds are being investigated. Materials capable of absorbing wound proteinases selectively from solutions have been developed. The pros and cons of their use in or as dressings for chronic wounds remain to be determined.

As well as degrading the provisional matrix and destroying the anti-proteinase shield, raised proteinase activity also inactivates endogenous growth factors such as vascular endothelial growth factor, an important stimulator of angiogenesis, a further indication of the problems produced by excess proteinase activity.

It is not surprising that pro-inflammatory cytokines and proteinases persist at elevated levels in chronic wounds. However, once such wounds begin to heal their levels fall. Whether the wounds begin to heal because the levels fall, or the levels fall because the wounds begin to heal, is unknown, though the former possibility is the more attractive of the two from the therapeutic viewpoint.

Clinically the most important action is to identify the causes or causes of the pro-inflammatory signals that result in neutrophils collecting within the chronic wound and, wherever possible, to remove them. If this cannot be done, then reduction of pro-inflammatory cytokines and selective reduction of proteinases by targeted therapies is appropriate.

It should be appreciated that although advanced age has been implicated as a cause of chronic inflammation, this should not be used as an excuse for lack of action. Although the clock cannot be turned back, it is science fact, not science fiction, that many of the problems associated with ageing that can result in chronic inflammation can be solved; the initiation of healing in chronically inflamed wounds by the application of topical oestrogen is a good example of what can be done.

REFERENCES AND FURTHER READING

Agren MS (1994) Gelatinase activity during wound healing. Br J Dermatol 131: 634–640.

Agren MS, Taplin CJ, Woessner JF (Jr), et al. (1992) Collagenase in wound healing: effect of wound age and type. J Invest Dermatol 99: 709–714.

Ashcroft GS, Horan MA, Ferguson MW (1998) Aging alters the inflammatory and endothelial cells adhesion molecular profiles during human cutaneous wound healing. Lab Invest 78: 47–58.

Barone EJ, Yager DR, Pozez AL, et al. (1998) Interleukin-1 alpha and collagenase activity are elevated in chronic wounds. Plast Reconstr Surg 10: 1023–1027.

Besdovsky H, Sorkin E, Felix D, Haas H (1977) Hypothalamic changes during the immune response. Eur J Immunol 7: 323–325.

Blalock JE (1989) A molecular basis for bi-directional communication between the immune and neuroendocrine systems. Physiol Rev 69: 1–32.

Borovikova LV, Ivanova S, Zhang M, et al. (2000) Vagus nerve stimulation attenuates the systemic inflammatory response to endotoxin. Nature 405: 458–462.

Bullen, EC, Longaker MT, Updike DL, et al. (1995) Tissue inhibitor of metalloproteinases-1 is decreased and activated gelatinases are increased in chronic wounds. J Invest Dermatol 104: 236–240.

Circolo A, Welgus HG, Pierce GF, et al. (1991) Differential regulation of the expression of proteinase/antiproteinases in fibroblasts: effects of interleukin-1 and platelet-derived growth factor. J Biol Chem 266: 1283–1288.

Clark RAF (1993) Biology of dermal repair. Dermatol Clin 11: 647–666.

Cohen IK, Diegelman RF, Dorne RY, et al. (1993) Wound healing. In: Greenfield LJ, Mulholland MK, Oldham KT, et al. (eds) Surgery: Scientific Principles and Practice, 3rd edn. Philadelphia: Lippincott-Raven, p. 86.

Davidson JM, Breyer MD (2003) Inflammatory modulation and wound repair. J Invest Dermatol 120(5): xi–xii.

DiPietro LA, Reintjes MG, Low QE, et al. (2001) Modulation of macrophage recruitment into wounds by monocyte chemoattractant protein-1. Wound Rep Regen 9: 28–33.

Dovi JV, He LK, DiPetro LA (2003) Accelerated wound closure in neutrophils-depleted mice. J Leukoc Biol 73: 448–455.

Dyson M, Lyder C (2001) Wound management: physical modalities. In: Morison MJ (ed). The Prevention and Treatment of Pressure Ulcers. Edinburgh: Mosby, pp. 177–193.

Edwards JV, Yager DR, Cohen IK, et al. (2001) Modified cotton gauze dressings that selectively absorb neutrophil elastase activity in solution. Wound Repair Regen 9: 50–58.

Engelhardt E, Toksoy A, Goebeler M, et al. (1998) GROalpha, MCP-1, IP-10 and Mig are sequentially and differentially expressed during phase-specific infiltration of leukocyte subsets in human wound healing. Am J Pathol 53: 1849–1860.

Fauci AS, Haynes BF (1994) Cellular and molecular basis of immunity. In: Braunwald E, Wilson J, et al. (eds) Harrison's Principles of Internal Medicine, 13th edn. New York: McGraw-Hill, p. 1552.

Folkman J, Brem H (1992) Angiogenesis and inflammation. In: Gallin JI, Goldstein IM, Snyderman R (eds) Inflammation: Basic Principles and Clinical Correlates, 2nd edn. New York: Raven Press.

Friedlander E (2002) Inflammation and Repair. www.pathguy.com/lectures/inflamma.htm.

Gharaee-Kermani M, Phan SH (2001) Role of cytokines and cytokine therapy in wound healing and fibrotic diseases. Curr Pharm Des 7: 1083–1103.

Grinnell F, Zhu M (1996) Fibronectin degradation in chronic wounds depends on the relative levels of elastase, alpha 1-proteinase inhibitor, and alpha 2-macroglobulin. J Invest Dermatol 106: 335–341.

Hall KL (2000) The Regulation of Wound Healing. University of Florida College of Medicine/Shands Health Care. Grand Rounds Online. www.medinfo.ufl.edu/cme/grounds/mast/intro.html.

Hart J (2002a) Inflammation 1: its role in the healing of acute wounds. J Wound Care 11: 205–209.

Hart J (2002b) Inflammation 2: its role in the healing of chronic wounds. J Wound Care 11: 245–249.

Herrick S, Ashcroft G, Ireland G, et al. (1997) Up-regulation of elastase in acute wounds of healthy aged humans and chronic venous leg ulcers are associated with matrix degradation. Lab Invest 77: 281–288.

Itoh Y, Nagase H (1995) Preferential inactivation of tissue inhibitor of metalloproteinase-1 that is bound to the precursor of matrix metalloproteinase 9 (progelatinase B) by human neutrophil elastase. J Biol Chem 270(28): 16518–16521.

Kerstein MD, Bensing KA, Brill LR, et al. (1998) The Physiology of Wound Healing. Philadelphia: The Oxford Institute for Continuing Education and Allegheny University of Health Sciences.

Kumar P, Clark M (2002) Clinical Medicine. London: Saunders.

Lauer G, Sollberg S, Cole M (2000) Expression and proteolysis of vascular endothelial growth factor is increased in chronic wounds. J Invest Dermatol 115: 12–18.

Lawrence WT (1998) Physiology of the acute wound. Clin Plast Surg 25: 321–340.

Li YQ, Doyle JW, Roth TP, et al. (1998) IL-10, and GM-CSF expression and the presence of antigen-presenting cells in chronic venous ulcers. J Surg Res 798: 128–135.

Martin CW, Muir IF (1990) The role of lymphocytes in wound healing. Br J Plast Surg 43: 655–662.

Minchenko A, Salced S, Bauer T, Caro J (1994) Hypoxia regulatory elements of the vascular endothelial growth factor gene. Cell Mol Biol Res 40: 35–39.

Monaco JL, Lawrence WT (2003) Acute wound healing an overview. Clin Plast Surg 30: 1–12.

Muller-Decker K, Hirschner W, Marks F, Furstenberger G (2002) The effects of cyclooxygenase isozyme on incisional wound healing in mouse skin. J Invest Dermatol 119: 1189–1195.

Murphy G, Docherty AJP (1992) The matrix metalloproteinases and their inhibitors. Am J Respir Cell Mol Biol 7: 120–125.

Nathan C (2002) Points of control in inflammation. Nature 420: 846–852.

Peschen M, Lahaye T, Hennig B, et al. (1999) Expression of the adhesion molecules ICAM-1, VCAM-1, LFA-1 and VFA-4 in the skin is modulated in progressing stages of chronic venous insufficiency. Acta Derm Venereol 79: 27–32.

Peterson JM, Barbul A, Breslin RJ, et al. (1987) Significance of T-lymphocytes in wound healing. Surgery 102: 100–105.

Rao CN, Ladin DA, Liu YY, et al. (1995) Alpha1-antitrypsin is degraded and nonfunctional in chronic wounds but intact and functional in acute wounds: the inhibitor protects fibronectin from degradation by chronic wound fluid enzymes. J Invest Dermatol 105: 572–578.

Roberts AB, Anzano MA, Wakefield LM, et al. (1985) Type beta transforming growth factor: a bifunctional regulator of cell growth. Proc Natl Acad Sci USA 82: 119–123.

Rogers AA, Burnett S, Moore JC, et al. (1995) Involvement of proteolytic enzymes, plasminogen activators and matrix metalloproteinases in the pathophysiology of pressure ulcers. Wound Repair Regen 3: 273–283.

Ross R (1987) Platelet-derived growth factor. Annu Rev Med 38: 71–79.

Scannell G, Waxman K, Kaml GJ, et al. (1993) Hypoxia induces a human macrophage cell line to release tumor necrosis factor-alpha and its soluble receptors in vitro. J Surg Res 54: 281–285.

Schaffer M, Barbul A (1998) Lymphocyte function in wound healing and following injury. Br J Surg 85: 444–460.

Seppa H, Grotendorst GR, Seppa S, et al. (1982) Platelet-derived growth factor is chemotactic for fibroblasts. J Cell Biol 92: 584–588.

Stevens A, Lowe J (2000) Pathology. Edinburgh: Mosby.

Sylvia CJ (2003) The role of neutrophils apoptosis in influencing tissue repair. J Wound Care 12: 13–16.

Tennenberg SD, Finkenauer R, Wang T (2002) Endothelium down-regulates Fas, TNF, and TRAIL-induced neutrophils apoptosis. Surg Infect (Larchmt) 3: 351–357.

Tracey KJ (2002) The inflammatory reflex. Nature 420: 853–859.

Underwood JCE (2000) General and Systematic Pathology. Edinburgh: Churchill Livingstone.

Wallace HJ, Stacey MC (1998) Levels of tumor necrosis factor-alpha (TNF-alpha) and soluble TNF receptors in chronic venous leg ulcers – correlations to healing status. J Invest Dermatol 110: 292–296.

Wexler BC, Dolgin AE, Tryczynski EW (1957) Effects of a bacterial polysaccharide (Piromen) on the pituitary-adrenal axis: adrenal ascorbic acid, cholesterol and histologic alterations. Endocrinology 61: 300–308.

Weyl A, Vanscheidt W, Weiss JM (1996) Expression of the adhesion molecules ICAM-1, VCAM-1 and E-selectin and their ligands VLA-4 and LFA-1 in chronic venous leg ulcers. J Am Acad Dermatol 34: 418–423.

Wilgus TA, Vodovotz Y, Vittadine E, et al. (2003) Reduction of scar formation in full-thickness wounds with topical celcoxib treatment. Wound Repair Regen 11: 25–34.

Witte MB, Barbul A (1997) Wounds healing: general principles of wound healing. Surg Clin North Am 77: 509–528.

Wysocki AB, Staiano-Coico L, Grinnell F (1993) Wound fluid from chronic leg ulcers contains elevated levels of metalloproteinases MMP-2 and MMP-9. J Invest Dermatol 101: 64–68.

Wysocki AB, Kusakabe AO, Chang S, Tian TL (1999) Temporal expression of urokinase plasminogen activator; plasminogen activator inhibitor and gelatinase-B in chronic wound fluid switches from a chronic to acute wound profile with progression to healing. Wound Repair Regen 7: 154–165.

Yager DR, Zhang LY, Liang HX, et al. (1996) Wound fluids from human pressure ulcers contain elevated matrix metalloproteinase levels and activity compared to surgical wound fluids. J Invest Dermatol 107: 743–748.

Diseases of the Immune System

Delva Shamley

2

THE IMMUNE SYSTEM

Pathogens

All living organisms are constantly exposed to the threat of invasion by disease-producing foreign agents and organisms, e.g. fungi, bacteria, viruses. The immune system is primed to defend the body against the threat of infectious organisms and consists of organs, cells and proteins. An infectious organism that causes disease is called a pathogen. Pathogens can be made up of anything from one to several different molecules which are recognized by our bodies as being foreign, these are called *antigens*. Many of our defence mechanisms depend on the body recognizing antigens and destroying them.

Sources and types of pathogens

Pathogens that can cause disease vary from single-celled microorganisms (viruses, bacteria, yeast) to multicellular parasites (fungi, parasitic worms). They vary in size from 20 to 400 nm (viruses) to 7 m in length (parasitic worms) and they vary with respect to how they enter and live inside the body (Table 2.1). Pathogens may enter the body via skin wounds and the lining of the gut, respiratory or genitourinary tracts. Once access to the body is achieved the ability of a pathogen to produce disease depends on its ability to multiply and spread in the body. Organisms that penetrate the skin by passing between or through epithelial cells are more easily spread through the body as the mucosa contains blood and lymph vessels both of which can disperse the organism to the rest of the body.

Pathogens can either multiply inside host cells (viruses, bacteria, protozoan parasites) or outside the cells (bacteria, yeast, parasites).

Single-celled organisms including bacteria, yeast and protozoan parasites multiply by cell division. Viruses multiply by replication, which results in the genetic material of the virus being duplicated within the infected cell. New viral particles assemble and then leave the cell, either when the infected cell bursts releasing the new viruses into the body and killing the infected cell, or when the infected cell gradually releases pockets of the virus ('budding') and the cell does not die.

Pathogen distribution

Extracellular organisms are spread via body fluids, e.g. blood, mucus and lymph. Intracellular organisms may need to be expelled from the cell first before they can be distributed by body fluids. Organisms can spread in the following ways:

- *Cell-to-cell contact*. Many organisms such as viruses move from one cell to the next without entering body fluids. This tends to result in localized infections, e.g. pneumonia where only the respiratory tract is infected. Symptoms, however, may be more widely felt, e.g. headache, fever.

Table 2.1.   Types of pathogen and how they differ

Organism	Habitat	Mode of multiplication
Virus:		
Poliovirus	Intracellular: pharynx, intestine, nervous system	Intracellular synthesis of viral components
Poxvirus	Intracellular: upper respiratory tract, lymph nodes, skin	Intracellular synthesis of viral components
Bacteria:		
Streptococcus pyogenes	Extracellular: pharynx	Cell fission
Mycobacterium leprae	Intracellular: macrophages, endothelial cells, Schwann cells	Cell fission
Fungi:		
Candida albicans	Extracellular: mucosal surfaces	Asexual budding
Histoplasma capsulatum	Intracellular: macrophages	Asexual budding
Protozoan parasites:		
Trypanosomes	Extracellular: in bloodstream	Binary fission
Plasmodium	Intracellular: red blood cells, hepatocytes	Asexually in hepatocytes (cell fission)
Metazoan parasites (worms):		
Ascaris lumbricoides	Intestine	Lays eggs
Taenia solium (tapeworm)	Gut	Releases body segments containing eggs

- *Via blood and lymphatic vessels.* Bloodborne pathogens are more speedily and effectively distributed throughout the body. However, specific pathogens tend to localize in specific tissues.

  Lymphatic transport of pathogens is different to blood transport owing to the fact that:
  - they depend on the contraction of local muscles to propel lymph fluid through the lymph vessels to the nodes
  - pathogens can enter lymphatic vessels via tissue fluid and be conveyed to local lymph nodes, thereby draining the site of the infection.
- *Via the nervous system.* Viruses can spread from central nervous system (CNS) to peripheral nervous system and vice versa. This may allow the virus to become more widespread in the nervous system, where it resides and causes disease (e.g. herpes simplex, Guillain–Barré). Since nerves enter the organs of the body they can also transmit viruses to these organs.

The rabies virus is a neurotropic virus found in the saliva of rabid animals. Following infection the virus moves along nerve axons at about 3 mm per hour. Signs and symptoms include CNS involvement, paralysis and eventually death.

Pathogenesis

Pathogens cause disease by one or more mechanisms. These include:

- *Secretion of toxins.* Many organisms, especially bacteria, cause disease by the production of toxins which have very specific toxic effects. These effects are responsible for the pathology that follows and the signs and symptoms subsequently seen. Examples include: the neurotoxin from the *Clostridium* family of bacteria responsible for tetanus and toxins of the bacterium *Shigella dysenteriae*, which causes dysentery.
- *Endotoxins.* Endotoxins are components of the cell wall of pathogens. These act on host cells resulting in the release of substances that may cause fever, a fall in blood pressure, inflammation and other effects.
- *Direct killing of host cells.* Some pathogens that replicate inside a cell kill the cell, which then breaks down releasing many replicates of the pathogen able to infect other cells. If the cell breakdown is extensive enough this can initiate a disease process.
- *Physical blockage.* This is the development of disease by virtue of the sheer size of the pathogen, e.g. elephantiasis caused by the filarial worm that blocks lymphatic vessels causing swelling of the limbs, genitals and breasts.

Defence mechanisms

The body has essentially three main mechanisms for dealing with the potential inflammation or infection that may ensue from pathogen invasion.

1. protective surface mechanisms
2. non-specific tissue defences
3. specific immune responses.

Both the protective and the non-specific mechanisms can be rapidly mobilized and require no previous contact with specific microorganisms to be effective in neutralizing them.

Protective surface mechanisms

This is the first line of defence. The keratinized epidermis of the skin offers relatively strong resistance except when burnt or abraded. The sero-mucous surfaces of the body, e.g. conjunctivae and oral cavity, are protected by a variety of antibacterial substances such as the enzyme *lysozyme*, which is secreted in tears and saliva and is capable of breaking down bacteria into component parts and thus destroying them. The respiratory tract is protected by continous turnover of surface mucus (produced by goblet cells) which traps particles and is moved by the motile cilia. The presence of an acidic environment in the stomach, vagina and to some extent the skin, inhibits growth of pathogens at these sites. Should these mechanisms fail, the non-specific mechanism is activated.

Non-specific tissue defences

Damage to tissue that incites a non-specific response results in *inflammation* which may be acute or chronic. Non-specific defences deny access to the body or destroy pathogens without distinguishing among specific types of pathogens. There are several components to this type of defence (Fig. 2.1):

Phagocytes are cells which engulf pathogens and debris from cell breakdown. *Macrophages* can be found in almost every tissue of the body either residing in that tissue or moving through. The equivalent cell in the blood is the *monocyte*. Together the system is known as the monocyte–macrophage system. An activated macrophage can respond to a pathogen in one of several ways:

- it may engulf and destroy the pathogen with lysosomal enzymes (enzymes responsible for breaking down proteins and some carbohydrates)
- it may bind to a pathogen in tissue fluids but only be able to destroy the pathogen with the help of other cells (discussed later)
- it may destroy the pathogen by releasing toxic chemicals, e.g. tumour necrosis factor (TNF), into the interstitial fluid.

Immunological surveillance is the rapid response and destruction of abnormal cells by natural killer (NK) cells in

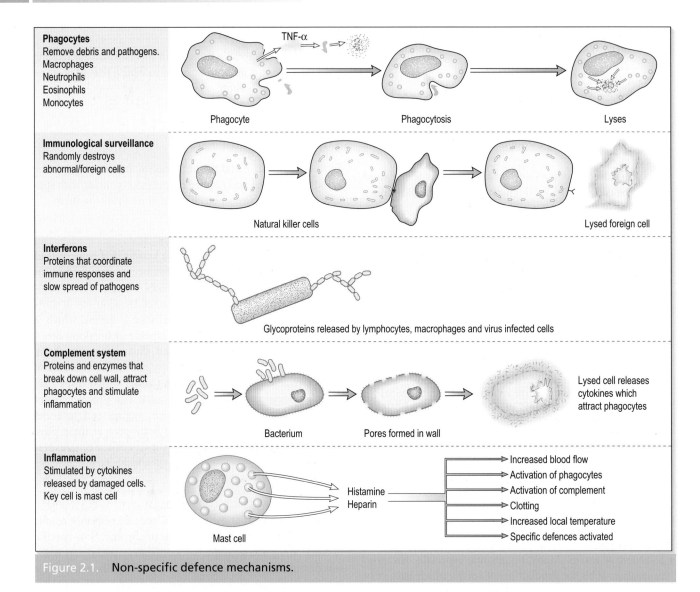

Phagocytes
Remove debris and pathogens.
Macrophages
Neutrophils
Eosinophils
Monocytes

Phagocyte   TNF-α

Phagocytosis

Lyses

Immunological surveillance
Randomly destroys
abnormal/foreign cells

Natural killer cells

Lysed foreign cell

Interferons
Proteins that coordinate
immune responses and
slow spread of pathogens

Glycoproteins released by lymphocytes, macrophages and virus infected cells

Complement system
Proteins and enzymes that
break down cell wall, attract
phagocytes and stimulate
inflammation

Bacterium   Pores formed in wall

Lysed cell releases
cytokines which
attract phagocytes

Inflammation
Stimulated by cytokines
released by damaged cells.
Key cell is mast cell

Mast cell   Histamine
Heparin

→ Increased blood flow
→ Activation of phagocytes
→ Activation of complement
→ Clotting
→ Increased local temperature
→ Specific defences activated

Figure 2.1.   Non-specific defence mechanisms.

peripheral tissues. These cells comprise 15% of all circulating lymphocytes and constantly monitor our tissues for abnormal cells. This is known as immunological surveillance. NK cells recognize abnormal cells by the presence of antigens on the surface of the abnormal cell. This recognition is not like the recognition of antigens by B- and T-lymphocytes discussed in detail later. B- and T-cells can only be activated by recognition of specific antigens at a specific site on the cell membrane. NK cells will respond to many antigens at many sites on the membrane. NK cell mechanisms are summarized in Figure 2.2. This type of response is very useful in slowing down viral infections. A virus reproduces inside cells and out of the reach of circulating antibodies. Viral proteins are, however, included in the membrane of the host cell and it is these proteins that are recognized by NK cells as being foreign. In the case of cancer cells, the *tumour-specific antigen* found in their membrane is unusual and is targeted by NK cells and destroyed. Some cancer cells, however, avoid detection either because they do not contain a tumour-specific antigen on their surface or because these antigens are covered in some way. Other cancer cells are able to destroy NK cells and thus continue to spread. NK cells respond to many *cytokines*. These are chemical messengers released by cells to coordinate local activity (see 'The role of cytokines in immune system' later in this chapter). NK cells respond to the cytokines interleukins (IL) and interferon (IFN), which increase their cytolytic, secretory, proliferative and anti-tumour functions.

Interferons are small proteins released by lymphocytes, macrophages and by tissue cells infected by viruses. The proteins migrate to normal cells, enter the cell and produce antiviral proteins. These antiviral proteins are not able to destroy the virus but are able to prevent it replicating in that cell. Thus the success of the infection spreading is reduced. As mentioned above, interferons are examples of cytokines able to stimulate the activity of macrophages as well as NK cells.

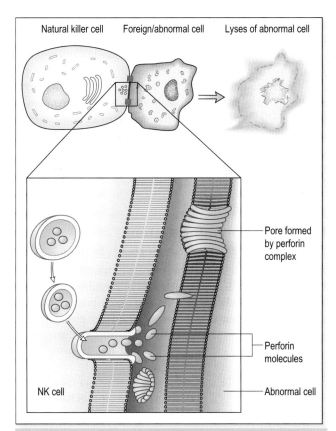

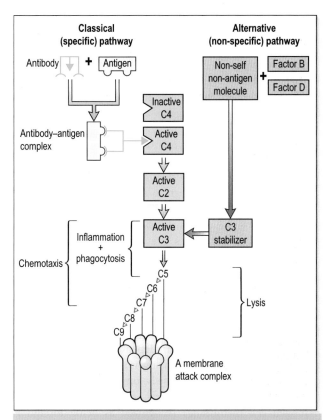

Figure 2.2.   Natural killer (NK) cell action on abnormal cells. The NK cell attaches itself to the target cell and releases vesicles of perforin molecules by exostosis. Perforin binds to the cell wall creating large pores which ultimately destroy the cell's integrity.

Figure 2.3.   The complement cascade. Activation of the cascade can be by the classical specific system or by the non-specific production of a C3-stabilizing combination of a non-antigenic but non-self molecule and factors B and D. Like all cascade systems, there is a multiplication of active molecules at each step, and these molecules cause inflammation, phagocytosis, chemotaxis and lysis of cells. (Reproduced with permission from Davies et al., 2001.)

The complement system   consists of complement proteins so called because they assist antibodies in the destruction of antigens. Complement proteins are a series of enzymatic proteins found in normal serum that, in the presence of a sensitizer, destroy bacteria and other cells. Figure 2.3 provides an overview of the complement system. Complement activation can be either antibody dependent (classical pathway) or antibody independent (alternative pathway).

1. *Classical pathway.* The pathway involves complement proteins C1–C9 and involves activation of the complement pathway starting with *complement fixation.* Complement protein (C1) binds to an antibody (immunoglobulins, Ig, of which there are five types – see later for details) which is already attached to its antigen (e.g. a bacterial cell wall). IgM is the most efficient at binding C1, with IgG1, IgG2 and IgG3 able to bind but not IgG4. Conversion of C1 protein produces an enzyme that catalyses a series of reactions involving other complement proteins (C2–C9). C3 is activated to C3b, which binds to the surface of the antigen triggering phagocytosis and inflammation. The final step in the process is the cleavage of C5. This contributes to the

formation of the membrane attack complex (MAC) and generates pores in the wall of the antigen. These pores are too small to allow the passage of proteins but large enough to allow ions and water to enter and leave the cell. There is therefore the movement of water into the cell and an ion imbalance which results in lysis of the cell.

2. *Alternative pathway.* This is a slower process that occurs in the absence of antibody molecules. The main difference between this and the classical pathway is that C1, C2 and C4 are not involved in the alternative pathway, but C3 and C5–9 are involved in all pathways. The body's own tissue is able to inactivate C3b but many microbes are not able to and go on to be opsonized or lysed by the alternative pathway. The pathway begins when several complement proteins, including *properdin (factor P), factor B* and *factor D*, activate C3 in the plasma. As with the classical pathway, C3b then activates C5, which in turn leads to the formation of the MAC from C5–9 proteins.

Effects of complement activation include:

- The formation of a *membrane attack complex (MAC)* as discussed above.
- *The stimulation of inflammation.* Activated complement proteins stimulate the release of histamine by mast cells and basophils which triggers an inflammatory reaction (see Ch. 1).
- *The attraction of phagocytes.* Activated complement proteins attract macrophages and neutrophils to the area.
- *The enhancement of phagocytosis.* Macrophage membranes have receptors that recognize and bind to complement proteins bound to antibodies. The complement–protein–antibody complex makes it easier for the pathogen to be engulfed. The antibodies are called *opsonins* and the process is called *opsonization.*

Inflammation   is another non-specific defence mechanism and is discussed in detail in Chapter 1.

Specific immune responses

This highly specific mechanism depends primarily upon the recognition of pathogens as being foreign to the body and discriminating these from those belonging to our own body. More commonly a particle (e.g. dust or component of pathogen cell membrane) recognized as being foreign is known as an *antigen.* However, some normal body components may also act as antigens in autoimmune reactions (see 'Autoimmune disorders' later in this chapter). This results in the activation of the immune system with the purpose of neutralizing or destroying the antigen with the production of a specific antibody. A second feature of the immune system is the recognition and enhanced reaction to an antigen at subsequent exposure and the ability to retain this memory for long periods of time. B- and T-lymphocytes (see below) are the key cells involved in the immune response. However, they often depend on phagocytic cells of the monocyte–macrophage system to *present the antigen* to the lymphocyte – these are called antigen-presenting cells (APC) (see 'T-lymphocyte activation' later in this chapter). Since a microorganism is usually made up of several different antigens an immunological response may be made up of a combination of responses; e.g. components of the non-specific defence system (complement, neutrophils, macrophages) are frequently employed in the final destruction of an antigen.

Cells of the immune system

B-lymphocytes are a type of white blood cell produced and matured in bone marrow. They circulate around the body via blood and lymph. B-lymphocytes are responsible for the production of antibodies, glycoproteins which bind to specific antigens with the aim of destroying them. These glycoproteins, also known as immunoglobulins, fall into five structural classes, namely IgG, IgA, IgD, IgM and IgE. In some cases, immunoglobulins are secreted into the blood. In others, they remain bound to the surface of the B-cell where they behave as antigen *receptors* (Fig. 2.4). Antigen receptors have a high affinity for specific antigen which when encountered will bind to the B-lymphocyte receptor. This process activates the B-cell to bind with the antibody in order to neutralize the antigen. Antigen receptors are able to recognize a number of foreign substances because their surfaces have a corresponding shape which allows them to bind together. For any one antigen there may be different regions with which a B-cell receptor can bind; these are called *antigenic determinants* or *epitopes*. As a rule, activation of B-cells requires the help of a T-helper cell

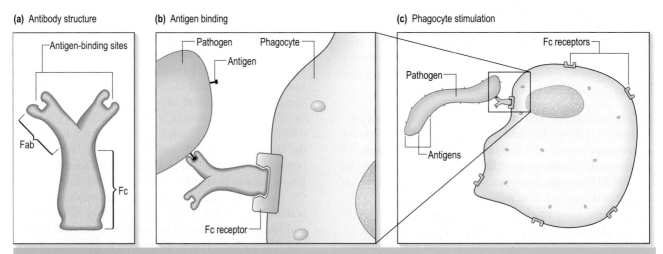

(a) Antibody structure

(b) Antigen binding

(c) Phagocyte stimulation

Figure 2.4.   Antibody binding to an antigen. (a) Structure of an antibody demonstrating the various binding sites for antigen (Fab) and phagocytes (Fc). (b) Antigen in the wall of a pathogen has many binding sites (epitopes), one of which is specific for an antibody and can therefore bind to the Fab portion of the antibody. (c) The free Fc portion of the antibody can also bind to phagocytes, inducing phagocytosis of the antigen or the pathogen.

responding to the same antigen (see 'B-lymphocyte activation' later in this chapter).

Once activated, the B-cell undergoes mitotic division to produce a clone of cells, able to synthesize immunoglobulin of the same specificity (but of more than one immunoglobulin class). Most of the B-cell clones mature into *plasma cells* which are capable of synthesis and secretion of large quantities of immunoglobulin or antibody. A few B-cells become memory cells.

T-lymphocytes are produced in bone marrow or the thymus. Those from bone marrow migrate to the thymus with the aid of chemotactic substances, so that all T-lymphocytes mature in the thymus (T = thymus). These lymphocytes have not yet had any contact with antigens. Clones of mature cells then travel via lymph and blood to populate the peripheral lymphoid tissue and from there continously circulate via the bloodstream in a constant quest for antigens. The surface of a T-cell has many binding sites called *T-cell receptors (TcR)* which recognize and bind to specific antigens, specifically microorganisms. T-cells can produce a wide variety of receptor molecules capable of recognizing over a million epitopes. Should some T-cells develop receptors that recognize our own body as being foreign, these cells are suppressed or destroyed in the thymus, resulting in *self-tolerance*.

The following are the types of T-lymphocytes discussed in detail in 'T-lymphocyte activation':

- Th – helper T-cells
- Tc – cytotoxic T-cells
- Ts – suppressor T-cells

Once mature lymphocytes have left the primary lymphoid tissues (bone marrow and thymus) via the blood, they then enter the secondary lymphoid tissues. These tissues include lymph nodes, spleen, thymus and mucosa-associated lymphoid tissue (MALT). After spending short periods screening these organs for antigens, they leave via blood or lymphatic capillaries and continue to circulate searching for antigens.

The lymphoid system

The lymphoid (immune) system consists of the secondary lymphoid tissues and lymphatic vessels connecting most tissues of the body to lymph nodes and ultimately to the bloodstream.

The lymphatic system

Lymphatic vessels can be found in the walls of most internal organs and in most tissues. They are similar in structure to blood vessels and transport lymphatic fluid around the body. Lymph has a similar constituent to blood except it is derived from interstitial fluid (fluid lying between cells and tissues) and has a lower protein content. Lymphocytes and tissue dendritic cells enter lymph from the tissues. Lymphatic vessels found in tissues are small and gradually increase in

size as they join up to form the largest vessels, the thoracic duct and right lymphatic duct, which drain into the right subclavian vein and left brachiocephalic vein (Fig. 2.5). As lymph leaves the tissues and travels around the body via the

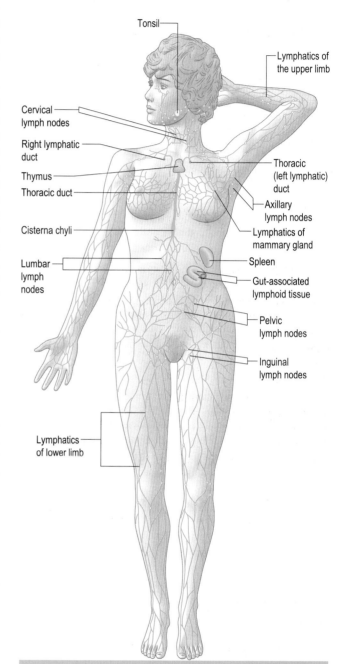

Figure 2.5. Lymphatic vessels and regions of lymph node aggregates. All lymph drained from tissues of the body ultimately reaches the venous system to enable cleaning and dispersal to the various lymph organs. The thoracic duct carries lymph from tissues inferior to the diaphragm and the left side of the body and drains into the left subclavian vein. The right lymphatic duct carries lymph from the rest of the body to the brachiocephalic vein.

larger lymph vessels towards the bloodstream, it passes through several lymph nodes in order to be filtered and screened for foreign substances.

Lymph nodes

Lymph nodes are small bean-shaped organs which, when relatively inactive, are only a few millimetres in length, and increase greatly in size when mounting an active immunological response. The lymph node (Plate I: see colour plate section between pp. x and 1) has an outer region, the cortex, which is highly cellular, and an inner region, the medulla, which is less cellular. The node is encapsulated in a dense collagenous connective tissue from which trabeculae extend for a variable distance into the node. *Afferent lymphatic vessels* divide into branches outside the node and then enter the node at the capsule to drain into a narrow space beneath the capsule known as the *subcapsular sinus.* The subcapsular sinus then opens into a system of channels that run from the cortex, via *cortical sinuses*, down into the medulla, via *medullary sinuses*, converging at the hilum in the concavity of the node. At the hilum an *efferent lymphatic vessel* leaves the node. Lymph fluid therefore enters at afferent vessels and courses through the node via the series of sinuses (leaving and entering the permeable walls of these sinuses to 'bathe' local cells in lymph) until it leaves the node via the efferent vessel at the hilum. This fluid will finally enter the circulation and be distributed to the rest of the body.

The parenchyma of the node consists of a mesh of reticulin fibres supporting a constantly changing population of lymphocytes. The cortex consists of densely packed lymphocytes lying on supporting reticulin fibres between trabeculae and sinuses (Fig. 2.6). These aggregates of lymphocytes then form cords of cells projecting into the medulla as *medullary cords*, lying between medullary trabeculae and sinuses. In the outer cortex lymphocytes are arranged as *lymphoid follicles* which may show a *germinal centre*. The number and size of germinal centres is dependent on the number and size of immune reactions taking place in a particular node and the individual as a whole at any one time. The germinal centre is the site for B-lymphocyte proliferation (hence 'germinal' centre). The inner cortex (paracortical zone) consists mainly of T-lymphocytes which are not arranged as follicles. The medullary cords have B-lymphocytes and plasma cells loosely arranged and producing immunoglobulins or antibodies in response to circulating antigens.

This specialized distribution of cells, together with the unidirectional flow of lymph, divides the node into specific functional regions, resulting in afferent lymph having a different composition to efferent lymph (Fig. 2.7).

Afferent lymph contains less than 10% of lymphocytes entering the node, particulate matter (including microorganisms), soluble antigens and some antigen-presenting cells migrating from peripheral organs. Efferent lymph contains little particulate matter or soluble antigens but contains large numbers of circulating T-lymphocytes,

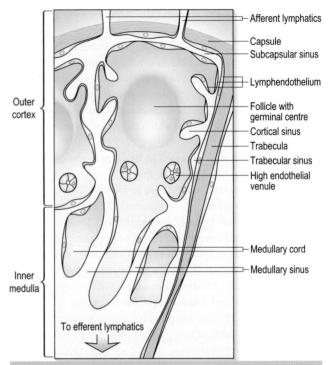

Figure 2.6. Schematic diagram of lymph node. (Reproduced with permission from Young and Heath, 2000.)

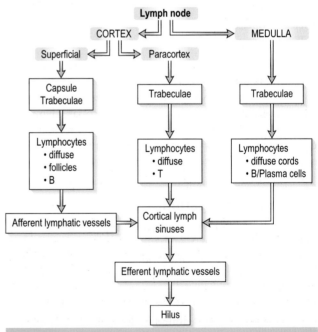

Figure 2.7. Summary of the structure and cell content of a lymph node.

varying numbers of B-lymphocytes, plasma cells and antibodies.

The blood supply of the lymph node is derived from one or more small arteries entering at the hilum of the node.

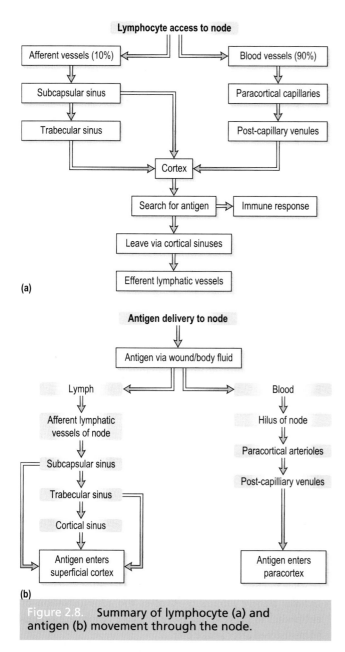

Figure 2.8. Summary of lymphocyte (a) and antigen (b) movement through the node.

These vessels divide into a network of capillaries branching into the substance of the node and ending as post-capillary venules. In the paracortex these venules permit the migration of lymphocytes across their cell walls. The post-capillary venules drain into small veins which leave the node at the hilum. Approximately 90% of lymphocytes and any circulating antigens enter the lymph node via these vessels.

Lymphocytes move through the lymph node in their quest to find antigens (Fig. 2.8a and b). Those not recognizing antigens leave the node within a few hours via the lymphatic sinuses and efferent lymph to rejoin the circulation. Antigens are phagocytosed by various types of antigen-presenting cells (APC) exposed to the lymph, processed and finally presented to lymphocytes.

Spleen

The spleen is a large lymphatic organ situated in the left upper part of the abdomen; it is supplied by a single large artery, the *splenic artery*, and drained by the *splenic vein* into the portal system. In the fetus the spleen is an important site for haemopoiesis, a function which may be resumed in the adult under certain disease conditions. However, in adult humans the spleen has two main functions:

- generation of immunological responses to bloodborne antigens
- removal from the circulation of particulate matter and old or defective blood cells, especially erythrocytes.

The spleen is similar to the lymph node except that the lymph circulation is replaced by blood circulation. The structure of the spleen provides for intimate contact between blood and immunologically active cells. The outer aspect of the spleen is surrounded by a connective tissue capsule which extends as trabeculae of connective tissue into the organ as support for the cellular and vascular components (Plate II: see colour plate section between pp. x and 1).

A single splenic artery divides into several large branches which enter the spleen at the hilum. These in turn divide into arterioles which enter the parenchyma of the spleen ending as a network of capillaries. Blood entering the spleen leaves these capillaries and passes into the parenchyma. While in the parenchyma old blood cells and particulate matter are phagocytosed and antigens are exposed to lymphocytes for antibody production. Healthy blood cells, lymphocytes and antibodies then enter the permeable interconnected sinuses which drain into tributaries of the splenic vein, finally joining the hepatic portal vein.

Splenic parenchyma (Fig. 2.9) therefore consists of lymphocytes, macrophages and erythrocytes. Lymphocytes are arranged as B-lymphocyte aggregates with varying numbers of germinal centres (white pulp), or more loosely arranged T-lymphocytes located around arterioles (red pulp). The loosely arranged lymphocytes and the large number of small vessels make up most of the organ.

It is thought that since aged or abnormal red blood cells are less deformable they cannot enter the slits in the sinusoidal membrane walls and are therefore removed, together with particulate matter, by macrophage activity in the parenchyma. Entering blood is therefore cleansed by the spleen before it enters the circulation again. Afferent blood contains mononuclear phagocytic cells, other macrophages, old/deformed blood cells, particulate matter and antigens. Efferent blood contains healthy blood cells, phagocytic cells, lymphocytes and antibodies.

Mucosa-associated lymphoid tissue (MALT)

The mucosa of the gastrointestinal and respiratory tracts contains a large amount of unencapsulated lymphoid tissue. MALT is formed during fetal development but is not activated

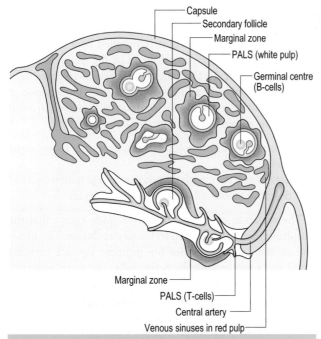

Figure 2.9. Schematic diagram showing organization of the spleen. (Reproduced with permission from Nairn and Helbert, 2002.)

until exposed to antigens at birth. The amount of MALT is maximal during childhood and reduces progressively in adulthood.

- The larger aggregates of lymphocytes, e.g. Peyer's patches in the gut, function in a similar way to the lymph node, where antigenic material entering the tract is recognized and both antibody-mediated and cytotoxic immune responses are initiated; they contain B- and T-lymphocytes and antigen-processing accessory cells.
- The diffusely scattered lymphocytes found just beneath the epithelia of the respiratory and genitourinary tracts are mostly B-lymphocytes some of which mature into antibody-secreting plasma cells. All classes of antibody are produced with IgA predominating. IgA is secreted either by diffusing through the epithelium or in specific secretions such as saliva, tears and in milk during lactation. Activated lymphocytes derived from the respiratory tract aggregations tend to move directly to the respiratory mucosa.

Summary of the immune system

- Both blood and lymph are the means by which particulate matter, microorganisms and other antigens reach the organs responsible for protecting us from infection.
- Lymph nodes, the spleen and MALT are the organs of the lymphoid system.
- The main cell types of the lymphoid system are lymphocytes. Lymphocytes are arranged either in aggregates, consisting mainly of B-lymphocytes with the potential to develop

germinal centres in response to antigenic stimulation, or loosely scattered and consisting of T-lymphocytes.
- Lymphoid organs also contain several other cell types which assist in the immune response.

The next step is the reaction that occurs when a pathogen/antigen encounters a cell from the immune system.

Acquiring specific immunity

The most effective way for the body to generate an immune response is to produce antibodies to specific antigens, to do so only when the antigen is present and to produce different classes of antibody with different functions. Antibodies to a specific pathogen can only be made *after* exposure to the pathogen. The following is a summary of the normal immune processes.

Forms of immunity

Immunity is either innate or acquired.

Innate immunity is present at birth and does not need previous exposure to the antigen.

Acquired immunity requires previous exposure to an antigen. There are several forms of acquired immunity:

- *Active immunity* is acquired after exposure to an antigen and after an immune response.
- *Naturally acquired immunity* begins after birth and continues through life as one encounters normally occurring antigens, e.g. flu viruses.
- *Induced-active immunity* is the artificially induced immunity achieved through immunization or vaccination. Vaccines consist of either a dead or inactive pathogen, or antigen derived from that pathogen, intended to induce an immune response, antibody formation and thus immunity.
- *Natural passive immunity* is the transfer of antibodies from mother to child via the placenta or breast milk.
- *Induced passive immunity* involves the administration of antibodies to prevent disease, e.g. snake venom antibodies administered after snake bite.

B-lymphocytes and antibody production

As mentioned previously surface immunoglobulins (antibodies) on B-cells are able to recognize free antigens (component of a pathogen), bind to and neutralize the antigens. Each B-lymphocyte recognizes and binds to specific antigen. This ability to recognize free antigens in the fluids of the body is known as *humoral immunity* (Fig. 2.10). By the time a lymphocyte is mature it has embedded in its membrane various immunoglobulin (Ig) molecules: IgM, IgD and either IgA or IgG. Once the B-cell Ig has bound to an antigen *sensitization* the B-cell undergoes cell division, producing lots of B-cells with the same specificity for that antigen (*clonal expansion*). This process requires additional stimulation by Th cells. Once proliferation has occurred the B-cell is able to

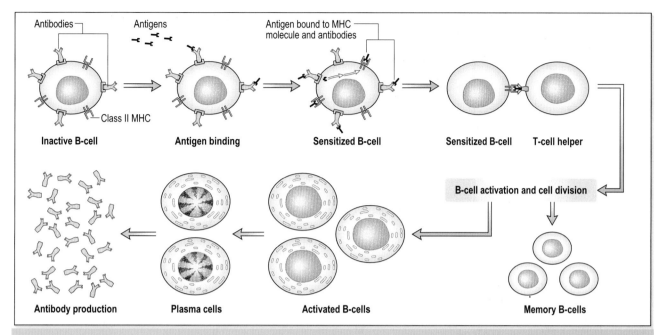

Antibodies — Antigens — Antigen bound to MHC molecule and antibodies

Class II MHC

Inactive B-cell   **Antigen binding**   **Sensitized B-cell**   **Sensitized B-cell**   **T-cell helper**

B-cell activation and cell division

Antibody production   **Plasma cells**   **Activated B-cells**   **Memory B-cells**

Figure 2.10. B-lymphocyte activation. Sensitization of the B-cell occurs with binding of the antigen to the antibody in the B-cell membrane. The antigen is then displayed by the MHC molecule on the B-cell membrane. Activated T-helper cells encountering the antigen release cytokines which activate the B-cell.

produce and secrete antibodies (*differentiation*). The antibody secreted has the same specificity for the antigen as the surface Ig molecule that initially bound to the antigen. The first antibody secreted by B-cells is IgM. B-cells then change the class of the surface Ig from IgM or IgD to either IgG, IgA or IgE. Random DNA mutations in the B-cell result in these Ig having a wide range of binding affinities enabling them to bind to several antigens on the one pathogen.

Differentiation of B-cells into plasma or memory cells

Some stimulated B-cells produce antibodies. These *plasma cells* may produce antibodies for a few weeks then die, while others secrete antibodies for months. Other B-cells (*memory B-cells*) continue to express the Ig on their cell membranes but return to the G0 phase (resting phase) of the cell cycle. Only cells expressing IgG, IgA or IgE can become memory cells. If the same antigen is encountered at a later point, the memory B-cell is activated and may then divide to form plasma cells and more memory B-cells. Secondary exposure to the same antigen results in the production of antibodies at a much faster rate than the initial exposure, largely due to the fact that proliferation, differentiation and class switch have already been done. This forms the basis of vaccinations discussed in 'Therapeutic applications of immunity' later in this chapter.

T-lymphocyte activation

T-lymphocyte activity depends on the class of T-cell involved (Fig. 2.11).

T-cell classes: CD nomenclature

T-cells are distinguished by the allocation of a *cluster determinant* number which defines the type of surface molecule found on the cell. Helper T-cells express a molecule called CD4 on their surface (CD4 Th or CD4+ Th), while suppressor and cytotoxic T-cells express CD8 on their surface (CD8 Ts/CD8 Tc or CD8+ Ts/CD8+ Tc). T-cells express either one or the other but not both. The CD molecules are believed to act cooperatively with T-cell receptors to mediate T-cell activation of a number of cellular functions, for example in the case of CD8 to help initiate cytotoxic or suppressor functions. T-lymphocytes can be divided into functional subpopulations. Subsets of CD4 T-helper differ in patterns of cytokine secretion and are designated Th1 and Th2 cells. Similarly, two CD8 T-cytotoxic cell subpopulations have been identified and designated Tc1 and Tc2. For the purposes of this chapter only the role of Th1 and Th2 cells will be discussed in subsequent sections.

T-cell receptor (TcR)

The TcR has a similar structure to the antibody produced by B-cells and can thus bind to specific antigen. However, the TcR is never secreted by the cell as are antibodies, but remains attached to the surface of the cell where it binds to antigen. Each TcR will bind with only one specific antigen. A TcR recognizes antigens only when they are associated with a specific molecule on the surface of a cell. In other words they do not recognize free antigen, only antigen-presenting cells (APC). T-lymphocytes are therefore involved in *cellular immunity*.

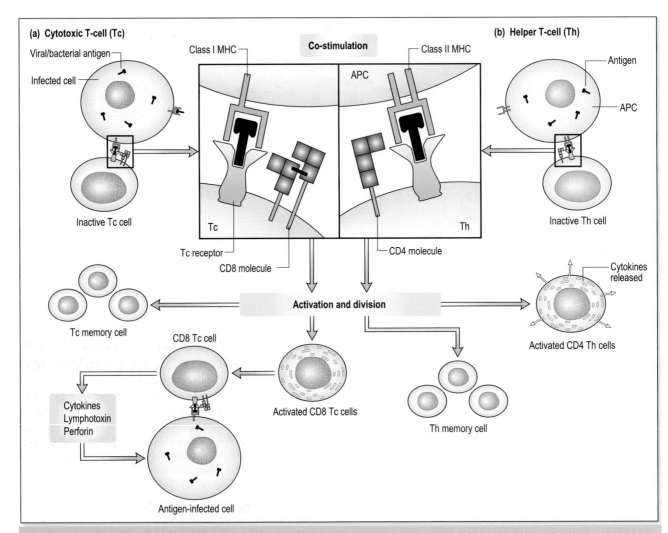

Figure 2.11. Cytoxic and helper T-cell activation. (a) Inactive Tc cells encounter infected cells displaying antigen bound to MHC class I molecules on their surface. This together with co-stimulation by the membrane of the infected cell activates the Tc cell to produce memory Tc cells and activated Tc cells. Activated Tc cells bind with other cells infected with the same antigen and release a number of substances inducing lysis of the infected cell. (b) Inactive T-helper cells encounter antigen-presenting cells displaying antigen bound to class II MHC molecules on the surface. Th cells are then activated to produce memory Th cells and activated Th cells. The latter release cytokines that induce cell-mediated and antibody-mediated immunities.

The specific molecules recognized by the TcR are referred to as *major histocompatibility complex (MHC) molecules.*

MHC molecules

The MHC is a group of glycoproteins expressed in every nucleated cell of vertebrates. The human MHC molecules are termed HLA (human leucocyte antigen)-A, B and C molecules. These are the major proteins that differentiate tissues of one individual from another and were first discovered in the context of human transplant rejection. Their task is to display the antigens of cells or microbes for recognition by T-cells. MHC proteins have been divided into three classes based on function. *Class I* (found on the surface of most

nucleated cells) and *Class II* (found primarily on monocytes, macrophages and B-lymphocytes) are similar and involved in T-cell recognition of antigen. MHC class I molecule expression is enhanced by inflammatory and immune stimuli. *Class III* consists of many types of proteins which are not related to each other and have many immune-related functions.

Both MHC class I and II molecules have a notch on top of the molecule to which an antigen could bind. When a cell that has an antigen attached to it comes into contact with a T-cell, part of the antigen/MHC molecule that is sticking out is recognized and bound by the TcR. The antigen/MHC molecule thus formed is then able to bind more efficiently to

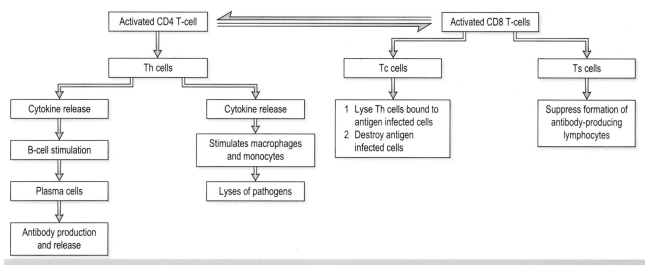

Figure 2.12. The role of CD4 T-cells and CD8 T-cells in the immune system.

other TcR. CD4 T-cells recognize antigen (endogenous) presented by self-class II MHC molecules and CD8 T-cells recognize antigens (exogenous) presented by self-class I MHC molecules.

When the antigen/MHC interacts with the TcR complex, signals are transduced to the T-cell nucleus, which leads to the proliferation of this clone and thus an amplification of the immune response (as with B-lymphocytes). T-cells not bearing the TcR corresponding to that antigen remain unresponsive. A summary of this mechanism is given in Figure 2.11.

Antigen-presenting cells
Antigen-presenting cells (APC) are specialized cells responsible for the activation of T-lymphocytes. Class II MHC proteins are found in the walls of APCs, allowing them to bind to antigens and present them to T-cells. APCs include:

- Phagocytic cells such as free and fixed macrophages in connective tissue, Kupfer cells of the liver and microglia in the central nervous system. Phagocytic APCs ingest and break down the antigen to smaller antigenic fragments. The fragments are then bound to MHC class II proteins and inserted into the membrane of the APC. The antigen/MHC complex is able to bind to TcR, resulting in T-cell activation.
- Non-phagocytic APC cells are bone-marrow derived *dendritic cells*. Dendritic cells are found in many tissues including lymph nodes, spleen and a specialized dendritic cell found in skin, called Langerhans cells. These cells remove antigenic materials from their surroundings by *pinocytosis* followed by binding of the antigenic fragments to MHC class II proteins and insertion into the APC cell wall.

Dendritic APCs are very efficient at presenting CD4 T cells with antigen and thus providing the co-stimulatory signal necessary for full CD4 T-cell activation.

- Both B-cells and macrophages are capable of expressing high levels of MHC class II in their membranes when stimulated by an ongoing immune response. Both cells are therefore capable of presenting antigen to T-cells and therefore stimulating new CD4 T-cell production.

The role of CD4 and CD8 T-cells
The role of these cells can be summarized as follows (Fig. 2.12):

- Once a CD4 T-cell has been stimulated by an antigen/ MHC molecule it proliferates and then differentiates into T-helper (Th) cells.

  Th cells control the process of B-lymphocyte activation, class switch and antibody secretion. T-cell stimulation of B-cells occurs with the release of an array of *cytokines* which act directly on the B-cell causing it to differentiate into a plasma cell and secrete antibodies. T-cell-independent response of B-lymphocytes to an antigen is limited compared to this mechanism.
- In addition to acting on B-lymphocytes, activated Th cells migrate to areas of infection and release specific cytokines. These stimulate the lytic activity of both monocytes and macrophages, allowing them to break down pathogens more efficiently.
- CD8 cytotoxic T-cells (Tc) destroy mature T-cells which have interacted with an antigen on a foreign cell and suppressor T-cells (Ts) cells suppress the formation of antibody-producing B-lymphocytes. Tc cells destroy antigen-containing cells either by releasing *perforin* which

ruptures the cell membrane, by secreting a poisonous *lymphotoxin* or by activating genes in the cell that tell the cell to die (genetically programmed cell death is known as *apoptosis*). Ts cells release *suppression factors*, cytokines that inhibit the responses of other B- and T-cells, thereby controlling the immune response.

- There is evidence to suggest that both CD4 T-cells and CD8 T-cells need to respond to the same antigen in order for the CD8 T-cytotoxic (Tc) cell to be effective in neutralizing the antigen.

Summary of immune system activation

There are several mechanisms for immunological activation:

1. Interaction of a B-cell with a protein or polysaccharide antigen which has a repeating chemical sequence, e.g. the polysaccharide coat of pneumococcus bacteria.
2. Antigen is taken up by an antigen-presenting cell (e.g. macrophage), 'processed' (e.g. protein broken down into peptides), and the elements of it bound to an HLA protein in the membrane of the presenting cell. An antigen–protein complex bound to class II HLA molecules induces a T-helper cell (Th) response. The Th cell is then able to 'help' B-cells to respond to the same antigen by producing antibodies. This help consists of the production of cytokines (interleukins, IL) which mediate activation, clonal expansion and maturation of the B-cell response.
3. Antigens produced within a cell of the body (e.g. tumour cell, virus-infected cell) are bound to a class I HLA membrane protein where it is available for recognition by CD8-bearing cytotoxic T-lymphocytes. Th activation is required for a Tc response to be activated. Both Th and Tc cells require processing and presentation of the antigen by a macrophage.
4. Cells bearing different HLA proteins, e.g. transplanted tissues, stimulate an immune response involving Th and either Tc cells or macrophages.

Overview of the lymphoid system

The previous sections can be summarized as follows. Antigen can enter tissue via the MALT, by draining into lymphatic vessels and then into lymph nodes or it can enter the circulatory system and enter the spleen. Antigen is taken up by dendritic cells in tissues, e.g. lymphatic tissue, and presented to CD4 T-cells which are then activated to become Th cells. Th cells move to the edge of lymphoid follicles (e.g. cortex of lymph node, white pulp of spleen) where they encounter and stimulate B-cells to produce antibodies. B-cells produce both memory B-cells and plasma cells. Antibodies secreted by plasma cells move around the body via lymph and blood. At the same time lymphocytes are circulating in the blood and lymph. This movement is controlled by adhesion molecules and chemokines which increase the chance of lymphocytes meeting their specific antigen. Once a B- or T-cell encounters an antigen, *neutralization* or *destruction* of the antigen will follow.

Neutralization and destruction of antigen

Antibody mechanisms

- *Neutralization.* Both viruses and bacterial toxins have binding sites on their membranes for binding to other cells. Antibodies bind to these sites, preventing the toxin from binding to cells of the body.
- *Agglutination.* Antibodies bind to more than one microbe, creating a large cluster of microbe and antibody. This is then phagocytosed.
- *Activation of complement.* Once bound to an antigen, portions of the antibody change shape, exposing areas that bind complement proteins. The bound complement molecules then activate the complement system, destroying the antigen.
- *Opsonization.* This is the coating of a pathogen in antibodies and complement proteins. The antibodies attract phagocytes and also assist phagocytes to hang on to the pathogen long enough to destroy it (see 'Complement system', earlier in the chapter).

T-cell mechanisms

- CD8 cytotoxic T-cells kill target cells containing antigen on their class I MHC molecules.
- Cytotoxic T-cells release granules of enzymes (perforin, granzyme) which enter the target cell and induce apoptosis (disintegration of cells into membrane-bound particles).
- Antigens residing in tissues activate CD4 T-cells to become Th1 cells. These then enter the blood and travel to infection sites where the pathogen is located. Th1 cells release cytokines which attract monocytes to the area from blood. Th1 cells activate monocyte and macrophage activity.

The role of cytokines in the immune system

Almost all of the above activites are controlled by cytokines. Cytokines are small proteins produced by cells in order to communicate with other cells in the local vicinity. Cytokines can either bind to receptors of a neighbouring cell (*paracrine activity*) or they can bind to receptors on the same cell that produced the cytokine (*autocrine activity*). These small proteins control proliferation, differentiation and many cell functions (Table 2.2). Cytokines have been divided into families and include interleukins, interferons, tumour necrosis factor, growth factors and chemokines. The function of some of these, particularly interleukins and chemokines, will be discussed again in appropriate sections of this chapter.

IMMUNE DISORDERS

A variety of clinical conditions can result from disorders of the immune system. *Hypersensitivity/allergic reactions* occur more commonly and are essentially an overreaction of the

Table 2.2. Cytokines of the immune system

Compound	Functions
Interleukins:	
Interleukin-1 (IL-1)	Stimulates T-cells to produce IL-2, promotes inflammation; causes fever
IL-2	Stimulates growth and activation of other T-cells and NK cells
IL-3	Stimulates production of mast cells and other blood cells
IL-4 (B-cell differentiating factor); IL-5 (B-cell growth factor); IL-6, IL-7 (B-cell stimulating factors); IL-10; IL-11	Promote differentiation and growth of B-cells and stimulate plasma cell formation and antibody production; each has somewhat different effects on macrophage and microphage activities
IL-8	Stimulates blood vessel formation (angiogenesis)
IL-9	Stimulates myeloid cell production (RBCs, platelets, granulocytes, monocytes)
IL-12	Stimulates T-cell activity and cell-mediated immunity
IL-13	Suppresses production of several other cytokines (IL-1, IL-8, TNF); stimulates class II MHC antigen presentation
Interferons (alpha, beta, gamma)	Activate other cells to prevent viral entry; inhibit viral replication; stimulate NK cells and macrophages
Tumour necrosis factors (TNFs)	Kill tumour cells; slow tumour growth; stimulate activities of T cells and eosinophils; inhibit parasites and viruses
Monocyte-chemotactic factor (MCF)	Attracts monocytes; activates them to macrophages
Migration-inhibitory factor (MIF)	Prevents macrophage migration from the area
Macrophage-activating factor (MAF)	Makes macrophages more active and aggressive
Growth-inhibitory factor (GIF)	Reduces or inhibits replication of target cells
Leukotrienes	Stimulate regional inflammation
Lymphotoxins	Kill cells; damage tissue; promote inflammation
Perforin	Destroys cell membranes by creating large pores
Transforming growth factor-β (TGF-β)	Stimulates production of IgA and of matrix proteins in connective tissues; inhibits macrophage activation and Tc maturation
Suppression factors	Inhibit Tc cell and B-cell activity; depress immune response
Transfer factor	Sensitizes other T-cells to same antigen
Chemokines	A cytokine that causes chemotaxis and attracts neutrophils, monocytes and T-lymphocytes to assist in destroying organisms

immune system to antigens. *Autoimmune disorders* develop when the immune system incorrectly targets normal body cells and tissues. *Immunodeficiency diseases* occur when the immune system fails to develop normally or when its action is blocked.

Hypersensitivity

Defined as 'an abnormal response to a stimulus of any kind', hypersensitivity reactions can be classified (types I–IV) according to which component of the immune system is involved.

Type I: immediate hypersensitivity (allergy)
Immune reaction
Invasion of host skin or mucosal tissues by relatively innocuous pathogens such as parasites, house dust or pollen granules should result in a normal immune response that rids the body of the pathogen. However, in some individuals the antigen-presenting cells capture and process the antigen (allergen), present it to B- and T-cells which then produce IgE antibodies (Fig. 2.13). Raised IgE antibodies are the key component

in immediate hypersensitivity reactions. IgE binds to Fc receptors on mast cells throughout the body, thereby sensitizing (priming) the mast cells for any future contact with the allergen. Subsequent exposure to the allergen results in the release of histamine from primed mast cells, creating an initial 5–30 minute response.

This may result in localized signs and symptoms including:

- an increase in vascular permeability
- constriction of smooth muscle of the bronchial tree and therefore bronchoconstriction
- increased mucus secretion from nasal, bronchial and gastric glands
- areas of inflamed, itchy skin (*urticaria* or *hives*)
- inflammation of the eyes (*conjunctivitis*)
- nasal cavity inflammation (*rhinitis*).

If, however, the result of contact with the allergen results in a systemic reaction, this is known as *anaphylactic shock* and can be fatal. In anaphylaxis the above effects are enhanced with severe asthma and/or severe hypotension due to loss of fluid from the blood to the tissues. The person

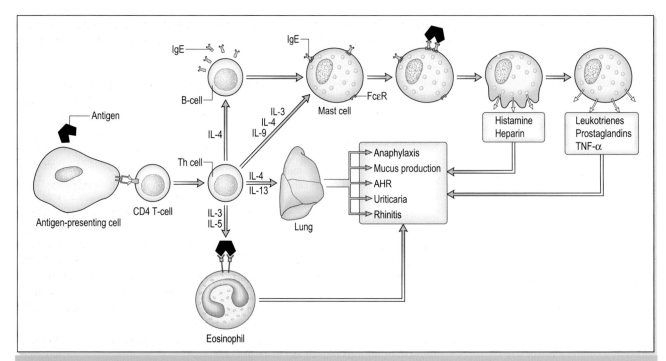

Figure 2.13.   Molecular and cellular events in atopic disease. Once activated by antigen presented by APC, Th cells release: IL-4 which induces B-cell maturation and release of antibody; Il-3, IL-4 and IL-9 required for mast cell activation; IL-4 and IL-13 suspected of direct action on lung tissue inducing atopic disease effects; IL-3 and IL-5 required for eosinophil growth differentiation.

develops pruritus (intense itching), urticaria, erythema (red rash), wheezing and dyspnoea (difficult breathing), vomiting, diarrhoea and cramps. The larynx may swell and if spasm develops this can be fatal. To reverse the reaction injections of histamine competitors (e.g. adrenaline (epinephrine), isoproterenol) and antihistamines are administered. If the reaction is not caught in time, patients can die from either respiratory or circulatory failure.

Late response. A subsequent, more extensive, allergic reaction occurs in 2–8 hours and can last for 2–3 days. This involves the formation and release of additional mediators which are responsible for the signs and symptoms of allergic reactions. These include cytokine (TNF-α) stimulation of the endothelium at the site resulting in the expression of adhesion molecules for the binding of eosinophils and neutrophils. Leukotrienes, prostaglandins, platelet-activating factor and protein-digesting enzymes are also stimulated by cytokines. Localized hypersensitivity can include asthma, hay fever, eczema and utricaria. The term *atopy* is used to describe an allergy for which there is a genetic predisposition.

People prone to allergic responses may therefore have:

1. elevated plasma IgE (particularly in allergic asthma)
2. an inherited general hyperresponsiveness
3. an inherited antigen-specific response
4. low numbers of suppressor T-cells.

The role of cytokines in allergic inflammation.   Figure 2.13 summarizes these mechanisms.

Atopic diseases are currently believed to be the result of type 2 T-helper cell (Th2) dominated responses to environmental allergens. Th2 cells have receptors (TCR) able to recognize and bind to allergen peptides. This interaction results in the release of cytokines, particularly interleukins (ILs), which in turn act on the following cells:

- IgE-antibody-producing B-cells (IL-4, IL-3).
- Mast cells (IL-4, IL-10). Mast cells are themselves an important source of IL-13 and IL-14. Mast cells are present in high numbers in the smooth muscle of the bronchial tree in asthmatic patients. Research is currently being conducted to determine whether this localization implicates them in the observed bronchoconstriction and airways hyperresponsiveness (AHR) seen in asthma.
- Eosinophil granulocytes (IL-5).

Th2 cell cytokines IL-4, IL-5, IL-9 and IL-13 are believed to account for the majority of pathophysiological manifestations of allergic patients. However, subepithelial fibrosis in asthma has been shown to result from growth factor (TGF-β), produced by T-cells, as well as IL-6 produced by several cell types. Current evidence suggests that T-cells play an important regulatory role in asthma, but that ongoing or chronic TGF-β production is responsible for the airway fibrosis and remodelling. Fibrosis and remodelling lead to thickened walls of the bronchial tree and contribute to the fixed airflow obstruction observed in many patients.

IL-4 and IL-13 in allergy. IL-4 facilitates the transfer of eosinophils into target tissues with the help of IL-5 and chemokines (discussed below) and stimulates mast cell growth and differentiation. IL-13 stimulates mucus hypersecretion by and metaplasia of mucus cells. IL-4 and IL-13 stimulate fibroblast growth and chemotaxis and the synthesis of extracellular matrix proteins. IL-4 activity appears to be largely responsible for the induction of the immune response, whereas, IL-13 appears to be critical in establishing the allergic inflammation.

IL-5 in allergy. IL-5 plays a role in eosinophil growth, survival and function. Animal studies have shown that in response to allergic stimulation in the lung, IL-5 regulates expansion of eosinophils in the bone marrow and enhances their mobilization into the circulatory system. Movement of eosinophils from the blood into other tissues, for example lung tissue, is therefore indirectly enhanced by IL-5. However, IL-5 works with eotaxin (a chemokine) to recruit eosinophils to the airways. IL-5 has also been shown to stimulate the maturation of eosinophils residing in lung tissue (Fig. 2.13).

Ultimately it is the coordinated expression of IL-5, other cytokines (particularly IL-4 and IL-13) and eotaxin that determines maximum lung pathology. The precise mechanisms involved are not yet clear, but not all asthma is associated with eosinophilic inflammation. In fact many asthmatics have raised neutrophils in their sputum. Identification of this group of patients is clinically important as early results have shown this patient group to be far less responsive to corticosteroids.

Summary of immune processes in allergy
1. Allergic responses are exaggerated molecular responses to specific stimuli, e.g. parasites, pollen.
2. Increased activity of Th2 cells marks the physiological onset of allergic reactions.
3. Th2 cells release cytokines causing a cascade of cellular events which contribute to the clinical picture of an allergic reaction.
4. The interleukin group of cytokines mediate communication between cells such as mast cells, eosinophils, T-cells and B-cells.
5. B-lymphocytes release IgE in response to the allergen.
6. In asthma the ongoing allergic response with subsequent fibrosis and myoplasia appears to be caused by increased TGF-β secretion.

Therapeutic strategies for allergic disease
1. Therapy at the onset. At the time of an allergic reaction use can be made of drugs that inhibit the release of histamine from mast cells. The use of histamine competitors and antihistamines serves to reduce the symptoms but does not address the underlying immune cause.

2. Preventative strategies. These include injecting the allergen in varying doses to reduce sensitivity. Injection tends to increase IgG, which binds with and removes antigen from the tissue fluids before it can interact with mast cells and produce a large allergic response. However, this does not always go according to plan and patients may experience a generalized or systemic anaphylaxis. Regardless of the triggering antigen (e.g. penicillin, bee venom, peanuts) the signs and symptoms are the same. However, in the case of asthma therapeutic strategies aimed at the immune origin of allergy are being explored and include neutralization of either the IL or the IL receptor. Early introduction of neutralizing IL-4 antibody shifts the balance from an initial Th2 cell response to a Th1 cell response, which in turn results in a weak allergenic phenotype (i.e. reduced airways hyperresponsiveness (AHR) and other allergic features).

Nuvance is a soluble form of IL-4Rα (one of the IL-4 receptor proteins) that binds to and neutralizes IL-4. Nuvance can be safely administered intravenously to asthmatic patients. Similarly neutralization of IL-13 has been shown to dramatically reduce many allergic indices, especially AHR. The possibility of delivering this therapeutic agent in aerosol form is currently being explored. Like soluble IL-4Rα, soluble IL-5 receptors may provide an alternative to anti-cytokine antibodies. However, antagonists of IL-5 have been developed to prevent airway eosinophilia. Alternative approaches such as the use of IL-12, which is directed at switching Th2 cells to Th1 cells, form part of ongoing trials.

Drug therapy utilizes the following compounds:

1. Adrenaline (epinephrine), a beta-adrenergic compound which can block mast cell degranulation by limiting the mast cell response.
2. Corticosteroids and non-steroidal anti-inflammatory agents which block the synthesis of leukotrienes and prostaglandins.

Type II: antibody-dependent cytotoxicity
Immune reaction
In this type of hypersensitivity antibodies (IgG or IgM) bind to cells or tissues and trigger a number of reactions. Natural killer (NK) cells attracted by the antibody will begin phagocytosing the 'infected' cell. The presence of the antibody provides an ideal site for precipitation of complement, activating the complement cascade (see 'Defence mechanisms' above). This process breaks down cell membranes, releasing chemicals that attract neutrophils, eosinophils and

macrophages. Death and phagocytosis of the cell then follows in earnest.

Type II hypersensitivity reactions can occur in autoimmune disease when the antibody is directed against self cells (discussed below). When the antibodies are directed against non-self cells then essentially three major syndromes are associated with type II hypersensitivity: blood transfusion reactions, haemolytic disease of the newborn and drug-induced hypersensitivity.

1. Blood transfusion reactions. Blood typing depends on the particular glycoproteins expressed in the red blood cells of an individual. There are three variants of the glycoprotein called A, B and O. An individual can be blood type O, A, B or AB. As these glycoproteins are similar to those expressed by bacteria normally encountered during a lifetime, individuals will have produced antibodies to the type of glycoprotein they do not have. Exposure to a foreign blood group via transfusion would also result in the development of antibodies to that blood group. This means that individuals with blood group O make antibodies to blood group A and B; blood group A make antibodies to blood group B; and blood group B make antibodies to group A. Blood group AB do not make antibodies to either A or B, which means they can receive either type A or B blood transfusions. The antibodies produced are usually IgM.

If an individual receives blood from a group against which they have antibodies, the antibodies bind to the red blood cells that have been transfused and the above process is activated culminating in the death of the donor cells and rejection of the transfusion. This results in the release of large amounts of haemoglobin, some of which is metabolized to bilirubin, which in large quantities, can be toxic.

2. Haemolytic disease of the newborn. Red blood cells from most people have a rhesus antigen on their surface (Rh+). However, a minority lack the antigen (Rh−). During childbirth blood passes from the baby to the mother's circulation. If the mother is Rh− and the baby is Rh+, the mother will produce antibodies to Rh as they will be seen as foreign antigens. The IgG antibodies can cross the placenta to the fetus and bind to the fetus's red blood cells. This can result in opsonization and phagocytosis of red blood cells in the liver and spleen, leading to enlargement of these organs and toxicity due to bilirubin. This can be prevented by injecting the mother with antibodies immediately after birth (to avoid cross-placental transfer). The antibodies will bind to the fetal antigens which are then destroyed before they can sensitize the mother.

3. Drug-induced hypersensitivities. A few drugs or their metabolites bind to red blood cells or platelets. The self-protein–drug complex that is formed in some cases creates a new antigen and is seen as foreign. Antibodies are made against the new complex and destroyed by either the complement system or opsonization. Examples of this include penicillin, which binds to red blood cells resulting in anaemia, and sedormid, which binds to platelets resulting in thrombocytopenia.

Therapeutic interventions

One approach is to desensitize the individual to the specific allergen. Small amounts of the allergen are given repeatedly to an allergic individual to stimulate the production of IgG specific to the allergen. The amounts of allergen given must, however, be small enough not to trigger an allergic response. If the individual is subsequently exposed to antigen, in sufficient quantity to stimulate an allergic response, then the antigen will bind to the IgG molecule and be neutralized. In this way the antigen is prevented from binding to the allergen-specific IgE on the mast cells which would lead to the release of histamine.

Type III: immune-complex-mediated hypersensitivity

Immune reaction

Aggregates of antigen bound to their antibodies are formed in a normal response to infection. If the concentration of both is equal, large complexes are formed which are transported in the bloodstream and quickly removed by the liver and spleen. If, however, antigen concentration is higher (as in lungs subjected to constant asbestos inhalation, dust inhalation and mould spore inhalation from hay,) or the antibody concentration is higher (*as in autoimmune disease*), smaller complexes are formed. These complexes are deposited in blood vessel walls, particularly those of the kidney, skin and joints where they trigger a variety of inflammatory processes resulting in increased permeability, vasodilatation and phagocyte chemotaxis. Disorders that result from immune-complex-mediated hypersensitivity include glomerulonephritis (kidney damage due to viral or bacterial infection) and rheumatoid arthritis (RA).

Type IV: cell-mediated delayed-type hypersensitivity

Immune reaction

This type of hypersensitivity only occurs after exposure to the antigen and sensitization. The antigen can be an intracellular bacterium (tuberculosis, leprosy), an immune complex (contact dermatitis), or a foreign tissue (see 'Tissue transplantation' below). Delayed-type hypersensitivity (DTH) is generally mediated by CD4+ T-cells and downregulated by CD8 T-cells.

Tuberculosis

Two billion people are infected with the aetiological agent *Mycobacterium tuberculosis* annually. Less than 10% develop the disease, the remainder harbour the pathogen in discrete lesions. The immune system is very successful at preventing the spread of the pathogen but not at eradicating it. The immune response to *M. tuberculosis* is T-cell dependent, comprising both CD4 and CD8 T-cells. However, in addition to the more familiar T-cells, the disease process also involves *gammadelta T-cells* and *CD1-restricted T-cells*. Gammadelta T-cells recognize phospholigands and CD1-restricted T-cells recognize glycolipids, which are abundant components of the mycobacterial cell wall. Acquired resistance is associated with two mechanisms:

- cytokine activation of macrophages
- direct cytolytic activity.

Protective granulomas are induced and sustained by cytokines, thereby preventing the bacterium from spreading to other parts of the body.

The only vaccine available against TB is the Bacillus Calmette Guérin (BCG). However, this does not provide consistent protection against TB and current investigations are exploring the potential to develop vaccines using newly identified antigen components.

Allergic contact dermatitis

The allergen in this case is a small chemical which comes into contact with the skin and results in an eczematous reaction of swelling, redness and severe itching. The reaction occurs 24–72 hours after contact. Skin cells transport the allergen (nickel, rubber, poison oak or ivy) from the skin via lymphatics to lymph nodes where it is presented to responsive T-lymphocytes. Activated T-cells proliferate and therefore sensitize the individual to that specific antigen. Subsequent exposure results in a faster and larger reaction due to the influx of effector T-lymphocytes to affected skin sites. Thus an inflammatory reaction is set up. Current evidence suggests that unlike other DTH, contact hypersensitivity is largely effected by CD8+ T-cells, with CD4+ T-cells playing a regulatory role. The primary pathophysiological role of CD8+ T-lymphocytes is the lysis of virally infected cells. The cytotoxic mechanisms are, however, most likely to include combined action of both CD8+ and CD4+ T-cells.

Autoimmune disorders

Autoimmune disorders affect 5% of adults in America and Europe. Autoimmune reactions involve a normal part of the body (usually proteins but occasionally carbohydrates, lipids or DNA), known as an autoantigen (self antigen), being targeted by an antibody (autoantibody) to create an autoimmune response. The immune response results in a *primary pathology* (the direct consequence of the immune reaction) and a *secondary pathology* (the subsequent effect of the primary pathology). These diseases are due to a combination of environmental and genetic factors, the precise nature of which is as yet unknown.

The diversity of autoimmune diseases means that we know more about some than others. Table 2.3 lists some of the more

Table 2.3. Examples of autoimmune diseases

Target tissues	Disease	Physiological effects
Endocrine glands:		
Thyroid	Hashimoto's thyroiditis	Thyroid destruction and underfunction
Thyroid	Graves' disease	Thyroid stimulation and overfunction
Islets of Langerhans (pancreas)	Insulin-dependent diabetes mellitus	Destruction of B-cells (insulin-producing cells)
Adrenal gland	Addison's disease	Adrenal insufficiency
Haematopoietic system:		
Red blood cells	Autoimmune haemolytic anaemia	Anaemia
Platelets	Autoimmune thrombocytopenia	Abnormal bleeding
Intrinsic factor (IF)	Pernicious anaemia	Autoantibody prevents absorption of vitamin B_{12}
Nervous system:		
Central nervous system	Multiple sclerosis	Progressive paralysis
Neuromuscular junction	Myasthenia gravis	Progressive muscle weakness
Skin:		
Nuclear antigens	Polymyositis-dermatomyositis	Fibrosis of skin
Joints:		
Synovium	Rheumatoid arthritis (RA)	Progressive destruction
Synovium	Systematic lupus erythematosus (SLE)	Deformity
Kidney:		
Basement membrane	Goodpasture's syndrome	Glomerulonephritis
Glomerulus	SLE	Glomerulonephritis

common diseases. Essentially diseases in which only one organ is affected by autoimmunity, e.g. insulin-dependent diabetes mellitus (IDDM), are called *organ-specific*, while those in which many tissues are involved, e.g. systemic lupus erythematosus (SLE), are called *non-organ-specific*. During an autoimmune response the immune system produces the same cells (cytotoxic CD4 T, effector CD4 T) and molecules (antibodies) discussed previously as necessary to produce an immune reaction. Not all diseases produce all components,

some are antibody-mediated autoimmune reactions (resulting in type II hypersensitivity) and others involve the generation of autoreactive T-cells.

Antibody-mediated autoimmune diseases

Most of the following conditions are discussed in other chapters of this book. However, a few will be discussed here.

Different autoantibodies with different functions have different effects on the body (Fig. 2.14).

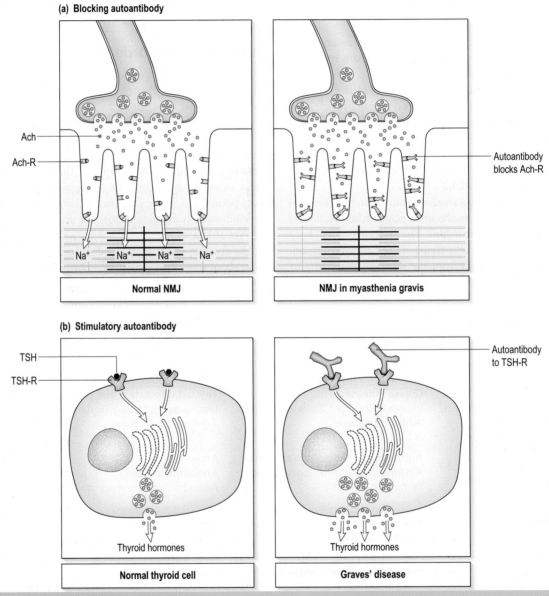

Figure 2.14.   Autoantibody action on receptors of self cells. (a) In myasthenia gravis autoantibodies bind to the acetylcholine receptors (Ach-R) at neuromuscular junctions (NMJ). This prevents Ach from binding, which in turn prevents the influx of sodium (Na$^+$) ions into the muscle cell. This, together with the destruction of Ach-R, disables the muscle contraction mechanism. (b) In the case of Graves' disease autoantibodies bind to thyroid-stimulating hormone receptors (TSH-R) and stimulate the thyroid cell to produce hormones, resulting in the excess production of T$_3$ and thyroxine.

Autoimmune haemolytic anaemia. Autoantibodies binding to red blood cells result in complement protein binding, resulting in death of the red cell.

Platelet deficiency (thrombocytopenia) and poor clotting. Autoantibody binds to platelets in the liver and spleen stimulating opsonization by phagocytes.

Myasthenia gravis. Autoantibodies bind to the acetylcholine (Ach) receptor at neuromuscular junctions, inhibiting Ach from binding and thus preventing the transmission of nerve impulses. This results in muscle disuse and weakness (discussed in Ch. 5).

Multiple sclerosis. This is a complex disease of the central nervous system resulting in demyelination of nerves, and characterized by functional disturbances of a relapsing and remitting nature (see Ch. 11). Current evidence suggests that a viral infection triggers an autoimmune attack against glial cells in genetically predisposed individuals. T-lymphocytes and macrophages may be sensitized to myelin antigens. Evidence suggests a role for pro-inflammatory cytokines in stimulating the macrophage-mediated demyelination. Similarly mast cells appear to play a crucial role in the induction and severity of the disease and research is currently investigating the potential for therapy aimed at mast cell function. The exact mechanisms are, however, still unclear. Future management of the disease is aimed at developing vaccines against the potential viral causes of multiple sclerosis and the potential genetic mechanisms.

Hashimoto's thyroiditis. Autoantibodies bind to antigen on the protein thyroglobulin, which is the protein in the thyroid gland that binds and stores thyroid hormones. These patients develop a goitre and hypothyroidism.

Graves' disease. Occasionally autoantibodies bind to a receptor and stimulate the receptor rather than block it. In Graves' disease autoantibodies produced against the thyroid-stimulating hormone (TSH) bind to their receptors on the epithelial cells of the thyroid gland (discussed in Ch. 4). This stimulates TSH, resulting in thyroid hyperactivity and symptoms of nervousness, tiredness, weight loss and proptosis (bulging eyes).

Type I insulin-dependent diabetes mellitus (IDDM). Autoantibody destruction of beta cells in pancreatic islets. Some evidence suggests pre-infection of beta cells which alters their antigenic make-up so that they are then recognized as non-self antigens and destroyed by self antibodies (discussed in Ch. 4).

Pernicious anaemia. Intrinsic factor, produced in the stomach, facilitates the absorption of vitamin B_{12} from the intestine. Autoantibodies bind to the intrinsic factor, preventing the binding and subsequent absorption of vitamin B_{12}. The vitamin deficiency leads to a lack of platelets and leucocytes and neurological damage.

Rheumatoid arthritis (RA). This disease is characterized by immune-mediated destruction of joints and is discussed in detail in Chapter 7. Some evidence suggest that a viral infection, e.g. Epstein–Barr virus, parvovirus and mycobacteria, inducing antigens, may precede the development of the disease. Other evidence suggests an autoimmune reaction. Autoantibodies, known as rheumatoid factor (RF), against self-IgG are found in most patients with this condition. The immune reaction results in a type III hypersensitivity reaction responsible for the pathology of RA. Recent evidence has demonstrated a key role for TNF-α in the regulation of pro-inflammatory mediators in the synovium of joints. This finding has led to the development of an antibody to TNF-α which is now in drug form (infliximab) and reduces the inflammatory reaction in the synovium.

Systemic lupus erythematosus (SLE). This condition results in systemic effects that manifest with periods of remission and intense exacerbation. Almost every patient with SLE has antinuclear antibodies (ANA) directed against many nuclear components including DNA. Detection of ANA in plasma is one of the 11 criteria for confirming diagnosis (Table 2.4). Immune complexes that are formed are not removed from the blood and deposit in tissues such as the kidney, skin, vessels and joints. The complexes attract complement proteins which lead to an inflammatory reaction and cell destruction in the affected tissue.

Aetiological factors include genetic, environmental and possibly hormonal (oestrogen).

Clinical manifestations: most patients experience chronic fatigue, weight loss and fever. Immune complex deposition in peripheral tissues results in:

- vasculitis (inflammation of arteries and arterioles)
- myocarditis and pericarditis secondary to acute vasculitis
- butterfly rash on the face
- raised, scaly, discoid rash on the scalp and other parts of the body
- alopecia (hair loss)
- proteinuria (loss of proteins) and haematuria (loss of cells) into urine as a result of damaged kidney walls (see Ch. 14.1).
- arthritis which does not damage joints, but the inflammation of synovial joints causes pain and discomfort.

Treatment: topical corticosteroids for easing symptoms and cytotoxic immunosuppressants such as cyclophosphamide and azathioprine can be used.

Progressive systemic sclerosis (scleroderma). This is a disease of connective tissues affecting females more frequently than males. Autoreactive B- and T-cells react to collagen.

Table 2.4.   Criteria for the diagnosis of SLE. The disease is deemed to be present when four of these eleven criteria are met

Criterion	Clinical manifestations
Malar rash	Erythema over the cheekbones
Discoid rash	Raised scaly patches of skin
Photosensitivity	Skin rash on exposure to sunlight
Oral ulcers	Ulcers in oropharynx and/or nasopharynx (usually painless)
Arthritis	Acute inflammation in two or more peripheral joints
Serositis	Acute inflammation in pleurae or pericardium
Renal disorder	Loss of protein in urine; blood cells or haemoglobin in tubule
Neurological disorder	Seizures or psychoses without other identifiable cause
Blood disorder	Deficiency of platelets or white cells, anaemia from red blood cell lysis
Immune disorder	Various antibodies identifiable
Antinuclear antibody	Antibodies to DNA in 50% of non-drug-induced SLE

The delayed type IV reaction generates cytokines that stimulate fibroblasts to secrete more collagen and the cycle starts again. There is increased deposition of collagen and also dysfunctional blood vessels. The reaction results in excess fibrosis of primarily the skin (hence scleroderma) but also of the kidneys, heart and vasculature and the gastrointestinal system.

Autoreactive Th cells

Immune tolerance of self tissues is maintained by a combination of genetic and environmental factors. Current knowledge suggests that to lose tolerance and develop autoreactive T-cells a combination of specific alleles from several genes is required. The environmental factor currently considered influential in developing autoreactive T-cells is the action of dendritic cells. Owing to the as yet undetermined causes of many of these diseases, it is often not clear whether the cause is autoantibody or autoreactive T-cell in nature (e.g. multiple sclerosis).

Immune deficiency syndromes

Previous sections have illustrated the complex interactions of the various components of the immune system necessary to defend the body. Deficiencies of one or more of these components can be divided into primary, secondary and acquired immunodeficiencies.

Primary immune deficiencies

These are usually of genetic origin, becoming apparent when an infant experiences recurrent infections. The genetic defect leads to the abnormal development of the immune system.

B-cell deficiencies

B-cell deficit results in lowered antibody production and thus reduced circulating antibody levels (*hypogammaglobulinaemia*) in response to infection. This means that viruses normally neutralized by antibodies will be able to survive and spread more easily. Similarly, bacteria requiring a coat of

antibody in order to be phagocytosed will escape detection and subsequent destruction.

> Bruton's agammaglobulinaemia – variable to very depressed antibodies. It is X-linked and thus affects primarily males. Lymph tissues are poorly developed, which affects the development of pre-B-cells into mature B-cells. T-cell numbers and function are normal. For unknown reasons affected individuals may develop autoimmune connective tissue diseases such as RA and SLE.

T-cell deficiencies

This deficiency affects the body's ability to deal with virally infected cells, yeasts/fungi (e.g. *Candida*) or intracellular bacteria (e.g. *Mycobacterium* producing tuberculosis). Once again these individuals experience recurrent infections against which they are ill equipped to defend themselves. Deficiency can be:

- *General T-cell deficiency*. Abnormal thymus development leads to a profound deficit of T-cells and can be treated by transplantation of fetal thymic tissue. However, the method of transplantation needs to consider the low immune system.
- *Specific T-cell deficiency*. In this case specific T-cell clones are absent, which means the T-cell population does not have a receptor for a specific antigen. For example, the condition *chronic mucocutaneous candidiasis* leads to *Candida* infections of the mucous membranes and skin.

Severe combined immunodeficiency (SCID)

This autosomal recessive or X-linked disease is serious and often fatal without successful bone marrow transplantation. Approximately half the children with autosomal recessive transmission of diseases lack the enzyme adenosine deaminase in their white blood cells. The result is the accumulation of substances toxic to lymphocytes and thus both T-cell and immunoglobulin production and function are affected, resulting in opportunistic infections in the first year of life.

Secondary immune deficiencies

Secondary immune deficiency may be due to the following factors.

1. *Age-related changes* – the thymus reaches peak T-cell production in the adolescent years and then gradually declines with age. Numbers of circulating T-cells remain relatively constant but T-cell-mediated responses are reduced with age. There is also an age-related increase in circulating autoantigens.
2. *Diet* – severe malnourishment leads to impaired T-cell, complement and neutrophil function. Similarly zinc loss in the diet, from burns or from diarrhoea, impairs both B- and T-cell function.
3. *Burns* – extensive burns can lead to generalized suppression of the immune system, depressed complement levels, reduced neutrophil chemotaxis and reduced cytotoxicity. Burn victims are more vulnerable to infection by bacteria (e.g. *Haemophilus influenzae, Staphylococcus*).
4. *Disease* – diabetes mellitus produces vascular changes which result in leucocyte dysfunction, poor immune responses and prolonged infections. Malignancies of bone and lymphoid tissues can suppress immune functions. In addition to the malignancy, tumour suppression treatments such as chemotherapeutic agents and radiotherapy can further suppress the immune system by blocking clonal expansion of antigen-specific B- and T-cells.

Acquired immune deficiency syndrome (AIDS)

The HIV virus belongs to the family of *Retroviridae*. These are RNA-containing tumour viruses which also contain the enzyme reverse transcriptase.

Viral structure

The virus lies in the centre of a protein envelope (Fig. 2.15). The viral envelope is a bi-layered membrane derived from the host consisting of two viral glycoproteins (gp120, gp41) which mediate viral entry and syncytium formation. One of these proteins (gp120) elicits a strong immune response. The HIV core consists of two RNA strands and viral enzymes. This is then surrounded by a protein *capsid*. The capsid protects the nucleic acid in the core of the virus from the destructive enzymes found in biological fluids and promotes attachment of the virus to susceptible cells.

Nucleotide sequencing on the RNA has led to the identification of three strains of HIV:

- M (majority) with 10 subtypes (clades A–J). Clade B is most common in the USA and western Europe. Clades A, B, C, D and E are most common in the developing world, with clade B being associated with heterosexual transmission.

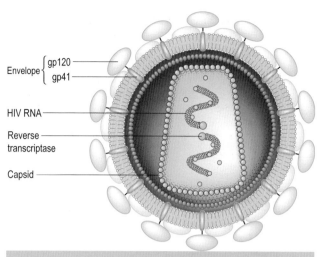

Figure 2.15.   **HIV viral protein structure.**

- O (outliers)
- N (non-M/non-O).

Regulation of transcription, replication efficiency of infection and nuclear transport is carried out by six regulatory proteins found on the virus.

Mechanisms of infection and replication

These mechanisms are summarized in Figure 2.16.

The HIV glycoprotein (gp120) recognizes cell surface CD4 molecules and specific surface receptors (CXCR4 or CCR5) found on lymphocytes and monocytes. Interaction of these proteins binds the virus to the host membrane. However, this is not sufficient and in order to release the capsid from the virus into the cytoplasm of the host cell the virus uses a chemokine receptor. HIV strains attracted to macrophages (M tropic) use CCR5 as a coreceptor and are referred to as R5 viruses. HIV strains attracted to T-lymphocytes use the CCX4 coreceptor, are referred to as X4 viruses, and induce the formation of syncytia (loss of cell wall) in infected cells. Knowledge on the exact mechanisms being used by the virus is constantly changing; for example, recent evidence has shown that the HIV virus is able to use alternative molecules (e.g. CD8) to enter primary T-cells.

Once in the cell the viral capsid releases the RNA genome and viral proteins into the cytoplasm of the cell. One of these proteins, *reverse transcriptase*, induces the reverse transcription of the viral RNA into cDNA with the resultant loss of the original RNA template. During this process an incorrect nucleotide is incorporated into the developing cDNA molecule every 1500–4000 bases. These rapid mutations partially explain the development of drug-resistant strains.

The resultant HIV-1 cDNA is transported to the nucleus where viral cDNA integrates into the host DNA randomly. This process is controlled by two HIV proteins and a viral enzyme, *integrase*.

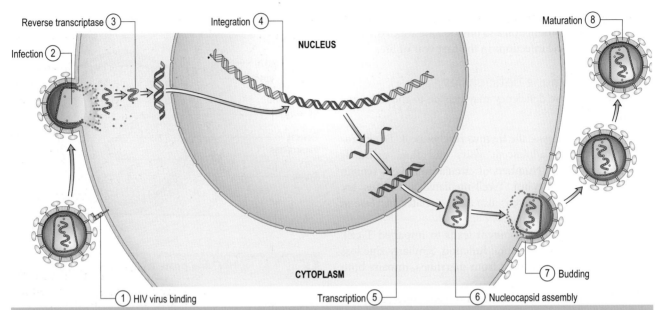

Reverse transcriptase ③   Integration ④   Maturation ⑧

Infection ②

NUCLEUS

CYTOPLASM

① HIV virus binding   Transcription ⑤   ⑥ Nucleocapsid assembly

⑦ Budding

Figure 2.16. The life cycle of HIV. 1, Gp120 binds to the CD4 molecule on cells; 2, nucleocapsid enters cell and releases viral RNA; 3, viral RNA is reverse transcribed to double-stranded DNA; 6, viral DNA integrates into the host genome where it may lie dormant as a provirus; 7, when cell activation occurs the viral DNA induces viral RNA production again which in turn is translated into viral proteins; 8, viral RNA assembles to form a nucleocapsid; and then 9, buds off; and 10, matures into an HIV virus capable of infecting more cells.

Drug therapy is aimed at:

- inhibiting the actions of reverse transcriptase
- inhibiting the action of the enzyme integrase
- inhibition of regulatory proteins Tat or Rev which have been shown to significantly impair HIV replication.

Once integrated into the host cell DNA, the virus is known as the *provirus*. This stage is known as the latent stage and the virus can lie dormant for a long time. At some point cellular transcription factors stimulate viral gene transcription resulting in many small mRNA molecules that are encoded for the viral regulatory proteins. These proteins regulate the subsequent speed and success of the spread of the viral mRNA transcribed from the original cDNA. Splices of the mRNA proteins and host cell proteins then form the envelope around the capsid, which protects the viral RNA genome. The viral RNA and the protective capsid assemble into particles which bud from the cell, taking part of the host cell membrane to form the viral envelope. These particles can then infect other cells and the process begins again.

Clinical course of HIV infection

HIV infection presents in the patient in three stages.

1. Infection. Approximately 15% of people demonstrate symptoms similar to influenza including: fever, malaise, painful throat, swollen lymph nodes and aching muscles. Following infection, antibodies to HIV antigens are produced, a process known as seroconversion. Blood levels of antibody are used to test for HIV infection.

2. Latency. During this period few clinical symptoms are apparent, yet HIV continues to replicate, possibly being controlled by cytotoxic CD8 T-cell activity and sequestered in lymph nodes.

Approximately 30–50% of patients present with lymphadenopathy (swollen lymph nodes) and no other symptoms. The length of the latency period is very variable, lasting from 1 year to as long as 15.

3. Development of AIDS. The clinical definition of AIDS includes major opportunistic infections or a drop in the CD4 T-cell count to below 200 cells/µl of blood. Symptoms include weight loss, persistent night sweats, long-lasting fever (3 months or longer) and diarrhoea. In the absence of treatment the infections will lead to death.

Immunology of HIV infection

Following HIV infection there is a period of rapid viral replication resulting in high levels of the virus in the blood (viraemia). This is followed by a combined antibody (B-cell) and cytotoxic T-cell response which is effective in eliminating 99% of the virus. The infection then enters the latent stage. The onset of AIDS results in a gradual loss of CD4 T-cells.

HIV infection results in comprehensive humoral and cellular immune responses including:

- increased production of Th1-type cytokines
- HIV-specific CD4+ T-cell proliferation activity and CD8+ T-cell cytotoxic activity
- increased synthesis of CD8+ T-cell suppressive factors and β-chemokines.

HIV counteracts this response by:

- downregulating the surface expression of MHC molecules
- reducing the number of specific CD8+ T-cells.

The humoral immune response

HIV infection results in B-cell dysfunction caused primarily by viral protein toxicity and cytokine dysregulation. This produces an initial response of:

- B-cell hyperplasia
- circulating immune complexes
- elevated autoantibodies
- polyclonal hypergammaglobulinaemia (large amounts of antibody in the blood from varying cell sources, of which approximately 20% are anti-HIV).

Ultimately B-cell depletion occurs with concurrent loss of specific antibody production to new or recall antigens.

Additional HIV effects on B-cells include a subpopulation of B-cells with enhanced immunoglobulin secretion but low antibody responses. This is thought to contribute to the high level of the virus present in the blood of HIV-infected patients (viraemia). HIV is able to activate complement pathways by using complement receptors. Complement is able to attach to HIV but seems unable to exert much of an attack.

The cellular immune response

HIV has several mechanisms in place to avoid the T-cell-mediated immune response. These include:

- HIV provirus latency
- viral strains switching from R5 to X4
- downregulation of MHC molecules
- viral protein mutations.

HIV infected CD4+ T-cells undergo induced apoptosis (apoptosis is normal programmed cell death), impaired production or redistribution into lymphoid organs. Patients present with accelerated destruction of CD4+ T-cells with death of both infected and non-infected cells.

This occurs in the thymus where the stroma is destroyed and cytokine production reduced. In bone marrow HIV causes lymphopenia, neutropenia, anaemia and thrombocytopenia.

With the aid of CD4+ T-cells, CD8+ T-cells destroy HIV-infected cells. When infection is acute these cells increase up to 20-fold, resulting in a strong HIV response and indicating progression of the disease in children and adults. These clinical observations are supported by animal models showing depleted CD8+ T-cell levels to be associated with viraemia. CD8+ T-cells control HIV activity by their HIV-specific cytotoxicity and by secreting soluble factors which inhibit HIV replication. Levels of CD8+ T-cells decline as the disease moves into the advanced stages, indicating the successful strategies the virus has to combat the immune system.

It is the success of HIV in suppressing the immune system that renders the body incapable of carrying out normal functions. HIV infections affect almost every system resulting in a host of clinical manifestations beyond the scope of this book. Since the use of antiretroviral drugs these signs and symptoms have been largely reduced. Some of the drugs do, however, have severe side effects.

HIV vaccine development

The development of HIV vaccines is currently at both the laboratory and clinical trial stage of investigation. One-third of vaccines develop anti-HIV cytotoxic T-cells and have weak neutralizing antibodies. Some of the approaches to vaccine development include targeting:

- dendritic cells – enhancing their role as antigen-presenting cells
- induction of specific CD8 T-cells which may protect against HIV infection
- DNA vaccines – DNA plasmids, subunits of the HIV gene, can be transferred into dendritic cells and administered to recipients where they might then induce strong T-cell responses as well as increased chemokine secretion.

TISSUE TRANSPLANTATION

The technique of transplantation is now an accepted form of treatment for many diseases. Tissues can be transplanted from one site on an individual to another site on the same individual (e.g. skin grafts) or from one individual to another (e.g. kidney transplant). Transplants between non-identical donors and recipients are rejected because the recipient body recognizes the tissue as foreign and correctly mounts a specific immune response. Rejection of transplanted tissue varies according to the tissue content of dendritic cells (e.g. skin and bone are richly supplied and therefore more reactive) and the MHC class (e.g. liver and kidney produce little antigen and therefore smaller reactions)(Fig. 2.17). Rejection can also occur if the recipient has had previous exposure, and is therefore sensitized, to the foreign antigens via blood transfusion or previous transplantation.

The degree to which tissue transplants are rejected forms the basis for three types of immune responses:

1. *Hyperacute rejection.* Pre-existing antibodies bind to the antigens on the graft and trigger either complement-mediated graft damage or antibody-mediated cellular

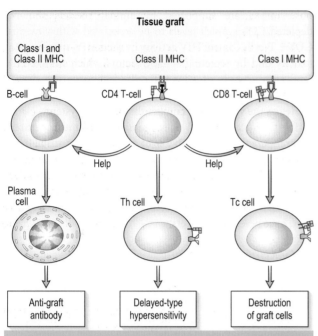

Figure 2.17.   Immune response to MHC molecules in transplanted tissues.

cytotoxicity. The antibodies in this case have been generated by MHC incompatibility and can be largely prevented by HLA cross-matching.

2. *Acute rejection.* In this instance a primary immune response occurs as described previously. Antigen-specific Th cells migrate to the graft and release lymphokines. These recruit macrophages, monocytes and Tc cells to the graft, where they destroy the tissue. This is similar to a delayed-type hypersensitivity reaction.

3. *Chronic rejection.* This usually occurs when a graft has been in place for approximately a year and is typically cell-mediated. The introduction of powerful immunosuppressive drugs has meant that chronic rejection is the leading cause of graft loss.

Graft rejection due to infection

In most cases graft or stem cell rejection is accompanied by infection. The reactivation, tissue invasion and continued proliferation of a number of viruses capable of causing infection and subsequent graft rejection is well described. Investigations have shown the presence of cytomegalovirus (CMV), adenovirus, enterovirus, parvovirus and herpes simplex virus in the endomyocardium of moderate to severe rejections. Similar viral findings, particularly the presence of CMV, have been shown in renal transplant rejection. However, a direct cause-and-effect relationship has yet to be shown and is the subject of ongoing research and debate.

Preventing graft rejection clearly forms the basis for successful transplants. There are three procedures that can be carried out to prevent graft rejection: (1) cross-match the blood type of donor and recipient and also check that the recipient does not have pre-existing antibody to the donor; (2) HLA tissue typing. Since MHC molecules have several sites, more than one HLA will be expressed. However, the aim is to match as many HLA molecules as possible between the donor and recipient tissue; (3) immunosuppression (see 'Therapeutic applications of immunity' below).

Graft versus host disease (GVHD)

This disease develops when donor cells mediate an immune response to recipient cells destroying them. GVHD can be divided into two forms based on timing of occurrence and clinical manifestations.

Acute GVHD

This occurs when a patient receives stem cells or tissues from an HLA-mismatched sibling or an HLA-identical unrelated donor. Donor T-cells recognize recipient HLA antigens as foreign, setting into motion cellular responses that increase the predisposition to infection. Potential effects include:

- atrophy of the lymphoid system
- thymic regression
- delayed B-cell reconstitution
- reversal of the CD4/CD8 ratio.

Clinical manifestations of acute GVHD include:

- maculopapular rash over trunk, face, extremities, palms and feet
- development of epidermal necrolysis
- hepatitis
- enteritis.

Chronic GVHD

This is a late development that is different to acute GVHD. Evidence suggests that the syndrome is mediated by donor T-lymphocytes recognizing minor histocompatibility complex differences and also by autoreactive T-cells destroying donor and recipient cells. The T-cells produce cytokines which lyse donor cells and may induce the production of autoantibodies frequently seen in patients with this syndrome. Clinical manifestations are similar to those of autoimmune disorders.

- Scleroderma – skin becomes taut, firm, and oedematous. It feels tough and leathery, may itch and later becomes hyperpigmented. Visceral involvement often follows these skin changes.
- 10–20% of patients develop bronchiolitis obliterans (inflammation and occlusion of bronchioles).

THERAPEUTIC APPLICATIONS OF IMMUNITY

Monoclonal antibodies

Because antigens have several different epitopes (sites for antibody attachment), resting B-cells can be activated by these antigens to produce several different antibodies, i.e. a *polyclonal* reaction. However, each antibody produced is specific for a particular antigen, i.e. a *monoclonal* antibody. This monoclonal antibody (Mab) can be labelled in a way that enables us to identify it amongst many other tissue components. In this way we are able to locate specific antigen (e.g. an antigen forming part of the cell wall of a bacterium or tumour cell) and study their production, storage and release. Mabs can be used therapeutically in a wide variety of ways:

* to identify tumour antigens and carry toxins to the tumour cells in order to destroy them
* to block receptor-mediated disease processes by binding the Mab to the receptor
* to neutralize a disease-producing substance being released into the body
* tissue and blood typing
* identifying hormones in the diagnosis of infectious diseases.

Immunization

This is a preventative measure used to protect us from infections by artificially inducing an immune response. The technique introduces either antigenic components or toxins which can induce an immune response but do not expose the body to an infection. The preparation containing these substances is called a vaccine. Vaccines may contain: *killed* or *inactivated* pathogen (particularly for viruses), *attenuated* pathogen capable of inducing antibody formation but not disease, *subunits* of pathogen, e.g. proteins or polysaccharides, and *toxoids* which immunize against specific toxins released by pathogens. All vaccines induce a primary immune response with long-term memory T- and B-cells. Subsequent infection will induce a faster and more effective secondary immune response.

Genetic engineering has introduced an entirely new approach to vaccines which is well into the investigative stage. New approaches to vaccines include:

* *Recombinant vector vaccines.* This approach involves introducing genes encoding antigens for a pathogen into the genome of an attenuated virus or bacteria. Vaccinating an individual with this solution would therefore result in the production of antigens specific to the vaccinia virus and also pathogen antigens. Because the vaccinia virus was attenuated it will not cause disease but the release of pathogen antigens into the recipients body would induce the production of antibodies to protect them against that specific pathogen in future infections.
* *DNA vaccines.* DNA containing antigen genes is introduced into muscle cells. This results in the production of pathogen proteins (antigens) which induce antibody and cell-mediated immunity.
* *Tumour vaccines.* Tumours have a number of mechanisms to avoid the immune system. There are two types of tumour vaccines undergoing investigation. The first approach is essentially the same as for microbial vaccines. Either the tumour cell antigens are injected into the patient to stimulate an immune response or the antigens are incubated in vitro with lymphocytes from the patient. These lymphocytes generate antibody-producing cells which are then injected back into the patient.

Antibiotic resistance

Antibiotic resistance presents an ongoing challenge in the fight against disease. Some bacterial species have an inherent ability to resist a number of antibiotics whereas others are normally highly susceptible to antibiotics (e.g. streptococci susceptibility to penicillin). Acquired resistance evolves via alterations in the pathogen's own genome (e.g. replacement of one amino acid with another) or by horizontal transfer of a *resistance gene* across the DNA. Mutations of this kind can occur at varying frequencies but generally occur initially as a low level resistance with the ability to become a stronger resistance. The main mechanisms of acquired resistance include:

1. decreased uptake of the drug
2. increased removal of drug from cells
3. inactivation or modification of the drug target
4. introduction of a new drug resistant target
5. hydrolysis of the antibiotic
6. modification, by enzymes, of the antibiotic.

It is clinically advantageous to identify organisms with low level resistance and develop drugs in time to halt that resistance. Despite advances in drug therapy there are and always will be microbes capable of lifelong resistance to antibiotics. Current gene research is looking at new drug therapies interfering with bacterial secretion of virulent proteins or with bacterial attachment and spread.

Oxazolidinones are a new class of antibacterial agents. These drugs inhibit the initiation step of protein synthesis and are not cross-linked to other classes of antibiotics. Clinical use is currently reserved for the treatment of antibiotic resistant Gram-positive infections.

Clinical immunosuppression

This is the use of drugs to suppress immune responses to transplants of tissues or stem cells. Ideally the drugs used should be specific to an antigen so that they do not suppress normal immune responses to other pathogens which might infect the body. However, specificity of drug action is currently at the investigative stage and drugs in use today inhibit the immune response to any antigen. As a result patients are prone to opportunistic infection which if unresponsive to antibiotics means they are withdrawn from drug treatment and may therefore experience graft rejection.

Immune tolerance

Tolerance-inducing therapies are designed to programme immune cells to eliminate pathogenic responses while at the same time preserving protective immunity. This form of treatment is advancing rapidly in development and could revolutionize the management of a number of diseases that require lifelong immunosuppression. Animal studies have demonstrated the feasibility of using tolerance-induced therapy for autoimmunity, allergy and graft rejection.

REFERENCES AND FURTHER READING

Normal structure and function

Davies A, Blakeley AGH, Kidd C (2001) Human Physiology. Edinburgh: Churchill Livingstone.

Guyton AC (2002) Textbook of Medical Physiology. London: WB Saunders.

Nairn R, Helbert M (2002) Immunology for Medical Students. St Louis: Mosby.

Wood P (2001) Understanding Immunology. London: Prentice Hall.

Young B, Heath JW (2000) Wheater's Functional Histology, 4th edn. Edinburgh: Churchill Livingstone.

Hypersensitivity reactions

Adachi T, Alam R (1998) The mechanism of IL-5 signal transduction. Am J Physiol 275: C623–633.

Bonecchi R, Biancchi G, Panina-Bordignon P, et al. (1998) Differential expression of chemokine receptors and chemotactic responsiveness of Th1 and Th2 cells. J Exp Med 187: 129–134.

Bradding P, Feather IH, Howarth PH, et al. (1992) Interleukin 4 is localized to and released by human mast cells. J Exp Med 176: 1381–1386.

Bradding P, Roberts JA, Britten KM, et al. (1994) Interleukin-4, -5 and -6 and tumor necrosis factor-alpha in normal and asthmatic airways: evidence for the human mast cell as a source of these cytokines. Am J Respir Cell Mol Biol 10: 471–480.

Burd PR, Thompson WC, Max EE, Mills FC (1995) Activated mast cells produce interleukin 13. J Exp Med 181: 1373–1380.

Cohn L, Tepper JS, Bottomly K (1998) IL-4-independent induction of airway hyperresponsiveness by Th2, but not Th1, cells. J Immunol 161: 3813–3818.

Cohn L, Homer RJ, Niu N, Bottomly K (1999) T helper 1 cells and interferon regulate airway inflammation and mucous production. J Exp Med 190: 1309–1317.

Corry DB, Grunig G, Hadeiba H, et al. (1998) Requirements for allergen-induced airway hyperreactivity in T and B cell-deficient mice. Mol Med 4: 344–355.

D'Ambrosia D, Mariani M, Panini-Bordignon P, et al. (2001) Chemokines and their receptors guiding T lymphocyte recruitment in lung inflammation. Am J Respir Crit Care Med 164: 1266–1275.

Emson CL, Bell SE, Jones A, Wisden W, McKenzie AN (1998) Interleukin (IL)-4-independent induction of immunoglobulin (Ig)E and perturbation of T cell development in transgenic mice expressing IL-13. J Exp Med 188: 399–404.

Finkelman FD, Katona IM, Urban JF Jr, et al. (1988) IL-4 is required to generate and sustain in vivo IgE responses. J Immunol 141: 2335–2341.

Finkelman FD, Shea-Donohue T, Goldhill J (1997) Cytokine regulation of host defense against parasitic gastrointestinal nematodes: lessons from studies with rodent models. Annu Rev Immunol 15: 505–533.

Foster PS, Hogan SP, Ramsay AJ, Matthaei KI, Young IG (1996) Interleukin 5 deficiency abolishes eosinophilia, airways hyperreactivity, and lung damage in a mouse asthma model. J Exp Med 183: 195–201.

Foster PS, Martinez-Moczygemba M, Huston DP, et al. (2002) Interleukins-4, -5 and -13: emerging therapeutic targets in allergic disease. Pharmacol Ther 94: 253–264.

Gavett SH, O'Hearn DJ, Li X, et al. (1995) Interleukin 12 inhibits antigen-induced airway hyperresponsiveness, inflammation, and Th2 cytokine expression in mice. J Exp Med 182: 1527–1536.

Grabbe S, Schwartz T (1998) Immunoregulatory mechanisms involved in elicitation of allergic contact hypersensitivity. Immunol Today 19: 37–44.

Henderson WR Jr, Chi EY, Maliszewski CR (2000) Soluble IL-4 receptor inhibits airway inflammation following allergen challenge in a mouse model of asthma. J Immunol 164: 1086–1095.

Hogan SP, Foster PS, Tan X, Ramsay AJ (1998) Mucosal IL-12 gene delivery inhibits allergic airways disease and restores local antiviral immunity. Eur J Immunol 28: 413–423.

Homann D, Teyton L, Oldstone MBA (2001) Differential regulation of anti-viral T-cell immunity results in stable CD8+ but declining CD4+ T-cell memory. Nature Med 7: 913–919.

Kimber I, Dearman J (2002) Allergic contact dermatitis: the cellular effectors. Contact Dermatitis 46: 1–5.

Kips JC, Brusselle GJ, Joos GF, et al. (1996) Interleukin-12 inhibits antigen-induced airway hyperresponsiveness in mice. Am J Respir Crit Care Med 153: 535–539.

Krasteva M, Kehren J, Horand F, et al. (1998) Dual role of dendritic cells in the induction and down regulation of antigen specific cutaneous inflammation. J Immunol 160: 1181–1190.

Leckie MJ, ten Brinke A, Khan J, et al. (2000) Effects of an interleukin-5 blocking monoclonal antibody on eosinophils, airway hyper-responsiveness, and the late asthmatic response. Lancet 356: 2144–2148.

McSharry C, Anderson K, Bourke SJ, Boid G (2002) Takes your breath away – the immunology of allergic alveolitis. Clin Exp Immunol 128: 3–9.

Mould AW, Ramsay AJ, Matthaei KI, et al. (2000) The effect of IL-5 and eotaxin expression in the lung on eosinophil trafficking and degranulation and the induction of bronchial hyperreactivity. J Immunol 164: 2142–2150.

Nelms K, Keegan AD, Zamorano J, Ryan JJ, Paul WE (1999) The IL-4 receptor: signalling mechanisms and biologic functions. Annu Rev Immunol 17: 701–738.

Ohno I, Nitta Y, Yamaucho K (1996) Transforming growth factor-β (TGF-β) gene expression by eosinophils in asthmatic airway inflammation. Am J Respir Crit Care Med 15: 4084–4090.

Palframan RT, Collins PD, Williams TJ, Rankin SM (1998) Eotaxin induces a rapid release of eosinophils and their progenitors from the bone marrow. Blood 91: 2240–2248.

Romagnani S (2000) The role of lymphocytes in allergic disease. J Allergy Clin Immunol 105: 399–408.

Romagnani S (2001) Cytokines and chemoattractants in allergic inflammation. Mol Immunol 38: 881–885.

Wang B, Fujisawa H, Zhuang L, et al. (2000) CD4+ Th1 and CD8+ type 1 cytotoxic T cells both play a crucial role in the full development of contact hypersensitivity. J Immunol 165: 6783–6790.

Wardlaw AJ, Brightling CE, Green R, et al. (2002) New insights into the relationship between airway inflammation and asthma. Clin Sci 103: 201–211.

Webb DC, McKenzie AN, Koskinen AM, et al. (2000) Integrated signals between IL-l3, IL-4, and IL-5 regulate airways hyperreactivity. J Immunol 165: 108–113.

Wills-Karp M (1999) Immunologic basis of antigen-induced airway hyperresponsiveness. Annu Rev Immunol 17: 255–281.

Wills-Karp M, Luyimbazi J, Xu X, et al. (1998) Interleukin-13: central mediator of allergic asthma. Science 282: 2258–2261.

Zhu Z, Homer RJ, Wang Z, et al. (1999) Pulmonary expression of interleukin 13 causes inflammation, mucous hypersecretion, subepithelial fibrosis, physiologic abnormalities, and eotaxin production. J Clin Invest 103: 779–788.

HIV

Chinen J, Shearer WT (2002) Molecular virology and immunity of HIV infection. J Allergy Clin Immunol 110(2): 189–198.

Moylett EH, Shearer WT (2002) HIV: Clinical manifestations. J Allergy Clin Immunol 110: 3–16.

Thomson MM, Pérez-Álvarez L, Nájera R 2002 Molecular epidemiology of HIV-1 genetic forms and its significance for vaccine development and therapy. Lancet ii: 461–471.

Autoimmune diseases

Boitard C (2002) The origin of type I diabetes: an autoimmune disease. Diabetes Metab 28 (4 pt 1): 263–265.

De Baets M, Stassen MH (2002) The role of antibodies in myasthenia gravis. J Neurol Sci 202(1–2): 5–11.

Looney RJ (2002) Treating autoimmune disease by depleting B cells. Ann Rheum Dis 61(10): 863–866.

Nevinsky GA, Buneva VN (2002) Human catalytic RNA- and DNA-hydrolyzing antibodies. J Immunol Methods 269(1–2): 235–249.

Salmaso C, Bagnasco M, Pesce G, et al. (2002) Regulation of apoptosis in endocrine autoimmunity: insights from Hashimoto's thyroiditis and Graves' disease. Ann N Y Acad Sci 966: 496–501.

Shanahan JC, St Clair EW (2002) Tumour necrosis factor-α blockade: A novel therapy for rheumatic disease. Clin Immunol 103(3): 231–242.

Stassi G, De Maria R (2002) Autoimmune thyroid disease: new models of cell death in autoimmunity. Nat Rev Immunol 2(3): 195–204.

Vincent A (2002) Unravelling the pathogenesis of myasthenia gravis. Nat Rev Immunol 2(10): 797–804.

Zauli D, Grassio A, Ballardini G, et al. (2002) Thyroid autoimmunity in chronic idiopathic urticaria: implications for therapy. Am J Clin Dermatol 3(8): 525–528.

Tissue transplant

Cainelli F, Vento S (2002) Infections and solid organ transplant rejection: a cause-and-effect relationship? Lancet Infectious Diseases ii: 539–549.

Rotrosen D, Matthews JB, Bluestone JA (2002) The immune tolerance network: A new paradigm for developing tolerance-inducing therapies. J Allergy Clin Immunol 10(1): 17–23.

Smyth MJ, Hayakawa Y, Takeda K, Yagita H (2002) New aspects of natural-killer-cell surveillance and therapy of cancer. Nature Revs – Cancer 2: 850–861.

Tabbara IA, Zimmerman K, Morgan C, Nahleh Z (2002) Allogenic hematopoietic stem cell transplantation: complications and results. Arch Intern Med 162: 1558–1566.

Antibiotic therapy

Henriques-Normark B, Normark S (2002) Evolution and spread of antibiotic resistance. J Intern Med 252: 91–106.

Malignancy: Malignant Neoplasms

Susan A. Brooks

Direct Endocrine Effects of Cancer 68

Paraneoplastic Effects 69

WHAT IS CANCER?

Neoplasm means 'new growth' or tumour. Tumours can be benign or malignant. Malignant tumours, or cancers, are a heterogeneous group of diseases that share the following characteristics:

1. Their growth has escaped the usual constraints and thus they are able to invade into surrounding healthy tissues.
2. Their cells have to a lesser or greater extent lost normal, differentiated organization. Some residual tissue architecture and function may remain.
3. Clinically, most significantly, they possess the ability to metastasize. Metastasis is the spread of tumour cells from the original site to other parts of the body through lymphatics and the bloodstream.

The metastatic cascade

Metastasis is often referred to as a 'cascade' in that it is believed that a series of many steps need to be achieved successfully in order for it to take place. Initially, the primary tumour must invade into local normal tissues. Cancer cells must then disengage from the primary tumour and find their way into blood vessels or lymphatics. They must travel around the body and escape destruction by the immune response. They must then escape from lymphatics or bloodstream, invade into surrounding tissue at the secondary site and grow there (Fig. 3.1.1).

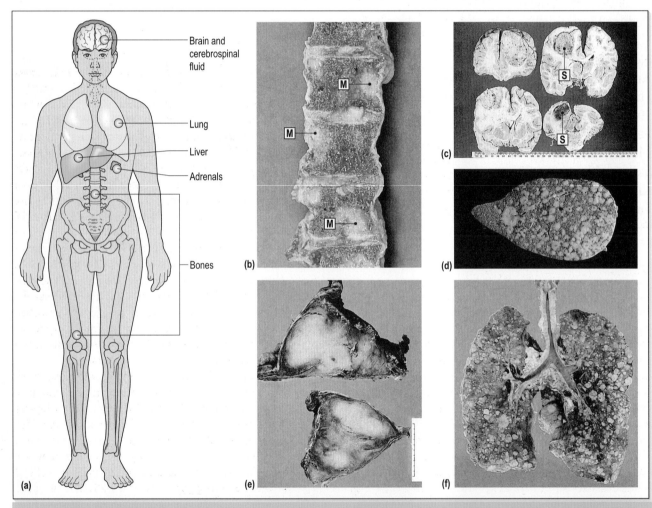

Figure 3.1.1.   Main sites of blood-borne metastasis. (a) Sites of haematogenous metastasis. (b) Metastasis in bone. (c) Metastasis in brain. (d) Metastasis in liver. (e) Metastasis in adrenals. (f) Metastasis in lungs. Blood-borne tumour metastasis leads to growth of secondary tumours in several main sites. The macroscopic appearances of bone metastasis are shown in (b), where lesions are seen in vertebrae (M). Numerous metastases from a neoplasm of the stomach (S) are seen in the brain in (c). The liver is the most common site for metastases from tumours in the gastrointestinal tract, as seen in (d), which arose from a colonic neoplasm. In (e) metastatic tumour has replaced both adrenal glands, as is commonly seen with spread from lung and breast tumours. The lung (f) is the most common site for blood-borne metastases from tumours outside the gastrointestinal tract, particularly mesenchymal tumours. (Reproduced with permission from Stevens and Lowe, 2000.)

The molecular events underlying this complex cascade are incompletely understood, but it is metastatic spread that is the most challenging aspect of cancer treatment and the most usual cause of eventual death in cancer patients.

Types of cancer

There are more than one hundred different types of cancer, which affect humans at every stage in life from early childhood to extreme old age. Common childhood cancers include leukaemia and Ewing's sarcoma and some of the most significant improvement in cancer survival rates are those seen in paediatric cancers. In adults, the commonest cancers are those of breast, lung and bowel (colorectum). In the UK, cancer affects one in three individuals and is the second most common cause of death after heart disease. With increasing public awareness, better diagnosis, screening programmes for some common cancers and ever improving treatment modalities increasing numbers of individuals are living with the long-term physical, psychological and psychosocial effects of diagnosis and treatment. They include those suffering the effects of immediate treatments for primary and metastatic disease, those in remission after treatment, long-term survivors and those cured of their disease, and those suffering its terminal effects. The disease itself, and the aggressive treatments aimed at controlling and irradicating it, are a leading cause of short- and long-term morbidity and impairment.

The clonal origin of cancer

It is believed that most cancers are monoclonal in origin – that is, they arise from a single transformed cell that develops the ability to escape the body's normal constraints and proliferates, passing its malignant phenotype on to its progeny. However, cancer cells appear to be genetically unstable and as they proliferate they give rise to daughter cells carrying more and more genetic aberrations in comparison to the original parent cell. Thus, clones of genetically distinct daughter cells proliferate, leading to great heterogeneity within the tumour mass. This may be reflected in the cytological appearance of cancer cells; as the tumour progresses, its cells become increasingly bizarre in appearance, and normal tissue architecture degenerates (see 'Histological grade' later in this chapter). This inherent genetic instability and heterogeneity has profound implications for therapy. Any treatment modality, such as radiation therapy (radiotherapy), immunotherapy or treatment with cytotoxic drugs (chemotherapy), will probably destroy some, even most, of the tumour mass, but there remains the potential for a subpopulation of cancer cells to be resistant, to survive, and to then proliferate again, resulting in a tumour that is immune to further attack by that approach.

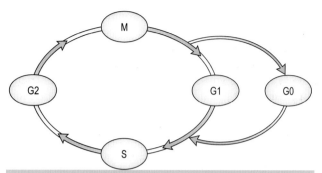

Figure 3.1.2.   The cell cycle. G0, resting phase; G1, first growth phase; G2, second growth phase; M, mitosis (two identical daughter cells produced); S, synthesis (DNA replication).

The cell cycle

It is helpful to understand the normal cell cycle in order to appreciate the biological mechanisms underlying malignancy, and the way in which some cancer therapies are designed to work. The cell cycle is illustrated in Figure 3.1.2.

Quiescent cells, or cells that are not undergoing active division, are said to be in G0, a resting phase. Cells that are about to divide first enter a 'growth' or 'gap' phase, called G1, which can persist for different lengths of time in different types of tissue, and under different circumstances. After G1, cells move into a 'synthesis' or S-phase, during which the genetic material (DNA) of the cell is replicated. The cell then passes into a second 'growth' or 'gap' phase, G2, and finally into a complex series of events termed mitosis, M, during which the DNA and cell contents are equally divided amongst the two new daughter cells. Mitosis takes about 30–90 minutes. Finally the two new daughter cells separate and either move immediately into another cycle of cell division by entering G1 again, or instead move into a longer or shorter period of quiescence by entering the resting phase G0.

The cells of normal healthy tissue vary in their rate of cell division, depending on their function and on circumstances. This may range from a cell cycle of a few hours in rapidly proliferating tissue to many years in quiescent cells. For example, the epithelial cells lining the digestive tract have a rapid cell cycle and are continually replaced as they are mechanically damaged by the passage of food. The cells of the bone marrow have a high rate of cell division as blood cells are continually replaced. In comparison, the cells of the brain, nervous tissue and the endothelial cells lining blood vessels have a very slow rate of turnover. Rapid cell division is also a feature of embryonic cells during development, of growing tissues during childhood development and during wound healing, for example after injury or surgery.

In normal cells and tissues, the cell cycle is carefully controlled and cell division is accurately balanced by cell loss. Thus, tissues and organs in the adult remain static in size, unless subjected to a changing environment, for example the healing of wounds or proliferation of glandular breast tissue during lactation. In cancer, this close regulation is lost and cell division outstrips cell death; thus the tumour increases in size. As a tumour grows, its cells require oxygen and nutrients supplied by the blood. Cancer cells die once they are more than 150 μm from a blood vessel as they are starved of these vital supplies. Many larger tumours contain patches of anoxia (areas starved of oxygen) and necrotic material where tumour cells have died. Successful tumours often synthesize and secrete angiogenic factors that stimulate blood vessels to grow into them.

At any one time, different cells within normal tissue, or a tumour, are at different stages in the cell cycle. Some are dying, some are quiescent and some are proliferating. The rate of cell division in cancers, as in normal tissues, varies. It is a popular misconception that cancer cells divide very rapidly in comparison to normal cells. Some cancers, for example acute lymphoblastic leukaemia, *do* exhibit very rapid cell division, typically every 3–5 days. Within most types of cancer it is usual to find individual tumours with very different rates of cell division. Typically, breast cancer cells divide every 25–500 days; lymphomas every 10–200 days; colorectal cancers every 50–250 days; and lung cancers every 25–350 days. To some extent, the rate at which cancer cells divide is related to the rate of cell division in the tissues from which they arise. Thus, the very rapid cell proliferation in acute lymphoblastic leukaemia reflects the rapid proliferation of normal lymphoblastic cells and the relatively long cell cycle of breast cancer cells reflects the long cell cycle of normal breast epithelial cells.

The rate of proliferation of cancer cells is of clinical significance because it determines both how rapidly a tumour will increase in size and how swiftly the disease will progress, but also how susceptible it is to chemotherapy, which specifically targets dividing cells (see 'Chemotherapy' later in this chapter). Some studies have suggested that the cells of small tumours divide more rapidly than those of larger ones. This would suggest that adjuvant (used in addition to surgery) chemotherapy directed against early (i.e. small) metastases should be more effective than palliative chemotherapy directed against later stage, clinically apparent disease.

Different chemotherapy drugs work in different ways. Some, for example *methotrexate*, only work on actively cycling cells. Others, like *alkylating agents*, act on quiescent cells (those in G0). Cycles of chemotherapy are planned to have the maximum biological effect. Thus, drugs such as *vinblastine*, which arrests cells in mitosis, may be used to temporarily halt the cell cycle, then, as the cells begin to recover, they will enter the next phase of the cycle synchronously and at this point another chemotherapy drug, such as *methotrexate*, which targets dividing cells, may be administered. Schedules are also subject to practical constraints, of course, such as clinic times and the ability of the patient to withstand continuing cycles of often very toxic compounds.

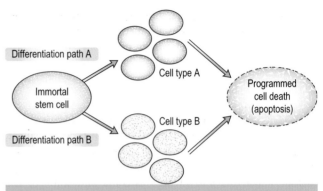

Figure 3.1.3.   The stem cell and tissue renewal.

Cellular differentiation

As illustrated in Figure 3.1.3, all normal tissues contain stem cells that give rise to daughter cells which themselves are committed to a certain path of differentiation. The daughter cells are pre-programmed to go on and divide a finite number of times and then to die. This programmed cell death, sometimes referred to as 'cell suicide', is termed apoptosis. One of the most common mutations found in cancer cells is a mutation to the gene coding for p53, a nuclear phosphoprotein that acts as a checkpoint in the cell cycle. If there is damage to the DNA, then during the cell cycle, p53 arrests that cell in the G1 phase of the cycle and directs the cell to death (apoptosis) instead of division. In normal tissues, therefore, cells with damaged DNA are not allowed to replicate themselves. In cancer, loss of p53 activity means that cells can continue to replicate themselves even when their DNA is damaged. Thus, potentially harmful mutations can accumulate.

In healthy tissues, stem cells continue to divide and replenish the cells of the tissue indefinitely. It is believed that cancers contain stem cells too. This has implications for therapy, because unless the cancer stem cells are destroyed, for example by chemotherapy or radiotherapy, the tumour will always have the capacity to regenerate.

The differentiated cells of healthy tissues exhibit the specialist functions associated with that tissue, for example hormone synthesis and secretion, production of certain enzymes or growth factors, or hormone responsiveness. Cancers arising from such tissues may retain some of these specialist features; for example, they may synthesize and secrete hormones and enzymes or be sensitive to the effects of such molecules. This may have implications for detection, symptoms and treatment, and this is discussed later.

As cancers progress, they become increasingly less differentiated. This is seen in their appearance under the microscope where normal tissue architecture is lost (see 'Histological grade'). However, in most cancers, remnants of original differentiation of the tissue is seen; for example, well-differentiated breast cancer cells exhibit an attempt to organize themselves into tubular duct-like structures reminiscent of those seen in normal breast.

WHAT CAUSES CANCER?

It is not a simple matter to define what causes cancer. There are many types of cancer, and their causes are multiple and complex, and not always understood. It is believed that in most cases, for cancer to arise, an 'initiation' event must be followed by a series of (probably several) 'promotion' events.

Initiators and promoters

Initiators are agents that cause permanent damage to the DNA of cells, but do not in themselves cause cancer. Damage by an initiator, such as a chemical carcinogen or a virus, must be followed by repeated transient effects on the initiated cell by *promoters*. The exact initiating and promoting substances or events will differ for different cancer types. An example might be a carcinogenic compound or a viral infection causing the initiating event, then ongoing dietary or hormonal factors causing repeated transient promotion events.

Cancer-associated viruses

A viral aetiology of cancer was first described by Rous in 1910 who showed that an infective agent, a virus, in a cell-free infiltrate from a chicken sarcoma could induce new sarcomas in healthy animals. There are a number of viruses associated with human cancers. For example, *HTLV-1* (human T-cell leukaemia lymphoma virus 1) is transmitted sexually, perinatally and through intravenous drug use and is associated with T-cell leukaemia. *Epstein–Barr virus*, which commonly causes glandular fever in the UK, is associated with *Burkitt's lymphoma* in immunosupressed individuals, particularly children, in parts of sub-Saharan Africa. It is relatively common in parts of Africa but uncommon in Western countries. Strains of human papilloma virus (HPV) which are transmitted sexually are also associated with cancer of the uterine cervix, penis, anus and other sites. Hepatitis B virus is associated with hepatocellular carcinoma.

Chemical carcinogens

Compounds that induce cancer, termed carcinogens, have been long recognized. In 1775 Sir Percival Pott first noted the high incidence of cancer of the scrotum in chimney sweeps and suggested that some agent in soot that was causing chronic irritation to the skin of the scrotum was responsible. Many proven chemical carcinogens are known, as indicated in Table 3.1.1. Common examples include polycyclic hydrocarbons (which are found in tobacco smoke, coal tar, vehicle exhaust fumes and charred foods such as barbecued meats), ultraviolet radiation in sunlight and radon gas emitted from the underlying rocky strata in some parts of the UK.

Table 3.1.1. Some examples of known chemical carcinogens

Aflatoxin
Alkylating agents
Aromatic amines
Arsenic
Asbestos fibres
Azo dyes
Benzene
Bis(chloromethyl) ether
Cadmium
Mustard gas
Nickel
Nitrosamines
Polycyclic hydrocarbons
Vinyl chloride

Ironically, alkylating agents which are used in cancer chemotherapy are themselves carcinogenic and their administration is associated with an increased risk of leukaemia in long-term survivors of cancer therapy.

Cancer inheritance

Some cancers appear to have a genetic basis. Xeroderma pigmentosum is an uncommon cancer syndrome where abnormality in a DNA repair protein means that sufferers are subject to development of multiple cancers, especially skin cancers associated with unavoidable ultraviolet light exposure. Breast cancer more commonly occurs in individuals who have a first degree relative who has suffered the disease, and although the majority of breast cancers are believed to be sporadic, at least two breast cancer-associated genes have been described (termed BRCA-1 and BRCA-2). Women with a very strong family history of breast cancer may seek screening for these genes, although the disease cannot be prevented in those carrying them. There are complex issues surrounding such screening and associated counselling.

THE IMMUNE RESPONSE AND CANCER

There has long been speculation that the immune response recognizes some, or perhaps most, very early cancers as 'foreign' and destroys them so that they never become clinically detectable. However, the immune response is generally ineffective in destroying clinically significant disease. This is probably because as cancer cells arise from the body's own normal cells, and cancer cells largely express the same antigens as are displayed by normal healthy cells, cancers are not recognized as a target. Some therapies, termed immunotherapy, are aimed at non-specifically enhancing the immune response in an attempt to limit the tumour (see 'Immunotherapy' later in this chapter).

CANCER-ASSOCIATED ANTIGENS

Much research has been aimed at identifying and mapping cancer-specific antigens as potential targets for immunotherapy. There are a few examples of cancer-associated antigens, some of which, like CEA (carcinoembryonic antigen), useful in colon cancer, are normally expressed by embryonic and fetal cells but not by normal cells of the adult.

Monoclonal antibodies (see also 'Monoclonal antibodies' later) against antigens expressed by tumour cells act as markers for cancer cells and have proved useful in classifying tumours, particularly lymphomas and leukaemias. They have also been used (largely experimentally) in imaging studies, in monitoring tumour load during and after treatment, to monitor success of treatment and predict relapse, and to target drugs and other cytotoxic compounds. Clinically, some markers have proved useful in clearing bone marrow of cancer cells for re-transplant back into patients following whole body irradiation in aggressive therapy of some tumour types.

PROGNOSIS AND PROGNOSTIC INDICATORS

At the time of initial diagnosis, it is difficult to accurately predict the likely prognosis of any individual patient. Prognosis is therefore often stated as overall 5- or 10-year survival rates for that particular type and stage of cancer. Different types of cancer have very different overall survival and cure rates. The life expectancy of a newly diagnosed cancer patient can therefore vary from a few weeks or months to many decades, and for any one type of cancer, survival rates may vary enormously.

Prognostic markers are useful in helping to predict individual patient prognosis, to advise and inform the patient of likely outcome, to identify individuals for whom treatment is likely to be worthwhile, those who would benefit from especially aggressive treatment in an attempt to prolong survival, and those for whom prognosis is poor and palliative care only may be appropriate.

GRADES AND STAGES OF CANCER

Possibly the most commonly used and most informative prognostic indicators are stage (a measure of tumour spread) and histological grade (a measure of tumour differentiation). The systems used vary slightly with individual tumour types, but generalized schemes are outlined below.

Staging by TNM classification

The TNM, or *t*umour, *n*odes, *m*etastasis, system is commonly used for solid tumours, but is less applicable to lymphomas and leukaemias. It is also of limited use in small cell carcinoma of the bronchus and ovarian cancer. 'T' indicates the size of the

Table 3.1.2. Summary of generalized criteria for TNM staging system

T, size of primary tumour
T0 = no evidence of tumour
Tis = carcinoma in situ
TX = tumour cannot be assessed
T1–T4 = progressive increase in tumour size or, in the case of melanoma, colon and bladder cancer, of depth of invasion

N, local/regional lymph node involvement
N0 = regional lymph nodes not involved
NX = regional lymph nodes cannot be assessed
N1–N4 = progressive increase in number of local/regional lymph nodes involved

M, distant metastases
M0 = no evidence of distant metastases
MX = distant metastases cannot be assessed
M1–M3 = increasing involvement of distant metastases

primary tumour, 'N' is a measure of local/regional lymph node involvement and 'M' a measure of distant metastatic involvement. Generally, the larger the primary tumour and the greater the extent of local and regional lymph node involvement, the poorer the prognosis. The presence of distant metastases is generally a very bad prognostic sign. A generalized scheme for TNM staging is given in Table 3.1.2 and Figure 3.1.4.

Solid tumours are then classified as stage I to IV on the basis of the TNM system. Stage I tumours have the most favourable prognosis and stage IV the poorest. The system varies slightly based on organ site, but generalized criteria are summarized in Table 3.1.3.

Histological grade

Histological grade is a measure of the histological or cytological characteristics of the cancer cells examined using a light microscope. It takes into account three features of the tumour cells:

1. The degree of differentiation of the tumour – that is, how much of the normal organization and architecture of the tissue is retained by the tumour, or conversely how disorganized it has become.
2. The rate of cancer cell division – assessed by the number of cells seen to be in mitosis, that is, actively dividing.
3. The appearance of the cancer cell nuclei – how regular and even sized, or conversely irregular and odd looking they are.

Grade I tumours are closest in morphological appearance to the normal tissues in which they arise, are thus said to be well differentiated and carry the most favourable prognosis. Grade II are moderately differentiated and have an intermediate prognosis, and grade III and IV tumours are the least differentiated and have the poorest prognosis.

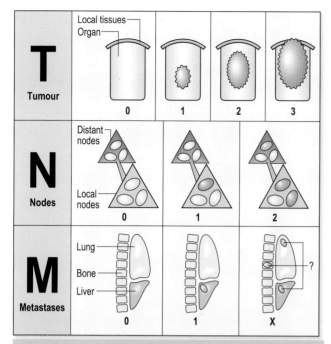

Figure 3.1.4. Staging of carcinoma by the TNM system. The general principles of TNM staging are as follows: T refers to primary tumour. The accompanying number denotes the size of tumour and its local extent. The number varies according to site. N refers to lymph node involvement, and a high number denotes increasing extent of involvement. M refers to the extent of distant metastases. As an example, the TNM system for staging malignant neoplasms of the breast is: T0 = breast free of tumour; T1 = lesion <2 cm in size; T2 = lesion 2–5 cm; T3 = skin and/or chest wall involved by invasion; N0 = no axillary nodes involved; N1 = mobile nodes involved; N2 = fixed nodes involved; M0 = no metastases; M1 = demonstrable metastases; MX = suspected metastases. (Reproduced with permission from Stevens and Lowe, 2000.)

Table 3.1.3. Generalized criteria for solid tumour staging based on the TNM system

Stage	TNM classification	Notes
I	Tis, or T1, N0 or N1, M0 or M1	In situ or limited to local site, small, resectable
II	T2, N0 or N1, M0 or M1	Locally invasive, medium-sized, invasion into local tissue and lymphatics, resectable
III	T3, N2, M1 or M2	Large, with regional and distant spread, operable but may not be completely resectable
IV	T4, N3, M2 or M3	Very large, regional and distant metastases, inoperable or incompletely resectable

IMAGING TUMOURS AND BIOCHEMICAL TESTS

At the time of diagnosis of primary tumour, it is usual for a battery of investigations to be carried out in an attempt to determine the extent of primary and metastatic disease. Similar investigations may also be employed to monitor response to treatment. Some commonly used investigations are outlined below.

X-rays

X-rays are useful for imaging tumour deposits in lung, pleura, lymph nodes or bone.

Ultrasonography

Ultrasound scans can be helpful in imaging tumour in soft tissues and the abdominal cavity. Ultrasonography is rapid, inexpensive, non-invasive and harmless. It works by imaging echo patterns from sound waves bounced back by tissues. These echoes are disrupted by bone and gas, and it is therefore not useful for tissues containing these substances. It is especially helpful in imaging tumours in the liver, gastro-intestinal tract, pancreas, ovary, kidney, thyroid, testes and prostate, and also lymphomas and sarcomas.

Biochemical tests

A range of biochemical tests may be performed, including blood count and liver function tests. Measurement of liver enzymes may provide evidence of primary or metastatic tumours in the liver. Blood count will reveal leuco-erythroblastic anaemia (where immature white cells and precursor red cells are present in the blood) typical of (usually metastatic) tumour in bone marrow, and also reveal normochromic anaemia (normal haemoglobin levels) associated with advanced cancer.

Bone marrow aspirate

Bone marrow aspirate is used for detection of metastases in the bone marrow that commonly arise from primary sites including small cell carcinoma of bronchus and *non-Hodgkin's lymphoma*.

CT (computed tomography) scan

CT scan visualizes the fat planes that surround normal tissues and reveals distortions or enlargement of organs or changes in their density, all of which may indicate the presence of tumour. Such investigations are especially useful in imaging lung cancers, lymphomas, testicular germ cell tumours, osteosarcomas, tumours of the brain, lymph node metastases from pancreatic and adrenal tumours, sarcomas, head and neck cancers, kidney tumours, and cancers of cervix, bladder, prostate and rectum.

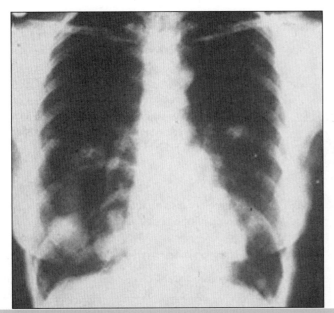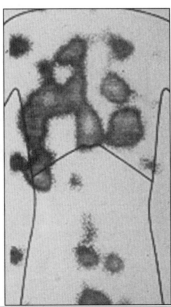

Figure 3.1.5.   Chest radiograph and immunoscintigraphy scan of a patient with carcinoma of the colon who has lung and liver metastases. The monoclonal antibody YPC2/12.1, raised against human colorectal cancer, binds to CEA. (A glycoprotein of 180 kDa.) The antibody was radiolabelled with ^{131}I and administered intravenously. Scintigrams were obtained after 48 hours. The image is that obtained after a subtraction procedure to eliminate background blood-borne antibody. (Courtesy of Professor K. Sikora. Reproduced with permission from Roitt, 2001.)

MR (magnetic resonance) imaging

In MR scanning, the patient lies in an intense magnetic field. It is non-invasive and harmless, though many patients find it frightening and unpleasant because of the claustrophobic nature of the enclosed and noisy chamber. It is expensive to perform because it is time-consuming and requires specialist and expensive machinery and experienced personnel. It is especially useful for imaging tumours in the brain and spinal cord and also sarcomas.

Imaging by lymphography

Lymph nodes of the pelvic, iliac, head and neck regions may be imaged by means of a contrast material injected into lymphatics. It may be useful in diagnosis of lymphoma and in imaging lymph node metastases. It is an invasive technique and lacks reliability. For example, lymph nodes that have been entirely replaced by tumour are not imaged at all and remain undetected. It has been largely superseded by MR and CT scans.

Radioisotope imaging

Low dose, and therefore relatively safe, radioactive compounds are injected systemically and used to image tumour deposits. They may be attached to monoclonal antibodies (see 'Monoclonal antibodies' later) directed against antigens

expressed by the tumour cells (Fig. 3.1.5). It is a useful technique for imaging tumour in bone and liver, but lacks sensitivity for most other sites.

Fine needle aspiration and fine needle biopsy

Diagnosis of primary or secondary deposits imaged at accessible sites may be made by means of a fine needle aspirate or fine needle biopsy. Examples of this are diagnosis of primary breast cancer or breast cancer metastases in axillary lymph nodes, which may be performed with mammographic guidance if the tumour is too small to detect by palpation, and diagnosis of lung tumours directed by chest X-ray.

TUMOUR MARKERS

As described previously, many cancers retain characteristics of the normal tissue in which they arise, such as synthesis of particular biochemicals. Others produce substances not synthesized by normal adult tissues at that site. In either case, these substances are often secreted into the bloodstream of the patient in detectable quantities and their presence can be used as a marker for the presence of tumour, an indication of its size, and to monitor response to treatment and to presage recurrence. Some examples of tumour markers are given in Table 3.1.4.

Table 3.1.4.   Some examples of tumour markers detectable in the blood of cancer patients

Cancer type	Marker
Choriocarcinoma, teratoma	Human chorionic gonadotrophin (hCG)
Ovarian cancer, seminoma	Placental alkaline phosphatase
Gut, breast and pancreatic cancer	Carcinoembryonic antigen (CEA)
Germ cell tumours, hepatoma	Alpha-fetoprotein (AFP)
Pancreatic cancer	Pancreatic oncofetal antigen
Ovarian cancer	CA-125
Thyroid cancer	Thyroglobulin
Medullary cancer of thyroid	Calcitonin
Small cell cancer of bronchus	Adrenocorticotrophic hormone (ACTH), alcohol dehydrogenase (ADH)
Osteosarcoma	Alkaline phosphatase
Neuroblastoma	Lactate dehydrogenase
Prostate cancer	Prostatic acid phosphatase (PAP), prostate-specific antigen (PSA)
Pancreatic cancer	CA-19-9

Tumour markers are not usually produced universally by every tumour of a particular type. Thus, they are not useful in screening or early diagnosis as their absence does not mean that tumour is not present. Tumours that do produce them do not necessarily do so in a predictable way, so serum level of tumour marker does not always indicate size of tumour. However, under certain circumstances, and for selected tumour types, they can be clinically useful. For example, if the primary tumour is shown to synthesize a certain marker substance, then the marker would be expected to disappear following successful primary treatment, and to reappear if the tumour recurs or if metastatic disease becomes apparent. A good example is *prostate-specific antigen* (PSA), which is normally produced by cells of the prostate and is also synthesized by most prostate cancers and their metastases. Raised levels are often detectable in the serum of patients with prostate cancers, and these levels will fall once the tumour is successfully removed, and reappear with the manifestation of metastatic disease. Serum levels of PSA may be useful in monitoring success of treatment in prostate cancer and in warning of early recurrence of tumour. In this manner, CEA is routinely used to monitor progress of colorectal cancer and CA-125 for ovarian cancer. AFP (alpha-fetoprotein) and hCG (human chorionic gonadotrophin) are clinically useful in early diagnosis of recurrence of teratoma. Sometimes serum levels may be raised for reasons other than cancer; for example, serum levels of PSA may be elevated in patients with benign prostate disease, and of CEA in patients with benign inflammatory bowel conditions.

CANCER TREATMENTS

Most patients suffering from either newly diagnosed primary cancer, or recurrent or metastatic disease face long-term, often very unpleasant, multimodal treatment. Typically, cancers are treated by combinations of surgery, radiotherapy, chemotherapy and immunotherapy. The precise treatment regimen for an individual patient will depend on the type of cancer, its stage and other prognostic information, the patient's overall health, the patient's wishes, plus practical considerations such as patient access to hospital/clinics, waiting lists, availability of specialist equipment and so on.

The goals of treatment may be:

- cure
- prophylactic treatment/destruction of early stage metastatic disease
- long-term control or suppression of primary or metastatic disease
- palliation of the symptoms of late stage disease to improve quality of life and possibly prolong survival.

Cure is only a realistic aim in the absence of clinically apparent metastatic disease. Once this is present, optimization of quality of life, and perhaps extension of survival become the treatment aims, but cure is unlikely.

Almost all cancer treatments are aggressive with significant unpleasant side effects. The severity and frequency of possible side effects vary from individual to individual. Fortunately, most treatment side effects are temporary and resolve with time once therapy is completed. However, it is usual for there to remain some long-term or permanent ill effects of the disease or its treatment in most patients.

Surgery

For many primary cancers, the first line of therapy is excision of the tumour mass, usually including a margin of apparently normal, healthy tissue. This is often accompanied by surgical excision of local lymph nodes for staging purposes. Surgical excision of metastases may be attempted in some cases if they are discrete and accessible.

Excision may be aimed at:

- cure, in the case of apparently early, localized cancers
- controlling primary or metastatic disease even if cure is unlikely
- the palliation of symptoms of late stage, incurable tumour.

All patients are likely to suffer from the types of problems associated with any type of surgery, such as deep vein thrombosis and muscle wasting arising from prolonged bed rest, postsurgical pain, problems associated with wound healing and infection, and phantom sensation. In addition, temporary or permanent physical impairment/loss of function may be expected in some patients, largely depending on the site and extent of the surgery. Examples include specific loss of function resulting from tissue or organ resection and lymphoedema from impaired lymphatic drainage if local lymph nodes have been excised. In addition, there may also be profound psychological effects resulting from changes in physical appearance, for example after loss of a breast following radical surgery for breast cancer, after disfiguring head and neck surgery for tumours at those sites, or limb amputation in the case of some bone tumours.

Radiotherapy

Radiotherapy is increasingly used as an alternative first-line therapy to surgery in treatment of many tumour types, including cancers of the larynx, head and neck, cervix, breast, bladder and prostate. It may also be given as an adjunct to surgery. For example, in patients treated by conservative surgery (lumpectomy or local excision) for breast cancer, it is usual practice to administer radiotherapy to the rest of the treated breast and axilla in an attempt to eradicate or control local recurrence of the disease. It is also frequently given in conjunction with chemotherapy in treatment of many tumour types either as part of the primary treatment or to treat metastatic or recurrent disease. It is often the treatment of choice for discrete bony metastases. As some chemotherapy drugs, for example *actinomycin D* and *doxorubicin*, are radiosensitizers this may exaggerate both the therapeutic and the adverse side effects of the radiation therapy.

Radiotherapy destroys the ability of any – both normal or cancer – cells that are exposed to it to grow and divide. It does this by directly damaging the cell's DNA. Many cells are killed outright, while others are able to recover over time (Table 3.1.5). Normal cells appear to be able to recover after radiation treatment more readily than cancer cells (see Part 2 of this chapter).

Permanent DNA damage to irradiated normal cells results in increased risk of tumours at the irradiated site after a long

Table 3.1.5. Relative radiosensitivity of some common human cancers

Largely insensitive	Sarcomas
	Melanoma
Intermediate sensitivity	Breast cancer
	Small cell lung cancer
	Squamous cancers of head and neck, skin and gynaecological sites
	Bowel cancer
	Glioma
Very sensitive	Lymphomas
	Leukaemias
	Seminoma
	Ewing's sarcoma
	Tumours of embryonal origin

latent period, usually of more than 10 years. Owing to the teratogenic effects of radiation, pregnant women should not receive radiotherapy until the last trimester when organogenesis is complete, and it should be avoided altogether during pregnancy if possible (see 'The treatment of cancer in patients who are pregnant' later in this chapter). Radiation therapy given early in pregnancy results in spontaneous miscarriage. Permanent DNA damage to ovaries or testes in both children and adults may adversely affect fertility and increases the risk of fetal abnormalities in any future conceptions.

Radiotherapy is commonly given in small, carefully calculated doses (referred to as 'fractions') as an outpatient procedure over a period of weeks or months. Normal, healthy tissues, especially vital organs, are shielded and the radiation beam angled to spare them as much as is possible. Some damage to normal structures is, however, almost inevitable. The nature and severity of local effects on normal tissue will depend on the type and duration of radiation, the total radiation dose, and the target tissue type.

Common short-term side effects include fatigue, especially in the latter weeks of treatment, and local skin reactions. Typically, damage to skin presents as redness and soreness of increasing severity, leading to first a dry then a moist desquamation (see Part 2 of this chapter for details).

Radiation therapy usually at least temporarily inhibits hair growth in the treated region. The treated area should not be shaved during treatment – for example, men should not shave facial hair if radiotherapy is being administered to the beard area; women should not shave the axilla during irradiation for breast cancer. Irradiation of the scalp may lead to temporary or permanent hair loss. Further irradiation of treated skin should be avoided because the area will remain permanently radiosensitive and, even if applied months or years later, will often result in tissue necrosis. As lymphocytes are highly radiosensitive, their incidental irradiation as they pass in the bloodstream through the treatment site also commonly results in general lymphopenia.

Other immediate side effects of radiation therapy include bone marrow aplasia, neurological, metabolic and cardiopulmonary damage, radiation myelopathy, mucositis and susceptibility of secondary infections. There may also be delayed effects due to radiation damage. Symptoms of pulmonary interstitial fibrosis often appear over 2 years after treatment has been discontinued.

Different types of cancer differ in their radiosensitivity, as indicated in Table 3.1.5. Also, it is thought that cells receiving a good oxygen supply are more radiosensitive than those starved of oxygen (anoxic). As described previously, many larger tumours outgrow their blood supply and contain significant anoxic, and necrotic, areas. This has implications for success of therapy as these parts of the tumour will be resistant to radiotherapy and provide a pool of surviving cancer cells from which the tumour may regrow once therapy has ceased. Even in the absence of anoxia and necrosis, tumours are shrunk, but rarely completely destroyed by radiotherapy. Any cancer cells remaining become insensitive to this form of attack and the remaining radioresistant cells can re-grow to form a new tumour that is resistant to further treatment by this approach.

Normal tissues also differ in their degree of radiosensitivity. Generally, as radiotherapy affects dividing cells, those tissues characterized by rapid cell division are most sensitive. This includes, for example, bone marrow, the stem cells of the gonads and the epithelial lining of gastrointestinal tract. Most normal tissues will apparently eventually recover once therapy ceases, but irradiation of the bone marrow usually results in long-term suppression as stem cells are destroyed and cannot be replaced, and irradiation of the gonads in both males and females usually results in permanent fertility problems for the same reason. Long-term bone marrow suppression means that further radiotherapy or chemotherapy may have drastic effects. The tissues of the nervous system are quite sensitive to radiation damage and do not readily regenerate. Thus, radiation damage to nerves is a special concern. Symptoms of tissue fibrosis around nerves may not appear for many months and up to around 3 years after treatment.

Radiotherapy in children poses special problems, as irradiation of the bone, especially the growth plates of the long bones, may interfere with subsequent normal growth. Administration of growth hormones will help, but stature may be permanently affected. High-dose irradiation of joints in patients of any age may result in damage to bone, cartilage or tendons and permanent stiffness and loss of flexibility.

Large brain tumours are commonly treated by radiation therapy. This may result in short-term oedema and consequent rise in intracranial pressure. Loss of hair in the irradiated area of scalp is expected and may be permanent. Radiotherapy is also commonly used to treat painful bony metastases, particularly in the spine. Doses must be carefully calculated because radiation damage to the spinal cord may lead to permanent partial paralysis.

> A late, but reversible, complication of radiotherapy to the spine is *Lhermitte's syndrome*, which is characterized by numbness of extremities and loss of flexion of the neck.

Acute lymphoblastic leukaemia, non-Hodgkin's lymphoma and myeloma are very radiosensitive. These diseases are usually widespread throughout the body and thus whole body irradiation followed by bone marrow transplant with healthy bone marrow is often the treatment of choice.

Radiotherapy is frequently used in treatment of cancers of the eyes (*orbital lymphomas*, *rhabdomyosarcomas* and *retinoblastomas*). Incidental irradiation of surrounding normal tissue may result in cataracts, which can be treated surgically, and damage to the lachrymal gland leading to corneal dryness and impaired tear formation. The latter can cause inflammation of the cornea and the conjunctiva.

Incidental irradiation of the healthy kidney in treatment of abdominal and retroperitoneal tumours causes damage that reduces glomerular filtration rate and renal plasma flow. This usually recovers over a period of a year or more once therapy ceases. However, the acute symptoms, which include proteinurea (the presence of protein in the urine), uraemia – symptoms of which include headache, vertigo, vomiting, loss of vision, convulsions, coma, sometimes partial paralysis and urinous odour of the breath – and hypertension, can be very dangerous. Long-term and sometimes permanent effects can be expected to some degree, and include albuminuria (the presence of albumin in the urine) and impaired glomerular and tubular function.

Irradiation of the lower abdomen in treatment of abdominal and cervical cancers may result in damage to the lower intestine and rectum. Acute symptoms include diarrhoea, tenesmus (painful straining of the bowels without evacuation of faeces) and rectal haemorrhage, but these usually resolve over time once treatment ceases and the bowel heals. There may, however, be long-term or permanent damage including fibrosis and oedema of the bowel resulting in diarrhoea, bleeding and pain. These symptoms are similar to those of primary or metastatic tumour of the colorectum and thus may cause concern and confusion. More extensive damage to the bowel, such as radiation-induced fistulas, abscesses and strictures, may occur and require surgical intervention.

Chemotherapy

Chemotherapy is therapy by means of toxic drugs that have a systemic effect. There are numerous chemotherapy drugs available, and treatment is usually much more effective when two or more are administered in combination (called combination chemotherapy) than when they are given alone or sequentially as single agents.

Chemotherapy is sometimes used as first-line therapy, for example, chemotherapy of some childhood leukaemias is extremely effective. It may also be administered to shrink a large primary tumour prior to its surgical excision, for example in large primary breast cancers. It is probably most often used as an adjuvant to surgery in treating presumed early metastatic disease and in systemic treatment of metastases in patients with later stage disease. It is often given in conjunction with radiotherapy. One of the rationales behind administering chemotherapy to patients immediately following surgery (adjuvant chemotherapy) is the idea that residual tumour regenerating after surgical excision should be particularly susceptible. Its aims may therefore be either curative, prophylactic, palliative, or to control metastatic disease with the aim of at least temporary remission.

Most chemotherapy drugs affect cells – both normal and cancer cells – undergoing division. Normal cells that divide rapidly are therefore most affected. These include the hair follicles, mucosal cells of the gastrointestinal tract, epidermal cells and haematopoietic cells. The distressing and unpleasant side effects of chemotherapy – such as hair loss, skin and mucosal membrane thinning, irritation and ulceration of the mouth and gut, nausea, vomiting, loss of appetite, anaemia, fatigue and decreased resistance to infection – are a result of the toxic effects of the drugs on these susceptible normal tissues. Healthy tissues that are characterized by a slower rate of cell division, such as those of the kidney, are adversely affected later in treatment. Eventual nerve damage following extended therapy may result in numbness/tingling sensations (paraesthesia), tinnitus (ringing in the ears) and hearing problems. Damage to very slow dividing cells may continue after chemotherapy has ceased, leading to long-term side effects.

As chemotherapy drugs are generally effective against dividing cells, therapy is most effective in rapidly growing tumours characterized by a high rate of cell division. Some types of cancer are intrinsically very sensitive to chemotherapy for this reason, for example lymphomas and germ cell tumours. Some chemotherapy drugs, notably those used in treatment of leukaemia, have been developed in conjunction with good animal models of the disease and are therefore extremely effective irrespective of the rate of cell division in those neoplasms. Chemotherapy has led to improved cure rates in some cancers, such as Ewing's sarcoma, rhabdomyosarcoma, Wilms' tumour, leukaemias, lymphomas and testicular cancers. In common cancers in adults, such as breast, colon and non-small cell lung cancer, more modest outcomes are expected. Other tumour types are intrinsically resistant, and not necessarily because they have a slow rate of cell division; these include pancreatic cancer and melanoma.

Different chemotherapy drugs act at different stages in the cell cycle (Fig. 3.1.2) and this has an influence on the timing of their administration, although, clearly, practical considerations such as clinic times and patient-specific considerations often play a role in planning treatment. *Vinblastine*, for example, has the effect of temporarily arresting cells in mitosis. As tumour cells recover from a dose of this drug they will therefore enter the next stage of the cell cycle synchronously and at this point a dose of a second drug, such as methotrexate, which affects cells in S-phase, will have maximal effect. Alkylating agents tend to be non-phase specific.

Consistent with the idea that most chemotherapy drugs affect cells undergoing active cell division, and as at any moment in time only a small proportion of cancer cells within a tumour will be dividing and therefore susceptible, chemotherapy is usually administered in intermittent pulses separated by rest periods over a long period of time, usually several months ('cycles'). Most patients receive chemotherapy on an outpatient basis. Patients will often be fitted with a Hickman catheter for long-term administration, and phlebitis at the site of administration can be a problem. The inherent heterogeneity of tumour cells mean that, almost inevitably, a subpopulation of cells will be inherently resistant to any given chemotherapeutic agent and be unaffected. They will form a residual pool of cells that once therapy has ceased will proliferate to form a new tumour resistant to this type of approach. Thus, over time, in most patients, the disease becomes resistant to chemotherapy.

Many chemotherapy drugs are highly toxic and cause unpleasant and sometimes severe side effects. A summary of some of the principal side effects of commonly used chemotherapeutic agents is given in Table 3.1.6. Systemic effects may include fatigue, weakness secondary to anaemia and weakness or aching of the muscles. Multiple neurological symptoms may occur with vincristine, vinblastine or procarbazine; cardiomyopathy may occur secondary to doxorubicin (adriamycin) or daunorubicin administration.

One of the commonest side effects of chemotherapy is nausea and vomiting, and the severity of this effect varies with different drugs, and between individual patients. The reason for the vomiting is not fully understood. Alkylating agents, doxorubicin and cisplatin, usually produce vomiting between 2 and 8 hours after administration, and symptoms typically persist for 8–36 hours. After repeated cycles of chemotherapy, some patients suffer anticipatory nausea and vomiting as they enter the hospital or at the sight of the needle. Anti-emetic therapy given well in advance can partially alleviate symptoms and a range of anti-emetics are available. However, none are completely effective, and all have side effects themselves including diarrhoea or constipation, headaches, dizziness and mood disturbances.

Another common and distressing side effect of many chemotherapy drugs is hair loss. This may be partial with some drugs, resulting in thinning or weakening and loss of condition of the hair, and in some cases, cooling the scalp

Table 3.1.6.   Examples of principal side effects of commonly used chemotherapy drugs

Drug	Side effect
Alkylating agents and nitrosoureas	
Mechlorethamine (mustine)	Nausea, vomiting, leucopenia, thrombocytopenia, thrombophlebitis, local tissue necrosis
Cyclophosphamide	Haemorrhagic cystitis, mild thrombocytopenia, nausea and vomiting, alopecia, pulmonary fibrosis, hyponatraemia, infertility in males
Ifosfamide	Renal dysfunction
Melphalan	Leucopenia, thrombocytopenia, long-term risk of leukaemia
Chlorambucil	Myelosuppression, thrombocytopenia
Busulphan	Bone marrow suppression, thrombocytopenia, pancytopenia, pulmonary fibrosis, skin pigmentation, glossitis, gynaecomastia, anhidrosis
BCNU (*bis*-chlororthyl-nitrosourea, carmustine)	Bone marrow suppression, nausea and vomiting, kidney and liver damage, oesophagitis and flushing, pulmonary fibrosis
CCNU (*cis*-chlororthylnitrosourea, lomustine)	Nausea and vomiting, delayed bone marrow suppression
DTIC (dimethyltriazenoimidazole carboxamide	Nausea and vomiting, myelosuppression, liver damage, nerve damage, myalgia
Folic acid antagonist antimetabolite drugs	
Methotrexate (amethopterin)	Toxic to gut, mucous membranes, oral ulceration, diarrhoea, skin rash, alopecia, bone marrow suppression, renal failure, pneumonitis, osteoporosis, pancytopenia
Pyrimidine and purine antagonist antimetabolite drugs	
5-FU (5-fluorouracil)	Diarrhoea, myelosuppression, nausea, stomatitis, alopecia, cardiac disturbances, cerebellar syndrome
Cytosine arabinoside (cytarabine, ara-C)	Bone marrow suppression, oral ulceration, nausea, vomiting, diarrhoea, CNS toxicity
6-Mercaptopurine (6-MP)	Cholestatic jaundice, nausea, vomiting, bone marrow suppression
Azathioprine (Imuran)	Bone marrow suppression
6-Thioguanine	Bone marrow suppression, nausea, diarrhoea
Vinca alkaloids and podophyllotoxin drugs	
Vincristine (Oncovin)	Neurological toxicity, loss of reflexes and paraesthesia, myalgic and neuritic pain, motor weakness, peripheral/sensory loss, cranial nerve palsies, autonomic neuropathy, constipation, alopecia, thrombocytosis
Vinblastine (Velbe)	Similar but less severe than vincristine: neutropenia, myelosuppression, some neurotoxicity, cellulitis, mucositis
Vindesine (Eldisine, Vinorelbine)	Similar and intermediate between vincristine and vinblastine
Paclitaxel (Taxol/Taxotere)	Mucositis, neutropenia, hypersensitivity, skin reactions, fluid retention, neuropathy, alopecia
Epipodophyllotoxin derivatives (e.g. etoposide)	Mucositis, bone marrow suppression, alopecia, leucopenia, nausea, vomiting, febrile reactions, peripheral neuropathy
Antibiotic drugs	
Actinomycin D (dactinomycin)	Nausea, vomiting, myelosuppression, mucositis, diarrhoea
Doxorubicin (adriamycin daunorubicin, cerubidin)	Liver toxicity, bone marrow depression, nausea, vomiting, mucositis, alopecia, gastrointestinal disturbances, cardiotoxicity leading to arrhythmia and heart failure
Mitoxantrone	Myelosuppression, alopecia, cardiotoxicity
Mithramycin	Nausea, stomatitis, thrombocytopenia, haemorrhages, impaired kidney and liver function
Bleomycin	Skin pigmentation, erythema, mucosal ulceration, pulmonary infiltrates and fibrosis, pyrexia, cardiac disturbances, respiratory problems
Miscellaneous agents	
cis-Diammine dichloroplatinum (cisplatin, DDP)	Nephrotoxicity, impaired renal function, nausea, vomiting, ototoxicity causing hearing problems, myelosuppression, peripheral neuropathy
Carboplatin (paraplatin)	Myelosuppression, nausea, vomiting, slightly nephrotoxic and neurotoxic
L-Asparaginase (Crasnitin, Elspar)	Anaphylaxis, pancreatitis, hyperglycaemia, impaired liver function, confusion, somnolence, coma, hypofibrinogenaemia, intense nausea
Procarbazine (Natulan)	Nausea, vomiting, leucopenia, CNS disturbances, psychological problems, flushing with alcohol, food reactions
Hydroxyurea (Hydrea)	Leucopenia and bone marrow suppression, gastrointestinal upset
Hexamethylmelamine (Hexalen)	Nausea, vomiting, neurotoxicity, abdominal cramps, diarrhoea, leukopenia, CNS effects including altered mental state, convulsions

during drug administration may minimize the effects. In many cases complete alopecia is an inevitable result, and this can be very upsetting for the patient. Normal hair regrowth should be expected once treatment is complete.

As chemotherapy drugs are so toxic, long-term side effects may be expected. These are of special consideration when there is a high probability of cure, for example in children treated for acute leukaemia or lymphoma and in men treated for testicular cancer. One significant effect is permanent damage to the gonads resulting in subfertility or infertility. Ovarian failure in females often results in early menopause, with sometimes severe and immediate menopausal symptoms. Chemotherapy-induced pulmonary fibrosis may result in permanently impaired lung function, and rarely there is permanent liver damage. Chemotherapy increases the risk of developing a second malignancy, particularly increasing the risk of developing acute myeloid leukaemia.

Hormonal therapy

Steroid hormones stimulate some cancer cells to grow and divide. The hormone, circulating in the blood, reaches the tumour, binds to a specific cell surface receptor, a message is sent to the nucleus of the cell, and the cell is stimulated to, for example, increase protein synthesis or enter the cell cycle and divide. The hormone sensitivity of a tumour can thus be assessed to a large extent by determining whether it expresses receptors for a particular hormone – for example, the oestrogen receptor (OR) and progesterone receptor (PR) are of particular relevance in breast cancer. Such cancers may be inhibited from growing and dividing by preventing them coming into contact with the stimulatory hormones. This may be achieved in a number of ways. It is often possible to physically ablate the site of hormone production and reduce the plasma concentration of circulating hormone. This may be achieved surgically or by the action of radiation or chemotherapy. Irradiating or surgically removing the ovaries (oophorectomy) or the administration of chemotherapy which will destroy ovarian function (sometimes called a medical oophorectomy) decreases oestrogen and progesterone production in the premenopausal woman. This approach appears to have beneficial therapeutic effect in about 50% of OR-positive patients and about 5% of OR-negative cases of breast cancer. Alternatively, hormone-inhibiting or hormone-blocking drugs may be used.

Breast cancer cells often express oestrogen (OR) and progesterone receptors (PR) and hormone therapy is employed in the treatment of OR- and PR-positive tumours. An oestrogen antagonist drug, tamoxifen, binds to the OR blocking the action of the steroid hormone. Tamoxifen is commonly prescribed as an alternative to ovarian ablation in breast cancer patients. It has a proven survival benefit and generally mild side effects which may include nausea and flushing. It does, however, increase the long-term risk of uterine cancer.

As androgens synthesized by the adrenal glands are converted into oestrogen in the liver, muscles and fat, ablation of the adrenal glands (adrenalectomy) may also have a therapeutic effect in breast cancer patients. Here, glucocorticoid replacement therapy is usually given. Aromatase-inhibiting drugs block conversion of androgens to oestrogen and depress synthesis of androgens and cortisol in the adrenal gland. They are often given in preference to surgical adrenalectomy. Aromatase inhibitors are especially useful in the treatment of advanced postmenopausal breast cancer, especially when there are metastases in bone. Their side effects include somnolence, skin rash, and muscle cramps.

In men, ablation of the testes (orchidectomy) reduces circulating testosterone levels and is a useful treatment for advanced prostate cancer. Drugs including *goserelin* and *leuprorelin* inhibit gonadotrophin release, which in turn suppresses plasma testosterone levels. They may be used in place of orchidectomy alone or in combination with anti-androgen drugs such as *megestrol acetate*. Megestrol acetate is a synthetic anti-androgen which lowers plasma testosterone levels and blocks the action of testosterone by binding to its receptor. Other anti-androgen drugs include *cyproterone* acetate and *flutamide*.

Occasionally, additive hormone therapies are useful in treating some types of cancer. Progesterone therapy is sometimes used in treatment of cancers of the uterus, and despite the generally beneficial effect of depriving breast cancers of steroid hormones, additive androgen, progestogen and glucocorticoid therapy is sometimes beneficial in the control of late stage disease. Additive progesterone therapy is sometimes useful in treating OR-positive and PR-positive cancers of the uterus.

The side effects of hormone therapy are usually directly related to the biological effect of administered hormone, or the biological consequences of its withdrawal from tissues. Oestrogen-blocking therapies in premenopausal women result in symptoms typical of the menopause such as amenorrhoea (lack of menstrual periods), hot flushes and mood changes. In some cases, hormonal manipulation may lead to distressing symptoms such as masculinization of a female patient (e.g. deepening voice or development of facial hair), or of feminization of a male patient (e.g. female-like breast development, termed gynaecomastia).

Immunotherapy

Immunotherapy most commonly involves the use of cytokines to stimulate, boost or enhance the immune system in the hope that it will recognize and destroy the cancer cells (Fig. 3.1.6). Cytokines have a number of biological effects,

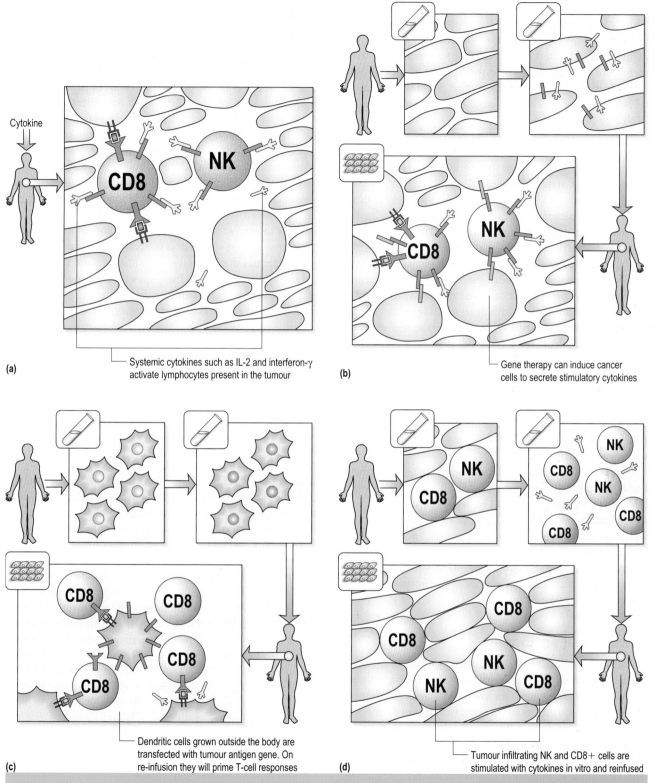

(a) — Systemic cytokines such as IL-2 and interferon-γ activate lymphocytes present in the tumour

(b) — Gene therapy can induce cancer cells to secrete stimulatory cytokines

(c) — Dendritic cells grown outside the body are transfected with tumour antigen gene. On re-infusion they will prime T-cell responses

(d) — Tumour infiltrating NK and CD8+ cells are stimulated with cytokines in vitro and reinfused

Figure 3.1.6(a–d).   Active immunotherapy for cancer. IL, interleukin; NK, natural killer, CD8 indicates CD8 + T-cells. (Reproduced with permission from Nairn and Helbert, 2002.)

including direct regulation of tumour growth, direct cyto-toxicity and mediation of the inflammatory response. Immunotherapy is generally not used routinely in treatment of most cancers, but is the subject of experimental treatments and clinical trials. The cytokines that have been most commonly employed in this context include interferons (IFNs), interleukin-2 (IL-2) and tumour necrosis factor (TNF) (see Ch. 2).

The interferons (interferon-α, interferon-β and interferon-γ), appear to have complex anti-tumour activity. They affect the immune response by stimulating the activity of effector T-cells, natural killer (NK) cells and lymphokine-activated killer (LAK) cells. In addition, they have a direct anti-proliferative effect on cells, including cancer cells, and induce differentiation. However, treatment with these agents has severe and unpleasant side effects reminiscent of influenza, with rigors, headache, muscle pains, chills, fever and leucopaenia. Other side effects of these and other cytokines may include loss of appetite, nausea, vomiting or diarrhoea, and a skin rash with dry and itching skin.

Interferon-α appears to have a therapeutic effect in chronic myeloid leukaemia, hairy cell leukaemia and follicular lymphoma, and may be useful in treatment of melanoma, Kaposi's sarcoma and renal cell carcinoma.

Tumour necrosis factor (TNF) is directly cytotoxic to leukaemia cells and B-cell lymphomas and is thus effective in their treatment; it also enhances the inflammatory response. However, as with other cytokine agents, there are significant side effects.

Interleukin-2 (IL-2) stimulates production of interferon-γ and TNF and thus activates LAK cells. It has been shown to have some therapeutic benefit in renal cell carcinoma and melanoma, but at the cost of significant side effects, some of which arise as a result of fluid retention, including fever, lethargy, hypotension, respiratory distress, nausea, vomiting, anaemia, neutropenia, disorientation and somnolence. Side effects are so severe that patients need to be hospitalized during its administration.

Monoclonal antibodies

Monoclonal antibodies (Mabs) are made by fusing an antibody-producing cell with an immortal, usually mouse, cultured myeloma cell. The result is an immortal hybrid cell that will secrete endless quantities of identical (monoclonal) antibody molecules all directed against exactly the same epitope, for example on a tumour-associated antigen. The antigen that the antibodies are directed against is unlikely to be tumour specific, i.e. unique to tumour cells, and will usually be expressed on some normal cells too (see 'Tumour markers' above).

Such monoclonal antibodies can be used in a number of ways. If they are attached to a label molecule (to facilitate their detection or monitoring within the body), such as a radioisotope, they may be injected into the patient and used to image tumours, such as occult metastases, although the

sensitivity of this approach is often poorer than with conventional techniques (see 'Radioisotope imaging' above). They may be attached to a cytotoxic compound, such as a radioactive isotope, drug or toxin, and used to direct the cytotoxin or dose of radioactivity preferentially to the tumour. In the case of radiotherapy directed in this way, in principle only a proportion of the cancer cells need to express the antigen recognized by the monoclonal antibody as the radioactivity will also kill other cells in the immediate vicinity. This concept of directing drugs or radiation directly to tumour cells is sometimes referred to as a 'magic bullet', but again the results in trials have often been disappointing and it is not an approach that is usually employed in mainstream treatment. Tumour heterogeneity is one problem – all tumour cells are unlikely to express the antigen that the monoclonal antibody is directed against – and there is usually significant uptake by normal tissues that share the same antigen, and non-specific uptake by tissues such as liver, spleen and bone marrow. In addition, as the monoclonal antibodies are usually derived from cultured mouse cells, they are quickly recognized by the immune response as being 'foreign' and destroyed. Attempts to 'humanize' monoclonal antibodies in order to overcome this obstacle are at least partially successful.

THE TREATMENT OF CANCER IN PATIENTS WHO ARE PREGNANT

Many types of cancer, including those of the breast, cervix, colorectum, and melanoma, lymphomas and leukaemias, all affect women of reproductive age, and it is not so unusual for cancer to be diagnosed in a pregnant woman. The treatment and outcomes depend upon the type of cancer, the stage of the pregnancy and the wishes of the patient.

Generally speaking, surgery is unlikely to affect the pregnancy unless the pregnancy is nearing term, or surgery to the abdomen is required. Radiotherapy to the abdomen carries a high risk of fetal abnormality at any stage in pregnancy and should be avoided. It may be considered in treatment of cancers in non-abdominal sites, but with caution. Chemotherapy in the first trimester carries a very high risk of fetal death, spontaneous abortion or fetal developmental abnormality, and should be avoided. It appears safer if administered during the second or third trimesters, with little chance of obvious fetal developmental abnormality, but the long-term effects on the unborn child remain largely unknown.

PSYCHOLOGICAL EFFECT OF CANCER

There are few diseases as feared, and which carry with them such strong and widely held associations of pain and death as cancer. The individual's first reactions to being told that they have cancer may be varied, and, of course, complex. A mixture of acceptance and denial, fear, panic, anxiety, grief and anger are not uncommon. Patients may have previous experience of the disease – because they or friends or family have been diagnosed, treated, cured, or are living with the disease or know someone who has died as a result of it – and these experiences, plus whatever knowledge they may have acquired from myriad sources, will all impact upon their reaction to their disease.

Cancer treatments, in particular radiotherapy and chemotherapy, have a frightening reputation, which, unfortunately, is generally well deserved. As described previously, these approaches have significant unpleasant effects and treatment often takes many gruelling weeks or months to complete. Patients may need considerable emotional as well as physical and practical support whilst undergoing therapy, and it is not uncommon for patients to find the experience so unpleasant as to wish to discontinue it. Under these circumstances, conflicting emotions of misery and depression at the thought of continuing treatment weighed against guilt and fear of the consequences of discontinuing treatment may be difficult to deal with.

Once primary therapy is finished, many patients find that although there is relief that unpleasant treatments are over, there is also considerable fear and anxiety about losing the support of the medical personnel that have been associated with those treatments. There is often an ongoing, and usually justified, fear of recurrence of the disease, and insignificant symptoms which prior to diagnosis would not have been noted are given unwarranted significance. Such anxieties may or may not be partially alleviated with the passage of time if the patient remains well. If the disease does recur after initial therapy, or if metastatic disease develops, the complex issues surrounding the reality of the situation are hard to deal with. Metastatic disease is rarely curable.

Honest advice, appropriate information, emotional and practical support are necessary at all stages of the disease and its treatment.

SPECIFIC PHYSICAL PROBLEMS FOLLOWING CANCER TREATMENT

Ileostomy and colostomy

Treatment of a number of primary cancers, including those of the colorectum, bladder, or uterus and cervix, and metastases to these sites, may result in the need for a temporary or permanent ileostomy or colostomy. This may result from either the direct effects of surgical resection, or because of local radiation damage. Appropriate stoma care is important. Significant fluid loss leading to electrolyte disturbances can cause problems in ileostomy patients.

Breast prostheses and implants

Patients who have lost a breast through surgery for breast cancer may either receive reconstructive surgery or be fitted with an external prosthesis that is normally worn with a specially adapted brassiere. In either case, a normal appearance

in clothes or swimwear is a realistic aim, although the cosmetic results of surgical reconstruction without clothes are variable. There are profound psychological issues surrounding loss of a breast, and breast reconstruction is a very important issue for some patients. Appropriate advice and counselling should be available whenever possible.

Reconstructive surgery may take place either at the time of the initial surgery to excise the cancer, or may be delayed until after the initial resection site has healed. Numerous reconstruction techniques exist, and may involve surgically implanting a prosthetic breast, or reconstructing the breast using fat and tissue taken from other parts of the body (commonly abdomen or buttocks).

Laryngectomy

Laryngectomy is a common surgical treatment for cancers of the larynx. It may be total or partial. In partial laryngectomy, if the vocal cords are spared, the voice may be retained but is often changed. Similarly, radiation damage to the larynx may adversely affect the voice. Speech therapy may be helpful in adapting to these difficulties. The voice is lost completely after total laryngectomy, and the patient needs to learn to create a voice either by using the oesophagus or by using an artificial larynx. Artificial larynxes are most commonly vibrating devices which are held against the throat externally, although occasionally permanent devices are implanted.

Prostheses for defects after surgery to the face

Mutilating surgery is often required to control cancers of the head and neck. Parts of the structure of the nose, jaws, teeth, eyes and eye sockets may be removed. Radiotherapy to head, neck and mouth may also cause permanent damage. Specialist facial prostheses designed to disguise the defects are available. There are clearly profound psychological issues involved in this type of mutilating treatment. Physical problems, including loss or impairment of sight, speech, taste and the ability to bite, chew, swallow or speak, may occur depending on the type and extent of surgery required.

Prosthetic limbs

Prosthetic limbs may be required after amputation of limbs in surgical treatment of primary bone cancers and soft tissue sarcomas or large metastases to these sites.

Depression of the bone marrow

Bone marrow depression may result from the systemic effects of chemotherapy or from the direct effects of radiotherapy to bone. It is especially a problem in high dose chemotherapy used in treatment of acute myeloblastic leukaemia and some solid tumours. Furthermore, the direct effect of primary disease (especially myeloma and leukaemia) or metastatic disease infiltrating bone marrow may destroy its function.

The most obvious treatment for bone marrow suppression is blood transfusion, or transfusion of preparations of blood cell fractions, such as platelet transfusion. Systemic treatment with growth factors, including granulocyte colony-stimulating factor (G-CSF), macrophage colony-stimulating factor (M-CSF), granulocyte-macrophage colony-stimulating factor (GM-CSF) and erythropoietin (EPO) increase blood cell counts and aid recovery during temporary bone marrow depression resulting from intensive courses of chemotherapy or radiotherapy.

Bone marrow depression may result in symptoms of anaemia, platelet count depression or granulocytopenia. Patients with anaemia complain of fatigue, malaise and breathlessness. Severe anaemia is not a usual side effect of chemotherapy and radiotherapy, as the red blood cells themselves are not killed and have a fairly long half-life. Moderate anaemia, resulting from killing of the progenitor cells that give rise to the red blood cells, is common. In severe cases, blood transfusion may be required.

A depleted platelet count increases the risk of haemorrhage, for example gastrointestinal bleeding.

Granulocytopenia only becomes symptomatic when infection is present. Here, fever, malaise, shaking and chills are common and oral ulceration and perineal inflammation are sometimes seen.

Infections

Patients with advanced cancer are often immunocompromised as a result of their disease, and aggressive anticancer treatments may also cause immunosuppression, so patients are more susceptible to infections than healthy subjects. Such infections can be fatal. Furthermore, microorganisms that are not pathogenic in healthy subjects may cause serious illness in cancer patients. The greatest danger is from the patient's own normal microflora, rather than from microorganisms carried by visitors, family or healthcare professionals. Long-standing, previously dormant infections that have long been held in check by the immune system, such as herpes and varicella zoster (the cause of chickenpox), may be reactivated. Shingles, a painful skin eruption caused by reactivation of previously dormant varicella zoster, is a common problem. The organism may also cause a potentially fatal pneumonia. Widespread herpes sores around the mouth and anus can cause misery. They may become infected with other organisms, particularly in the perianal area, and infection may become life-threatening. For this reason, attention to personal hygiene and avoidance of constipation (which can cause anal tearing) is important.

Respiratory infections with a variety of microorganisms including bacteria (e.g. *Streptococcus pneumoniae*, *Mycobacterium*, *Legionella*), fungi (e.g. *Aspergillus*, *Candida*, *Cryptococcus*), viruses (e.g. cytomegalovirus, herpes virus, measles virus), protozoa (e.g. *Pneumocystis*) are common. Diagnosis may require chest X-ray and possibly bronchoscopy with culture of the microorganism.

Oral thrush caused by *Candida albicans* is a very common problem in patients undergoing chemotherapy. Patients complain of a sore mouth and white plaques on an erythematous base are obvious in the mouth and pharynx. In extreme cases, the infection may extend into the oesophagus, stomach and bowel.

Generalized fever may indicate bacteraemia and septicaemia caused by *Escherichia coli*, *Pseudomonas aeruginosa*, *Staphylococcus* species and *Streptococcus* species. These are usually effectively combated by appropriate antibiotic treatments.

Urinary tract infections are common in patients with obstructive bladder outflow or atonic bladder. These conditions may arise as a direct result of the physical effects of tumour in the region, or from damage after aggressive local radiotherapy. Urine culture is required for diagnosis.

Staphylococcus epidermidis is a common pathogen in sites of subcutaneous infusion lines. If this occurs, the cannula should be removed and the site treated appropriately.

Leukaemia and lymphoma patients are sometimes subject to meningitis caused by *Cryptococcus neoformans* infecting the central nervous system. The first symptom is often a persistent headache.

Effects of inactivity and bed rest

Inactivity and prolonged bed rest may occur in long duration treatments of primary or recurrent disease, and may be necessary in patients with advanced or terminal cancer. This may result in significant impairment of physical function. Therapy should be aimed at optimizing and improving, as much as possible, physical function and psychological wellbeing. This may include a programme of appropriate physical exercises to improve circulation, pulmonary function, muscle strength and flexibility and to maintain bone density. If this is not possible, passive mobilization of joints and body segments and frequent posture change may be appropriate to prevent deterioration in joint flexibility and motion and to prevent pressure sores. Support hose may be indicated to prevent thrombosis.

Appropriate exercise also has a positive effect on mood. Social support and mental stimulation should also be encouraged to prevent sensory deprivation and depression. Professional psychological support and/or drug therapy may be helpful in dealing with feelings of depression, anxiety and nervousness, anger, agitation or irritability, with mental confusion or hallucinations and insomnia. This may be especially important in patients with late stage disease.

Other signs and symptoms of disease should be monitored. These may include hypotension, nausea, vomiting or diarrhoea, fatigue and lethargy, weakness, dizziness, blurred vision, laboured breathing, fever or chills, facial flushing, confusion or disorientation, claudication or cramping. Appropriate intervention should be instigated.

DIRECT PHYSICAL EFFECTS OF A PRIMARY OR METASTATIC TUMOUR MASS

The tumour mass itself, whether a primary cancer or metastatic disease, may exert direct physical effects on organs and tissues. This may result from replacement or destruction of normal tissue, for example liver failure resulting from healthy liver being replaced by cancer, or bone destruction from growth of bony metastases. Tumour growth may result in local haemorrhaging, for example into the gastrointestinal tract, liver or the brain. Destruction of brain, haemorrhaging into brain tissue or pressure on brain tissue can cause a variety of neurological symptoms, such as blurred vision, dizziness, numbness, limb weakness and stroke symptoms. Obstruction of organs associated with the respiratory system, such as bronchus and lungs, will cause respiratory problems; obstruction of any part of the gastrointestinal tract, such as oesophagus, stomach or large or small bowel, will cause problems ingesting or digesting food or excretion.

Bones

Prolonged bed rest or periods of inactivity may result in a decrease in bone density, as will the indirect effects of the disease (e.g. hypercalcaemia – see 'Paraneoplastic effects' later in this chapter) and its treatment. There is therefore increased risk of fracture, especially after falls, which patients with late stage disease and/or elderly patients may be more subject to. In elderly patients, there is also the likelihood of coexisting bone disease, such as osteoporosis. In addition to primary tumours of the bone, many soft tissue tumours metastasize to bone, including cancers of the breast, lung, prostate, pancreas, stomach, bladder and Hodgkin's lymphoma. Bony tumours are often painful, bones may crumble, affected vertebrae may collapse, and involved bone is more likely to fracture. Fractures of bones that are caused by a tumour may be resistant to healing.

Vascular and lymphatic system

Excision of lymph nodes for staging of primary cancers, for example breast cancer, or to remove bulky lymph node metastases as part of treatment may result in defective drainage of lymph and thus local lymphoedema, which can be extreme. In the case of lymphoedema of the limbs, compression bandage and elevation may alleviate the symptoms.

Direct compression of blood vessels by tumour will cause stasis, with an increased risk of clotting and infection. Surgical resection of tumours, and fibrosis after healing, may increase the risk of vascular complications such as deep vein thromboses, emboli, thrombophlebitits and ischaemia. Symptoms of cancer effects on the vascular and lymphatic system may include pain or tenderness, oedema, local heat or coolness of the skin to touch, and reduced or absent peripheral pulses.

Skin

Therapy, including surgical excision and radiotherapy, of primary cancers of the skin or nodules of metastatic tumour from other sites will have local effects. Surgical excision will result in wounds which will require time to heal, and may leave extensive scarring. Skin grafting or reconstruction may be required after excision of large lesions. Radiotherapy may result in radiation fibrosis and burns (see 'Radiotherapy' above). Damaged skin and treatment sites may be prone to opportunistic infection. Paraneoplastic syndrome (see 'Paraneoplastic effects' later) sometimes includes a wide range of skin problems including erythema (redness), pigmented and non-pigmented lesions and ichthyosis (scaly skin).

Lungs and heart

Primary lung cancers and metastatic tumour in the lungs and bronchus cause direct effects on respiration, including coughing, chest pain, laboured breathing and spitting blood. Systemic changes in general metabolism from most types of cancer and immunosuppression as a result of treatment increase the risk of opportunistic respiratory infections. Other treatment side effects may include radiation fibrosis of lung and heart.

Genitourinary system

The direct effects of primary and metastatic tumours in the genitourinary system and their treatment may result in a wide range of problems. Urinary problems may include increase in urinary frequency, urinary incontinence or urinary retention, pain with urination and haematuria (blood in the urine). Effects on the female reproductive system may include infertility, amenorrhoea in the childbearing years, early menopause, pain on intercourse and fistulas. Male patients may suffer from infertility and impotence.

Metastases in the liver

Many common cancers, including small cell carcinoma of the lung, cancer of the breast and lymphoma, commonly metastasize to the liver. Symptoms include fatigue, anorexia and weight loss and abdominal distension from ascites (see 'Malignant ascites' below). There may be persistent pain in the right upper quadrant of the abdomen, and/or sudden episodes of acute intense pain which is caused by sudden haemorrhage in the liver. Advanced liver metastases will disturb liver function causing jaundice and nausea, patients will become increasingly cachexic (see 'Paraneoplastic effects'), and skin itching and steatorrhoea (fatty stools) may be reported.

Patients with liver metastases are usually suffering from widespread metastatic disease at other sites, and prognosis is poor. The average life expectancy of a patient with liver metastases is usually only a few months. Treatment is therefore palliative rather than aimed at cure. Liver metastases are often responsive to chemotherapy and this is usually considered the first line of treatment. However, if the patient has already received chemotherapy earlier in their treatment regime, then repeated chemotherapy is not usually indicated. If the metastases are discrete tumours, radiotherapy or even surgical excision may be offered. Corticosteroid drugs such as prednisolone, anti-nausea drugs and analgesics for pain may provide some relief from symptoms.

Malignant pleural effusion

Pleural effusion is very common in patients suffering from primary and metastatic cancer of the bronchus/lung and mesothelioma, or with pleural metastases arising from primary tumours from a number of common sites, such as those from breast and ovary and lymphoma. It may occasionally have a cause other than malignancy. The volume of fluid may be very large, up to 5 litres, and causes significant discomfort. It may be accompanied by a persistent unproductive dry cough caused by irritation of the phrenic nerve.

Pleural effusion is usually indicative of advanced disease, and is a poor prognostic sign. Treatment is aimed at relieving symptoms, rather than cure. The commonest approach is aspiration, which relieves immediate discomfort from fluid build-up. However, rapid aspiration of very large volumes of fluid may result in local pulmonary oedema so gradual aspiration of extensive effusion, often over several days, may be indicated. Systemic treatment of pleural tumours may also provide palliation and prevent, or at least slow down, reaccumulation of fluid. For this reason, chemotherapy or endocrine treatment (depending on the type of tumour) may be offered. Physical sclerosing agents such as talcum powder, antibiotic drugs like tetracycline, cytotoxic drugs or radioactive colloids may be directly introduced into the site of effusion, and may be effective, although at the expense of significant unpleasant side effects. Occasionally, surgery to excise metastatic disease may be appropriate.

Malignant ascites

Metastatic disease in the peritoneal cavity often results in the accumulation of fluid which is unable to drain owing to mechanical blockage of lymphatics by tumour. It is a common condition in patients with advanced disease, including metastatic cancer of the breast, ovary, bronchus, colorectum, stomach, pancreas and also melanoma especially when liver metastases are present. It can also arise quite commonly from non-malignant disease, including portal hypertension, hepatic vein thrombosis and raised systemic blood pressure. It is thus common in patients suffering from heart failure.

The overwhelming symptom of ascites from any cause is uncomfortable abdominal distension sometimes accompanied by peripheral oedema, especially noticeable as swollen ankles. Malignant ascites are usually cloudy and straw coloured. They contain large numbers of cancer cells. As with malignant pleural effusion, the presence of malignant ascites indicates late stage, poor prognosis disease, and treatment is aimed at relief of symptoms rather than cure. Most patients will be expected to live for only a few months. Gradual drainage of ascites over a period of several days will relieve symptoms. Systemic chemotherapy to shrink the tumours producing the fluid may limit or slow down reaccumulation of fluid and diuretics may also give some relief. Radioactive colloids may be introduced into the peritoneal cavity, again to target the tumour. If ascites are particularly distressing, extreme or recurrent, a surgical shunt may be considered to redirect the fluid away from the peritoneum and into the blood circulation.

Pericardial effusion

Malignant pericardial effusions are uncommon, but sometimes accompany malignant pleural effusion in patients with metastatic disease arising from carcinomas of the breast and bronchus, and lymphomas. Pericardial effusion in cancer patients sometimes occur as a result of other, non-malignant causes including infection, myxoedema, collagen disorders and rheumatoid arthritis. The treatment of pericardial effusion is quite similar to the approaches taken in treatment of pleural effusion. Drainage of the effusion is usually through a surgical window created to direct the fluid into the mediastinum. This may be accompanied by systemic chemotherapy, antibiotics or endocrine therapy, radiotherapy or local radioactive implants.

DIRECT ENDOCRINE EFFECTS OF CANCER

Cancers arising in the endocrine organs, such as those of the pancreas and adrenal gland, are very likely to produce and secrete the hormones characteristically made by the normal tissues at those sites. Furthermore, cancers arising in normally non-hormone-producing tissues may also synthesize and secrete hormones as a result of genes being inappropriately switched on. The hormone molecules synthesized by cancer cells may have full biological function, may be partially defective or abnormal (e.g. aberrantly glycosylated) and have impaired or partial biological activity, or be completely defective and inactive. They may therefore have unpredictable and often dramatic effects. A large number of cancer-related syndromes caused by ectopic hormone production by cancer cells have been described. The effects of cancer cell secretion of some specific hormones are described briefly below.

Human chorionic gonadotrophin (hCG)

Ectopic hCG induces breast development in males, oligomenorrhoea (an insufficiency of the menstrual flow) in females, and precocious puberty in infants. It may occur with hepatoblastoma, hepatoma, teratoma, seminoma, carcinoma of bronchus, pancreatic tumours, bone metastases from any source, squamous cancers, renal and ovarian cancers.

Corticotrophin (adrenocorticotrophic hormone)

Cancers of the lung, ovary, pancreas, adrenal and thymus sometimes release corticotrophin, resulting in elevated serum levels. The symptoms are hypertension, muscle weakness, hyperglycaemia, hypokalaemia (abnormally low levels of potassium in the blood), oedema and weight loss. These are different to the presenting symptoms of corticotrophin elevation found in association with other diseases. Corticotrophin production is a feature of late stage cancer, and is therefore a bad prognostic sign.

Ectopic expression of adrenocorticotrophic hormone gives rise to the symptoms of *Cushing's syndrome*, which are hyperkalaemia (abnormally high levels of potassium in the blood), glucose intolerance, hypertension and muscle weakness. It occurs with small cell carcinoma of the bronchus, carcinoid tumours of the bronchus, thymoma and neuroblastoma. It is indicative of poor patient prognosis.

Insulin and substances with insulin-like activity

Insulin elevation resulting in symptoms of insulin shock are sometimes seen in cancers of the bronchus and liposarcoma.

Some tumours produce other hormones with insulin-like activity. They too result in hypoglycaemia (abnormally low blood glucose levels) leading to severe hypoglycaemic attacks either associated or unassociated with fasting. This is most usually seen with large thoracic and abdominal sarcomas, hepatomas, mesotheliomas, adrenal carcinomas and lymphomas.

Antidiuretic hormone (ADH)

Elevated serum levels of antidiuretic hormone (ADH) inhibits urine production leading to haemodilution and hyponatraemia (abnormally low concentrations of sodium in the blood). This in turn causes neurological changes which eventually lead to aberrations in the electrical conduction of the heart and brain.

Arginine vasopressin

Ectopic production of arginine vasopressin results in the syndrome of inappropriate ADH secretion (SIADH). Symptoms are confusion and tiredness or drowsiness. It is associated with small cell lung cancer, thymoma, lymphoma and pancreatic cancer.

PARANEOPLASTIC EFFECTS

Patients with cancer commonly suffer from a variety of non-specific, bewildering symptoms and disturbances that cannot be explained by the direct effects of the tumour or its treatment. These are referred to as paraneoplastic effects or paraneoplastic syndrome. Anorexia, weight loss, cachexia and hypercalcaemia (abnormally high concentrations of calcium in the blood) are common features of paraneoplastic syndrome. Other less well-defined problems such as mood disturbances and fever also occur. These, and other, symptoms may partially be explained by hormonal and metabolic disturbances caused directly or indirectly by the tumour, as described in previous sections.

Special concerns of patients with advanced disease and the dying may include, primarily, analgesia to control pain from the disease, but also considerations not directly concerned with the tumour, such as appetite, constipation, mobility and other symptom control.

Anorexia, weight loss and cachexia

Loss of appetite and reduction in consumption of food leading to sometimes dramatic weight loss often accompanies cancer. It may result from the direct effects of the (primary or metastatic) tumour, especially head and neck tumours, colorectal cancers, pelvic masses or tumours in the liver. Direct causes include difficulties in swallowing food and narrowing or obstruction of the gastrointestinal tract which will have the effect of reducing food intake. It may also result directly from the metabolic or endocrine effects of substances synthesized and secreted by the tumour. Sometimes even small tumours may cause dramatic weight loss. Often effective removal of the tumour will result in the return to normal weight.

Anorexia and weight loss may also arise as a result of the side effects of radiotherapy and chemotherapy, such as changes in perception of taste, soreness of the mouth or inflammation of the mucous membranes lining the mouth, throat and gastrointestinal tract. Many chemotherapy drugs cause intense nausea and vomiting (see 'Chemotherapy' above). Nausea and vomiting may also be an unpleasant symptom of late stage disease. It is a common cause of suppression of appetite and weight loss, and can be treated by a variety of drugs. Endocrine disturbances arising from the effects of either tumour or treatment may lead to pancreatitis or hepatitis which will affect food intake and nutrient absorption.

Taste disorders and food aversions are not uncommon, especially with advanced disease, as is early satiety. Changes in dietary patterns and reduced overall food intake may result in dietary deficiencies. Vomiting may result in bile salt deficiency, and electrolyte and fluid disorders.

In patients with advanced disease the problems of anorexia and vomiting are compounded by defects in the protein-sparing mechanisms that would normally be activated during starvation to preserve muscle mass and energy levels. Glucose metabolism may be directly affected. Furthermore, the tumour itself will demand and use energy for growth. Metabolic products of the tumour may affect appetite, perception, consumption and absorption of food. An overall increase in metabolic rate, in spite of reduced calorific intake, also often occurs. These culminate in extreme weight loss termed cachexia. Cachexia is accompanied by decreased serum albumin levels, hyponatraemia (abnormally low concentrations of sodium in the blood) and consequent elevation in intra- and extracellular water causing oedema. Nutritional support, such as enteral nutrition, parenteral nutrition or hyperalimentation, will limit its effects, but cachexia may still be unavoidable. In terminal illness, the cachexic patient is wasted, weak and lethargic. At this stage it is probably inappropriate to attempt to control or reverse weight loss.

In cases of anorexia and weight loss in patients where there is realistic hope of long-term survival or cure, for example those undergoing therapy for early/primary disease, appropriate nutritional support is indicated as good nutrition will reduce morbidity and aid recovery. In more advanced disease, nutritional support may be appropriate, but it is important to strike an appropriate balance between palliation of symptoms and the sometime unpleasant or uncomfortable means by which adequate nutrition may need to be delivered. The simplest nutritional support is enteral (by mouth), taking into account patient food preferences and adding supplements if necessary. Loss of appetite is common in terminal disease and weight loss can be extreme. Steroid drugs sometimes help, as does a common-sense approach of offering small, regular meals and snacks of nutritious and tempting foods, perhaps accompanied by a glass of sherry or wine to stimulate appetite. Liquid diets may help if patients have difficulty coping with solid food, but have the disadvantage of delivering a high solute load for renal excretion which can have the unwanted effect of causing nausea and diarrhoea. Short-term feeding through a nasogastric tube may be considered in some cases. In extreme cases, intravenous feeding (parenteral nutrition) through a deep vein catheter may be the only option.

Weakness and fatigue

Most patients report feeling fatigued during radiotherapy and chemotherapy treatments, especially towards the end of extended courses of therapy. This fatigue may persist long after treatment ends, and probably arises from a complex mixture of physical and psychological causes. Myopathy (muscle weakness) is a side effect of prednisone treatment. Muscle weakness may also be caused by prolonged bed rest, nerve and muscle damage from the direct effects of tumour or its treatment. Surgical resection of muscle or soft tissue and radiation fibrosis will all cause these problems. Endocrine disturbances from tumour or treatment may also result in fatigue. Anaemia causes fatigue and may result from chemotherapy or radiation therapy induced bone marrow suppression, tumour-induced bleeding into tissues or poor diet (see 'Anorexia, weight loss and cachexia' above). In some cases, weakness and fatigue may be extreme, causing significant morbidity and loss of function.

Reduced immunity

As described previously, the immune response may be suppressed by both the effects of the disease itself and the side effects of therapies such as radiotherapy and chemotherapy.

Pain

Bone tumours are typically very painful. Pain is not usually present in at least the early stages of most other types of cancer. As disease progresses, the level of pain experienced by patients is very variable, ranging from little or no pain even in the extremes of terminal disease to chronic, severe and debilitating pain. Pain is perhaps the most feared of all symptoms of advanced and terminal stage disease. Appropriate pain control is paramount, and approaches to pain control may change as the disease progresses and symptoms worsen. In addition to the obvious physical suffering it causes, uncontrolled pain results in psychological distress, anxiety and depression, and in social isolation. Pain management in cancer is thus extremely important.

Pain may be caused by the effects of the disease itself or as a side effect of treatment, for example postsurgical pain. The tumour itself may cause pain by infiltrating and destroying surrounding tissue, from compressing tissues including nerves, distending or stretching viscera or tissues, and obstructing organs. Primary or metastatic tumour in bone may cause fracture. Distension of pleura as a result of malignant pleural effusion, local infection, or irradiation of the pleura in lung cancer causes chest pain.

Analgesic drugs provide systemic pain control. A summary of commonly prescribed analgesics and their side effects is given in Table 3.1.7.

Non-drug-based approaches to pain relief such as acupuncture and transcutaneous nerve stimulation may be helpful in some patients. Continuous or intermittent epidural infusion of

Table 3.1.7.   Analgesics for pain relief in cancer, and their side effects

Analgesic	Side effects
Mild analgesics	
Aspirin	Gastrointestinal pain and bleeding
Paracetamol	Skin rash, liver toxicity
Ibuprofen	As aspirin
Indole derivatives	As aspirin
Moderately powerful analgesics	
Codeine/dihydrocodeine	Constipation, excitement
Oxycodone	Constipation, hypotension, nausea, dysphagia
Pentazocine	Nausea, dizziness, palpitations, hypertension, dysphagia
Dipipanone	Constipation, mental confusion, respiratory depression
Very powerful analgesics	
Morphine sulphate	Constipation, hypotension, nausea, dysphagia
Diamorphine	As above
Methadone	As above
Dextromoramide	Dizziness, sweating, constipation, respiratory depression
Pethidine	Nausea, dry mouth, respiratory depression

Table 3.1.8.   Some paraneoplastic neurological syndromes

Syndrome	Symptoms	Pathology
Distal sensory and motor neuropathy	Generalized peripheral neuropathy ranging in severity from mild to severe	Segmentational demyelination of distal nerves, axonal degeneration
Sensory neuropathy	Slowly progressive, pains and paraesthesia in limbs spreading to trunk and face. Eventually patient unable to walk	Degeneration of dorsal root ganglia, with mononuclear cell infiltrate
Carcinomatous myelopathy	Acute onset flaccid paraplegia with loss of sphincter control. Occasional less severe form with progressive onset	Spinal cord necrosis in the presence of little inflammation
Cerebellar degeneration	Rapidly progressing unsteadiness of gait, truncal ataxia, vertigo, diplopia	Spinal cord degeneration, abnormal cerebrospinal fluid, cell loss in cerebellum with inflammatory infiltrate
Limbic encephalitis	Rapid onset of confusion, memory loss, agitation	Temporal lobe degeneration with perivascular infiltrate
Progressive multifocal leucoencephalopathy	Aphasia, dementia, coma, visual field loss, blindness, focal paralysis, fits	Patchy demyelination in brain white matter, abnormal oligodendroglia
Lambert–Eaton myasthenic syndrome	Weakness, aching, fatigue in shoulder and pelvic muscles	IgG antibody impairing calcium flux and acetylcholine release

analgesics using an external pump can provide medium-term relief of more extreme pain, but tolerance is likely to develop over a period of weeks or months and infection at the catheter site is a risk. Localized pain that is not well controlled by other approaches may be tackled by surgical nerve block, although this will result in loss of all sensation in that part of the body. Bone cancers and bony metastases are often extremely painful and relief may be obtained by local radiotherapy.

Neurological symptoms

Neurological symptoms including generalized or specific muscle weakness, pain, paralysis, numbness, changes in balance, dizziness, changes in mental state such as mood changes, confusion, anxiety, depression, anger, hostility, insomnia, restlessness, and behavioural changes may all accompany progression of cancer. They may arise from the direct effects of tumour, such as compression of nerves or parts of the brain, or from systemic endocrine effects of disease (see 'Direct endocrine effects of cancer' above).

As cancer progresses, tumour may cause haemorrhage, infarction or emboli and lead to a stroke, which, clearly, also carries with it a spectrum of physical problems.

A very wide range of neurological disorders with no obvious direct cause are also a feature of paraneoplastic syndrome. Some are listed in Table 3.1.8.

Anxiety and depression

It is not surprising that patients suffering from advanced or terminal stage disease may be subject to anxiety and depression. The social support of friends, relatives and carers is important. Antidepressant drugs may provide some relief.

Haematological effects

Anaemia

Almost all patients with advanced cancer suffer from anaemia, the principal symptom of which is fatigue (see 'Weakness and fatigue' above). Fatigue resulting from anaemia is an almost universal feature of paraneoplastic syndrome. Anaemia arises as a result of a combination of factors including poor nutrition (see 'Anorexia, weight loss and cachexia'), blood loss through internal haemorrhaging as a result of advanced tumour, shortened half-life of red blood cells and disturbances in iron metabolism. If fatigue is severe or chronic, blood transfusion may be indicated.

Autoimmune haemolytic anaemia is sometimes associated with B-cell leukaemias and Hodgkin's lymphoma. Erythropoiesis (the production of red blood cells) is sometimes suppressed in carcinoma of the bronchus.

Clotting disorders

A number of blood clotting disorders are caused by factors associated with the normal blood clotting cascade being synthesized and secreted by tumour cells. In thrombophlebitis multiple small migratory thromboses occur in superficial veins, such as those of the arms and legs. It is seen in a variety of different types of adenocarcinomas, most notably pancreatic cancer. Disseminated intravascular coagulation is a clotting disorder sometimes induced by cancers of the prostate, breast, pancreas, ovary and neuroblastomas and rhabdomyosarcomas. It is sometimes associated with red cell fragmentation or with chronic renal failure that leads to haemolytic uraemic syndrome.

Other haematological disorders

The presence of opportunistic infections (e.g. *Staphylococcus* and *Streptococcus*, upper respiratory tract infections, pulmonary tuberculosis, *Pneumocystis carinii* pneumonia) or bleeding disorders are also indicative of haematological disturbances in cancer.

Kidney and adrenal tumours, some lung, ovarian and thymus tumours and, unusually, cerebellar haemangioblastoma, hepatoma and uterine leiomyosarcoma can be associated with erythrocytosis (excessive formation of red blood cells). This is caused by erythropoietin-like substances (erythropoietin stimulates red blood cell production) secreted by the cancer cells.

Leukaemia patients may suffer from granulocytosis. Eosinophilia sometimes occurs in Hodgkin's lymphoma and other lymphomas, some brain tumours and melanomas, and is often associated with mycosis fungal infections.

Thrombocytopenia (reduction in blood platelet count) is seen in patients with cancers of lung, breast, rectum, testes, gall bladder, some leukaemias and Hodgkin's lymphoma. Granulocytosis occurs in paraneoplastic syndrome in patients with cancers of the lung, brain, pancreas, gastrointestinal tract and lymphomas and melanomas.

Hypercalcaemia

High serum levels of calcium (hypercalcaemia) occur in up to 20% of advanced cancer patients, especially those suffering from cancers of the breast, bronchus and kidney and their metastases. It occurs as an indirect humoral effect of the disease on bone by complex hormonal mechanisms, which result in the delicate balance of bone synthesis/resorption being upset. There is a net breakdown of bone with release of calcium into the bloodstream. Bones of the thorax, the long bones and the skull are most commonly affected. Parathyroid hormone elevation associated with cancers of the lung, colon, uterus, bladder, kidney, liver and pancreas result in hypercalcaemia. It is especially common in patients with metastases to bone, as these tumours often directly release factors such as transforming growth factor alpha (TGF-α), transforming growth factor beta (TGF-β), epidermal growth factor (EGF) and interleukin-1 (IL-1) which promote bone dissolution. Symptoms, which can be so severe as to be life-threatening in extreme cases, include lethargy, anorexia, abdominal pain, proximal muscle weakness, excessive urine production, excessive thirst, severe dehydration, gastrointestinal disturbances such as nausea, vomiting, diarrhoea or constipation, depression, pain, confusion, coma and cardiac arrhythmia.

Hypercalcaemia also disturbs kidney function, as high levels of calcium in the distal tubules make the kidney unresponsive to antidiuretic hormone (ADH). This results in salt and water loss and consequent uraemia (retention of substances in the blood that would normally be excreted in the urine – symptoms include headache, vertigo, vomiting, loss of vision, convulsions, coma, sometimes partial paralysis and urinous odour of the breath). There is also loss of potassium in the urine leading to hypokalaemia (low blood concentrations of potassium). Hypercalcaemia also decreases glomerular filtration rate. Elderly patients, those with already impaired renal function and myeloma patients are at high risk of renal failure. Therapy includes salt and water replacement with isotonic saline, bisphosphonates to inhibit bone resorption, oral prednisolone and intravenous hydrocortisone. Sometimes phosphate or calcitonin therapy is also indicated.

Fever

In cancer patients, fever is most usually a symptom of infection. However, the activity of the cancer itself may induce fever,

Table 3.1.9. Examples of paraneoplastic skin disorders

Skin problem	Symptoms	Tumour
Acanthosis nigricans	Velvety, papillary, darkly pigmented eruptions in armpit, groin and on trunk	Adenocarcinomas of gastrointestinal tract, lymphomas
Hypertrichosis	Lanugo (fine downy facial hair), sometimes associated with acanthosis nigricans	Adenocarcinoma of lung, breast, gut, bladder
Erythroderma	Red, maculopapular rash, may progress to exfoliative dermatitis	Lymphoma
Pyoderma gangrenosum	Red nodules that expand rapidly, centre becomes necrotic to yield painful ulcers that can become infected	Lymphoma or myeloproliferative tumours
Alopecia	Patchy hair loss	Lymphomas, particularly Hodgkin's lymphoma
Pruritus	Itching without rash, worse at night or in warm conditions	Hodgkin's lymphoma, carcinomas of lung, colon, breast, stomach, prostate

especially in Hodgkin's lymphoma and other lymphomas, sarcomas, primary liver cancer and metastases in the liver and bone marrow arising from a variety of solid tumours. It is usually a poor prognostic sign, being associated with advanced and aggressive disease. The fever may be short-lived, or recur intermittently. Treatment includes steroidal and non-steroidal antipyrogenic and anti-inflammatory agents including aspirin.

Muscle and joint problems

Some of the muscle fatigue, aching joints and general weakness experienced by patients with advanced cancer can be explained by muscle loss arising from anorexia and weight loss (see 'Anorexia, weight loss and cachexia' above). There are, however, specific joint and muscle problems experienced by cancer patients, and non-specific paraneoplastic effects.

Polymyositis (the simultaneous inflammation of many muscles) with dermatomyositis (inflammation of both skin and muscles) is characterized by progressive, symmetrical proximal muscle weakness accompanied by facial erythema (redness) and oedema or puffiness around the eyes and nose.

Metastatic cancer of the bronchus may cause thickening and inflammation at the ends of the long bones, with clubbing, swelling and local hotness, called hypertrophic pulmonary osteoarthropathy.

Arthritis-like conditions may sometimes occur in paraneoplastic syndrome.

Skin problems

Cancer patients suffer a variety of skin problems which may be caused either by infiltration of the skin by metastatic tumour, or as a side effect of the metabolic effects of tumour on other organs and systems (see also 'Skin' earlier in this chapter).

Some skin problems are a non-specific feature of paraneoplastic syndrome with no obvious cause. Some specific skin disorders seen in cancer patients are summarized in Table 3.1.9. Occasionally, skin problems are the presenting symptom of

cancer. There are also relatively unusual problems associated with advanced disease, such as thrombophlebitis (see 'Clotting disorders' above) and dermatomyositis (see 'Muscle and joint problems' above) that indirectly affect the appearance of the skin. An SLE (systemic lupus erythematosus)-like condition, characterized by flat, slightly raised red skin patches on the face, neck, trunk and sometimes the extremities, is seen in lymphoma patients.

Some genetic disorders that have skin problems as a symptom predispose sufferers to a high risk of cancer. Patients with Gardner's syndrome, for example, suffer from epidermal cysts and multiple polyps in the colon. The polyps are associated with high risk of colorectal cancer. Sufferers of the genetic disorder *ataxia-telangiectasia* have telangiectases (hard, elevated, red, wart-like spots composed of dilated groups of blood capillaries) on their face and neck and behind their elbows and knees; other symptoms are cerebellar ataxia (lack of coordination of muscle action) and IgA deficiency. These patients are at high risk of lymphoma and leukaemia.

Kidney problems

The kidney may be affected directly by primary renal cancer and by metastatic tumour from a number of different primary sites. Glomerular damage often occurs in patients with advanced cancer from many sites, especially breast, colon, stomach cancers and Hodgkin's lymphoma, and it may result in glomerulonephritis. Myeloma patients are sometimes subject to amyloid degeneration of the kidney.

Tumour lysis syndrome

When chemotherapy is effective in killing large numbers of cancer cells, their death and breakdown (lysis) results in the release of many potentially toxic by-products such as urea, urate and phosphate. Metabolism of these substances results in uraemia (substances normally excreted in the urine being retained in the blood), hyperuricaemia (excess uric acid in the blood), hyperphosphataemia (excess phosphate in the blood) and hyperkalaemia (high blood levels of potassium), which can cause quite severe symptoms. This is referred to as tumour lysis syndrome. It is more common, and more severe, after chemotherapy treatment of especially chemosensitive tumours including acute lymphoblastic leukaemia and non-Hodgkin's lymphoma, especially in children. Hyperuricaemia leads to deposition of urate in renal tubules (urate nephropathy) reducing glomerular filtration rate, which exacerbates the condition. Renal failure may result in extreme cases, and is more problematic in patients with existing kidney problems such as renal obstruction or tumour in the kidney. Hyperphosphataemia has the effect of lowering serum levels of calcium causing tetany (intermittent, bilateral, painful, tonic muscle spasms). In patients with highly chemosensitive tumours, prophylactic treatment with a xanthine oxidase inhibitor to limit urate formation, plus adequate, possibly intravenous, fluids may prevent or limit the problem. If symptoms are severe, chemotherapy may need to be stopped while the condition is treated. Treatment includes administration of intravenous fluids, alkalinization of the urine to promote urate excretion and administration of a xanthine oxidase inhibitor. Peritoneal dialysis may also relieve acute symptoms.

REFERENCES AND FURTHER READING

Fulton C (1999) Patients with metastatic breast cancer: their physical and psychological rehabilitation needs. Int J Rehabil Res 22(4): 291–301.

Grond S, Radbruch L, Meuser T, et al. (1999) Assessment and treatment of neuropathic cancer pain following WHO guidelines. Pain 79(1): 15–20.

Harris SR, Hugi MR, Olivotto IA, Levine M (2001) Steering Committee for Clinical Practice Guidelines for the Care and Treatment of Breast Cancer. Clinical practice guidelines for the care and treatment of breast cancer: 11. Lymphedema. CMAJ 164(2): 191–199.

Naim R, Helbert M (2002) Immunology for Medical Students. St Louis: Mosby.

Penson J, Fisher RA (eds) (2002) Palliative Care for People with Cancer, 3rd edn. London: Edward Arnold.

Price P, Sikora K (eds) (1995) Treatment of Cancer, 3rd edn. London: Chapman & Hall Medical.

Ripamonti C (1999) Management of dyspnea in advanced cancer patients. Support Care Cancer 7(4): 233–243. [Review]

Roitt I (2001) Immunology. St Louis: Mosby.

Souhami R, Tobias J (1995) Cancer and its Management, 2nd edn. Oxford: Blackwell Science.

Stevens A, Lowe J (2000) Pathology. St Louis: Mosby.

Thompson N, Chittenden T (1998) The sepsis syndrome and the cancer patient: respiratory management and active physiotherapy. Eur J Cancer Care (Engl) 7(2): 99–101. [Review]

Malignancy: Radiation Injury to Normal Tissues

Mohi Rezvani and Delva Shamley

IONIZING RADIATION AND CANCER

Ionizing radiation was employed in medicine for diagnostics and therapy soon after the discovery of X-rays by W.R. Roentgen in 1895. The first cancer treatment by X-rays was carried out in 1896 by Grubbe. Understanding of the physics and biology of radiation helped the development of different radiation qualities and relatively safer methods of radiotherapy planning. Radiotherapy became the treatment of choice for the eradication of several malignant tumours and despite new developments in the treatment of cancer by other modalities radiotherapy has not lost its importance. Radiotherapy is still considered to be an important modality in the treatment of malignant diseases and in fact it is employed in more than 50% of cases, either as a treatment of choice or as an adjuvant to other forms of treatment. Radiotherapy is used only palliatively in most advanced cases of cancer.

Despite vast developments in the understanding of the physical processes involved in the interaction of radiation with matter, the complex mechanisms of the interaction between ionizing radiation and biological systems and subsequent development of radiation-induced pathologies are far from being completely understood. However, there is ample evidence to suggest that the percentage of cells surviving irradiation is inversely related to the dose of radiation. The greater the radiation dose the greater is the cell kill. This implies that the greater the radiation dose the greater is the probability of tumour control (Fig. 3.2.1). Therefore, it must be possible, at least theoretically, to eradicate a localized tumour if a large enough dose of radiation could be delivered to that tumour. However, practically, there is always the danger of damaging normal tissues adjacent to the tumour. Two hypothetical dose–effect curves are shown in Figure 3.2.1. Increasing the dose of radiation increases the probability of tumour cure (left). However, parallel to this runs the dose–effect curve for the incidence of normal tissue injury (right). Increasing radiation dose increases the probability of developing normal tissue reaction. The vertical line shows that a dose of radiotherapy designed to produce 95% tumour cure can be associated with a significant level of normal tissue reactions. In radiotherapy of laryngopharyngeal tumours 95% of patients might experience an early transient reaction and more than 60% suffer more persistent late reactions.

Fortunately, there are some differences in the response of tumours to radiation in comparison with that of normal tissues. Overall, normal tissues tolerate radiation more than tumours. These subtle differences have enabled radiotherapists to develop methods of treatment within the normal tissue tolerance limit with acceptable levels of therapeutic gain. Therapeutic gain can be enhanced either by sensitizing the tumour or by protecting the normal tissues. This is represented by shifting the tumour cure curve to the left or by shifting the normal tissue curve to the right in Figure 3.2.1. The greater the separation of the two curves the bigger the therapeutic gain. Advances in the administration of radiation such as dose fractionation, low dose-rate irradiation, application of radiosensitizers or radioprotectors and better localization techniques have increased the therapeutic gain. In the planning of radiation treatment for a cancer patient, consideration has to be given to the risk of any morbidity arising from damage to healthy normal tissues unavoidably included within the treatment volume or in the path of the radiation beam. Recently, interventional treatments after radiotherapy and application of various biological response modifiers (BRMs) have been suggested.

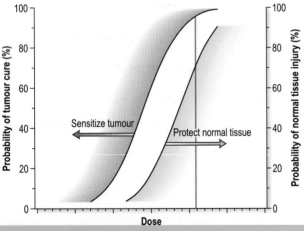

Figure 3.2.1. Hypothetical dose–effect curves showing that increasing the dose of radiation increases the probability of tumour cure (left). However, parallel to this runs the dose–effect curve for the incidence of normal tissue injury (right). Increasing radiation dose increases the probability of developing normal tissue reaction too. The vertical line shows that a dose of radiotherapy designed to produce 95% tumour cure can be associated with the incidence of a significant level of normal tissue reactions. The greater the separation of the two curves the bigger the therapeutic gain. This can be achieved either by sensitizing the tumour or by protecting the normal tissues.

DIAGNOSIS

Radiation injury to normal tissues is non-specific and generally it produces no pathognomonic morphological changes. The combined alterations in the structure of parenchyma and supportive tissues characterize the radiation damage. Therefore, a history of radiation exposure is most helpful in diagnosis.

The severity of radiation damage is dose and tissue dependent. While local irradiation of a specific tissue produces a localized lesion characterized by that tissue, total body irradiation produces a more generalized syndrome. In cases of exposure to large doses (such as those in radiation accidents) radiation syndrome starts within 2 hours of exposure, with anorexia, nausea, malaise and fatigue. Normal tissue reactions associated with radiotherapy of cancer are those induced by much lower therapeutic radiation doses and mainly by localized irradiations. In any event characteristics of radiation-induced lesions change with dose of radiation, time after irradiation and type of tissue involved. Precursor cells in almost all tissues, such as stem cells of the haematopoietic system, intestinal crypts, basal epithelial cells of the skin, are more radiosensitive than differentiated cells of that tissue. Therefore, radiation lesions do not fully develop until the differentiated cells reach the end of their lifespan. Then radiation lesion develops due to the lack or inability of precursor cells to replace the lost mature cells. The latency period for radiation-induced lesions varies from tissue to tissue and for acute lesions it is determined by the turnover time of the cells comprising that tissue.

Development of late effects of radiation is more complex and is determined not only by the damage to parenchymal cells but the extent of damage to vascular and other supportive tissues as well.

HAEMATOPOIETIC SYSTEM

Bone marrow is the organ at risk in the event of total body irradiation for therapeutic purposes or in unfortunate cases of radiation accidents. Total body irradiation produces severe granulocytopenia (loss of granular leucocytes, e.g. neutrophils, eosinophils, basophils) with subsequent infection and thrombocytopenia (loss of blood platelets) with haemorrhage (*bone marrow syndrome*). Bone marrow depletion, which occurs after large doses of radiation to marrow, begins with a rapid necrosis and lysis of nucleated cells of the marrow within the first 24 hours of exposure with a lowest point at 3–5 days. Lymphocytes undergo inter-phase death and rapidly lyse. Non-nucleated cells, erythrocytes and platelets are the most resistant of the haematopoietic cells. A lethal total body dose reduces haematopoietic cells to a level that normally will not support survival. Survival after such doses of total body irradiation requires renewal of haematopoietic stem cells and production of functional end-cells within a critical time period before the body succumbs to haemorrhage and infection from opportunistic pathogens. Doses of 2.4–7.5 Gy to whole body result in death through the mechanism of bone marrow failure within 60 days of exposure. (Gy is abbreviation for gray, the SI unit for absorbed dose; 1 Gy is one joule of energy absorbed by a kilogram of tissue.) The radiation dose sufficient to bring about 50% mortality (LD_{50}) within this period in an exposed group is about 3 Gy or about 4.5 Gy if the patient receives optimal supportive care. The LD_{90}, radiation dose sufficient to bring about 90% mortality, is about 7 Gy.

RADIATION-INDUCED SKIN DAMAGE

Radiation injury to skin (summarized in Fig. 3.2.2) starts with a transient early erythema that may appear at the time of exposure or a few hours afterwards. It may be due to capillary dilatation that may be associated with an increase in vascular permeability. This erythema is thought to be caused by the release of histamine or serotonin. However, it has been shown, in experimental animals, that during the early erythema the increase in permeability was not caused by serotonin or histamine but by a protease system. The early erythema often indicates a severe evolution and it might be of prognostic significance. True erythema reaction begins from a few days to one week after exposure and peaks around 2–3 weeks after irradiation. The skin becomes red, warm, oedematous and the patient might complain of itchy skin. This phase of erythema is due to the release of proteolytic enzymes from damaged epithelial cells. The severity of erythema is dose related. Histologically, the blood vessels of the upper dermis (Fig. 3.2.3) are dilated and larger vessels, particularly arterioles, may be obstructed by fibrin thrombi at later stages. Around this time, epilation might be present and the skin becomes dry due to the suppression of sebaceous glands.

If the dose of radiation delivered to cutaneous tissue is large enough, the skin might show moist desquamation around

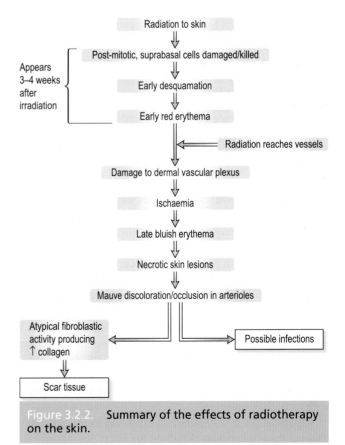

Figure 3.2.2.   Summary of the effects of radiotherapy on the skin.

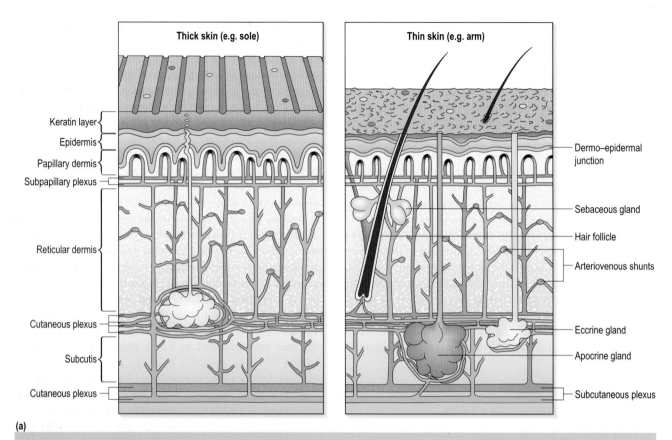

Figure 3.2.3.   (a) Architecture of the skin. The most superficial layer of the skin is the epidermis. This varies in thickness from site to site and is covered by acellular keratin, which is thick in thick skin and thin in thin skin. Beneath the epidermis is the dermis, which has two components: a more superficial loose papillary dermis and a denser reticular dermis, which comprises the bulk of the layer. The dermis is mainly composed of collagen with some elastic fibres. The deepest layer of the skin, the subcutis, has a variable structure; when prominent it is composed largely of adipose tissue intersected by fibrocollagenous septa. The subcutis contains the main subcutaneous network of arteries and veins from which vessels extend upwards and form a network (the cutaneous plexus) at the dermo-subcutaneous junction. From here, smaller vessels penetrate the dermis, giving branches to the skin appendages and culminating in a superficial network of small venules and arterioles (the subpapillary plexus). Capillary loops from this plexus extend upward into the dermal papillae to lie close to the dermo-epidermal junction. Blood vessels do not penetrate the epidermis.

3–4 weeks after irradiation. Moist desquamation or epithelial erosion is usually associated with oedema, fibrinous exudate and leucocyte infiltration. This gives the skin inflammatory characteristics comparable to that of a second-degree burn. Moist desquamation is a transient reaction caused by depletion of clonogenic epidermal stem cells and may heal within 2 weeks by proliferation of the surviving cells or by the migration of epidermal cells from the adjacent healthy tissues. Moist desquamation is histologically characterized by eroded epidermis and leucocyte infiltration. Inflammatory reaction may subside by week 5–7. Third-degree radiation dermatitis refers to severe moist desquamation with denuded dermis and intense hyperaemia and oedema of deep tissues, possibly with secondary infection.

Repopulation of the epidermis, following irradiation with doses at the approximate threshold for moist desquamation,

is predominantly by the proliferation of surviving clonogenic basal cells from within the irradiated area. Cell colonies could easily be recognized in histological sections at 21 days after single doses of 15 Gy and 20 Gy, in a pig model. This was prior to the peak of the skin reaction. The labelling index of cells in colonies after the injection of [^{3}H] thymidine was between 30% and 40%. A high proportion of regenerating colonies has been found to be associated with the canal of hair follicles. The rapid rate of healing of moist desquamation after thulium-170 as compared with strontium-90 (maximum energy = 2.27 MeV) irradiation, for doses producing the same incidence of moist desquamation, has been attributed to the greater survival of clonogenic cells within the canals of hair follicles after thulium-170 irradiation. Beta rays from thulium-170 (maximum energy = 0.97 MeV) are less penetrating than relatively high energy beta rays from

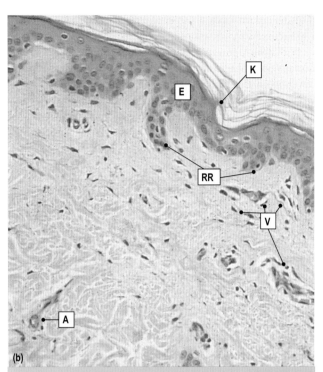

Figure 3.2.3.   (b) Thin skin. Micrograph showing the thin epidermal (E) and keratin (K) layers of thin skin, which is also characterized by a poorly developed rete ridge system (RR), small numbers of hair follicles, and variable numbers of eccrine glands, venules (V) and arterioles (A). (Parts (a) and (b) reproduced with permission from Biophoto Associates.)

strontium-90 (maximum energy = 2.27 MeV). If there are sufficient surviving cells within the irradiated area then moist desquamation will heal quickly without any secondary structural damage to the dermis.

While the severity of moist desquamation is dose dependent the timing of the occurrence of moist desquamation is defined by the total turnover time of the epidermal structure exposed and is not influenced by radiation dose. Earlier denudation of the epithelium, i.e. shorter than the normal turnover time, can only occur if basal cells and more specifically post-mitotic suprabasal cells are killed directly by irradiation, usually after very high-dose exposures. High-dose localized irradiation of the epidermis, without comparable effects on deeper dermal layers, can only occur as a result of exposure to low energy β-emitters or to α-particles. In this situation the primary energy absorption will be in the viable layers of the epidermis above the basal layer. Exposure of the skin to β-emitting isotopes such as ^{147}Pm or ^{60}Co results in highly non-uniform irradiation with respect to the variation in doses with depth in tissue. There may be an ~80% reduction in dose across the epidermis. Cells in the post-mitotic, but

viable, upper layer of the epidermis will receive a significantly higher dose than stem cells in the basal layer and within the shaft of hair follicles. Histological investigations in pig skin after ^{147}Pm exposure have shown that the very early but very transient epithelial response that is produced is related to the interphase death of suprabasal cells; this initiates an inflammatory reaction with the subsequent disruption of all cell layers in the epidermis.

If a substantial dose of radiation is received by dermal vasculature another phase of erythema might appear at around 8–9 weeks after irradiation. Unlike the early erythema, this late erythema usually has a bluish appearance and suggests damage to dermal vascular plexus. This brings about a state of ischaemia and a necrotic skin lesion develops at a relatively later time of 9–16 weeks after irradiation. Dermal necrosis may develop as a late lesion even without an acute dermatitis. This is usually preceded by a dusky or mauve coloration of the skin. At this stage focal occlusions might be found in arterioles, particularly those in the deep dermal plexus, and necrosis would appear to develop as a result of vascular insufficiency. The rate of healing will depend on the surface area of the original skin site involved and the depth of necrosis. The depth of necrosis depends to a large extent on the radiation dose and radiation quality. Necrosis may take several months to heal and be replaced by a large block of scar tissue.

Additional factors, such as infection, may exacerbate the extent of the lesion. If the radiation field is small and the exposure is localized, necrotic cells will shed off and the tissue will possibly heal with scar tissue. In subcutis, normal adipose tissue might be replaced by collagen. The number of fibroblasts is usually reduced but the surviving fibroblasts are prominent and some are atypical. Atypical fibroblasts are not specific to irradiated tissues as they can be found in unirradiated human tissues, e.g. pressure ulcers. Necrosis of large fields will leave an open wound, prone to infection.

Beyond one year the skin acquires characteristics of late radiation damage that manifest as dyspigmentation, atrophy, fibrosis and telangiectasia (dilation of a group of small blood vessels). Dyspigmentation, which can be in the form of hypo- or hyperpigmentation, is usually observed within the first 2 years. Impairment of lymphatics develops usually in a biphasic manner and telangiectasia can manifest as late as 10 years after irradiation.

For skin sites that do not develop ischaemic dermal necrosis after irradiation, dermal thinning may be a late consequence. Serial measurements of changes in skin thickness in a pig model, using an A-scan ultrasound technique, have indicated that the thinning of dermal tissue developed in two distinct phases after single doses of both X- and β-rays. The first phase of reduction in dermal thickness developed between 14 and 20 weeks after irradiation, the second phase after 52 weeks. The mean reduction in dermal thickness in the period 20–51 weeks and 76–129 weeks after irradiation was dose related after both ^{90}Sr/^{90}Y and ^{170}Tm irradiation.

However, based on skin surface doses in this model the magnitude of the response was less after irradiation with the lower energy ^{170}Tm source. When radiation dose was expressed in terms of the dose at 900 μm depth, the mid-dermal depth, comparable results were obtained for both radiation energies. This implied a possible target depth for the development of skin thinning.

RADIATION-INDUCED CNS DAMAGE

The central nervous system (CNS) is an important dose-limiting factor in radiotherapy of cancer. Approximately one-third of all cancers in childhood are leukaemias, of which 80% are acute lymphoblastic leukaemia (ALL) that require the irradiation of CNS. Brain and spinal tumours account for 24% of cases. Overall, the central nervous system is involved in more than half of childhood cancers. Prior to 1970, children diagnosed with acute lymphoblastic leukaemia (ALL) had a life expectancy of less than 1 year. Death often resulted, not from the original disease of the blood, but from progression of the disease within the central nervous system. Administration of cranial irradiation, in conjunction with intrathecal methotrexate, has dramatically improved the life expectancy of these children. A majority of children, ~70%, survive ALL but there has been an increasing awareness in recent years of neurological deficits, with particular reference to memory and learning deficits, as a result of treatment in a considerable number of these patients. The treatment of ALL involves irradiation of the entire craniospinal axis with 24 or 18 Gy (in 4-weekly fractions) radiation in addition to intrathecal chemotherapy and steroids. Some investigators attribute cognitive deficits primarily to cranial irradiation while others consider intrathecal methotrexate equally neurotoxic. A study of the cognitive and educational performance of 150 cancer patients 7–16 years of age has demonstrated that children receiving chemotherapy alone performed similarly to controls, while children treated with cranial irradiation and chemotherapy performed more poorly compared with non-irradiated patients. It appears that cranial irradiation has been responsible for the decline in intellect, particularly memory and learning deficits. This deficit appears to be more prominent in younger (<7 years) patients.

Although some reports indicate a higher tolerance in adults some studies suggest that cranial irradiation-induced intellectual deficit, memory loss and dementia also occur frequently in adults. Radiation-induced dementia can be as high as 20–50% in long-term surviving brain tumour patients who received cranial irradiation after the age of 50.

Obviously with the development of more effective treatments and the resultant prolonged survival of ALL patients and application of radiotherapy in the treatment of arteriovenous malformations (AVMs), epilepsy and other non-malignant

disorders of the CNS, late complications of cranial irradiation will become a more common problem.

Radiation damage to CNS, as a consequence of radiotherapy, is progressive and, based on its time of expression, develops in three different phases: acute, early delayed and late delayed. Transient symptoms usually develop relatively early after irradiation, but permanent and often disabling nervous damage may develop, progressively, within months to years after radiotherapy.

Radiation-induced encephalopathy

Acute radiation-induced encephalopathy is expressed within days to weeks after irradiation and it is associated with headache, somnolence, nausea and vomiting. It develops mainly due to an increase in intracranial pressure and usually responds to corticosteroid therapy. Acute encephalopathy is fairly uncommon under current radiotherapy protocols.

Early-delayed encephalopathy occurs 2–4 months after radiotherapy and in children who receive prophylactic whole-brain irradiation for leukaemia this phase is associated with somnolence syndrome, which improves spontaneously over days to weeks.

Late-delayed radiation encephalopathy develops within months to years after irradiation of brain either prophylactically for leukaemia in children or treatment of brain tumours in adults. It is usually irreversible, progressive, with no effective treatment available at present and have been causally associated with the mortality of radiation-induced CNS injury.

Radiation-induced myelopathies

Myelopathies induced by irradiation of human spinal cord are subdivided into acute transient radiation myelopathy (ATRM) and delayed radiation myelopathies. Transient radiation myelopathy is characterized by paraesthesia and electric-like shocks that radiate down the spine to the extremities often brought on by flexion of the neck (Lhermitte's sign). It presents usually between a few weeks and a few months after irradiation of the spinal cord with a median latency period of 4 months and average duration of 5.3 months. The mechanism of ATRM is not well understood but it is suggested that it may result from transient demyelination in the posterior column and lateral spinal tracts within the radiation field. However, since it is reversible it is likely that lesions other than demyelination may mediate this myelopathy. Changes in the capillary permeability of irradiated spinal cord have been reported.

Delayed myelopathies are less common but more severe. They present with a history of progressive neurological signs and symptoms such as paraesthesia, decreased pain and temperature sensation, changes in gait, difficulty in walking, hemiparesis, various degrees of incontinence and eventually paraplegia. Babinski signs are common. Lhermitte's sign is rare in delayed radiation myelopathy but it is suggested that this syndrome accompanies this type of myelopathy more often than is appreciated. The first signs such as unilateral sensory deficit and clumsiness are hardly noticed by the patient. The patient might complain when the signs and symptoms have intensified. Generally, the various signs and symptoms of radiation myelopathy can occur in almost any combination, depending on the site and severity of the lesion.

Delayed radiation myelopathy is considered to be irreversible and even partial recovery is exceptional. The probability of dying of radiation myelopathy is approximately 25% at 18 months for thoracic cord injuries and 55% for cervical cord injuries. Latency period of delayed radiation myelopathy ranges from 4 months to 4 years. A bimodal frequency distribution for latency periods with modes at 52 and 120 weeks after radiotherapy has been reported. In severe cases of long survival, atrophy of the irradiated part of the spinal cord might be recognized radiologically by myelography. Cerebrospinal fluid pressure is usually normal. Mild elevation in cerebrospinal protein concentration may be observed and spinal conduction might be impaired. A dose-dependent latency period has been observed for the development of radiation myelopathy in animal models and humans. The higher the radiation dose the shorter the time till development of myelopathy.

Histopathology of radiation-induced CNS injury

The response of both brain and spinal cord to irradiation has been extensively studied and documented. The histological appearance of radiation-induced CNS damage is nonspecific and changes are seen in all tissue elements but the lesions are prominent in the white matter. Loss of myelin (demyelination) from individual nerve fibres or a group of nerve fibres (spongiosis) and complete loss of demyelinated axons (malacia) are consistent and dominant morphological features of radiation myelopathy. Delayed radiation-induced lesions in brain develop from several months to many years after exposure and while all regions of brain can be affected damage tends to be more prominent in the white matter. Histologically, white matter lesions are characterized by frank necrosis and vascular changes. Single doses of about 20 Gy of X-rays have been found to produce predominantly vascular lesions after a latent period of about 12 months in rats. With higher single doses, damage was more pronounced in white matter and the latency for the development of such lesions was significantly shorter than 12 months. The fimbria, internal capsule and corpus callosum are especially vulnerable to delayed radiation-induced injury and these sites exhibit both dose- and time-related progression to necrosis. A single dose of 25 Gy induces necrosis of white matter in all

three of these areas (fimbria, corpus callosum and internal capsule). The fimbria-fornix appears to be more responsive to radiation than other major myelinated bundles. For example in the rat, necrosis of the fimbria-fornix occurs with a latency of 36 weeks after a single dose of 25 Gy, whereas the latency for the necrosis of internal capsule and the corpus callosum is 47 and 49 weeks, respectively. Necrotic areas are devoid of cells and blood vessels, showing only marks of pre-existing structures with myelinated fibres around the area of necrosis. Grossly dilated blood vessels may be present in the vicinity of the necrotic areas. In a rat model of radiation-induced CNS injury white matter necrosis was seen in the fimbria-fornix in 78% of the irradiated animals, whereas lesions of the corpus callosum were seen in 33% and of the internal capsule in only 11% of the irradiated brains at 41 weeks. At 46 weeks after irradiation all of the animals showed marked necrosis in both the fimbria and corpus callosum but degeneration of internal capsule remained at 10%. In contrast to this substantial necrosis following 25 Gy, animals irradiated with 20 Gy and killed 46 weeks later showed no evidence of demyelinating lesions.

Progressive vascular lesions are characterized by varying degrees of endothelial swelling in small arteries and arterioles, endothelial proliferation, adventitial fibrosis and occlusion of the blood vessels. Vasculopathies associated with radiation myelopathy occur in both arteries and veins but monkeys with radiation myelopathy symptoms have consistently shown lesions in the lateral corticospinal motor tract, which is an area affected by venous lesions. This zone of blood supply is considered the most vulnerable site to ischaemia. White matter necrosis in the dorsal column and the adjacent dorsal horns of the spinal cords of rats has been reported. In the spinal cords of cats irradiated with X-rays, small infarcts in the white matter of the irradiated areas of the spinal cord accompanied neural death and oedema of the grey matter close to the central canal. Ultrastructurally, the infarcts were shown to stem from necrosis and thrombosis of small blood vessels. A biphasic change in the capillary permeability of irradiated rat spinal cord has been reported. The first increment was observed at 30 days and the second increment was after 60 days after irradiation that was progressive even after animals became paraplegic. After a transient peak of early changes in capillary permeability of the irradiated rat spinal cord, there was progressive damage to the endothelium that might play a primary role in delayed radiation myelopathies. On the basis of the data from irradiation of the spinal cords one can conclude that less severe lesions such as focal fibre loss and scattered white matter vacuolation are not usually associated with neurological signs. However, the three most severe lesions, white matter necrosis, massive haemorrhage and segmental parenchymal atrophy, have been consistently associated with abnormal neurological signs. Radiation-induced vascular damage has been considered as to the most likely cause of these three lesions. Microglia and astrocytes have been considered as target cells for the development of radiation myelopathy. On the other hand, the role of vasculature has been extensively emphasized in the development of radiation-induced CNS injury.

Despite substantial data on histological development of radiation-induced CNS injury, classical radiobiology has failed to identify a target cell responsible for the development of this lesion. There is still controversy over whether the endothelium or the parenchyma is the prime target for radiation damage. This has divided the investigators into two groups. Those who support the *glial hypothesis* view the parenchyma, and more specifically the oligodendrocytes, the cells responsible for myelination in the CNS, as a prime target. This group considers the lesion to be a consequence of a direct effect on parenchymal cells. The glial hypothesis gained strength with the identification of the *oligodendrocyte type-2 astrocyte (O-2A)* progenitor cells and the reports that irradiation resulted in loss of reproductive capacity of the O-2A progenitor cells. However, depletion of glial cells has been detected in the brain of both animals and humans after relatively low radiation doses which are not usually associated with the late necrosis. The other school of thought, those who support the *vascular hypothesis*, considers the endothelium as the critical target and views radiation myelopathy as a lesion mediated by vascular damage. The end lesion, radiation-induced malacia, is considered as an ischaemic phenomenon secondary to the impaired blood supply to the nervous tissue. However, radiation-induced necrosis has also been reported in the absence of vascular changes. This argues against the absolute dependence of white matter necrosis on vascular damage.

The tolerance dose for the adult human brain, based on an iso-effect analysis of brain necrosis, is established as a total dose of 52 Gy given in conventional 2 Gy fractions, 5 daily fractions per week. The estimated rate of brain necrosis at that dose level is 0.04–0.4%. Assuming an α/β ratio of 2 Gy, this fractionated dose will be equivalent to ~13.4 Gy single dose. However, an immediate increase in electroencephalogram activity, with spontaneous spike discharges, has been observed in the hippocampus and cortex of cats after irradiation with doses as low as 2 Gy.

The molecular hypothesis on the development of radiation-induced CNS injury suggests that the cellular response to radiation is cytokine derived. According to this hypothesis molecular changes are part of a well-coordinated healing process and radiation-induced symptoms of CNS damage might result not only from direct cell loss but from several mechanisms such as the side effects of the healing process or a failure to restore homeostasis. Involvement of pro-inflammatory cytokines such as TNF-α, IL-1α and IL-1β and their receptors has been indicated. TNF-α expression has been indicated in both acute and late radiation-induced brain damage.

A recent hypothesis views the cellular interactions as an important factor in the development of radiation-induced CNS injury. This hypothesis indicates the contribution of a persistent oxidative stress in addition to direct cell death and molecular changes. This hypothesis views the latent period, the time preceding the clinical manifestation of damage, as an active phase where cytokines and growth factors play important roles in inter- and intracellular communication.

RADIATION DAMAGE TO PERIPHERAL NERVES

The incidence of peripheral neuropathy is directly associated with total radiation dose and fraction size. The use of a large fraction size increases the risk of neuropathy and with conventional 2 Gy fraction radiotherapy the risk of neuropathy increases with total doses in excess of 60 Gy. The latency period can be within 5–30 months after treatment. However, some animal studies have shown peripheral neuropathies clustered around 6–18 months after intraoperative radiotherapy. Peripheral neuropathy is considered irreversible although recovery has been reported in some cases. Radiation-induced peripheral neuropathy has been rarely reported as a complication of conventional radiotherapy. However, it is one of the important limiting factors in intraoperative radiation therapy. In particular, when intraoperative radiotherapy is used on the abdomen, pelvis and retroperitoneal region, peripheral nerves are frequently irradiated beyond the tolerance dose. Peripheral neuropathy as high as 32% has been reported in the management of primary or recurrent pelvic tumours by intraoperative radiotherapy.

Animal studies have shown enzyme changes, abnormal microtubule formation, bioelectrical dysfunction and altered vascular permeability, within 2 days of irradiation of nerves. Single doses of 15 Gy result in a loss of predominantly large myelinated fibres (as much as 50% reduction in axons and myelin). Fibrosis occurs in the endoneurium, but not the perineurium, and it is the fibrosis which is believed to cause nerve entrapment with secondary demyelination. Loss of axons and demyelination with increased levels of endoneurial, perineurial and epineurial connective tissue have been reported at later times of 2 years after intraoperative radiotherapy. This was associated with necrosis, thrombosis of small vessels and areas of haemorrhage and telangiectasia around nerve fibres after higher radiation doses. These findings have been confirmed at a cellular level in neurons of patients treated for breast cancer. Altered neural dynamics is known to create secondary problems such as pain referral and altered muscle function. Most studies report injury to the vessels supplying the nerve, which has the potential to create an ischaemic environment further altering neural dynamics. It has been suggested that surgical release of nerve from fibrotic surroundings may help selective patients since separation from surrounding tissues might prevent demyelination and vessel damage.

Peripheral neuropathy, while relatively low, is still a recognized clinical entity. However, long-term follow-up studies need to be carried out to confirm and quantify the extent of neural damage and the effects on functional activities and quality of life.

RADIATION-INDUCED VASCULOPATHIES

The controversy involving the issue of whether the parenchymal or the vascular tissue is the prime target for radiation damage is not unique to the CNS. This controversy exists in the study of the effects of ionizing radiation on almost every kind of tissue. It must be borne in mind that radiation is an indiscriminate agent that hits every component of the target tissue. It is equally likely to hit both the parenchymal and vascular components of the irradiated tissues. Damage to any tissue component initiates a series of changes leading to an organ-specific radiation lesion. Therefore, there is always an element of parenchymal damage which is augmented by vascular damage. However, the extent of the contribution of different components of tissue in the development of late radiation damage is not fully understood. The degree of importance of each tissue component is determined by the radiosensitivity of that tissue component and its role in preserving the functional integrity of the irradiated tissue. Blood capillaries and sinusoids are the most radiosensitive components of vascular tissue. This reflects the radiosensitivity of endothelial cells, which constitute a major proportion of the capillary wall.

Manifestation of the effects of irradiation on endothelium varies with time after irradiation and the size of blood vessel. An increased cell permeability after irradiation of endothelial cells and before cell death, irregularity of endothelial cytoplasm, formation of pseudopodia, detachment of endothelium from basal lamina, rupture of plasma membrane, rupture of capillary wall, and loss of entire capillary segment have been observed after irradiation of different tissues.

Reduction in the number of endothelial cells lining the walls of the blood vessels has been observed after irradiation of mouse mesentery, pig skin and choroid plexus of the rat brain. Loss of endothelium results in a reduction of the microvascular network. Dilatation is very common in the remaining microvasculature and when superficially located it can be clinically detected as telangiectasia of skin or mucous membrane. Also, irradiation enhances the proliferation of endothelial cells. Therefore, after irradiation a few reproductively viable surviving cells would proliferate in response to cell loss and produce large clones of cells and develop areas where the vasculature diameter is reduced. This phenomenon together with reduction of the microvascular network eventually brings about a state of ischaemia in irradiated tissue and subsequent ischaemic necrosis. This structural damage to the vasculature and loss of functional capability of endothelial cells might initiate the development of arteriosclerosis, as it has been shown that radiation increases the risk of the development of arteriosclerosis.

Endothelium is no longer considered a non-adherent inner lining of the blood vessels which acts as a passive barrier between blood and parenchyma. The endothelial cell is involved in various physiological functions that may include:

- angiogenesis, coagulation
- inflammation and immune response
- synthesis of stromal components and
- vascular tone regulation.

In addition, endothelial cells play an important role in determining the distribution of circulating leucocytes, their adhesion to injured blood vessel wall and modulation of acute inflammation.

Normal blood vessels are leakage proof and non-adherent to blood cell elements. The endothelial monolayer lining the inner surface of the blood vessels and the heart acts as a non-adherent protective surface which controls the transport of various substances from or into the bloodstream. Platelet–endothelium interaction consists of rolling of platelets in the bloodstream and along the vascular wall. Only under certain, inflammatory, conditions platelets adhere to endothelial cells. An important component of the inflammatory response is the localization of leucocytes at the sites of inflammatory lesions (see Ch. 1). Adhesion molecules present on the surface of the endothelial cells and leucocytes play a major role in endothelium–leucocyte interactions. Before polymorphonuclear leucocytes are attracted to the endothelium, they must first adhere to the vascular endothelium. In vitro studies have demonstrated the neutrophil-recruiting capacity of the endothelial cells and suggested them as the initiators and modulators of the inflammatory response. Increased adhesion of human granulocytes to the surface of endothelial cells after irradiation has been shown and a dose-dependent release of chemotactic agents for human neutrophils by irradiated endothelial cells has been reported (Fig. 3.2.4). Inflammatory cytokines induce a number of adhesion molecules which bind endothelium to leucocytes and lymphocytes. The nature of molecules such as endothelial leucocyte adhesion molecule-1 (ELAM-1), intercellular adhesion molecule-1 (ICAM-1) and vascular cell adhesion molecule-1 (VCAM-1) and their role in intercellular interactions is becoming clear and it appears that we are beginning to unravel the structure of various adhesion molecules and their role in the process of vessel occlusion. Nowadays we understand that platelets, either stimulated or unstimulated, do not adhere to intact endothelial cells but to injured endothelial cells, denuded basal lamina or to the stroma surrounding a ruptured basal lamina. This process was observed as early as 1857 by Ernst Brucke, who stated that 'In sound and living vessels the blood remains fluid, but it coagulates in dead ones'.

Endothelial cells synthesize many active substances including prostacyclin (PGI_2) and prostaglandin E_2 (PGE_2). PGI_2 is a potent vasodilator and inhibitor of platelet adhesion and participates in the regulation of platelet–blood vessel wall interactions (Fig. 3.2.5). It is able to depress the enhanced mitotic activity induced by irradiation. Its balancing action on thromboxane A_2 (TXA_2), a promoter of platelet aggregation and vasoconstrictor produced by platelets, regulates haemostasis and the formation of intra-arterial plugs. Irradiation causes an initial increase in prostacyclin production followed by a long-term reduction. The initial increase in PGI_2 production is counterbalanced by a temporary increase in TXA_2 formation. Then TXA_2 formation returns to normal and appears to be unaffected but PGI_2 formation stays suppressed for a long time. This suppressed production of PGI_2 might be responsible for thrombotic and degenerative lesions induced by irradiation.

RADIATION DAMAGE TO SKELETAL MUSCLE

Muscle is a relatively radioresistant tissue in human body. However, damage to muscular tissue which can impair the normal movement contributes significantly to the quality of life of cancer patients. This in turn necessitates thorough physical medicine and rehabilitation programmes during and post-treatment, as these could reduce late complications in patients receiving soft tissue irradiation. An understanding of the physiopathology, histological and molecular development of muscle damage is crucial to the development of such rehabilitation programmes.

The incidence of muscle complications (atrophy, weakness) is as high as 58% in breast cancer patients, between 77% and 100% for muscles of the pelvis in prostate cancer, and moderate to severe muscle weakness occurs in 20% of patients with soft tissue sarcomas of the limbs. The extent of muscle damage is both dose dependent and related to the time since irradiation. Clinical observations support the finding that symptoms of muscle dysfunction can remain for years after cessation of radiation therapy.

MRI scans have allowed some detailed macroscopic studies of damage to tissues in men irradiated for prostate cancer and men and women irradiated for musculoskeletal sarcomas. Observed changes to muscle include the presence of

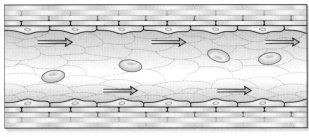

(a)

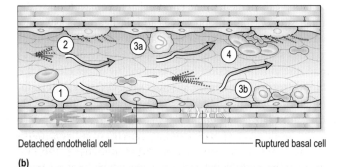

Detached endothelial cell ———————   ——————— Ruptured basal cell

(b)

Figure 3.2.4.   Radiation-induced endothelial inflammation. 1, Damaged endothelial cell and basal lamina. 2, Release of cytokines and chemotactic agents from damaged endothelial cells. 3a and 3b, Cytokines induce adhesion of leucocytes and lymphocytes to endothelial cells. 4, Adherence of platelets to damaged endothelial cells, creating plaque formation.

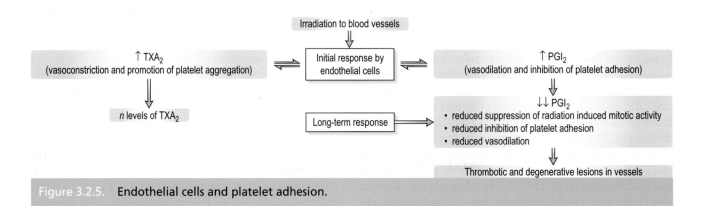

Figure 3.2.5.   Endothelial cells and platelet adhesion.

Reported incidence of shoulder dysfunction following treatment for breast cancer varies from 17% to 85%. There is evidence to suggest that those undergoing both surgery and radiotherapy demonstrate an increased effect, and that the severity of shoulder dysfunction appears to vary over time. A few studies have highlighted, but not quantified, winging of the scapula, weakness in serratus anterior, pectoralis major and latissimus dorsi. If in fact there is reduced shoulder movement due to thickening of connective tissue, constricted and/or shortened muscles that lie in the path of surgery and/or radiation, the resultant effect could be altered biomechanics of the entire shoulder complex, particularly the scapula. The effect of a muscle imbalance on the functioning of the shoulder complex has been a topic of many recent studies. Altered shoulder biomechanics is thought to result in scapular substitution patterns.

oedema in intramuscular septae for longer periods than in fat or muscle, and decreases in muscle size.

Histological changes

Histological studies of muscle changes are mainly in animal models and have seldom gone beyond the first year after irradiation. In rats focal areas of increased collagen content, death of myocytes, muscle degeneration and vacuolization associated with a loss of capillaries, were found 2–4 months after a single dose of 20 Gy. Irradiated gastrocnemius muscles of rats with 80 Gy in 40 fractions of 2 Gy resulted in progressive changes beginning from day 1 after final exposure and still seen at 12 months of assessment. Morphological changes were characterized by haemorrhage, lymphocyte infiltration, vascular damage and increased collagen content. Significant changes were seen in the number, size and structure of mitochondria as late as 12 months after final exposure. No muscle recovery was seen in 12 months. Early changes (3–10 months) from large single doses in various species of animals result in muscle necrosis, atrophy and fibrosis accompanied by vessel lesions as discussed above. Later progressive changes to muscle are thought to occur as a result of vascular lesions resulting in ischaemia. However, the precise nature of these changes to total muscle size, sarcomere structure and function following radiation therapy are currently unknown.

Molecular changes

Increased amino acid release, suggesting protein breakdown, has been reported in rats immediately after irradiation. The later fibrotic phase is usually associated with an increase in type III collagen and an increase in production of sulphated glycosaminoglycans (GAGs) for up to 7 months after irradiation.

Recently, molecular research into the fibrotic changes associated with muscle tissue damage from radiation therapy has focused on the role of transforming growth factor (TGF-β1) and β-Actin. A twofold to fourfold increase in TGF-β1 expression was found within 3 weeks after 35 Gy and up to 1 year later. TGF-β1 was localized to all the cells involved in the fibrotic process in muscle (myofibroblasts, mononuclear inflammatory cells and endothelial cells). For most cell systems TGF-β1 produced by irradiated cells acts to inhibit cell proliferation. The regulation and expression of TGF-β1 in fibroblast populations is the subject of ongoing research. Less is known about its expression and effect in muscle cells following irradiation. However, the increased production of TGF-β1 may act via other mechanisms (Fig. 3.2.6). Muscle differentiation is controlled by four regulatory genes: *Myf5* and *MyoD* in the early stage and *MRF4* and *myogenin* in the late. *Myf5* and *MyoD* are involved in the determination of satelite cells into myocytes, with *MyoD* known to be critical for muscle regeneration. *Myogenin* is involved in differentiation of the myotube and *MRF4* in myotube maturation. Both *MyoD* and *myogenin* have been shown to be inhibited by TGF-β, thereby decreasing the cells' ability for differentiation and regeneration.

GENERAL CONSIDERATIONS

According to accepted concepts of cellular radiobiology, based on target theory for single cells, it is assumed that radiation kills cells at random and the dose of radiation and the radiosensitivity of irradiated cells determine the probability of cell kill. This concept was extended to tissues by viewing normal tissue radiation injury as a result of the sterilization of clonogenic cells within that tissue. According to this concept, tissue-specific function is restricted to functional non-proliferative cells derived from clonogenic cells. Failure of clonogenic stem cells to replace the functional cells, which continue to be lost at a normal rate, results in a gradual depletion of functional cells. When the number of functional cells gets to a critical level, the tissue cannot sustain its function and radiation-induced injury is expressed. This reductionist view is no longer tenable. Radiation indiscriminately affects every component of the irradiated tissue. It is

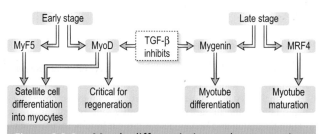

Figure 3.2.6.   Muscle differentiation and regeneration.

naive to assume that while a sole component of the irradiated tissue is suffering radiation damage the other components are passive bystanders. Tissues are complex integrated systems and their function relies on their integrity. Radiation injury to normal tissues should be seen as a dynamic, multifaceted process that develops from interactions between different tissue components. It has been shown that priming rats with 7 Gy partial body irradiation renders their foot skin more radioresistant. This indicates that development of radiation lesions is not simply determined by the reduction of target cells.

The latent period, the time prior to the clinical manifestation of damage, should be viewed as an active phase where biochemical processes such as persistent oxidative stress and molecular components such as cytokines and growth factors play important roles in inter- and intracellular interactions. This new paradigm offers an exciting new approach to radiation-induced normal tissue morbidity, i.e. the possibility that radiation injury can be modulated by the application of therapies directed at altering steps in the cascade of events leading to the clinical expression of injury. Since such a cascade of events does not occur in tumours, where direct clonogenic cell kill predominates, these treatments should not negatively impact anti-tumour efficacy. Thus, targeting potential mediators and/or pathways involved in the cascade of events leading to expression of radiation-induced injuries might alter the severity or the incidence of normal tissue reactions to irradiation. Although the exact identity of the specific biological mediators involved in the development of radiation-induced normal tissue injury remains unknown, application of a number of modalities has successfully modified these lesions. These include treatment with diverse modalities such as vasoactive drugs, intervention with oxidative stress, growth factors and stem cell transplantation.

Furthermore, the function of organs should be seen as an integrated function of component tissues; therefore, in physical medicine directed at treating irradiated organs the role of components of that organ and the extent of damage to each component should be taken into account. For example, restriction in movement caused by irradiation should not be seen as a result of damage to muscular fibres but as a combination of damage to the peripheral nerves, vasculature and connective tissue involved.

REFERENCES AND FURTHER READING

Haematopoietic system

Baverstock KF, Ash PJND (1983) A review of radiation accidents involving whole body exposure and the relevance to the LD50/60 for man. Br J Radiol 56: 837–849.

Champlin R (1990) Medical assessment and therapy in bone marrow failure due to radiation accidents. Role of bone marrow transplantation and hematopoietic growth factors. In: Browne D, Weiss JF, Macttie TJ, Pillai MV (eds) Treatment of Radiation Injuries. New York: Plenum Press, pp. 3–6.

Skin

Ackerman AB (1978) Histologic Diagnosis of Inflammatory Skin Diseases. Philadelphia: Lea & Febiger, pp. 201–202.

Hamlet R, Hopewell JW (1988) A quantitative assessment of changes in the dermal fibroblast population of pig skin after single doses of X-rays. Int J Radiat Biol 54: 675–682.

Mortimer PS, Simmonds RH, Rezvani M, et al. (1991) Time-related changes in lymphatic clearance in pig skin after a single dose of 18 Gy of X rays. Br J Radiol 64(768): 1140–1146.

Panizzon RG, Goldschmidt H (1991) Radiation reactions and sequelae. In: Modern Dermatologic Radiation Therapy. New York: Springer-Verlag, pp. 25–36.

Rezvani M (2002) The response of skin to acute, protracted and fractionated irradiation. BJR Special issue 26: 226–232.

Stevens A, Lowe J (1996) Human Histology. St Louis: Mosby.

Nervous system

Anderson V, Smibert E, Ekert H, Godber T (1994) Intellectual, educational, and behavioural sequelae after cranial irradiation and chemotherapy. Arch Dis Child 70: 476–483.

Asai A, Matsutani M, Kohno T, et al. (1989) Subacute brain atrophy after radiation therapy for malignant brain tumor. Cancer 63: 1962–1974.

Blakemore WF, Palmer AC (1982) Delayed infarction of spinal cord white matter following x-irradiation. J Pathol 137: 273–280.

Burns RT, Jones AN, Robertson JS (1972) Pathology of radiation myelopathy. J Neurol Neurosurg Psychiatry 35: 888–898.

Calvo W, Hopewell JW, Reinhold HS, van den Berg AP, Yeung TK (1987) Dose-dependent and time-dependent changes in the choroid plexus of the irradiated rat brain. Br J Radiol 60: 1109–1117.

Calvo W, Hopewell JW, Reinhold HS, Yeung TK (1988) Time- and dose-related changes in the white matter of the rat brain after single doses of X-rays. Br J Radiol 61: 1043–1052.

Chiang C-S, Hong J-H, Stalder A, et al. (1997) Delayed molecular responses to brain irradiation. Int J Radiat Biol 72(1): 45–53.

Conomy JP, Kellermeyer RW (1975) Delayed cerebrovascular consequences of therapeutic radiation. Cancer 36: 1702–1708.

Daigle JL, Chiang C-S, McBride WH (2001) Radiation-induced gene expression in brain. Jpn J Cancer Clin 47(1): 26–30.

DeAngelis LM, Delattre J-Y, Posner JB (1989) Radiation-induced dementia in patients cured of brain metastases. Neurology 39: 789–796.

Delattre JY, Rosenblum MK, Thaler HT, et al. (1988) A model of radiation myelopathy in the rat pathology, regional capillary permeability changes and treatment with dexamethasone. Brain 111: 1319–1336.

Dorfman LJ, Donaldson SS, Gupta PR, Bosley TM (1982) Electrophysiologic evidence of subclinical injury to the posterior columns of the human spinal cord after therapeutic radiation. Cancer 50: 2815–2819.

Dowell RE, Copeland DR, Francis DJ, Fletcher JM, Stovall M (1991) Absence of synergistic effects of CNS treatments on neuropsychologic test performance among children. J Clin Oncol 9: 1029–1036.

Dynes JB (1960) Radiation myelopathy. Trans Am Neurol Assoc 85: 51–55.

Eiser C (1991) Cognitive deficits in children treated for leukaemia. Arch Dis Child 66: 164–168.

Fike JR, Cann CE, Turowski K, et al. (1988) Radiation dose response of normal brain. Int J Radiat Oncol Biol Phys 14: 63–70.

Fogarty K, Volonino V, Caul J (1988) Learning disabilities following CNS irradiation. Clin Pediatr 27: 524–528.

Friedman WA, Bova FJ (1992) Linear accelerator radiosurgery for arteriovenous malformations. J Neurosurg 77: 8332–8841.

Glosser G, McManus P, Munzenrider J, et al. (1997) Neuropsychological function in adults after high dose fractionated radiation therapy of skull base tumors, Int J Radiat Oncol Biol Phys 38: 231–239.

Hochberg FH, Slotnick B (1980) Neuropsychological impairment in astrocytoma survivors. Neurology 30: 172–177.

Hodges H, Katzung N, Sowinski P, et al. (1998) Late behavioural and neuropathological effects of local brain irradiation in the rat. Behav Brain Res 91: 99–114.

Hong JH, Chiang CS, Campbell IL, et al. (1995) Induction of acute phase gene expression by brain irradiation. Int J Radiat Oncol Biol Phys 33: 619–626.

Jannoun L (1983) Are cognitive and educational development affected by age at which prophylactic therapy is given in acute lymphoblastic leukaemia? Arch Dis Child 58: 953–958.

Kamiryo T, Kassell NF, Thai Q-A, et al. (1996) Histological changes in the normal rat brain after gamma irradiation. Acta Neurochir 138: 451–459.

Maire JP, Coudin B, Guerin J, Coudry M (1987) Neuropsychologic impairment in adults with brain tumors. Am J Clin Oncol 10: 156–162.

Mastaglia FL, McDonald WI, Watson JV, Yogendran K (1976) Effects of x-radiation on the spinal cord: An experimental study of the morphological changes in central nerve fibres. Brain 99: 101–122.

Mulhern RK, Wasserman AL, Fairclough D, Ochs J (1988) Memory function in disease-free survivors of childhood acute lymphocytic leukemia given CNS prophylaxis with or without 1,800 cGy cranial irradiation. J Clin Oncol 6: 315–320.

Myers R, Rogers MA, Hornsey S (1986) A reappraisal of the roles of glial and vascular elements in the development of white matter necrosis in irradiated rat spinal cord. Br J Cancer 53 (suppl VII): 221–223.

Powers BE, Beck ER, Gillette EL, Gould DH, LeCouter RA (1992) Pathology of radiation injury to the canine spinal cord. Int J Radiat Oncol Biol Phys 23: 539–549.

Raff M, Miller R, Noble M (1983) A glial progenitor cell that develops in vitro into an astrocyte or an oligodendrocyte depending on culture medium. Nature 303: 390–396.

Regis J, Bartolomei F, Metellus P, et al. (1999) Radiosurgery for trigeminal neuralgia and epilepsy. Neurosurg Clin N Am 10: 359–377.

Schultheiss TE, Stephens LC (1992) Invited review: Permanent radiation myelopathy. Br J Radiol 65: 737–753.

Schultheiss TE, Higgins EM, El-Mahdi AM (1984) The latent period in clinical radiation myelopathy. Int J Radiat Oncol Biol Phys 10: 1109–1115.

Schultheiss TE, Stephens LC, Peters LJ (1986) Survival in radiation myelopathy. Int J Radiat Oncol Biol Phys 12: 1765–1769.

Schultheiss TE, Stephens LC, Maor MH (1988) Analysis of the histopathology of radiation myelopathy. Int J Radiat Oncol Biol Phys 14: 27–32.

Sheline GE, Wera WM, Smith V (1980) Therapeutic irradiation and brain injury. Int J Radiat Oncol Biol Phys 6: 1215–1218.

Tofilon PJ, Fike JR (2000) The radioresponse of the central nervous system: A dynamic process. Radiat Res 153: 357–370.

van der Kogel AJ (1991) Central nervous system injury in small animal models. In: Gutin RH, Leibel SA, Sheline GE (eds), Radiation Injury to the Nervous System. New York: Raven Press, pp. 91–111.

van der Maazen RWM, Verhagen I, Kleiboer BJ, van der Kogel AJ (1991) Radiosensitivity of glial progenitor cells of the perinatal and adult rat optic nerve studied in an in vitro clonogenic assay. Radiother Oncol 20: 258–264.

Vasculature

Archambeau JO, Ines A, Fajardo LS (1984) Response of swine skin microvasculature to acute single exposures of x rays: Quantification of endothelial changes. Radiat Res 98: 37–51.

Archambeau JO, Ines A, Fajardo LS (1985) Correlation of the dermal microvasculature morphology with the epidermal and the endothelial population changes produced by single x-ray fractions of 1649, 2231 and 2619 rad in swine. Int J Radiat Oncol Biol Phys 11: 1639–1646.

Baillet F, Housset M, Michelson AM, Puget K (1986) Treatment of radiofibrosis with liposomal superoxide dismutase. Preliminary results of 50 cases. Free Radic Res Comms 1: 387–394.

Bloomer WD, Hellman S (1975) Normal tissue response to radiation therapy. N Engl J Med 293: 80–83.

Cliff WJ (1966) The acute inflammatory reaction in the rabbit ear chamber with particular reference to the phenomenon of leukocytic migration. J Exp Med 124: 543–556.

Cotran RS (1987) New roles for the endothelium in inflammation and immunity. Am J Pathol 129: 407–413.

Dunn MM, Drab EA, Rubin DB (1986) Effects of irradiation on endothelial cell–polymorphonuclear leukocyte interactions. J Appl Physiol 60(6): 1932–1937.

Dustin ML, Springer TA (1988) Lymphocyte function-associated antigen-1 (LFA-1) interaction with intercellular adhesion molecule-1 (ICAM-1) is one of at least three mechanisms for lymphocyte adhesion to cultured endothelial cells. J Cell Biol 107: 321–331.

Eldor A, Vladovsky I, Fuks Z, Matzner Y, Rubin DB (1989) Arachidonic metabolism and radiation toxicity in cultures of vascular endothelial cells. Prostaglandins Leukot Essent Fatty Acids 36: 251–258.

Fajardo LF (1989) Special report, the comlexity of endothelial cells. Am J Clin Pathol 92: 241–250.

Hirst DG, Denekamp J, Travis EL (1979) The response of mesenteric blood vessels to irradiation. Radiat Res 77: 259–275.

Lazorthes G (1972) Pathology, classification and clinical aspects of vascular diseases of the spinal cord. In: Vinken PJ, Bruyn GW (eds) Handbook of Clinical Neurology, vol. 12. NHPC, p. 492.

Matzner Y, Cohn M, Hyam E, et al. (1988) Generation of lipid neutrophil chemoattractant by irradiated bovine aortic endothelial cells. J Immunol 140: 2681–2685.

Mercandetti AJ, Lane TA, Colmerauer MEM (1984) Cultured human endothelial cells elaborate neutrophil chemoattractants. J Lab Clin Med 104: 370–380.

Narayan K, Cliff WJ (1982) Morphology of irradiated microvascular: a combined in vivo and electron-microscopic study. Am J Pathol 106: 47–62.

Osborn L, Vassallo C, Benjamin CD (1992) Activated endothelium binds lymphocytes through a novel binding site in the alternately spliced domain of vascular cell adhesion molecule-1. J Exp Med 176: 99–107.

Phillips TL (1966) An ultrastructural study of the development of radiation injury in the lung. Radiology 87: 49–54.

Povlishock JT, Roseblum WI (1987) Injury of brain microvessels with a helium-neon laser and Evans blue can elicit local platelet aggregation without endothelial denudation. Arch Pathol Lab Med 111: 415–421.

Rubin DB, Drab EA, Ward WF (1991) Physiological and biochemical markers of the endothelial cell response to irradiation. Int J Radiat Biol 60: 29–32.

Sinzinger H, Cromwell M, Firbas W (1984) Long-lasting depression of rabbit aortic prostacyclin formation by single-dose irradiation. Radiat Res 97: 533–536.

Muscle

Brosius FC, Waller BF, Roberts WC (1981) Radiation heart disease: analysis of 16 young (aged 15 to 33 years) necroscopy patients who received over 3500 rads to the heart. Am J Med 70: 519–530.

Carmel RJ, Kaplan HS (1976) Mantle irradiation in Hodgkin's disease. An analysis of technique, tumor eradication and complications. Cancer 37: 2813–2825.

Hsu H-Y, Chai C-Y, Lee M-S (1998) Radiation-induced muscle damage in rats after fractionated high-dose irradiation. Radiat Res 149: 482–486.

Powers BE, Gillette EL, McChesney SL, LeCouteur RA, Withrow SJ (1991) Muscle injury following experimental intraoperative irradiation. Int J Radiat Oncol Biol Phys 20: 463–471.

General considerations

Delanian S, Baillet F, Hurat J, et al. (1994) Successful treatment of radiation fibrosis using liposomal Cu/Zn superoxide dismutase: Clinical trial. Radiother Oncol 32: 12–20.

Dörr W, Noack R, Spekl K, Farrell CL (2001) Modification of oral mucositis by keratinocyte growth radiation exposure. Int J Radiat Biol 77: 341–347.

Fajardo LF (1982) Pathology of Radiation Injury. New York: Masson.

Fajardo LF (1989) Morphologic patterns of radiation injury. In: Vaeth JM, Meyer JL (eds) Radiation Tolerance of Normal Tissues. Frontiers of Radiation Therapy and Oncology, vol. 23. Basel: Karger, pp. 75–84.

Hopewell JW, van den Aardweg GJMJ, Morris GM, et al. (1994) Unsaturated lipids as modulators of radiation damage in normal tissues. In: Horrobin DF (ed.) New Approaches to Cancer Therapy: Unsaturated Lipids and Photodynamic Therapy. London: Churchill Communications, pp. 88–106.

Hornsey S, Myers R, Jenkinson T (1990) The reduction of radiation damage to the spinal cord by post-irradiation administration of vasoactive drugs. Int J Radiat Oncol Biol Phys 18: 1437–1442.

Imperato JP, Paleologos NA, Vick N (1990) Effects of treatment on long-term survivors with malignant astrocytomas. Ann Neurol 28: 818–820.

Lefaix JL, Delanian S, Leplat JJ, et al. (1996) Successful treatment of radiation-induced fibrosis using Cu/Zn-SOD and Mn:SOD: an experimental study. Int J Radiat Oncol Biol Phys 35: 305–312.

Moulder JE, Fish BL, Cohen EP (1998) Angiotensin II receptor antagonists in the treatment and prevention of radiation nephropathy. Int J Radiat Biol 73(4): 415–421.

Plowman PN, McElwain T, Meadows A (1991) Complications of Cancer Management. Oxford: Butterworth-Heinemann.

Reinhold HS, Calvo W, Hopewell JW, van den Berg AP (1990) Development of blood vessel-related radiation damage in the fimbria of the central nervous system. Int J Radiat Oncol Biol Phys 18: 37–42.

Rezvani M, Alcock CJ, Fowler JF, et al. (1989) A comparison of the normal-tissue reactions in patients treated with either 3F/Wk or 5F/Wk in the BIR trial of radiotherapy for carcinoma of the laryngo-pharynx. Int J Radiat Biol 56: 717–720.

Rezvani M, Alcock CJ, Fowler JF, et al. (1991) Normal tissue reactions in the British Institute of Radiology study of 3 fractions per week versus 5 fractions per week in the treatment of carcinoma of the laryngo-pharynx by radiotherapy. Br J Radiol 64: 1122–1133.

Rezvani M, Birds DA, Hodges H, et al. (2001) Modification of radiation myelopathy by the transplantation of neural stem cells in the rat. Radiat Res 156: 408–412.

Endocrinology

W. John Kalk

Adrenal Cortex

Calcium Homeostasis

OVERWEIGHT AND OBESITY

Energy homeostasis and factors influencing the development of obesity

Body weight is regulated by a series of physiological processes, including appetite and satiety controls energy expenditure and disposition, which are substantially influenced by external societal and environmental factors. Neuronal circuits within the hypothalamus, which converge in the arcuate nucleus, seem to be the primary regulators of energy balance. Two groups of neurons are involved: those which stimulate appetite and inhibit energy expenditure, and others which do the reverse – inhibit appetite and enhance energy expenditure. Modulating influences are

- Central nervous system:
  - input from higher (psychological) centres provide information about, for example, the palatability of food and about the environment
  - input from lower centres, such as sleep–awake, pain.
- Autonomic nervous system: via vagal impulses.
- Gastrointestinal hormones, which appear to act both on the vagus nerve and in the hypothalamus
  - stimulates appetite: ghrelin
  - inhibit appetite: cholecystokinin, glucagon-like peptide 1 oxyntomodulin, and Peptide YY. The latter is probably the most important regulator of appetite and energy expenditure.
- Other hormones, such as leptin (from adipocytes) and insulin. In rodents leptin is a powerful suppressor of appetite, but its role in humans is unclear.

In a sedentary individual whose weight is stable over time energy intake (food) is equivalent to energy expenditure, which is made up from

- *resting metabolic rate* (RMR) (~60% of energy expenditure) (RMR varies between individuals of similar weight by up to 25%, but is constant in any individual)
- all *physical activity* (~30%) (the proportion of energy expended by physical work is obviously variable and can rise to 50% of daily energy output in those who do heavy manual work)
- *dietary induced thermogenesis* (~10%) (±constant).

Weight gain

Regular energy consumption which exceeds energy output results in a *positive energy balance* – a proportion of the excess food, whether carbohydrate, protein or fat, is converted into storage lipid (triglycerides) and stored in adipocytes to be potentially available in times of reduced food intake, when energy consumption is less than expenditure – *negative energy balance*. Weight gain leading to obesity is the result of a *small positive energy balance occurring over years and decades*. For example, the daily consumption of 50 Cal a day (one small bar

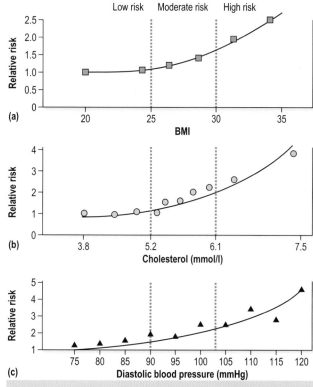

Figure 4.1.   Illustration of the similar continuous graded increase in relative risk of mortality as body mass index (BMI), blood pressure and serum cholesterol rise. (Reproduced with permission from WHO, 1998.)

of chocolate) in excess of daily energy expenditure amounts to 18 250 Cal over one year, and would result in a 2 kg gain of fat.

The ability to ensure the continuous availability of energy, stored as fat, in the face of variable food supplies has probably been a major determinant of the survival of mammals, including humans. An assured supply of food, amplified by diminishing needs for physical activity, has led to the worldwide epidemic of human obesity.

Obesity is currently classified by the World Health Organization (WHO) as a disease, with health connotations similar to high blood cholesterol or hypertension (WHO, 1998). It is a condition in which body fat has accumulated to an extent that health may be adversely affected. In the United States, for example, obesity-related conditions account for some 300 000 deaths each year.

Figure 4.1 illustrates the effects of increasing obesity on the relative risk of mortality in comparison with cholesterol and blood pressure.

Measures of 'fatness'

Body mass index (BMI) is a crude but useful and widely used estimate of total body fat content. BMI is calculated:

$$\text{body mass (kg)} \div [\text{height (m)}]^2$$

Table 4.1. Classification of overweight according to BMI

BMI (kg/m²)	Classification	Co-morbidity risk
<18.5	Underweight	Low (but risk of other health problems increased)
18.5–24.9	Normal range	Average
≥25	*Overweight*	
25.0–29.9	Pre-obese	Increased
30.0–34.9	Obese class I	Moderate
35.0–39.9	Obese class II	Severe
>40	Obese class IV	Very severe

Adapted from WHO (1998).

Table 4.2. Risk of obesity-associated metabolic complications in white men and women

	Normal	Increased	Greatly increased
Men	<94 cm	≥94 cm	≥102 cm
Women	<80 cm	≥80 cm	≥88 cm

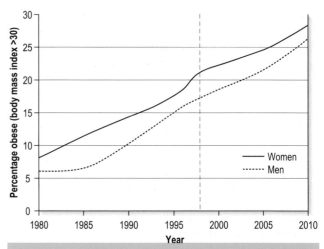

Figure 4.2. Trends in the prevalence of adult obesity in England. (Reproduced with permission from *British Medical Journal*, 2001.)

BMI is used to estimate the degree of 'fatness' in individuals and populations, and the associated risks to health. The WHO (1998) classification of BMI according to health risks is shown in Table 4.1.

Waist circumference measurements, and the ratio of the waist to hips (*WHR*) assess fat distribution and are better predictors of health status than BMI. *Body fat distribution* helps define the health impact of overweight not accounted for by BMI alone. Obese subjects with a disproportionately increased accumulation of intra-abdominal *visceral adipose tissue* (*VAT*) – those with '*central obesity*' – are at high risk from the adverse effects of obesity, higher than in individuals with a similar BMI but a smaller VAT mass.

Health risk and waist circumference

Table 4.2 illustrates the risk levels for waist circumference measurements in white men and women (WHO, 1998).

The 'risk cut points' are likely to be lower in South Asian (and probably in Chinese and Japanese) populations who seem to be more 'metabolically sensitive' to VAT accumulation than Northern Europeans, and higher in sub-Saharan African people who have substantially less VAT than Europeans for comparable waist circumferences.

Prevalence of obesity

The prevalence of obesity and overweight in populations varies among countries. In the WHO MONICA study of 48 countries in the 1980s (mainly in Europe and North America)

overweight and obesity prevalence ranged from 50 to 75% in populations aged 34 to 64 years, indicating the international nature of the epidemic. In many countries, both developed and developing, there is good evidence that the prevalence of obesity is increasing rapidly in adults; in some societies there is data that overweight and obesity are becoming a serious problem in children. Figure 4.2 illustrates the progressive rise in the prevalence of obesity in England.

Factors influencing prevalence of obesity in a population

- Obesity: women > men.
- Overweight: men > women.
- Increasing age, to about 65–70 years.
- Lower socio-economic status (and are more vulnerable to adverse effects of obesity).
- Method of assessment (BMI or waist). For example, a recent Australian survey found a higher prevalence of unhealthy overweight in men when waist measurements were used rather than BMI; and nearly 20% of subjects in an Indian study had central obesity yet were not overweight according to BMI.
- Genetic influences.

Genes and obesity

There is a significant *genetic influence* on body weight (25–40% of variance), but nutrient intake and physical activity influence 'weight gene' expression. Genes probably act as *predisposing* rather than causative factors in weight gain.

- Rare single genetic mutations have been identified as causes of obesity in humans. For example, the absence of functioning leptin (a hormone produced by adipocytes) because of mutations in the leptin gene, or its receptor gene, have been described in a handful of very obese individuals.

- In contrast to the small number of single gene mutations which cause polyphagia (greatly increased appetite) and obesity, most obesity is likely to be associated with multiple genes (polygenic).
- The '*thrifty genotype*' hypothesis. During human evolution food shortages may have been frequent. Periods of famine positively selected for genes which enhanced survival by promoting efficient energy storage, as fat, in times of food availability. In modern populations with permanent access to food and little daily energy expenditure such genes would still promote efficient energy storage, leading to excessive fat accumulation and obesity.

Epidemiological trends over the past 20 years indicate that the rate of increase in the prevalence of obesity has been too rapid to be explained by changes in human genes. Rather genetic factors interacting with personal influences also contribute to abnormal weight gain:

- ethnicity
- sex and age
- socio-economic conditions
- smoking
- population behavioural changes – eating patterns (consumption of high fat, energy dense foods) and the modern environment with reduced need for daily physical activity (sedentary lifestyles).

For example, associations have been shown between:

- childhood obesity and time spent watching television
- continued weight gain in children and consumption of sweetened soft drinks
- stopping cigarette smoking.

In summary, overweight and obesity are already common in both children and adults in wealthy and many developing countries. There are clear secular trends demonstrating that its prevalence is rising steeply in many societies. Since obesity may affect the health of millions it has major health economic implications.

Development of obesity

There are *three stages* in the development of obesity:

- A *pre-obese static phase* (long-term energy balance – weight constant).
- This is followed by a *dynamic phase* of gradual weight gain (small long-term positive energy balance) during which the rate of weight gain gradually diminishes as energy expenditure increases as a consequence of the increase in body mass (from a rising RMR and the increased energy cost of all weight bearing activities).

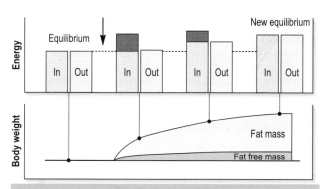

Figure 4.3.   The effects on energy expenditure, energy balance and body weight of an increase in energy intake relative to energy requirements. Note that rise rate of rise in body weight gradually slows down and reaches a plateau – the 'set point' (see text). (Reproduced with permission from WHO, 1998.)

- After some years an *obese static phase* is attained, in which the obese individual reaches a new equilibrium of energy balance.
- In some way the body comes to recognize this new energy equilibrium as 'normal' – a new, higher, *set point* for body weight has developed. This new set point is defended against weight loss: underfeeding results in a decline in RMR and an unconscious physiological drive to increase food consumption to regain the acquired, obese, steady state (Fig. 4.3). Normal weight people also have a body weight *set point* – after several weeks of voluntary increases or decreases in food intake the reintroduction of a free diet results in the return of weight to 'normal' for each individual.

Visceral adipose tissue (VAT)

VAT is made up of adipose tissue within the abdominal cavity (e.g. omental and perinephric fat). In addition to its anatomical site and venous drainage (part directly into the portal vein), VAT is in some respects distinct from subcutaneous adipose tissue.

Compared to subcutaneous adipose tissue, VAT:

- has more cells per unit mass
- has higher blood flow
- has more β-1 and β-2 adrenergic receptors
- is *more sensitive* to the lipolytic effects of catecholamines
- is *less sensitive* to the anti-lipolytic effects of insulin
- has increased concentrations of glucocorticoid receptors
- has increased concentrations of androgen receptors (stimulate β-adrenergic receptor expression; enhance lipoprotein lipase activity and hence lipolysis).

Excessive accumulation of intra-abdominal fat, VAT, is a marker of cardiovascular risk, independent of obesity as defined by BMI. Increased VAT mass is associated with a cluster of interrelated metabolic abnormalities, labelled the 'metabolic syndrome', which comprises some or all of the following:

- *Insulin resistance* (higher than normal plasma insulin levels required to maintain normal plasma glucose concentrations). Insulin resistance is central to the other listed disorders.
- *Dyslipidaemia*, characterized by
  - elevated serum *triglyceride* levels (fasting and sustained high concentrations after a fatty meal)
  - low levels of *high density lipoprotein cholesterol (HDL-C)*
  - usually normal low density lipoprotein cholesterol (LDL-C) levels, but a raised proportion of atherogenic *small, dense LDL-C* particles.
- *Higher blood pressures* and an increased prevalence of hypertension.
- *Plasminogen activator inhibitor-1 (PAI-1) and fibrinogen* concentrations raised.
- *Vascular endothelial dysfunction* (e.g. impaired vasodilatation, increased endothelial adhesiveness).
- Raised plasma levels of *inflammatory markers* (e.g. C-reactive protein) and some *cytokines* (e.g. interleukin-1 (IL-1), tumour necrosis factor-α (TNF-α).
- *Microalbuminuria* (small increases in urinary albumin excretion which indicate glomerular (and probably widespread endothelial) dysfunction.

Combinations of these abnormalities substantially raise the risk of cardiovascular diseases.

Insulin resistance (IR)

Insulin resistance is reflected in an impaired metabolic response to endogenous insulin secretion and to exogenous insulin administration, i.e. reduced insulin-stimulated glucose uptake and metabolism by skeletal muscle and fat, and impaired insulin suppression of hepatic glucose production (Fig. 4.4).

Factors influencing insulin resistance

- Genes
- Increasing age
- Increasing fatness (especially VAT)
- Low levels of physical activity
- Race/ethnicity
- Some medications.

Possible mechanisms causing insulin resistance

- Free fatty acids (FFA) and IR:
  - enhanced uptake of FFA by muscle inhibits glucose oxidation and glycolysis, hence decreasing muscle glucose uptake (the Randle cycle hypothesis)
  - high circulating concentrations of FFA reduce the insulin-dependent transport of glucose into cells, necessitating

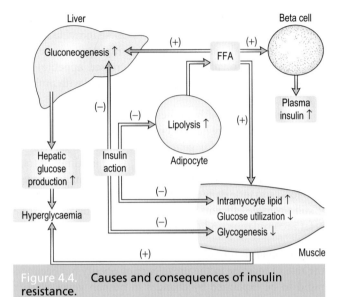

Figure 4.4.   Causes and consequences of insulin resistance.

higher levels of insulin to maintain normal plasma glucose concentrations.
- Skeletal muscle and IR:
  - increased amounts of intra-myocyte triglycerides, a consequence of a mismatch between FFA uptake and metabolism, correlate with the degree of IR.
  - a deficit in non-oxidative glucose disposal – a defect in glycogen synthesis.
- Hyperinsulinaemia and IR. High circulating insulin concentrations characteristic of IR states downregulate insulin receptors on cell membranes and so impair insulin action – its ability to synthesize glycogen. (This mechanism is of minor significance.)
- Post-receptor abnormalities in IR. These are complex intracellular mechanisms of insulin action which ultimately impair glucose transport across cell membranes and its intracellular disposal.
- As a consequence of an increased VAT mass and high rates of lipolysis in VAT, portal plasma concentrations of FFAs entering the liver are elevated; these contribute to hepatic insulin resistance, manifest as increased hepatic glucose output.

Other factors associated with obesity-related insulin resistance seem to be the consequence of an increased total body fat mass per se. Adipocytes are endocrine cells which secrete a number of products that contribute directly to insulin resistance:

- increased production of FFA
- tumour necrosis factor-α (TNF-α)
- interleukin-6 (IL-6)
- resistin (a recently described peptide hormone which inhibits insulin-mediated glucose uptake)
- adiponectin (a potent insulin sensitizer; levels are reduced in insulin-resistant states.

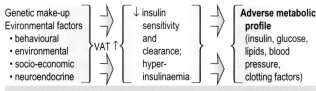

Figure 4.5. VAT and the metabolic syndrome.

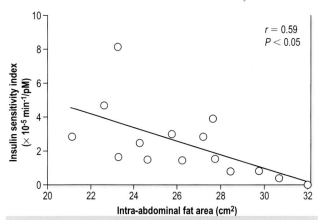

Figure 4.6. The relationship between VAT mass (assessed as cross-sectional area on abdominal scan) and insulin sensitivity index. (Reproduced with permission from Kahn et al., 1993.)

Factors influencing body fat distribution

- Obesity tends to run in families, suggesting the possibility of either genetic or environmental influences, or both, on excessive weight gain. With central obesity – high VAT mass – the *genetic influence* is stronger (accounting for 50–60% of inter-individual variation) than for obesity assessed as BMI (see above).
- *Individual metabolic factors* also seem to play a part. For example, in women VAT mass correlates strongly with circulating androgenic activity, and VAT tends to increase after the menopause, perhaps related to falling oestrogen levels.
- Recent research suggests that *perceived stress-related perturbations of the hypothalamic-pituitary-adrenal axis* (HPA) are associated with increased VAT accumulation (Fig. 4.5). It has been hypothesized that subjective life stresses lead to chronic, small (within the range of normality) HPA hyperactivity – slight increases in circulating cortisol levels – which stimulate visceral adipocyte fat accumulation.

The amount of VAT correlates directly with measured IR (Fig. 4.6).

Health consequences of obesity

Overweight and obesity impact on health in both adults and children (Tables 4.3, 4.5).

Table 4.3. Health consequences of obesity in adults

Greatly increased risk (RR > 3×)	Moderately increased risk (RR 2–3×)	Small risk (RR 1–2×)
IGT Type 2 diabetes	Hypertension	Some cancers, e.g. breast, endometrium, colon
Dyslipidaemia	Coronary heart disease	Polycystic ovary syndrome
Breathlessness	Stroke	Reduced fertility
Sleep apnoea	Osteoarthritis	Fetal defects
Gall bladder disease	Hyperuricaemia/ gout	Low back pain
NASH		Increased anaesthetic risk

IGT, impaired glucose tolerance; NASH: non-alcoholic steatohepatitis.
Adapted from WHO (1998).

Table 4.4. Prevalence of overweight[a] in children aged 6–8 years

	USA 1988–1991	China 1993	Russia 1994	South Africa 1994
Boys	21	14	25	25
Girls	24	12	18	20

[a] Defined as BMI > US reference NHES 85th centile.
Adapted from Popkin et al. (1996).

In addition to these physical disorders obesity may be associated with psychosocial problems, some of which may be culturally dependent:

- higher rates of unemployment for medical reasons
- discrimination – social and in employment
- eating disorders more prevalent.

Overweight and obesity in children

Excessive weight gain in children has become a worldwide phenomenon (Table 4.4).

Childhood obesity is associated in poor populations with *stunting* (i.e. children are short for age and may be overweight), and in affluent societies with physical inactivity and consumption of sugary drinks. Some researchers have found an association between parental neglect and later overweight.

Overweight in pre-adolescent children is also associated, in industrialized countries, with poor social functioning and impaired academic success. In adolescents obesity is associated with low self-esteem and later, in early adulthood, with social problems and lower incomes.

Table 4.5.   Health consequences of obesity in children

High prevalence	Intermediate prevalence	Low prevalence
Faster growth (early tall stature)	NASH (non-alcoholic steatohepatitis)	Orthopaedic problems
Psychosocial problems	Abnormal glucose metabolism (rarely type 2 diabetes)	Sleep apnoea
Dyslipidaemia		Polycystic ovary syndrome
Higher blood pressure persists into adulthood		Hypertension

From WHO (1998).

Other influences on obesity-related disorders

- The age at which weight is gained (worse consequences with adult onset obesity).
- The amount of weight gained (the greater the degree of overweight, the greater the health risks).
- The cardiovascular risks of obesity are modified by the degree of physical fitness of individuals. Across a range of adiposity, cardiovascular mortality is lower in fit than in unfit cohorts.
- The 'Barker hypothesis': Intrauterine growth retardation probably a reflection of intrauterine malnutrition, has been linked in epidemiological studies to the development in middle age of the metabolic syndrome with its associated cardiovascular risk profile, including hypertension and type 2 diabetes.

Benefits of weight loss

Modest weight loss (5–10% loss):

- improves glucose homeostasis
- reduces blood pressure
- lowers cholesterol
- improves lung function and breathlessness
- decreases the frequency of sleep apnoea
- may reduce back pain.

Substantial weight loss (sustained 20–30 kg loss) (usually achieved by surgical treatment of severe obesity – gastroplasty) results in greater risk reductions in otherwise healthy subjects and in patients with existing obesity-related diseases, such as ischaemic heart disease, dyslipidaemia, diabetes and polycystic ovary syndrome:

- marked fall in serum lipids and blood pressure
- smaller future incidence of the metabolic syndrome.

Management of obesity

Management involves a range of interdependent strategies – prevention of excessive weight gain, weight maintenance, promotion of weight loss in overweight and obese in individuals, and management of obesity related co-morbidities.

Prevention

- Populations: aim for a beneficial influence on eating habits. For example, the draft WHO dietary guidelines (2003) recommend that sugar (sucrose) should provide no more than 10% of daily energy intake.
- Children; adolescents; high risk adults (e.g. pregnant women) could be targeted for public programmes for weight control.

Treatment

Reduction of food energy intake creates a negative energy balance; regular physical exercise helps weight loss and may promote weight stabilization after loss.

A few medications are available to help treat obesity; many are being tested for use in humans:

- orlistat, which reduces fat digestion in the gut – fewer fat calories are absorbed
- sibutramine, which reduces appetite

Both are successful in increasing the weight loss of strict diets, but weight stabilizes after 4 to 6 months at about 5 kg less than the effect of the diet alone. If therapy is discontinued weight is regained.

For very obese patients surgically reducing the volume of the stomach has proved to be the most reliable and long-lasting treatment modality – 20 to 30 kg weight loss can be maintained for many years.

How much weight loss?

Experience has shown that in obese subjects sustained weight loss, to reach normal or ideal weight, is seldom achieved. Thus the attainment of normal body weight is an unrealistic goal in obesity management. Rather perceived attainable weight targets should be set which are likely to be beneficial over time. Thus a loss of 5 to 10% of weight usually reduces the cardiovascular risk profile significantly. Since weight gain so frequently occurs as individuals age, even weight maintenance can be considered a partial management 'success' (Fig. 4.7).

GLUCOSE HOMEOSTASIS AND DIABETES

Normal glucose homeostasis

Plasma and tissue glucose is derived from three sources:

- the gastrointestinal tract after carbohydrate digestion
- from glycogenolysis (breakdown of glycogen)

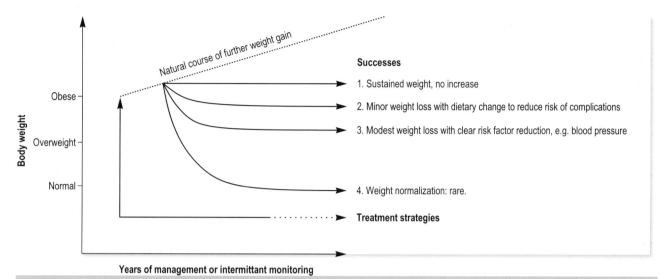

Figure 4.7. Indicators of 'success' in the management of obesity. (Reproduced with permission from WHO, 1998.)

- from gluconeogenesis (from precursors – predominantly lactate, alanine, glutamine, glycerol).

Most cells can synthesize and break down glycogen. Only the liver and kidney release glucose into the circulation.

Fate of intracellular glucose
- to glycogen
- to pyruvate – acetyl CoA – energy cycle
- to fatty acid synthesis – triglyceride
- to ketone body synthesis
- to cholesterol synthesis
- released into the circulation.

Plasma glucose regulation
Plasma glucose concentrations are maintained within a narrow range by a physiological balance between glucose utilization and glucose entering the circulation from the liver between meals and from the gastrointestinal tract during and after meals. This balance is maintained by hormonal and neural influences.

Hormones
- Increase glucose concentration: *glucagon*, adrenaline, growth hormone, cortisol.
- Decrease glucose concentration: *insulin*.

Glucagon is produced by the α-cells of the pancreatic islets; high levels are found in portal blood entering the liver. Glucagon increases hepatic glucose production by activating glycogenolysis.

Adrenaline increases hepatic glycogenolysis, and limits glucose utilization, e.g. by muscle.

Insulin, in high concentrations in portal blood, reduces hepatic glucose production, and stimulates glycogen synthesis.

Autonomic neural influence on liver
- Sympathetic – increases glucose release.
- Parasympathetic – reduces glucose release.

Insulin secretion
Fasting state: ± constant insulin secretion and plasma concentrations.

After carbohydrate ingestion and digestion: rapid release of insulin, from β-cell stores, and a sharp rise in plasma concentration in response to rising glucose levels. Glucose-stimulated insulin secretion is enhanced by the release of gastrointestinal hormones in response to food ingestion – 'incretins', which stimulate the β-cells in the presence of rising plasma glucose levels. The major physiological incretins are:

- gastrointestinal inhibitory polypeptide (GIP)
- glucagon-like peptide 1 (GLP-1).

Additional factors which regulate insulin secretion are outlined in Figure 4.8.

Insulin secretory phases
In response to glucose ingestion, or to intravenous glucose infusion, circulating insulin levels rise sharply, within minutes – the *first phase* insulin release. Subsequently there is a slower, lower but sustained, *second phase* release of insulin which gradually declines as glucose concentrations decline to normal. Figure 4.9 illustrates the biphasic insulin response to an intravenous infusion of glucose.

Diabetes: diagnosis and classification
(Table 4.6)

The American Diabetes Association Expert Committee defines diabetes as: 'a group of metabolic diseases characterized by hyperglycaemia resulting from defects in insulin secretion, insulin action, or both. The chronic hyperglycaemia is associated with damage, dysfunction and failure of various organs, especially eyes, kidneys, nerves, heart and blood vessels'.

Classification of diabetes

Type 1 diabetes: β-cell destruction leading to absolute insulin deficiency:

- autoimmune
- idiopathic.

Type 2 diabetes: ranges from:

- predominant insulin resistance with relative insulin deficiency
- to predominant insulin deficiency ± insulin resistance.

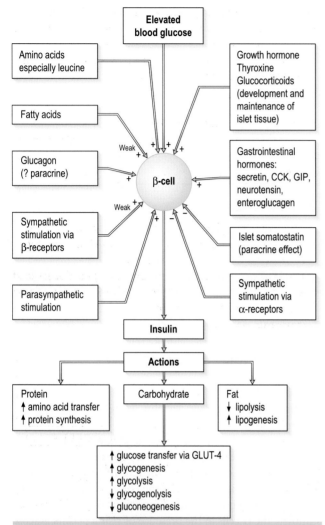

Figure 4.8.   Factors affecting insulin secretion and an outline of the actions of insulin. GLUT-4, glucose transport protein-4. (Reproduced with permission from Davies et al., 2001.)

Table 4.6.   Diagnosis of diabetes: fasting glucose concentrations and response to a 75 g oral glucose tolerance test

	Fasting plasma glucose (mmol/l)		2-hour plasma glucose (mmol/l)
Normal	<6.1		<7.8
Impaired glucose tolerance[a]	<7.0		7.8–11.0
Diabetes	≥7.0[b]	and/or	≥11.1[b]
Impaired fasting glucose	6.1–6.9		–

[a] A potentially prediabetic state associated with ~2-fold increased risk of cardiovascular diseases.

[b] Approximate plasma glucose concentrations above which the population prevalence of diabetic retinopathy rises.

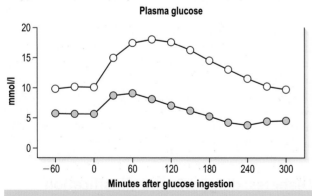

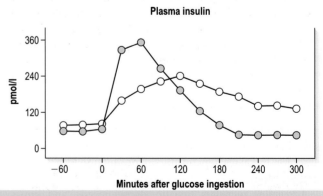

Figure 4.9.   The changes in plasma concentrations of glucose and insulin in diabetic (open circles) and normal subjects (closed circles). Note both the absence of the early insulin rise and the delayed decline in insulin levels, both characteristic of type 2 diabetes. (Adapted with permission from Mitrakou et al., 1992.)

Other specific types (rare)
- genetic defects of β-cells
- genetic defects of insulin action
- disease of the exocrine pancreas
- endocrinopathies
- drug/chemical induced
- infections
- rare forms of autoimmune-mediated diabetes
- rare genetic syndromes sometimes associated with diabetes.

Gestational diabetes: diabetes occurring for the first time during pregnancy.

Type 2 diabetes

Type 2 diabetes is the predominant form of diabetes, accounting for >90% of cases in the world. Its prevalence is increasing in both the developed and developing countries and is reaching epidemic proportions: the estimated global prevalence in 1995 was 150 million, and is predicted to reach 300 million by 2025.

Epidemiological determinants of type 2 diabetes

Genetic predisposition (polygenic)	Obesity (degree, duration, VAT mass)
Race/ethnicity	Physical inactivity
Sex	Stress
Increasing age and life expectancy	Urbanization, Westernization

---

Pathogenesis

The pathogenesis of type 2 diabetes is complex: genetic predisposition and environmental factors interact. Fundamentally, in type 2 diabetes the β-cells are unable to adapt to, or keep pace with, increasing demands for greater insulin secretion as insulin resistance persists or worsens with increasing age and/or fat mass (Fig. 4.10). Eventually the capacity of the β-cells to produce 'first phase' insulin is exceeded, glucose intolerance starts (initially impaired glucose tolerance (IGT) and postprandial hyperglycaemia), fasting plasma glucose

---

Risk factors for type 2 diabetes

Family history (parents, siblings)	Hypertension
Overweight/Obesity (especially big VAT mass)	Insulin resistance
	History of gestational diabetes
Physical inactivity	Polycystic ovary syndrome
Race/ethnicity	

---

levels rise, and eventually diabetes supervenes. The combination of insulin resistance and reduced insulin secretion is found in most subjects with type 2 diabetes.

Insulin resistance in type 2 diabetes has the same pathogenesis as in 'uncomplicated' obesity (see 'Overweight and obesity', above).

Insulin secretory abnormalities

Abnormalities in insulin secretion can be detected before the onset of overt diabetes, in subjects with IGT and in siblings of patients with type 2 diabetes but normal glucose tolerance. The defects are more pronounced in the presence of overt diabetes:

- loss of the 'first phase' of insulin secretion in response to rising plasma glucose levels, without which glucose tolerance deteriorates (Figs 4.9 and 4.10)
- delay in the peak insulin response after an oral glucose load
- loss of coordinated β-cell responsiveness to changing plasma glucose concentrations
- increase in proinsulin secretion.

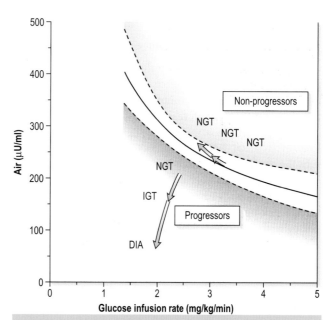

Figure 4.10.   The relationship over time between the acute (first phase) insulin response (AIR) to intravenous glucose and insulin action (insulin sensitivity – resistance), assessed as the rate of glucose infusion (mg/kg/min) required to keep plasma glucose concentrations normal in the face of a constant intravenous infusion of insulin. With ageing and weight gain subjects who progressed to diabetes lost the first phase insulin response, developed IGT and 'progressed' to overt diabetes. Subjects who retained normal glucose tolerance ('non-progressors') continued to produce increasing amounts of insulin as their insulin resistance increased. NGT, normal glucose tolerance; IGT, impaired glucose tolerance; DIA, diabetes. (Reproduced with permission from Weyer et al., 1999.)

Complications of type 2 diabetes

These are similar to those of type 1 diabetes (see 'Complications of type 1 diabetes' below), except that the presence of type 2 diabetes reflects long duration or a more severe form of the metabolic syndrome. Thus cardiovascular diseases are frequent. In comparison with matched populations without diabetes, in those with type 2 diabetes the risk of coronary heart disease is increased twofold in men and fourfold in women; stroke risk is doubled; and the frequency of peripheral arterial disease is greatly increased. The pathogenesis of the vascular complications is the same as in type 1 diabetes.

Management of type 2 diabetes

- Lifestyle changes
  - weight loss (at least 5–10%)
  - diet adjustments (low fat (<30% energy), 15–20% energy from protein, high fibre carbohydrates)
  - increased physical activity for sedentary individuals.
- Pharmacotherapy
  - insulin sensitizers (biguanides, thiazolidinediones)
  - insulin secretagogues (sulphonylureas, meglitinides).
- Inhibitors of intestinal glucose absorption
  - glucosidase inhibitors.
- Insulin therapy (with or without continued oral agents).

Recent research indicates that the loss of β-cell function is progressive and that most subjects with type 2 diabetes require increasing amounts and combinations of medication over time in order to maintain reasonable glycaemic control.

Prevention of type 2 diabetes

- In the general population: up to 90% of type 2 diabetes is potentially preventable if populations remained lean and physically fit with advancing age.
- High risk populations with IGT: three recent studies have shown that modest weight loss plus increased exercise reduced the risk of developing diabetes by about 50%. Pharmaceutical interventions were less effective.

Type 1 diabetes

Incidence

The incidence varies among countries, from ~0.1 cases/100 000/year (China) to 49/100 000/year (Finland):

- is increasing in most countries
- peak age of onset – 10–14 years, but increasing incidence at age <5 years; ~20 years in sub-Saharan Africans
- family clustering
- accounts for <10% of diabetes in most countries.

Aetiology

Type 1 diabetes is caused by cell-mediated autoimmune destruction of pancreatic β-cells. There appears to be a genetic predisposition, but unknown environmental 'triggers' initiate the autoimmune process, which is characterized by a chronic

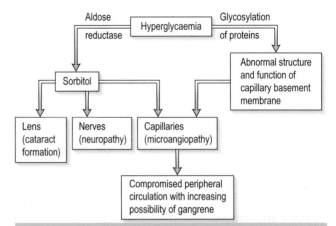

Figure 4.11. Physical changes caused by persistent hyperglycaemia. Glycosylation of proteins causes swelling of the basement membrane, and sorbitol produced by abnormally high levels of glucose exerts a damaging osmotic effect on nerves and the lens of the eye. (Reproduced with permission from Davies et al., 2001.)

inflammatory cell 'insulitis' of the islets of Langerhans, and one or more of several circulating islet cell autoantibodies. The β-cell mass gradually diminishes. When insufficient insulin is secreted for normal glucose homeostasis, hyperglycaemia supervenes – diabetes (Fig. 4.11).

Principles of therapy

There is an absolute deficiency of insulin; thus insulin administration is necessary to sustain life – insulin dependence. Usually combinations of short- and longer-acting insulins are injected into subcutaneous fat 2–4 (or more) times a day to maintain blood glucose control. The aim of insulin treatment is to maintain plasma glucose levels as close to the normal ranges as is safely possible: the limiting factor is the increasing risk of hypoglycaemia as glycaemic control approaches normality.

Complications of type 1 diabetes

Acute complications

Insulin-induced hypoglycaemia (develops in minutes). Treatment involves glucose administration, orally if patient is able to swallow, or by intravenous injection if in coma, or by the subcutaneous injection of glucagon.

Symptoms and signs of hypoglycaemia	
Symptoms	*Physical signs*
Anxiety	Sweating
Palpitations	Tachycardia
Sweating	Tremor
Hunger	Confusion
Headaches, blurred vision	Neurological signs (may be bizarre)
Behavioural changes	Stupor, coma

Diabetic keto-acidosis (DKA): a life-threatening 'metabolic emergency' (due to profound insulin deficiency) which develops over hours to days, and which results in:

- usually severe hyperglycaemia (plasma glucose >20 mmol/l)
- dehydration, from osmotic diuresis
- excessive lipolysis
- increased rates of fatty acid oxidation
- increased production of β-hydroxybutarate, aceto-acetate (both acidic) and acetone
- metabolic acidosis
- electrolyte disturbances, notably acidosis-related egress of intracellular potassium into plasma and potassium loss via the kidneys (total body potassium depletion)
- patients with severe and prolonged DKA may become stuporose, even comatose.

Treatment of DKA:

- rehydration
- intravenous insulin administration
- intravenous infusion of potassium.

Chronic complications of diabetes

These develop over years and decades and are a consequence of 'diabetic' injury to the organs, mediated by damage to their microcirculation. There is good evidence that the duration and intensity of hyperglycaemia are causative mechanisms.

Eyes: diabetic retinopathy
- background
- proliferative (new vessel formation: requires laser treatment).

Kidneys: diabetic glomerular disease occurs in about one-third of poorly controlled patients with type 1 and type 2 diabetes – there may be genetic determinants which render a subgroup susceptible to chronic hyperglycaemia.

Stages of diabetic kidney disease:

- normal protein excretion and normal or increased glomerular filtration rate (GFR)
- micro-albuminuria (albumin excretion rate (AER) increased to above normal, i.e. 20–200 µg/min)
- macro-albuminuria (AER >200 µg/min): associated with rising blood pressure, declining GFR, and other severe diabetic complications.

Neuropathy: damage to nerves
- sensory-motor polyneuropathy: affects nerves in the feet – loss of sensation and deformities (liable to painless trauma and abnormal pressures which can lead to ulceration, infection, amputations)
- autonomic neuropathy: cardiovascular neuropathy, gastro-intestinal neuropathies – gastroparesis, 'diabetic' diarrhoea, chronic constipation, genitourinary neuropathies – impotence, neurogenic bladder with urinary retention.

Mechanisms of hyperglycaemic organ damage

1. Increased polyol pathway
   - hyperglycaemia → increased sorbitol production and accumulation → decreased NADPH → cell damage.
2. Increased production and accumulation of advanced glycation endproducts (AGEs):
   - hyperglycaemia → raised intracellular dicarbonyls react with amino groups of proteins → AGEs
   - potential effects of AGEs
     - altered function of intracellular proteins
     - AGE-modified extracellular proteins, which may interfere normal matrix-cell functions
     - AGE-modified plasma proteins bind to receptors, e.g. on macrophages, increasing reactive oxygen species.
3. Activation of protein kinase C (PKC).
4. Increased hexosamine pathway flux.

Recent research has identified a potential *common pathway for hyperglycaemia induced damage* – 'oxidative stress' – which may explain each of the above mechanisms.

Hyperglycaemia induces mitochondrial superoxide overproduction, via the tricarboxylic acid cycle, which results in increased formation of reactive oxygen species (ROS). Experimental blockade of ROS formation inhibits each of the pathophysiological consequences of hyperglycaemia. Thus it can be deduced that ROS overproduction:

- adversely affects the polyol pathway
- initiates the increased formation of intracellular AGEs
- indirectly activates PCK
- stimulates the hexosamine pathway.

ANTERIOR PITUITARY GLAND

The anterior pituitary gland is physiologically part of the *hypothalamic-pituitary 'peripheral target organ' axis* (Figs 4.12 and 4.13). The peripheral endocrine target organs are the

- thyroid
- adrenals
- gonads
- breast
- liver and other tissues responsive to growth hormone.

The hypothalamus secretes its hormones into the hypothalamic-pituitary portal system. In the pituitary they stimulate or inhibit secretion of the various pituitary trophic hormones. The peripheral target endocrine glands are stimulated to secrete their hormones, which exert a *negative feedback effect*, usually at both the hypothalamic and pituitary levels (Table 4.7).

Recently a new pituitary glycoprotein hormone has been described – *thyrostimulin* – which appears to be active at the

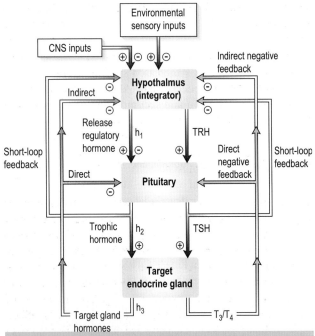

Figure 4.12.   Indirect (and direct) negative feedback. The pathway on the left illustrates the general principle. That on the right illustrates the principle as applied to the hypothalamo-pituitary-thyroid axis. The relative importance of the direct negative feedback at the pituitary and indirect negative feedback at the hypothalamus varies with each axis. (Reproduced with permission from Davies et al., 2001.)

Table 4.7.   The hypothalamic, pituitary and target organs' feedback hormones

Hypothalamic	Pituitary	Target gland	Feedback hormones
TRH (+)	TSH[a]	Thyroid	T_3/T_4
CRF (+)	ACTH	Adrenal cortex	Cortisol
GnRH (+)	LH[a] and FSH[a]	Gonads	Oestrogen, testosterone, inhibin
Dopamine (−)	Prolactin	Breast	Prolactin
GHRH (+) Somatostatin (−)	Growth hormone	Liver	IGF-1

TRH, thyrotrophin-releasing hormone; TSH, thyroid-stimulating hormone; GnRH, gonadotrophin-releasing hormone; LH, leuteinizing hormone; FSH, follicle stimulating hormone; CRH, corticotrophin-releasing hormone; ACTH, adrenocorticotrophic hormone (corticotrophin); GHRH, growth hormone releasing hormone; IGF-1, insulin-like growth factor-1.
[a] Glycoproteins consisting of two linked subunits. The α-subunit is common to the three hormones and to the placental human chorionic gonadotrophin (HCG); the β-subunits differ and determine the specificity of each hormone.

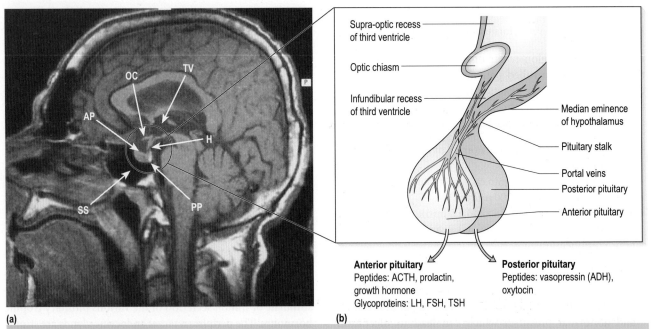

(a)   (b)

Figure 4.13.   (a) An MRI of the brain through the midline illustrating the position of the hypothalamus and the pituitary gland, and (b) a diagram outlining the anatomy of the pituitary and the organs above it. SS, sphenoid sinus; AP, anterior pituitary; OC, optic chiasm; TV, third ventricle; H, hypothalamus; PP, posterior pituitary. (Reproduced with permission from Haslett et al., 2002.)

TSH receptor on thyroid follicular cells (stimulates cAMP production). It may also be synthesized by other tissues. Its precise physiological role has yet to be determined.

Pituitary diseases

The most frequent disorders of the pituitary gland are tumours, nearly always benign adenomas. They often secrete one or more intact hormones, or fragments of hormones (e.g. glycoprotein hormone α-subunits), but some are non-secretory. The *clinical manifestations* of pituitary tumours depend on the hormone, if any, they secrete, or on the mass effect of an expanding tumour which may damage or destroy the surrounding normal pituitary, leading to pituitary and therefore peripheral endocrine organ failure. Large tumours often expand upwards and impinge on the optic chiasm, which is situated a few millimetres above the pituitary, and cause visual field defects.

The management of pituitary tumours may be with medication, e.g. for prolactin or growth hormone secreting adenomas, surgery or radiotherapy, or therapeutic combinations. For pituitary failure the end-organ hormone is replaced, e.g. thyroxine, cortisol, sex steroids.

THE THYROID

The function of the thyroid gland is to synthesize, store and release thyroid hormones for utilization by peripheral tissues.

Thyroid hormones are:

- thyroxine (T_4 with four iodine atoms)
- triiodothyronine (T_3, with three iodine atoms; biologically more active than T_4).

Thus dietary *iodine* is an essential micronutrient for normal physiological functioning. For normal iodine balance and thyroid homeostasis 100–150 μg dietary iodine is required to replace faecal and urinary losses. During pregnancy daily iodine requirements increase to about 250–300 μg.

Dietary iodine deficiency is common. Some one billion people live in iodine-deficient areas in the world, and are at risk for iodine deficiency disorders (see below).

Regulation of thyroid function

The hypothalamic-pituitary-thyroid axis

Thyrotrophin releasing hormone (TRH) is synthesized in the hypothalamus and released into the hypothalamic-pituitary portal system; it stimulates the pituitary to release thyroid stimulating hormone (TSH, thyrotrophin) into the systemic circulation. TSH binds to specific receptors on thyroid follicular cells (thyrocytes) and stimulates the synthesis and release of thyroid hormones, predominantly T_4 (Fig. 4.14). In peripheral tissues, e.g. liver and kidney, some T_4 is enzymatically deiodinated to T_3. About 70–80% of circulating T_3 is derived from the peripheral deiodination of T_4. T_4 and T_3 exert negative feed back control at the levels of the hypothalamus and pituitary.

In the circulation both T_4 and T_3 are highly protein bound; less than 1% is unbound. The plasma carriers are thyroxine binding globulin (transports 70% of circulating thyroid hormones), transthyretin (thyroxine binding pre-albumin) (15%) and albumin (15%).

Action of thyroid hormones

Cells of most tissues have thyroid hormone receptors. T_3 binds to specific nuclear receptors: cell function is altered so mediating the physiological effects of thyroid hormones.

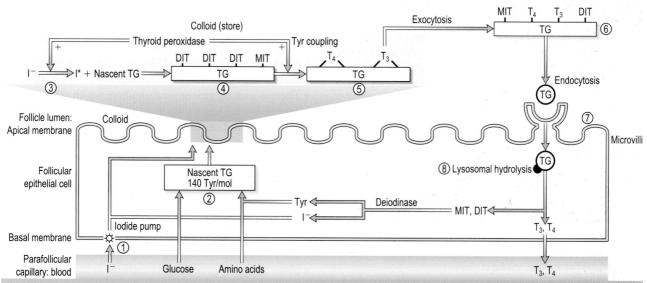

Figure 4.14.   Thyroid hormone synthesis and secretion. (Reproduced with permission from Davies et al., 2001.)

Physiologic effects of thyroid hormones

- Fetal development – brain and skeletal development.
- Oxygen consumption and heat production – partly through the stimulation of Na^+-K^+ ATPase.
- Cardiovascular – increases myocardial contractility and β-adrenergic receptor numbers; positive ionotrophic and chronotrophic effects.
- Sympathetic nervous system effects – increases β-adrenergic receptor numbers on skeletal muscle and adipose tissue and increases sensitivity to catecholamines.
- Haemopoietic effects – increases production of erythropoietin by the kidneys.
- Gastrointestinal effects – increases gut motility.
- Skeletal effects – increases bone turnover.
- Neuromuscular effects – increases speed of muscle contraction and relaxation, and protein turnover.
- Effects on lipid and carbohydrate metabolism – increases lipolysis and gluconeogenesis, and turnover of cholesterol.
- Endocrine effects – modulate the metabolic turnover of several hormones.

Abnormalities of thyroid function

Hyperthyroidism

The normal metabolic effects of thyroid hormones are exaggerated – a hypermetabolic state.

Causes

- Autoimmune hyperthyroidism (Graves' disease). Specific autoantibodies bind to the TSH receptors and stimulate thyrocytes in an unregulated fashion.
- Multinodular toxic goitre. Commonly an activating mutation of the TSH receptor is found in relatively hyperfunctioning thyroid nodules. The mutation results in increased activity of the receptor, independent of circulating TSH levels, so that post-receptor events are overactive. As the thyroid gland enlarges, so more thyroid hormones are secreted in an uncontrolled fashion: when concentration exceed normal a hyperthyroid state develops.

Symptoms and signs of hyperthyroidism

Symptoms	Signs
Anxiety	Tachycardia
Heat intolerance	Goitre
Palpitations	Skin changes
Fatigue	Tremor of hands
Weight loss	Eye signs
Dyspnoea	
Weakness	
Eye symptoms	

Diagnosis: measurement of T_4 (elevated) and TSH (undetectable).

Therapy: antithyroid medications; radio-active iodine therapy; surgery.

Hypothyroidism

This is a hypometabolic state in which the functions of thyroid hormones are diminished. This condition affects about 2% of women and 0.1–0.2% of men.

Aetiology: autoimmune thyroid destruction; surgery; radio-iodine therapy; some medications.

Symptoms and signs of hypothyroidism

Common symptoms	Common signs
Cold intolerance	Bradycardia
Dry skin	Dry skin
Constipation	Facial puffiness
Weight gain	Slow tendon reflex
Deafness	relaxation
Muscle stiffness and cramps	Anaemia

Diagnosis: elevated TSH; low T_4.

Treatment: thyroxine: the dose is titrated to achieve a normal TSH concentration.

Multinodular goitres

Goitres with normal function are common, being clinically evident in some 7% of iodine-replete adult populations, especially in women from middle age. At autopsy the prevalence ranges from 30 to 60%. The prevalence is higher in iodine-deficient populations.

- Most are *multinodular* and *benign* – about 7% may contain malignancy.
- There is a strong *genetic predisposition*, which interacts with *environmental factors* such as iodine deficiency, dietary goitrogens and smoking.
- Most benign nodules seem to arise from *genetic mutations* which result in *monoclonal or polyclonal* overgrowth of thyrocytes with a growth advantage, independent of TSH.
- *Activating mutations of the TSH receptor* are found in most hyperactive thyroid nodules (see above).

  Management includes:

- observation for growth and function
- surgery
- radio-iodine therapy.

Iodine deficiency disorders (IDD)

IDDs occur in populations which are deficient in dietary iodine – about one billion people worldwide. They include a spectrum of disorders affecting neonates, older children and adults.

Spectrum of IDD: increased frequencies in iodine-deficient compared with iodine-replete populations

Pregnancy and infancy	Children and adolescents	Adults
Abortion and stillbirth	Psychomotor defects	Goitre
Perinatal mortality	Impaired mental function	Hypothyroidism
Infant mortality	Slow physical growth	Impaired mental function
Congenital anomalies	Neurological deafness	Cretinism
Neonatal goitre	Strabismus	
Neonatal hypothyroidism	Hypothyroidism	
Cretinism – neurological – myxoedematous	Goitre Cretinism	

Prevention of IDD is achieved by ensuring an adequate dietary iodine intake by the population as whole. Dietary iodine supplementation is most often achieved by adding iodate to table salt.

ADRENAL CORTEX

The adrenal cortex of the adrenal glands secretes the steroid hormones which are synthesized from cholesterol and have the same basic structure (Fig. 4.15).

Adrenal steroid hormones:

- glucocorticoid – cortisol
- mineralocorticoid – aldosterone
- sex steroids – mainly weak androgens.

Regulation of adrenal steroids

Cortisol is secreted (10–20 mg per day) by the *zona fasciculata* of the adrenal cortex. Secretion and synthesis is controlled by pituitary adrenocorticotrophic hormone (ACTH) which is subject to negative feedback loops acting at both the pituitary and hypothalamic levels (see above).

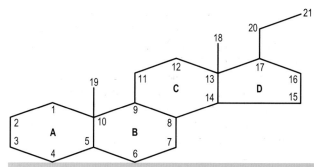

Figure 4.15.   The basic structure of the steroid nucleus. Additions at carbon atoms 3, 11, 17 and 18, 21 and various double bonds in the rings alter biological function.

ACTH and cortisol secretion exhibit a *circadian rhythm* with peak plasma concentrations at about 5 to 9 a.m., and a nadir at about midnight. This rhythm is dependent on both day–night and sleep–wake cycles, and is disrupted by day–night shift work and by rapid travel across time zones. About 2 weeks of adaptation are required to reset a new circadian rhythm.

ACTH and cortisol rhythms are overcome by the *stress responses* – inflammatory, physical and emotional stresses:

- inflammatory cytokines such as interleukin-1 (IL-1), interleukin-6 (IL-6) and tumour necrosis factor-α (TNF-α) augment ACTH secretion
- physical stress such as trauma or surgery via neuronal pathways to the hypothalamus
- clinical depression, via higher brain centres to the hypothalamus.

Each of these stresses overcomes the normal CRF-ACTH-cortisol secretory patterns and causes circulating cortisol levels to rise.

Cortisol effects

- Carbohydrate and fat metabolism
  - liver: increases glycogen synthesis and increases gluconeogenesis and hepatic glucose output
  - muscle: glucose uptake and utilization inhibited (insulin resistance)
  - adipose tissue: adipogenesis stimulated; increases lipolysis with a resulting rise in circulating FFA levels, contributing to insulin resistance.
- Sodium, potassium and blood pressure control: cortisol increases renal tubular *Na retention* and *K loss*; and increases vascular sensitivity to catecholamines. With high cortisol levels blood pressure tends to rise, and vice versa.
- Bone: cortisol inhibits osteoblast action (high levels cause bone loss).
- Skin, muscle and connective tissue: high cortisol levels cause atrophy.

- Anti-inflammatory effects: cortisol modulates immune responses: high levels
  - decrease circulating lymphocyte and eosinophil numbers
  - decrease immunoglobulins
  - increase circulating neutrophils.
- central nervous system: chronically high or low cortisol concentration can affect mood (see below).

Diseases of the adrenal cortex

Under physiological circumstances and normal functioning of the hypothalamo-pituitary-adrenocortical axis, cortisol contributes to the body's normal homeostasis. Cortisol excess or deficiency causes disease.

Glucocorticoid excess can be caused by prolonged pharmacological use of high dose 'steroids' (e.g. prednisolone), or from chronic endogenous overproduction of cortisol. Both result in *Cushing's syndrome.*

Endogenous over-secretion of cortisol arises from excessive secretion of ACTH, from pituitary tumours or from malignancies ('ectopic ACTH production') or from cortisol-secreting adrenal tumours (usually benign).

Typical clinical findings in Cushing's syndrome

Symptoms	Clinical signs	Other findings
Weight gain	Obesity (mainly central)	Hypertension
Menstrual irregularities	'Moon face'	Glucose intolerance
Hirsutism	Hypertension	Osteoporosis
Psychiatric dysfunction	Easy bruising	
Muscle weakness	Red striae (stretch marks)	
Balding	Muscle weakness Increased pigmentation	

Management consists of surgical removal of ACTH-secreting pituitary adenoma or adrenal tumour; stop glucocorticoid medication.

Glucocorticoid deficiency can be caused by destruction of the adrenal glands (autoimmune, infection e.g. tuberculosis, infiltration: *Addison's disease*); or by ACTH deficiency from destruction of the pituitary gland (by tumour, surgery, trauma, infiltration); or by inherited enzyme defects in the biosynthesis of cortisol and aldosterone – *congenital adrenal hyperplasia* (the adrenals become hyperplastic because of high ACTH levels in the absence of the cortisol negative feedback).

Typical clinical and laboratory findings in hypo-adrenal states

Symptoms	Clinical signs	Laboratory tests
Weakness, fatigue	Weight loss	Hyponatraemia
Anorexia, nausea	Hyperpigmentation (not in pituitary disease)	Hyperkalaemia
Weight loss	Postural hypotension	Azotaemia
Postural faintness	Depression	Anaemia
Salt craving		Hypoglycaemia
Muscular aches		

Management involves replacement therapy with glucocorticoids and aldosterone analogues. The latter are not replaced in adrenal failure due to pituitary disease as the renin-angiotensin-aldosterone axis remains intact.

CALCIUM HOMEOSTASIS

Calcium (Ca) and phosphorus (P), together with magnesium and collagen, are the principal constituents of bone.

Ninety-nine per cent of body Ca resides in bone, and 99% of bone calcium is localized to the crystal structure of bone. The remaining 1% of body Ca is part of a rapidly exchangeable pool of which half is intracellular and half extracellular. Calcium ions are involved in cellular functions within the mitochondria and are essential for some cellular functions such as muscle contraction and endocrine and exocrine secretion. In plasma about 50% of Ca is protein bound, principally to albumin, and the remainder circulates in ionized form.

Calcium homeostasis (Fig. 4.16) is determined by four organs functioning in concert:

- parathyroid glands, which secrete *parathyroid hormone (PTH)*
- kidneys, which reabsorb Ca filtered by the glomeruli and produce the active form of vitamin D – *1,25-dihydroxy cholecalciferol (1,25D)* – both actions stimulated by PTH
- intestinal mucosa, which absorbs dietary Ca – stimulated by 1,25D
- bone – PTH stimulates bone turnover.

Regulation of PTH secretion

- Short term
  - the Ca-sensing receptor in the parathyroid cells
  - amplification of this regulation by intracellular degradation of PTH

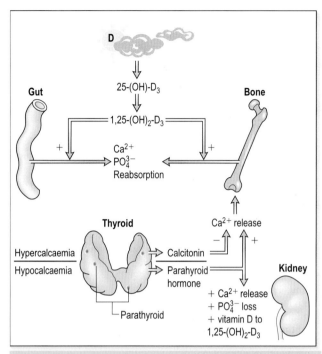

Figure 4.16. Calcium homeostasis. The actions of parathyroid hormone, calcitonin, vitamin D and its products 25-hydroxycholecalciferol (25-(OH)-D$_3$) and 1,25-dihydroxycholecalciferol (1,25-(OH)$_2$-D$_3$) on calcium homeostasis. (Reproduced with permission from Davies et al., 2001.)

  – plasma Ca concentration: a fall in ionized Ca increases PTH messenger RNA (mRNA) in the parathyroid cells.
● Long term
  – parathyroid cell regulation of PTH gene expression
  – 1,25D suppression of PTH gene transcription.

Actions of PTH
● Kidney:
  – stimulates renal tubular cell Ca reabsorption from the glomerular filtrate
  – inhibits tubular phosphate reabsorption
  – stimulates proximal tubular synthesis of 1,25D (from 25D) which in turn stimulates intestinal absorption of ingested calcium.
● Bone:
  – increases bone formation by increasing the numbers of osteoblasts and osteocytes
  – its predominant action – increases bone resorption by stimulating osteoclast formation.

Parathyroid diseases

Parathyroid gland diseases occur if there is too much PTH – *hyperparathyroidism* – or too little functioning PTH – various forms of *hypoparathyroidism*.

Hyperparathyroidism
● Parathyroid adenoma (80% of cases); caused by a clonal genetic mutation in usually one gland (parathyroid cancers are rare).
● Parathyroid polyclonal hyperplasia, occurring in all four glands.

In both these conditions the PTH secreting cells proliferate *and* are less sensitive to the negative feedback effects of a rising Ca level, resulting in *hypercalcaemia.*

Management of hyperparathyroidism is controversial. Current guidelines suggest observation in older individuals (>50 years) *provided that* the serum Ca is minimally elevated and if urinary Ca excretion and bone density are normal. All other patients should undergo parathyroidectomy.

Hypoparathyroidism: the absence of functioning PTH
● Congenital and inherited forms of inactive PTH (rare).
● Autoimmune destruction of the parathyroid glands (rare).
● PTH-Receptor abnormalities – 'pseudohypoparathyroidism' in which PTH levels are not low (rare).
● Surgical destruction of the parathyroid glands (most commonly during thyroid surgery).

Management of hypoparathyroid states: pharmacological doses of 1,25D, and calcium supplements.

Osteoporosis

Osteoporosis is defined as 'a disease characterized by low bone mass and micro-architectural deterioration, leading to enhanced bone fragility and a consequent increase in fracture risk' (US Consensus Development Conference, 1993) (Fig. 4.17). It is a very common disorder: in a recent epidemiological study 40% of women and 13% of men were at risk of osteoporotic fractures after the age of 50 years. Common sites of fracture are the spinal column, neck of femur and the wrist.

Pathogenesis of osteoporosis
● Failure to achieve optimal peak bone mass as a young adult.
● Bone loss from increased rates of bone resorption.
● Inadequate replacement of lost bone because of reduced bone formation.

Contributing causes include:

● genetic predisposition
● hypogonadism, especially premature menopause
● glucocorticoid excess: long-term pharmacological 'steroid' therapy; Cushing's syndrome
● hyperthyroidism, especially after the menopause.

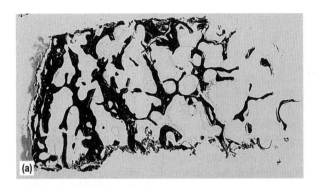

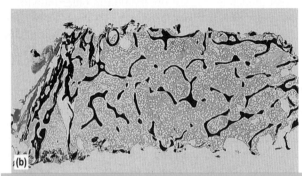

Figure 4.17.   Comparison of normal and osteoporotic bone architecture. (a) Micrograph of a resin section of a bone biopsy from the iliac crest, showing normal cortical and trabecular bone. It has been stained with a silver method, which stains calcified bone black. (b) Micrograph of bone from a patient with osteoporosis. When compared with (a), which shows bone mass of a normal patient of the same age, it is obvious that the cortical zone is narrower, and that the trabeculae are thinner and less numerous. (Reproduced with permission from Stevens and Lowe, 2000.)

Diagnosis

Osteoporosis may be diagnosed by bone densitometry; X-ray changes are seen late.

Prevention and treatment

- Nutrition – adequate dietary Ca intake.
- Exercise and the prevention of falls in the elderly.
- Hormone replacement therapy in postmenopausal women – oestrogen (and in hypogonadal men – testosterone).

- Bisphosphonates: increase bone density and reduce fracture rates.
- Calcitonin therapy.
- PTH supplements (currently under investigation).

REFERENCES AND FURTHER READING

British Medical Journal (2001) 24 February.

Davies A, Blakeley AGH, Kidd C (2001) Human Physiology. Edinburgh: Churchill Livingstone.

Dunn JT Guarding our nation's thyroid health. J Clin Endocrinol Metab 87: 486–488.

Fashauer M, Pashke R (2003) Regulation of adipocytokines and insulin resistance. Diabetologia 46: 1618–1628.

Hales CN, Ozanne SE (2003) Fetal and early postnatal growth restriction lead to diabetes, the metabolic syndrome and renal failure. Diabetologia 46: 1013–1019.

Haslett C, Chilvers ER, Boon NA, et al. (2002) Davidson's Principles and Practice of Medicine, 19th edn. Edinburgh: Churchill Livingstone.

Kahn SE, Prigeon RL, McColough DK, et al. (1993) Quantification of the relationship between insulin sensitivity and beta-cell function in human subjects. Evidence for a hyperbolic function. Diabetes 42: 1663–1672.

Mitrakou A, Kelley D, Mokan M, et al. (1992) Role of reduced suppression of glucose production and diminished early insulin release in IGT. N Engl J Med 326: 22–29.

Nishikawa T, Edelstein D, Du XL, et al. (2000) Normalizing mitochondrial superoxide production blocks three pathways of hyperglycemic damage. Nature 404: 787–790.

Pickup JC, Williams G (eds) (2003) Textbook of Diabetes. Oxford: Blackwell Publishing.

Popkin, et al. (1996) Williams Textbook of Endocrinology. Philadelphia: Saunders.

Reaven GM (ed.) (2003) Type 2 Diabetes: The Fatty Acid Story (a compendium of classic papers). Cambridge Medical Publications, UK.

Reed Larsen R, Kronenberg HM, Melmed S, Polonsky KS (eds) (2003) Williams Textbook of Endocrinology, 10th edn Philadelphia: Saunders.

Stevens A, Lowe J (2000) Pathology. Edinburgh: Mosby.

Weyer C, Bogardus C, Mott DM, et al. (1999) The natural history of insulin secretory dysfunction and insulin resistance in the pathogenesis of type 2 diabetes mellitus. J Clin Invest 104: 787–794.

WHO (1998) Obesity. Preventing and Managing the Global Epidemic. Report of a WHO Consultation on Obesity, 3–5 June, 1997. Geneva: WHO.

WHO (2003) WHO Technical Report, series 916. Diet, nutrition and the prevention of chronic diseases. Geneva: WHO.

ALTERED MOBILITY AND IMMOBILITY

Muscle and Connective Tissue – Key Concepts for Rehabilitation

Mel C. Siff (Posthumously prepared for publication by Dr Delva Shamley and Mr S. Porter)

INTRODUCTION

Healthcare professionals must possess a detailed knowledge of the properties and behaviour of skeletal muscle if they are to plan and execute the most effective rehabilitation regimes for their clients, whether that be a person on bed rest, a person with a limb in plaster cast, or an elite athlete.

In this chapter we will examine the structure and function of muscle, ligament and tendon, and how these tissues respond to rehabilitation. Throughout the chapter, valuable practice points are highlighted.

Muscle integrity may be affected by many disorders, such as muscular dystrophy, cerebral palsy, central nervous problems, other neuromuscular diseases or local muscle infection (see Ch. 6). Injury in the physical activity setting, including all manual tasks, recreation and sports training, may be due to either biomechanical or physiological causes, including tissue deterioration, inherent tissue weakness, fatigue, accident or inefficiency of movement. This chapter will discuss the structure and function of the soft tissues involved with producing mobility and stability, then deducing how this information can be used to enhance the rehabilitation process.

In addressing the issue of muscle rehabilitation, all components of the muscle complex and other components of the musculoskeletal system involved in human movement must be considered. For example, all movements, especially those executed at high speed, depend on the storage and release of elastic energy from the tendons. Moreover, passive stability, flexibility and protection of the joints depends on the integrity of the ligaments and other connective tissues around the joint. These provide a structural framework for the muscles and a network of connections between many parts of the musculoskeletal system, which both stabilizes and transmits forces throughout the body.

STRUCTURE AND FUNCTION OF THE MUSCLE COMPLEX

We cannot discuss muscle action or rehabilitation without considering the normal structure of muscle and the connective tissues associated with muscle (Fig. 5.1). Any model of muscle structure and function needs to be a complex one which includes both the contractile and the non-contractile tissues. This is vital because some muscle disorders may involve deterioration of or damage to the connective tissues associated with muscle. These tissues occur in the form of sheaths around muscle (epimysium) and its subunits (perimysium, sarcolemma) at all levels, and as tendons at the ends of muscles. Not only do they protect, connect and enclose muscle tissue, but they play a vital role in determining the range of joint movement (i.e. flexibility), and improving the efficiency of movement by providing essential damping of vibration, as well as storing and releasing elastic energy derived from muscle contraction.

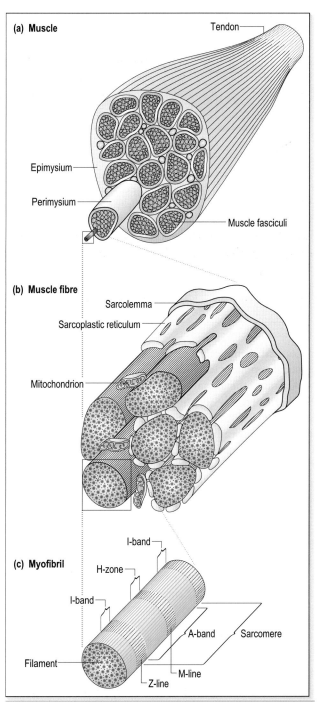

Figure 5.1.   The parts of a muscle. The component parts of a voluntary muscle, from the functional units (myofibrils) to the epimysium which contains the whole muscle and is continuous with the tendons of origin and insertion. (a) Muscle. (b) Muscle fibre (cell). (c) Myofibril. (Reproduced with permission from Davies et al., 2001.)

All muscle comprises a contractile component, the actin–myosin system, and a non-contractile component, the connective tissue. In mechanical terms, muscle may be analysed further in terms of a contractile component in series with a

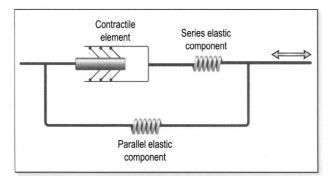

Figure 5.2.   A physical model of the components of skeletal muscle. The model shows the contractile element made up of actin and myosin and the elastic components which explain the behaviour of a whole muscle. Although the elastic components are shown outside the contractile element, a substantial proportion of both resides within the contractile mechanism. (Reproduced with permission from Davies et al., 2001.)

series elastic component (SEC) and in parallel with a parallel elastic component (PEC), as illustrated in Figure 5.2.

Although the anatomical location of these elements has not been precisely identified, the PEC probably comprises sarcolemma, rest-state cross-bridging (Fig. 5.3), and tissues such as the sheaths around the muscle and its subunits. On the other hand, the SEC is considered to include tendon, the cross-bridges, myofilaments and the Z-discs. Of these elements, the myofilaments apparently provide the greatest contribution to the SEC. The PEC is responsible for the force exerted by a relaxed muscle when it is stretched beyond its resting length, whereas the SEC is put under tension by the force developed in actively contracted muscle. The mechanical energy stored by the PEC is small and contributes little to the energy balance of exercise. Considerable storage of energy occurs in the SEC, since an actively contracted muscle resists stretching with great force, particularly if the stretching is imposed rapidly.

Muscle fibres can also stretch passively and store elastic energy, like tendons. In this respect, the myosin cross-bridges that are considered to pull the actin filaments between the myosin filaments during muscle contraction are known to be compliant structures which may stretch considerably before they detach from the activated sites on the actin filaments. It is believed that this compliance may be caused by rotation of the meromyosin heads of the cross-bridges and by elongation of its tail, which appears to have a helical structure that would promote extensibility (Figs 5.4 and 5.5). In other words, even a contracted muscle can stretch, not only due to its collagenous component, but also due to its contractile tissue. Thus, we can see that the traditional advice to impose stretch only on relaxed muscles may be seen to be misplaced if the goal is also to stretch contractile elements in the muscle,

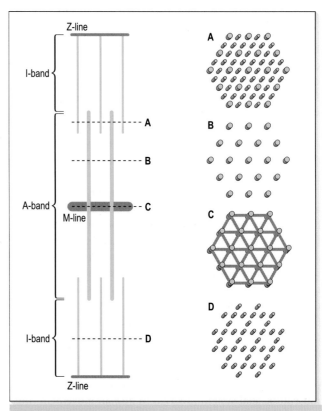

Figure 5.3.   Structure of a sarcomere. Longitudinal (left) and cross-sectional (right) diagrams showing the arrangement of actin (thin) and myosin (thick) filaments. The light and dark bands of a sarcomere, extending between two Z-lines, are the result of the presence of: actin filaments only (I-band; section D); actin and myosin filaments (A-band; section A); myosin filaments only (H-zone; section B). (Reproduced with permission from Davies et al., 2001.)

which should be part of the process of all-round muscle rehabilitation.

COLLAGENOUS TISSUE

Connective tissues comprise essentially three types of fibres, namely collagen, elastin and reticulin, with the former two fibres constituting approximately 90% of the whole. The collagen fibres (of which there are at least 10 distinct types) impart strength and stiffness to the tissue, elastin provides compliance or extensibility under loading, and reticulin furnishes bulk. The elastic fibres occur in small concentrations in the intercellular matrix of tendons and most ligaments, but their function is not entirely clear. It has been suggested that they may play a role in restoring the crimped collagen fibre configuration after stretching or muscle contraction. The response of collagenous tissue to mechanical stress depends on the structural orientation of the fibres, the properties of the

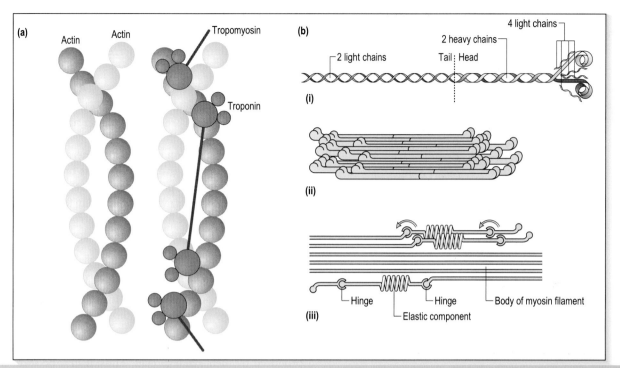

Figure 5.4.   Filaments. (a) The actin 'thin filament' consists of a 1 μm long double-stranded helix of F-actin made up of molecules of G-actin with strands of tropomyosin stretched between troponin complexes covering units of 7G-actin molecules. Ca^{2+} interacts with the troponin complex to alter the configuration of tropomyosin and allow the bridging of actin and myosin. (b) The myosin 'thick filament' is 1.5 μm long and 15 nm diameter. It is made up of about 200 myosin molecules shaped like golf clubs with double heads. (i) Each myosin molecule consists of a tail of two coiled peptide chains of 'light meromyosin' and a head of two units of 'heavy meromyosin' and four light chains which exert regulatory functions. The ATPase activity of the molecule appears to be concentrated in the head. (ii) The myosin molecules are set in the filament with their tails toward the centre so that the heads are concentrated towards two ends leaving the centre portion bare. (iii) It is suggested that there are two 'hinges' in the molecule, one where the light and heavy meromyosin of the tail meet and one below the head. The light meromyosin of the tail is thought to be fixed to the body of the thick filament and the heavy component of the tail can tilt out to allow the head to engage the actin filament. (Reproduced with permission from Davies et al., 2001.)

collagen and elastin fibres, and the relative proportions of collagen and elastin.

In particular, the tendon fibres are closely packed and virtually parallel, but for a slight waviness in the relaxed state.

This simplicity of structure suffices for tendon, since the latter usually has to transmit forces linearly from one point to another. In ligaments and joint capsules the fibre organization, though still generally parallel, is less uniform and often oblique or spiral, its exact structure depending on the function of the particular ligament. Most ligaments are purely collagenous, the only elastin fibres being those associated with the blood vessels. Virtually the only ligaments that are mostly elastin are the ligamentum flavum of the human spine and the ligamentum nuchae of the cervical spine, both of which are composed of about two-thirds elastin fibres and therefore display almost completely elastic behaviour. Permanent deformation of such ligaments by traditional stretches, therefore, would be unlikely. In general, the structure of ligament has to be more complex than that of tendon, because joint ligaments have

to control forces over a larger number of degrees of freedom. Thus, the conditioning, rehabilitation and stretching of ligaments require a more extensive variety of techniques, which involve both linear, rotational and spiral patterns of action.

The structure and function of ligaments and tendons

Both ligaments and tendons are similar in the manner in which their structures gradually alter as they approach their attachment sites to bone. For instance, the transition from ligament to bone is gradual, with rows of fibrocytes in the ligament transforming into groups of osteocytes, then gradually dispersing into the bone matrix by way of an intermediate stage in which the cells resemble chondrocytes. Some authorities have divided the insertion region of ligament into four zones (Fig. 5.6):

● the collagen fibres at the end of the ligament (zone 1) intermesh with

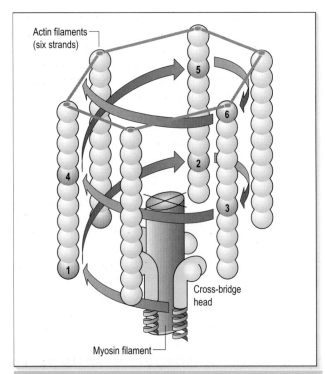

Actin filaments (six strands)

5

6

4

2

3

1

Cross-bridge head

Myosin filament

Figure 5.5. A myosin head 'climbing' its six actin filaments. The myosin cross-bridge binds with alternate actin filaments of the six that surround its myosin filament. The cross-bridges on the myosin come in pairs at 180° to each other (like a nail driven right through a rod of wood), at 14.3 nm intervals along the filament, and with each pair turned through 120°. Therefore, in a straight line along the myosin filament, cross-bridges occur directly underneath each other at every third interval ($3 \times 14.3 = 42.9$ nm). (Reproduced with permission from Davies et al., 2001.)

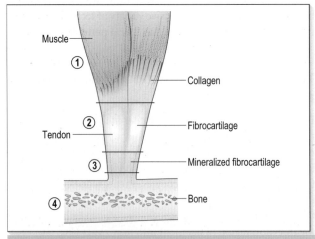

Muscle

①

Collagen

Tendon

②

Fibrocartilage

③

Mineralized fibrocartilage

④

Bone

Figure 5.6. The structural transition of typical collagenous tissue to bone.

- fibrocartilage (zone 2), which gradually becomes
- mineralized fibrocartilage (zone 3), and
- the latter complex finally merges with cortical bone (zone 4).

Thus, the stress concentration at the insertion of the ligament into the more rigid bone structure is decreased by the existence of these three progressively stiffer transitional composite materials.

Transition from tendon into bone is generally not quite as distinct as in ligament, and tendon inserts broadly into the main fibrous layer of the periosteum. Nevertheless, as in ligaments, the same type of gradual transition in four zones from collagen to bone may be identified. This structure, as before, minimizes the detrimental effects of sudden stretching or loading which would occur if there were abrupt transitions from muscle to collagen and then to bone.

Whereas ligaments are often closely associated with joint capsules, tendons occur in two basic forms: those with sheaths (called paratenons) and others without sheaths. Sheaths generally surround tendons where large frictional forces are found and provide lubrication by means of synovial fluid produced by their synovial cells. Thus, it may be seen that tendons with sheaths have a larger PEC than unsheathed tendons and any stretching in the relaxed state will probably have a greater effect on the sheath. The tendon itself comprises primarily the SEC, which is tensed only when its attendant muscle is active. This again emphasizes that different conditioning and stretching techniques are necessary for enhancing the strength and extensibility of the different tissues.

Some research has indicated that the long-term use of anabolic-androgenic steroids (AAS) may compromise the relative strengths of these various zones and thereby increase the likelihood of tissue rupture. Similar problems may occur if any corticosteroids are injected near the musculotendinous transition zones, because, if they fail to enter the paratenon, as stipulated by standard procedure, and instead are injected outside this region or diffuse into the neighbouring transition zones, the tendon may be severely weakened or damaged.

Loading of collagenous tissue

Since stretching is a particular type of mechanical loading, application of stretching can be more effectively applied if the effects of loading on collagen are studied carefully. In fact, physiological stretching is possible because collagen is a viscoelastic material; that is, under rapid loading it behaves elastically, while under gradual loading it is viscous and can deform plastically.

At slow loading rates, the bony insertion of a ligament is the weakest component of the ligament–bone complex, whereas the ligament is the weakest component at very fast loading rates. These results imply that, with an increase in loading rate, the strength of bone (which also contains collagen) increases more than the strength of the ligament. Of added relevance is the finding that the tensile strength of healthy tendon can be more than twice the strength of its associated muscle, which explains why ruptures are more common in muscle than in tendon. These facts are directly relevant to appreciating the difference between static, passive and ballistic modes of stretching, with slow and rapid loading rates having different effects on each of the soft tissues of the body.

Despite the widespread opinion that the muscles act as efficient synergistic stabilizers, it should be remembered that the musculature cannot respond quickly enough to protect a joint against injury if large impacts are applied rapidly, particularly if they are torsional. Since joint stability involves three-dimensional actions over several degrees of freedom, the necessity for appropriately conditioning all the interacting soft tissues becomes obvious. Moreover, muscle rehabilitation will be seen to be incomplete unless loading to enhance tissue structure is also accompanied by concurrent neuromuscular rehabilitation which improves the ability of the nervous system to produce and control muscle action. This more integrated approach to rehabilitation will also improve reaction times, motor decision-making skills, and other psychophysiological factors which enable the body to produce efficient stabilizing and mobilizing muscle actions. Joint stabilization and flexibility are discussed in greater detail later.

The role of stored elastic energy

It has been found that the energy cost of running for animals with heavy limbs is about the same as those with light limbs. This is the case because much of the energy involved is stored from step to step as elastic energy in the tendons. Throughout this process there is significant change in length of the tendons, but not in the muscle itself.

Considerable storage of energy can occur in the SEC during dynamic exercise, since an actively contracted muscle resists stretching with great force, particularly if the stretching is imposed rapidly. The tendons play a major role in storing this energy. The traditional view of tendons serving to attach muscle to bone presents only part of the picture. Tendons, together with other series elastic components, particularly after termination of powerful isometric or eccentric contractions, play a vital role in storing elastic energy during locomotion and other motor acts, thereby saving energy and increasing muscular efficiency. For example, it has been found that much of the muscle activity in running is associated with tensioning of the tendons, which thereby store energy for successive cycles of movement. This tensioning or rewinding of the tendon fibres by largely isometric muscle contractions is achieved with very little change in the length of the muscle fibres themselves. The fact that the forces involved are derived mainly from isometric contractions means a decreased energy expenditure because isometric contractions thermodynamically are considerably less expensive than dynamic contractions. For these reasons, it is important that any stretching manoeuvres or medications do not compromise the strength or ability of the tendons to store elastic energy throughout their range of movement. This implies again that tendon stretching exercises should be accompanied by strength conditioning against adequate resistance. Similarly, ligaments should not be overstretched to the point of diminished joint stability.

The ability to use stored elastic energy depends on:

1. the velocity of stretching
2. the magnitude of the stretch and
3. the duration of the transition between termination of the eccentric and initiation of the concentric phases of the movement. This delay between the two phases should be minimal or the stored elastic energy will be rapidly dissipated, because a more prolonged delay will allow fewer cross-bridges to remain attached after the stretch. The increase in positive work associated with rapid eccentric-concentric (or plyometric) contractions is usually attributed to the storage and utilization of elastic energy, but some of this enhanced work output is probably caused by preloading (or prestretch) of the muscle complex. This is due to the fact that, during an impulsive eccentric–concentric action, the tension at the beginning of the concentric contraction is much greater than if the contraction had started from rest.

Studies of the mechanical and biochemical properties of tendon reveal a close relationship between tensile strength and the amount of collagen. Similarly, the concentration of total collagen is higher for slow muscle than for fast muscle. This difference also appears at the level of individual muscle fibres, with the concentration of collagen in slow twitch fibres being twice that in fast twitch fibres. The type, structure and amount of collagen determine the tensile properties of collagenous tissues. There are at least ten distinct types of collagen, each with a different chain composition and occurring in various forms in different subsystems of the body. At a microscopic level, the characteristic mechanical strength of collagen depends largely on the cross-links between the collagen molecules. It has been shown that the type of exercise can affect the properties of muscle (Fig. 5.7), a fact which relates to these collagen cross-links, rather than merely to the actin–myosin complex. For example, muscle endurance training increases the tensile strength of both slow and fast muscles, as well as the elasticity of the former. Prolonged endurance activity such as running also increases the concentration of collagen in tendon and the ultimate tensile strength of tendon. This finding is most relevant to the prescription of all rehabilitative exercise.

In contrast with this finding, the concentration of collagen in muscle is not altered by muscle endurance training. However, the increase in elasticity and tensile strength of the more collagenous slow muscles after exercise suggests that

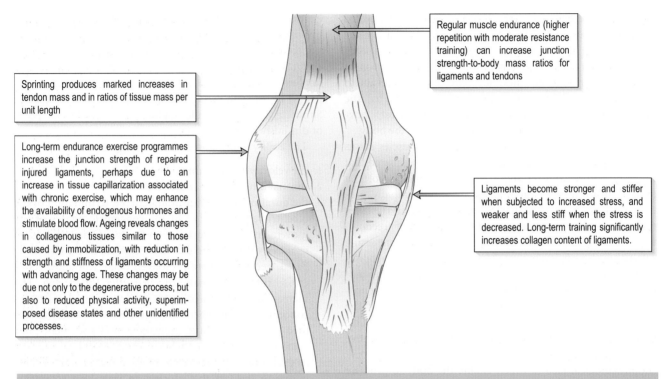

Sprinting produces marked increases in tendon mass and in ratios of tissue mass per unit length

Long-term endurance exercise programmes increase the junction strength of repaired injured ligaments, perhaps due to an increase in tissue capillarization associated with chronic exercise, which may enhance the availability of endogenous hormones and stimulate blood flow. Ageing reveals changes in collagenous tissues similar to those caused by immobilization, with reduction in strength and stiffness of ligaments occurring with advancing age. These changes may be due not only to the degenerative process, but also to reduced physical activity, superimposed disease states and other unidentified processes.

Regular muscle endurance (higher repetition with moderate resistance training) can increase junction strength-to-body mass ratios for ligaments and tendons

Ligaments become stronger and stiffer when subjected to increased stress, and weaker and less stiff when the stress is decreased. Long-term training significantly increases collagen content of ligaments.

Figure 5.7.   Some effects of exercise or inactivity on the connective or collagenous tissues.

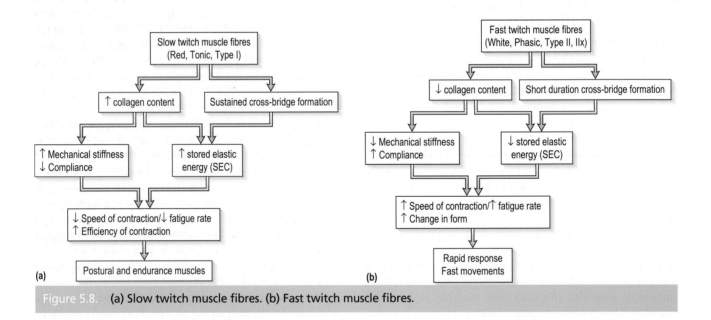

Figure 5.8.   (a) Slow twitch muscle fibres. (b) Fast twitch muscle fibres.

collagen must undergo some structural changes. In this respect, it is possible that these changes in the mechanical properties of slow muscles are related to stabilization of the reducible cross-links of collagen. With specific reference to muscle tissue, it has been proposed that slow twitch (ST) fibres may be able to sustain cross-bridge attachments for a longer period than fast twitch (FT) fibres. Therefore, the former would utilize the elastic energy stored in their cross-bridges more efficiently during slow movements. In addition, this process may be augmented by the behaviour of the connective tissue in each given muscle in determining the ability of the slow and fast muscles to perform different types of work. Slow muscles with their greater content of strongly cross-linked collagen would then be more adapted to slow contraction, since the fairly rigid collagenous connective tissue would resist fast contraction. The less rigid connective tissue in fast muscle, on the other hand, would facilitate fast movements with greater changes in form. The differences noted in the collagenous components of different muscle types could also imply that a slow muscle can store relatively more elastic energy in its collagenous tissue than fast muscle, thereby explaining the efficiency of slow muscle in postural and endurance tasks (Fig. 5.8a and b). This research into the structure and function of muscle fibre stresses that all-round rehabilitation necessitates the use of a wide variety of concurrent and sequential slow, rapid and ballistic, endurance and non-endurance exercises chosen to condition the different types of muscle fibre and connective tissue.

TYPES OF MUSCLE FIBRE

Muscle fibres may be classified in terms of factors such as colour, contractile properties, content of myoglobin (the pigment which binds oxygen in the blood, relative content of metabolic enzymes, and the content of mitochondria.

Slow and fast twitch muscle fibres

Earlier we discussed the actin and myosin components of muscle. We now note that the myosin plays a special role in determining the contractile characteristics of the muscle via one of its specific components, namely the myosin heavy chain (MHC). This chain appears in three different varieties or isoforms, referred to as type I, IIa and IIx isoforms, as are the muscles fibres which contain them (i.e. I, IIa and IIx). Type I fibres are also referred to as slow fibres, while the other two fibres are known as fast fibres, because the latter contract far more rapidly than the former (type IIx fibres contract approximately 10 times faster than type I fibres, with the contraction velocity of IIa fibres lying intermediate to types I and IIx).

The type I, IIa and IIx fibres, or pure fibres, are not the only form in which the various isoforms express themselves: there are also hybrid fibre types, which contain mixtures of slow and fast myosin isoforms. Interestingly, these hybrid fibres are scarce in young people, with vastus lateralis studies showing that the latter exhibit less than 5% of this variety. On the other hand, in older adults this value rises to over 30% and hybrid fibre becomes the dominant fibre type in very old adults.

All muscle fibres appear to lie on a continuum, which extends between the slow contracting, slow fatiguing fibres at one extreme and the fast contracting, fast fatiguing fibres at the other. Most classification schemes refer to these extremes as type I red, slow twitch (ST) fibres and type II white, fast twitch (FT) fibres, where the difference in colour is due to the fact that red fibres have a higher content of myoglobin. Since slow fibres rely largely on aerobic metabolism and fast fibres depend more on anaerobic metabolism, low intensity endurance activities are heavily reliant on a large percentage of slow fibres, and high intensity, short duration or strength activities require a large percentage of fast fibres. In general, ST (type I) fibres are slow contracting, slow fatiguing reddish fibres with a small diameter, high oxidative capacity and low glycolytic capacity (ability to rely on stored glycogen as an energy source for resynthesizing ATP). They are efficient in maintaining posture and sustaining prolonged, low intensity activity such as distance running, particularly since they usually contain a large number of mitochondria and use ATP slowly. These fibres may be tonically or phasically active for prolonged periods, being known to fire at fairly low rates for as much as 20–35% of the day.

FT (type II) fibres have usually been subdivided into several subclasses, the most frequently mentioned being FTa (type IIa) and FTb (type IIb or IIx in humans). Type IIa (FTa) fibres are also called fast twitch, oxidative-glycolytic (FTOG), since they are able to draw on oxidative and glycolytic mechanisms for energy. They are apparently suited to fast, repetitive, low intensity movement and are recruited next after type I (ST) fibres. They possess fairly large numbers of mitochondria and therefore tend to be reasonably resistant to fatigue and can recover fairly rapidly after exercise. Some authorities believe that the type IIa (FT) fibres are adapted for endurance activity. In the world of sport, bodybuilders often tend to have a high relative percentage of these fibres, which has led some researchers to propose that these fibres may be especially able to adapt to hypertrophy in response to suitable training stimuli.

Type IIx (IIb or FTb) fibres are fast contracting, whitish, low myoglobin fibres with a large diameter, high glycolytic capacity, low oxidative capacity and few mitochondria. They are suited to high power output and are usually recruited only where very rapid or very intense effort is required, as in field athletics and weightlifting, where athletes in these sports exhibit high percentages of these fibres. They fatigue rapidly and replenish their energy supplies mainly after exercise has ceased. (The properties of muscle fibre types are summarized in Table 5.1.)

Some controversy still surrounds skeletal muscle fibre nomenclature and classification (see the next section, 'Muscle protein isoforms'). For instance, the slow twitch fibres have been subdivided into types I and Ic, while the fast twitch fibre population has been subdivided into types IIa, IIb, IIc and even types IIab and IIac to form part of an entire fibre continuum. The possible transformation between fibre types or characteristics by specific types of exercise is currently an area of prolific research. Every muscle group contains a different ratio between fast and slow twitch fibres, depending on their function and training history. For example, muscles such as the soleus of the calf usually have a higher content of

Table 5.1.   Properties of muscle fibre types

II (slow twitch)	IIa (FTa) Also known as fast twitch oxidative glycolytic (FTOG)	IIx (FTb)
Slow contracting	Suited to fast, repetitive low intensity movement Recruited after type I fibres	Fast contracting
Slow fatiguing Reddish in colour	Fatigue resistant (high numbers of mitochondria); recover rapidly after exercise	Fatigue rapidly Whitish colour, low myoglobin
Small diameter High oxidative capacity Low glycolytic capacity Phasically or tonically active for 20–35% of the day	High proportions found in bodybuilders may be especially able to hypertrophy	Large diameter Low oxidative capacity High glycolytic capacity Suited to high power output recruited in weight lifting
Useful in maintaining posture		

ST fibres than gastrocnemius, whereas the arm triceps generally have a higher proportion of FT fibres.

Muscle fibres usually tend to be surrounded by fibres of a different type rather than concentrating in the immediate neighbourhood of one other. The superficial layers of muscle tend to contain a greater percentage of faster fibres, whereas slower fibres seem to predominate in the deep muscle layers. It has been suggested that the separation of muscle fibre types in the same and different layers of muscle may enhance mechanical efficiency during demanding activities. Interestingly, as one grows older, type II fast twitch fibres seem to preferentially atrophy, but it is not yet known whether this is due to physical inactivity or biological ageing. The responsiveness of these fast fibres to strength training supports the value of this type of exercise and rehabilitation to older adults. Recent technological advances have facilitated research into the microstructure of muscles, with analysis focusing on the adequacy of the original sliding filament model, the cross-bridging process and the structure of the actin and myosin subunits. The myosin molecule has now been recognized as comprising several different heavy myosin chains (MHC) and several light myosin chains (MLC), each chain consisting of various polypeptides. Other work has suggested that there may not just be a single binding state between the actin and myosin filaments, but there may be distinct weak and strong binding states, with the myosin powerstroke being driven by the release of a strained linear elastic element.

Muscle protein isoforms

All muscle fibres contract according to the same cross-bridging or sliding filament action. The distinction between the different fibres lies in the rate at which cross-bridging occurs and their ability to sustain a cross-bridging cycle. Cross-bridging takes place far more rapidly and consumes more ATP in fast twitch muscle fibres than in slow, postural muscles. Apparently, the difference in response between fibres lies in the diversity of forms in which muscle fibre is synthesized. Instead of occurring in one identical form for all muscle fibres, many of the protein building-blocks of muscle exist in a variety of subtly different forms, known as protein isoforms. Research reveals that a muscle will manifest itself as 'slow' or 'fast' on the basis of precisely which protein isoforms it is manufacturing, in particular which isoform of the heavy myosin filament is being formed. The role of the myosin is very important, not only because of its size, but also because of its diversity of function. Besides providing muscle fibres with cross-bridges, it also reacts with ATP to harness the energy released by the mitochondria for contraction. Geneticists have discovered that different members of the myosin gene family are activated at different stages of human development from embryo to adult. The reason for this is not yet known, but the fact that embryonic muscle continues to grow in the absence of contraction or mechanical stimulation suggests at least one hypothesis. It is possible that the embryonic form of the myosin heavy chain liberates muscle fibres from dependency on mechanical stimulation for growth. Evidence for this proposal comes from the observation that the cells of damaged muscle fibres revert to synthesizing the embryonic form of the myosin protein in an apparent attempt to assist in tissue repair.

Four myosin heavy chain (MHC) isoforms, MHC I, MHC IIa, MHC IIb, and MHC IId(x), have been identified in small mammals and are regarded as the building blocks of the histochemically defined muscle fibre types I, IIa, IIb, IId(x) respectively. These fibres express only one MHC isoform and are called pure fibre types. Hybrid fibres expressing two

MHC isoforms are regarded as hybrid or transitional fibres between the different pure fibre types. The existence of pure and hybrid fibres even in normal muscles under steady state conditions creates a wide spectrum of possible fibre types. The variety of fibre types is even greater when myosin light chains are taken into account. A large number of isomyosins result from the combinations of various myosin light and heavy chain isoforms, thereby further increasing the diversity of muscle fibres. As shown by comparative studies, different fibre types vary in a muscle-specific and a species-specific manner. Furthermore, research has shown that the previously classified IIb muscle fibres in human muscle should more accurately be classified as IIx fibres, with the analogous IIb fibres being present in species other than humans.

Genetic mechanisms and plasticity

The laboratory of Goldspink and others have found several members of the sarcomeric myosin heavy chain (MHC) gene family in the human genome, but many of them have not yet been identified. The distribution of beta/slow, IIa, and IIx MHC transcripts defines three major muscle fibre types – either beta/slow, IIa, or IIx MHC mRNA, and two populations of hybrid fibres co-expressing beta/slow with IIa or IIa with IIx MHC mRNA. Fibre typing by histochemistry shows that IIa MHC transcripts are more abundant in histochemical type IIa fibres, whereas IIx MHC transcripts are more abundant in histochemical type IIb fibres. The IIa, IIx and IIb MHCs were first detected in the muscles of newborn babies, with their expression in developing and adult muscle being regulated by neural, hormonal and mechanical factors. The functional role of MHC isoforms has been in part clarified by biochemical-physiological studies on single-skinned fibres which indicate that both MHC and MLC isoforms determine the maximum velocity of shortening of skeletal muscle fibres. The existence of numerous forms of the myosin chain endows muscle fibres with an inherent plasticity, thereby enabling them to modify their myofibrils to produce muscles with different contractile properties. Unlike other genes, which are generally switched on and off by the indirect action of signalling molecules such as hormones or growth factors, muscle genes are regulated largely by mechanical stimulation.

Passive stretching and electrical stimulation separately have only a mild effect on the myosin genes, but together they virtually halt synthesis of the fast myosin chain, thereby reprogramming fast twitch muscles to express themselves as slow twitch muscles. Immobilization has been shown to cause the normally slow twitching soleus muscle to become fast twitching: apparently it requires repeated stretching to sustain synthesis of the slow myosin chain. In other words, the 'default' option for muscles seems to be the fast myosin chain. Moreover, training apparently can alter the contractile properties of muscle by modifying one type of fibre to act like or become another type of fibre or by enhancing the selective growth of a particular fibre type.

MUSCLE FIBRES AND EXERCISE

Fibre types

Fibre types differ considerably between individuals, especially between endurance and strength athletes. For instance, vastus medialis biopsies reveal that the proportion of FT fibres in field athletes and weightlifters can be over three times (i.e. over 60% FT fibres) greater than that of marathon runners (approximately 17% FT fibres) and 50% greater than that of bodybuilders, cyclists and race walkers (all about 40% FT fibres). The importance of fast fibres in short duration explosive or maximal strength efforts is underscored by the fact that fast type IIx fibres contract 10 times faster than slow type I fibres.

Although research indicates that fibre distribution is strongly determined by genetic factors, it appears as if these differences may also be strongly influenced by the type, intensity and duration of training, as well as the pre-training status of the individual.

Near-maximal and explosive resistance exercise also produces greater hypertrophy of FT fibres than ST fibres. In this respect it is noteworthy that maximal muscle power output and potential for explosive movement is determined strongly by the proportion of FT fibres in the relevant muscles. Moreover, endurance training reduces vertical jump power, explosive speed and similar FT fibre activities, possibly because endurance training may degrade FT fibres, replace them with ST fibres or cause enzymatic and neuromuscular changes more appropriate to slow endurance activities.

Heavy resistance training causes a decrease in the percentage of type IIx/b and an increase in the percentage of type IIa fibres in vastus lateralis, suggesting that resistance training had caused transformation among the fast twitch fibre subtypes. This is confirmed by the fact that neither MHC I composition nor type I muscle fibre percentage changes with training. In addition to this, heavy resistance training enlarges type II fast twitch fibres twice as much as in slow fibres, which shows that strength training can increase the relative cross-sectional area of FT fibres without increasing the relative proportion of FT fibres in the muscle. Since the velocity of muscle contraction depends on the area covered by fast fibres, we may use intense strength training to increase strength and power, even if we cannot change the actual proportion of fast fibres in the muscles.

Another interesting finding is that, after a period of resistance training, MHC IIx content decreased from 9.3% to 2.0%, with a corresponding increase in MHC IIa from 42.4% to 49.6%. After a detraining period of 3 months, the amount of MHC IIx reached values that were 17% higher than before and after resistance training, revealing what the researchers call MHC IIx overshoot. This seems to suggest that, if we wish to increase the relative amount of fast muscle fibre isoforms, a logical method would be to decrease the training load and allow the fastest fibres to express themselves a few weeks later. This finding appears to lend some support to the practice of training 'tapering' that has been implemented for many years among strength and sprint athletes.

Some researchers have suggested that there may be an optimal or maximum size for individual muscle fibres undergoing training hypertrophy, since efficiency of strength, power and work production decreases if muscle cross-sectional area is too small or too large. The existence of possible optimal fibre size, the limited ability of advanced athletes to experience muscle hypertrophy and the lack of correlation between hypertrophy and strength gain stresses the futility of prescribing hypertrophy training for highly qualified athletes. This may be suitable for rehabilitation of novices or non-athletes, but its regular use may be detrimental to the strength and power development of elite athletes.

There is also considerable evidence to indicate that cardiovascular ('aerobic') endurance exercise performed at low intensity for long periods during the same stage of a conditioning programme as strength training seriously compromises the development of strength and power. This is probably partly due to the fact that it is relatively easy for the faster twitching fibres to become or behave like slow twitch fibres with prolonged low intensity training. Furthermore, studies of the gastrocnemius muscles of distance runners have shown that prolonged distance training produces muscle necrosis and inflammation, which can be detected at least 7 days after a marathon. Comparative muscle biopsy studies of weightlifters, sprinters and rowers after strenuous training sessions do not show any of these abnormalities. These findings have important ramifications for the design of sport-specific rehabilitation programmes, since some therapists and machine manufacturers maintain that continuous circuit training (CCT) regimes simultaneously develop cardiovascular endurance and strength. Research does not support this belief. On the contrary, it shows that it is more appropriate to prescribe cardiovascular exercise separately in limited amounts during the early off-season and high intensity resistance exercise at a later stage. In addition, interval circuit training (ICT) using high intensity loading and regular rest intervals is more suitable for development of strength and strength-endurance.

Fibre recruitment

The sequence of recruitment of muscle fibres by exercise also has important consequences for rehabilitation. The ST (type I) fibres are recruited first for muscle tensions up to about 25%, the FTa (type IIa) are recruited next and type IIx fibres last, as the intensity of the activity increases towards a maximum or as the ST fibres become seriously energy depleted (Fig. 5.9). Therefore, if the intention is to train FT fibres for a particular form of physical activity or sport, it is vital that high intensity training be concentrated upon.

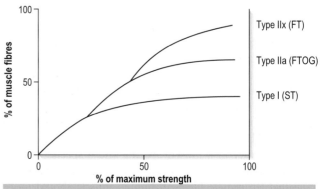

Figure 5.9.   Dependence of the recruitment sequence of the different muscle fibres on intensity of exercise.

Further research reveals that this high intensity is not necessarily dependent on the use of maximal or near-maximal loads, but the degree to which the relevant muscle fibres are recruited during the effort. In this respect, the terms fast twitch and slow twitch do not necessarily mean that fast movements recruit exclusively FT fibres and slow movements ST fibres. To analyse the involvement of different fibre types, it is vital to determine the force that needs to be produced. If large acceleration of the load is involved, Newton's second law of motion decrees that the resulting force will be large. Thus, the maximal force generated during rapid acceleration of a 100 kg load can easily exceed the maximal force produced during a slowly accelerated 150 kg load for the same exercise. Both a small load accelerated rapidly and a heavy load accelerated slowly, strongly involve the FT fibres. Likewise, explosive movements rely heavily on the action of FT fibres.

Moreover, rapid movements often recruit the muscle stretch (myotatic) reflex, which can elicit a powerful contraction. Relevant to this process is Starling's law, which states that the strength of contraction is proportional to the original length of the muscle at the moment of contraction. The ideal relationship between tension and length in a sarcomere occurs when the muscle is slightly stretched and the actin and myosin filaments just overlap slightly. However, in applying this law, it has to be remembered that the advantage offered by the stretching may be diminished in cases where this stretching occurs at large joint angles, which provide poor leverage. The well-known prestretch principle in proprioceptive neuromuscular facilitation (PNF), bodybuilding training and many throwing, kicking, lifting and thrusting movements in sport relies on this phenomenon. Many exercise machines are seriously limiting in that they do not allow the user to begin a movement with a prestretch. Not only does this diminish the force which can be generated, but it also exposes joints to a greater risk of injury, because the movement begins without muscular assistance for the ligaments.

The development of strength is related to the number of appropriate muscle fibres firing simultaneously, which is entirely a function of the nervous system. An additional finding is that, if the nerve which normally supplies an ST muscle fibre is surgically interchanged ('cross reinnervated') with one which supplies an FT fibre, the ST fibre will behave like an FT fibre. These studies, carried out on rabbits, suggest that sensitivity to motor innervation increases from the glycolytic to oxidative types of fibre, in the order: IIb > IIx/IId > IIa > I (where the IId, like the IIb fibre types, occur in small mammals as analogues of the human IIx type). In other words, the behaviour of muscle would appear to be determined by the activity of the nerve fibres that supply it. This is discussed further in the next section.

The rate and number of fibres firing depends on voluntary and involuntary processes, the voluntary ones being related to personal motivation and biofeedback techniques, and the involuntary ones to feedback information from the proprioceptive system, including the various stretch reflexes. Thus, the simple act of motivating or emotionally willing oneself, through methods such as self-talk or guided imagery, to produce greater or faster efforts can recruit a greater number of muscle fibres at an increased rate of firing. Encouragement by the therapist can also play a useful role in this regard, if done at appropriate stages during rehabilitation. Interestingly, the method of training with progressively heavier loads or at larger accelerations is a valuable way of learning how to motivate oneself at progressively higher levels of performance. The carry-over of this may well benefit one in all aspects of daily life.

Further aspects of muscle plasticity

Ongoing research is investigating the plasticity, or structural-functional change, of muscle in response to various conditions, such as active and passive loading, different types of neural activation, lack of loading and electrical stimulation. Some of this work has been reported elsewhere in this chapter, but it is relevant to include some further information on other recent findings in this regard.

Neural activation

One of the prominent hypotheses is that the pattern of neural activation determines the quantity and quality of contractile proteins (myosin and actin isoforms) and metabolic proteins (glycolytic and oxidative enzymes) which the muscles express. This thesis emerged from studies which showed that typical FT muscle after very prolonged daily low frequency stimulation (24 hours a day) produces physiological, biochemical and structural changes which resemble those found in ST. The neural influence on muscle speed may not only be exerted by nerve impulses, but may also be due to neural growth processes associated with hormonal factors (e.g. thyroid hormone and testosterone).

Hormonal activation

Hormonal effects generally seem to depend on the type and level of activity of the muscle fibres involved. The muscle fibre types involved in the anabolic properties of oestrogens have not yet been clearly described, but in the case of growth hormone and insulin, mainly the ST type is affected, partly via an increased secretion of somatomedins (insulin-like growth factors – IGFs) or by interaction on IGF receptors. The other hormones in the body tend to produce a shift toward more vigorous fast contracting activity, which increases the percentage of fast glycolytic fibres. Anabolic hormones such as the androgens, catecholamines and beta-agonists enlarge these fibres, whereas excess quantities of thyroid hormones or glucocorticoids promote their catabolism ('breakdown'). The powerful influence of androgenic and anabolic steroids such as testosterone on muscle hypertrophy and function are well known, which has led to their huge abuse in sport. Less well known is the potent effect of thyroid hormone in this same regard, a fact which is most relevant if one is rehabilitating patients with thyroid disorders.

Hypothyroidism:

- Decreases the normal shortening velocity by 60%, while hyperthyroidism increases this velocity by 20%.
- Completely suppresses the expression of FT fibres in soleus. Even though soleus comprises only about 15% of FT fibres, this FT to ST conversion produces significant changes in the soleus force–frequency curve, which implies that the small relative population of FT fibres in soleus plays a vital role in determining the mechanical properties of this muscle. Thyroid state, however, has far less effect on FT muscles such as plantaris.
- Also retards the rate and extent of muscle growth, although the change in maximal muscle tension per unit cross-sectional area is insignificant.

Hyperthyroidism:

- Converts some slow type I fibres to the faster type IIa and IIx fibres.

Another aspect of this work is the fascinating discovery that there appears to be a subset of the ST fibre group which is unresponsive to hormonal, mechanical or electrical stimuli and these have been called refractory type I fibres. In summary, this research, which is part of an effort to understand altered gene expression for specific isofoms as a central process in muscle adaptation, shows that thyroid hormone and mechanical activity can produce rapid qualitative and quantitative changes in muscle protein expression and possibly also on overall muscle function.

Other research concerning the plasticity of muscle has shown that:

1. Muscle atrophy produced by lack of stimulation, nerve damage or reduced gravity proceeds in the following

order: atrophy in the slow extensors is greater than in the fast extensors, which in turn is greater than in the fast flexors. Conversely, regular progressive overloading increases the mass of fast muscle more than slow muscle, with fast extensors hypertrophying more than fast flexors. Possibly this is a rational manifestation of some survival mechanism, since rapid extensor actions, which are associated with striking an assailant or thrusting him away, generally are involved more in self-defence processes than are flexion activities.

2. Typically, the deeper regions of the muscle, namely those with the highest proportion of oxidative (ST) fibres, tend to atrophy more than the superficial regions, while the same regions also seem to show the greatest hypertrophy after functional overload.

3. Fast FT (type II) fibres are assumed to consistently have larger diameters than slow type II, an observation which seems to be borne out in the superficial muscle regions, but not in deeper regions, where the two fibre types have similar diameters. Moreover, in predominantly slow muscles such as soleus, vastus intermedius and adductor longus, animal studies show that the fast fibres are consistently smaller than the slow fibres. In human males, the type II (FT) fibres of vastus lateralis are larger than the ST fibres, but the opposite tends to occur in females.

4. The largest muscles tend to atrophy and hypertrophy the most, irrespective of fibre type. When this change is calculated in the form of a relative percentage, it is often the same in slow and fast muscle.

5. The fastest rate of muscle atrophy takes place in the initial 1–2 weeks of inactivity, especially regarding the degradation of contractile proteins (like slow myosin in soleus), after which this rate progresses more slowly. The situation concerning hypertrophy is more complicated. Muscle mass increases markedly within a few days of functional overload (despite the assumptions that all initial changes are mainly neural), but, during the first week or so, this increase in cross-sectional area offers little or no increase in strength. After this initial latency period during which relative muscle strength decreases, this trend reverses and normal concurrent increases in hypertrophy and strength proceed for several weeks or months. After 2–3 months, the rate of increase slows down, as is the case with atrophic changes after a similar period.

6. Prolonged muscle stimulation does not increase muscle strength and hypertrophy, but can actually decrease both after several weeks of electrical stimulation. Moreover, fibres that are the least active, as based on the sequence of accepted recruitment patterns, usually are the largest fibres in normal mammals. This raises questions about the practice of continued long periods of intense resistance training. These findings suggest that excessive amounts of strenuous training can produce stagnation or decrease of hypertrophy and muscle function.

7. There is a close association between enzymes associated with myosin ATP metabolism and those involved with glycolysis, suggesting that there may be some functional advantage for the maximal rates of glycogen and ATP breakdown to coincide, as happens during intense muscle contraction. Since this would match the rate of energy expenditure during myosin activity with an immediate replacement of energy by glycolysis, this concept seems logically compelling. This idea is supported further by the fact that fast myosin hydrolyses ATP twice as rapidly as slow myosin, which is reflected by a very marked increase in the flux of energy substrates via the process of glycolysis. It would not be unexpected to find that the expression of proteins associated with specific myosin type and the glycolytic capabilities of a fibre indeed are closely linked.

8. Muscles and motor units can atrophy without altering their fatiguability, with slow muscle fibres showing prolonged capacity to metabolically support the amount of contractile proteins left in the atrophying muscle cells. However, if the whole body is involved in producing strength output, the atrophied muscles will become more easily fatigued because of recruitment of larger numbers and types of muscle fibres, many of which may well be susceptible to fatigue.

9. Although most research has stressed that training increases the size of muscle fibres, some studies show that muscles adapt sarcomere number and rest length in response to different patterns of use. For instance, fixing a joint in a flexed or extended position that lengthens some muscles and shortens others causes the muscle fibres to lengthen or shorten to establish a new mean sarcomere length which ensures that active force production is maximal at the maintained joint position. These findings collectively add further support for the view (expressed by Goldspink and others) that the relative expression of isoforms of myosin in skeletal muscle is strongly influenced by the degree of mechanical or gravity-related stress imposed on muscle, a fact that obviously relates directly to the use of regimes of rehabilitation.

High versus moderate intensity rehabilitative exercise

Besides the adaptive effects of the different regimes of rehabilitation training discussed above, there are other effects worthy of mention which refer to the different outcomes produced by high intensity versus moderate or submaximal resistance training. Besides enhancing muscle hypertrophy, low volume high intensity resistance exercise also increases the cross-sectional area of fast and slow twitch fibres, with a greater relative hypertrophy occurring in the fast twitch fibres (Fig. 5.10). Transitional muscle fibres exhibit contraction times similar to those of fast fibres, but with fatigue resistance more like slow fibres. Thus, the capacity for strength-endurance seems to increase. A mechanism for this muscle

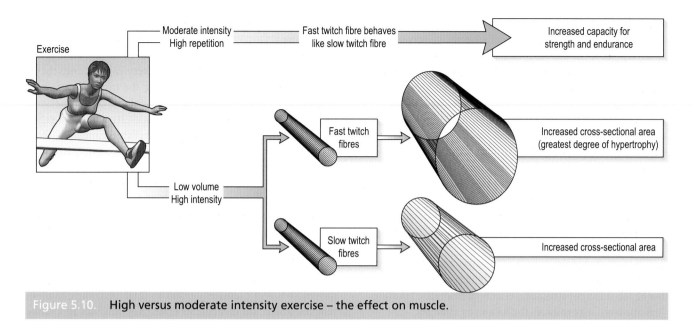

Figure 5.10.   High versus moderate intensity exercise – the effect on muscle.

adaptation may be that the fast isoforms of myosin disappear and are replaced by isomyosins that are characteristic of slow muscle after chronic overloading. The fibre transformation caused by chronic stimulation is regulated primarily at the genetic transcriptional level of regulation. This process is associated with the presence in fast twitch muscle of a myosin light chain component that is usually observed only in slow twitch fibres. For these reasons, it would appear that high volume, moderate resistance training is actually high intensity, general endurance training.

THE MECHANISM OF MUSCLE GROWTH

Living tissue grows by increase in the size of its components (hypertrophy) or by increase in the number of its components (hyperplasia). This growth in structure is an adaptation to the functional demands placed on the given system, where adaptation occurs at a molecular level within the genetic structure of the cells.

Research by Meerson discovered a link between the volume of loading imposed on the cells and their genetic structure. He learned that stimulating cellular function activates the genetic apparatus and increases the speed of transcription, translation, protein synthesis and build-up of certain structures. He propounded the concept of *intensity of functioning of structures* (IFS), which posits that the functional capacity of a system is related to its mass. Thus, the more intense the required function, the greater the mass of the working structure needed to perform the function. Here, the mass involved should be understood to be the 'active mass'.

We are now in a position to examine the increase in muscle mass as an adaptation to resistance exercise. In the case of muscle fibres, the occurrence of hypertrophy in response to strength training is a well-established fact, but there is considerable debate concerning muscle hyperplasia. Recent evidence suggests strongly that fibre hyperplasia may also contribute to muscle mass increases in mammals under certain extreme conditions. Research involving direct counts of muscle fibres using nitric acid digestion techniques has shown that both exercise and stretch overload result in significant increases in the number of muscle fibres; furthermore, indirect fibre counts using histological measurements of muscle cross-sections have suggested fibre hyperplasia. In addition, the expression of embryonic myosin isoforms has furnished indirect evidence for the formation of new fibres in bird flight muscles subjected to long-term stretch overloading (with weights attached to their wings). Moreover, satellite cells, which can activate new cell formation, have been shown to be involved in muscle fibre hyperplasia in stretching and dynamic exercise. Hyperplasia may also occur due to the splitting of large fibres that subdivide into two or more smaller fibres.

It has been suggested that muscle hyperplasia may occur with extremely intense resistance training, but current evidence from human subjects is still by no means unequivocal.

The prolific amount of evidence which shows that increase in muscle mass most commonly is associated with an increase in muscle cross-sectional area certainly emphasizes that hyperplasia does not take place as a simple matter of course, but under very special conditions which warrant further research. Although the existence of hyperplasia of muscle fibre may be uncertain or rare, hyperplasia of structures within the muscle fibre and cell does occur. Increase in muscle diameter is due to enlargement of individual muscle fibres by an increase in the number and size of individual myofibrils, accompanied by an increase in the amount of connective tissue. This increase in muscle protein is produced by increased protein synthesis and decreased protein degradation. Growth of any living structure is related to the balance between its volume and its surface area. When muscle hypertrophy occurs, the surface of the fibres grows more slowly than their volume and, according to Hartwig and Mezia, this imbalance causes the fibres to disintegrate and restructure in a way which preserves their original thermodynamic state. It would appear that light and medium increases in loading require less energy, facilitate cell repair, minimize the occurrence of destructive processes and stimulate the synthesis of new, non-hypertrophied organelles.

The fact that conventional isometric training improves performance in static, rather than dynamic, exercise may be due to the different structural effects of isometric training.

Static training produces the following changes:

- the sarcoplasmic content of many muscle fibres increases
- myofibrils collect into fascicles
- nuclei become rounder
- motor end-plates expand transversally relative to the muscle fibres
- capillaries meander more markedly
- and the layers of endomysium and perimysium thicken.

In the case of dynamic training:

- the transverse striations of the myofibrils become very pronounced
- the nuclei become oval and fusiform (spindle-shaped)
- motor end-plates extend the length of the muscle fibres
- the layers of endomysium and perimysium become thinner.

The above work seems to corroborate the hypothesis referred to earlier that there may be an optimum size for muscle fibres undergoing hypertrophy. The importance of prescribing resistance exercise regimes which produce the optimal balance between hypertrophy and specific strength then becomes obvious. Thus, it is not only prolonged cardiovascular training which can be detrimental to the acquisition of strength, but multiple, fairly high repetition sets of heavy bodybuilding or circuit training routines to the point of failure may also inhibit the formation of contractile muscle fibres.

Neurophysiological aspects of muscle rehabilitation

The central nervous system is the complex central computing facility of the brain and spinal column which processes incoming information and sends out commands to the rest of the body (including the muscles) via the peripheral nervous system.

At the outset it should be noted that in certain emergency situations the muscles have to react very rapidly and, therefore, time cannot be spent in having the input signals pass through the entire computing facility of the central nervous system. The body provides for this with its system of reflex loops. During voluntary movements reflex action also occurs at the level of the motor cortex and not merely at the level of the spinal cord. The Russian scientist Pavlov was the first researcher to recognize that conditioned reflexes could be learned by proper methods of reinforcement. In other words, programmes of correctly repeated movements can eventually enable these movements to become automatic. This is particularly important in the case of all manoeuvres which have to be executed rapidly and cannot accommodate delays caused by active thinking about the process. Repetition of incorrect movements will eventually result in their becoming built-in reflexes which are difficult to erase. Any attempt to change faulty technique usually results in a feeling of awkwardness and an inability to perform as comfortably as before. This is because the body has adapted to its inefficient movement patterns, and the emotional distress caused by apparently useless new techniques can prevent the patient from implementing any changes. It is rare for any movement sequence to be controlled entirely by reflex loops; instead, reflexes operate together with the entire control system depicted in Figure 5.11.

The motor cortex is at a lower level of control, more directly connected to spinal-cord motor neurons than either the cerebellum or the basal ganglia. In addition the cerebellum, the basal ganglia and the motor cortex all become active before any movement begins. There is also an increase in muscle tone and other changes in activity of the cerebral cortex (such as the 'orientation response' and 'expectancy waves') preceding the commencement of a motor response. It is also known that the cerebellum does not initiate movement, but corrects or reorganizes motor commands before they reach the muscles, thereby implementing inner feedforward mechanisms to ensure maximum external muscular efficiency. The cerebellum can even coordinate movement in the absence of all information from the periphery of the body.

Since brain activity precedes movement, it is vital that correct patterns of movement are correctly visualized even before exercise begins. In fact, the technique of visualization by observation of practical demonstrations or even videos, combined with proper mental rehearsal, should form an integral part of rehabilitation and training. The motor cortex determines the amount and pattern of muscular contraction, rather than the displacement produced. Moreover, the motor cortex is involved with both slow and fast movements, whereas the basal ganglia seem to be preferentially active in slow movements. It has further been suggested that the major role of the cerebellum is to preprogramme and initiate rapid ballistic movements.

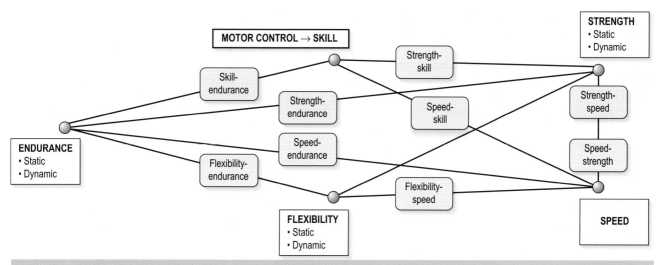

Figure 5.11.   Pyramidal model comprising the major elements of musculoskeletal fitness.

In the overall scheme of events, the basal ganglia and the cerebellum receive information from the intero-receptors (proprioceptors and other inner sensors) and the exteroceptors (eyes, ears and other external receptors) of the cerebral cortex (the supreme thinking control centre), transform this information and then send an appropriate pattern of signals to the motor cortex. Information about the state of the muscles is constantly fed back from the proprioceptors to the central nervous system (CNS); otherwise control of movement would be impossible.

The primary function of the cerebellum in fine motor control has recently been challenged by research showing that it may also be involved in perception, cognition, visualization and memory storage. An alternative hypothesis is that the lateral cerebellum is not activated by the control of movement per se, but is strongly engaged during the acquisition and discrimination of sensory information. These findings suggest that the lateral cerebellum may be active during motor, perceptual and cognitive performances specifically because of the requirement to process sensory data.

The cerebellum also appears to play a role in the visualization of movement and feedforward processes. Analysis of cortical activity has already supported the hypothesis that motor imagery and motor performance possess similar neural substrates. The differential activation in the cerebellum during executed and imagined movements is in accordance with the assumption that the posterior cerebellum is involved in the inhibition of movement execution during imagination.

The thalamus and reticular activating system situated deep within the brain play a vital role in activating different parts of the brain acting as relay stations, and in integrating emotional and hormonal responses with the more mechanical functions. It is at this level that the hypothalamus generally becomes involved. Even though the same muscles may be involved in a movement, they may be controlled by different parts of the brain, depending on the speed of movement. Yet, it is not only speed that may determine the brain mechanisms required. There is strong evidence that two different control mechanisms are involved in the cardiovascular response to exercise. This means that isometric and dynamic exercise recruit different brain mechanisms, because isometric exercise causes a marked increase in blood pressure, but little increase in blood flow. Dynamic exercise, however, generates an oxygen demand that is met largely by an increase in the volume of blood pumped and a decreased resistance to its flow.

SOFT TISSUE FLEXIBILITY

Earlier the relative contributions to joint stiffness by the different soft tissues was discussed. To understand and apply the principles of judicious stretching to these various tissues, we will now examine their biomechanical characteristics. It is useful to recall the model of the muscle complex discussed earlier. It divided the soft tissues into a contractile system, comprising the actin–myosin muscle fibre complex, and a viscoelastic non-contractile system, comprising mainly the connective tissue of tendons, ligaments and capsules. The viscoelastic component of muscle was further analysed in terms of a series elastic component (SEC) and a parallel elastic component (PEC).

Current knowledge of soft tissue stretching may be summarized as follows:

- Different methods are necessary for conditioning muscles, tendons and other soft tissues.
- Slow twitch muscle groups contain a greater proportion of connective tissue than fast twitch muscle groups.

- The high stiffness and low strain of slow muscle is most appropriate for muscle function intended for continuous support of posture.
- Different brain and spinal cord mechanisms control high speed, low speed, and topological patterns of muscle activity.
- All conditioning is primarily functional, since functional stimulation precedes structural change (Wolff's law) – thus, it is erroneous to refer to any exercises as purely 'structural'.
- Rapid ballistic stretching of contracted muscle (plyometric loading) should not be avoided by serious athletes, since the ability to use elastic energy is vital to all high level performance.
- Static stretching of a relaxed muscle has a more pronounced effect on the PEC than ballistic stretching of a contracted muscle, which has a greater effect on the SEC (essential for any fast activities).
- Static and cyclic stretching, as commonly performed by athletes (up to 90 seconds duration each), increase joint range of motion by increasing stretch tolerance while the viscoelastic characteristics of the muscle remain unaltered.
- Different rates of loading and stretching have different effects on bone, tendon and muscle.
- Prolonged slow stretching can cause permanent viscous deformation of connective tissue and high levels of strain in muscle.
- Physiotherapeutic proprioceptive neuromuscular facilitation shows that rapid or powerful recruitment of the different stretch reflexes can be safely applied to rehabilitate and strengthen.
- There is generally no such thing as an unsafe stretch or exercise: only an unsafe way of executing any movement for a specific individual at a specific time.
- Elastic fibres occur in small concentrations in the intercellular matrix of tendons and most ligaments, and may help restore the crimped collagen fibre configuration after stretching or muscle contraction.
- Multi-directional stretching is important, since the structural orientation of the fibres is different for the different collagenous tissues and is specifically suited to the functions of each tissue.
- The stress concentration at the insertion of the ligament and tendon into the more rigid bone structure is decreased by the existence of three progressively stiffer transitional composite materials – a system which can be disrupted by ingestion of anabolic steroids.
- At slow loading rates, the bony insertion of a ligament or tendon is the weakest component of the bone–soft tissue complex, whereas the soft tissues are the weakest components at very fast loading rates.
- Tendons, unlike ligaments, are not simply passive stabilizers of joints – instead, together with strongly contracted muscle fibres (particularly during phases of eccentric contraction), they play a vital role in storing elastic energy during running and other impulsive motor acts, thereby saving energy and increasing the efficiency of muscular activity.
- No stretching manoeuvres must compromise the strength or ability of the tendons to store elastic energy throughout their range of movement; thus, tendon stretching exercises should be accompanied by strength conditioning against adequate resistance.
- Since tendons and ligaments are viscoelastic, they exhibit sensitivity to loading rate, and undergo stress relaxation, creep and hysteresis.

Flexibility, stability and muscle activity

The musculature alone cannot respond quickly enough to protect a joint against injury if large impacts are applied rapidly, particularly if they are torsional. It is probably more accurate to state that joint stabilization takes place in the following manner: the contractile element of muscle activated by the stretch reflex complex, together with the SEC of that muscle, act as primary stabilizers of the joint if the loading rate permits the muscles to respond rapidly enough. If the joint reaches the physical limits of muscle length, strength or endurance, it has to rely on protection by ligaments and the SEC of its muscles. If, at the same time, the inverse stretch reflex signals the muscles to relax at their maximum length, then the PEC of the muscle will also contribute to joint stabilization. However, it should be noted that receptors resembling Golgi tendon organs have been located on the surface of cruciate ligaments and that muscles will show reflex contraction if ligaments are stretched until pain results. If the joint is extended to its limits without sufficient muscle contraction becoming possible, primary stabilization is afforded by the ligaments and the PEC of the muscles. As soon as the initial latency period for muscle excitation is over, the contracting muscles and their SEC will contribute as secondary stabilizers.

The influence of exercise on connective tissue

Regular resistance exercise produces not only muscle hypertrophy, but also an increase in the collagen content of the ligaments and the connective tissues that surround the muscle fibres. It should be noted, however, that moderate intensity treadmill training of rats produces neither muscle hypertrophy nor increased growth of intramuscular connective tissue. Prolonged, low intensity training evidently suffices to condition the cardiovascular system significantly, but not the musculoskeletal system. Apparently it is anaerobic, muscle endurance training which has the most pronounced effect on enhancing the concentration and strength of collagenous tissue and its junction zones. Progressive stretching regimes in conjunction with this type of training would then be seen to be especially valuable as a component of all patient rehabilitation programmes.

Rehabilitation considerations:

- Static and passive stretches increase passive flexibility. Increases in passive and active flexibility are the same and the difference between them remains unchanged.
- Full range strength exercises increase passive flexibility and decrease the difference between active and passive flexibility.
- Concurrent strength and flexibility exercises increase passive and active flexibility and decrease the difference between them.

Thus, dynamic stretching executed while one deliberately concentrates on progressively contracting and relaxing the muscle complex being stretched can prove invaluable in enhancing active flexibility.

Proprioceptive neuromuscular facilitation (PNF) techniques using phases of contraction and relaxation can be both safe and effective. Application of the PNF principles of spiral and diagonal patterns of movement can also produce three-dimensional functional range of movement superior to standard static stretches. It is interesting to note that many conventional stretches are executed in only one plane at a time and very few rotational stretches about the longitudinal axes of the limbs are ever used. Thus, many of these stretches could be enhanced if they included elements of rotation and twisting, especially if they followed some of the patterns encountered in daily activities. The use of quasi-isometric activity can be especially useful in developing active flexibility. This requires one to exercise a limb through a full range of movement against a resistance that is allowed to stretch a joint gently beyond its limit of static flexibility without producing any sudden movement which may recruit the myotatic reflex. Free weights, pulley (e.g. the familiar 'Westminster' pulley systems that have been used in physiotherapy for many years) and other functional training machines can be particularly versatile in allowing one to execute natural patterns of movement against resistance. In addition, longer periods of progressive isometric or quasi-isometric activity in full range movement produce greater gains in active flexibility.

Low flexibility versus non-functional muscle tension

Limitations in functional range of movement (ROM) should not automatically be attributed to joint stiffness alone, because this can lead to an unnecessary emphasis on stretching. Limitations to full ROM can also be caused by various forms of spurious tension or excessive muscle tension such as co-ordination tension, which may accompany the appropriate muscle tension required by the given movement. This non-functional tension can occur in both phasic and tonic muscles before, during and after the movement. It is of little consequence to have highly flexible joints with well-conditioned, supple connective tissues and large ROM, if action is limited by any spurious muscle tension. Flexibility exercises, therefore, should always be combined with neuromuscular training to produce efficient, functional ROM.

Methods of improving the ability to relax muscles are:

- Contract–relax, hold–relax and other PNF methods which use the different stretch reflexes to promote muscle relaxation.
- The change of muscle groups from a state of tension to relaxation in a controlled, gradual manner or in a series of stages (e.g. Jacobsen's progressive relaxation method).
- The use of controlled visualization of the muscles progressing from contraction to relaxation and back.
- The use of autogenic training, progressive relaxation, meditation or massage.
- The use of breathing patterns on the basis that tension is associated with breath inhalation and holding, with breath holding (the Valsalva manoeuvre) being used where maximal force and spinal stabilization must be produced. Conversely, relaxation is associated with gentle, controlled exhalation. Appropriate techniques of breathing should always be combined with all phases of movement to enhance mobility, stability and relaxation.
- The execution of exercises against a background of exhaustion of selected muscle groups, provided that movement technique does not suffer.
- The use of distracting or focusing activities which cause the individual to concentrate on stimuli other than those associated with the given rehabilitative or sporting action (e.g. music, talking to a training partner while running, thinking of something pleasant). These methods may involve internalization or externalization of focus, the suitability of any method being determined on an individual basis.
- The gentle use of rhythmic cyclical, swinging, shaking or circling movements of the body and limbs to relax muscles which have just been strongly contracted (e.g. some of the movements of dance, swimming or tai chi).

ADAPTATION AND THE TRAINING EFFECT

The phenomenon of increase in strength and all other motor and fitness factors in response to training is clear evidence of biological adaptation to stress. In fact, fitness may be defined as the ability of the body to cope with a specific task under specific conditions, where the task is characterized by a set of particular physical and psychological stressors. Musculoskeletal rehabilitation may thus be defined as the process of imposing physical loading in a particular way to achieve a specific type of functional fitness. One has to distinguish between the related factors of work capacity, fitness and preparedness, as introduced earlier. Training and environmental factors affect all of these abilities.

As is well known, physical training is highly specific to the methods being used, a fact which has been formulated as the well-known SAID principle (specific adaptation to imposed demands). Simply stated, this means that the body adapts with a specific type of fitness to any demands which may be regularly imposed on it, provided the loading does not exceed the adaptive capabilities of the body at that time.

A MODEL OF PHYSICAL FITNESS

The definition of fitness given earlier needs to be expanded to incorporate all the essential factors which contribute to this state. Fitness comprises a series of interrelated structural and functional factors which conveniently may be referred to as the basic S-factors of fitness: Strength, Speed, Stamina (general systemic endurance or local muscular endurance), Suppleness (flexibility), Skill (neuromuscular efficiency), Structure (somatotype, size, shape) and Spirit (psychological preparedness). Within the scope of skill, there is also a fitness quality known as Style, the individual manner of expressing a particular skill. A comprehensive model of physical fitness may be constructed from the functional motor elements of fitness, as shown in Figure 5.11. The model may be developed in two stages: firstly, as a triangular model which interrelates strength, stamina (muscular endurance), speed and suppleness (flexibility), and secondly, as a more complete pyramidal model which interrelates all of these factors with the process that makes all movement possible, namely neuromuscular control or skill.

Figure 5.11 illustrates that strength, endurance and flexibility may be produced statically or dynamically, unlike speed, which changes along a continuum from the static (speed = 0) to the dynamic state. However, this convenient picture could be complicated by including the quasi-isometric state, which can influence production of any of the motor qualities at very slow speeds. For this and other reasons, this model should be viewed as one that is representational or descriptive rather than scientifically analytical.

The quality of flexibility has been placed at the centre of the base of the pyramid, because the ability to exhibit any of the other qualities depends centrally on ROM. It should be noted that static or dynamic flexibility refers to the maximum ROM that may be attained under static or dynamic conditions, respectively. The line joining all adjacent pairs of primary fitness factors depicts a variety of different fitness factors between each of the two extremes.

Alterations in this model reflect damage to muscles and their associated soft tissues. Chapter 6 discusses the various muscle disorders whereas injury due to overtraining is discussed below.

A physiological framework for overtraining/overuse injuries

The insidious road to overtraining is signposted, not necessarily very clearly, by unexplained drops in performance, residual fatigue or soreness, persistent minor injuries, loss of motivation, compromised motor control, sleeplessness, lengthened reaction time, longer recovery heart rate, changes in blood pressure, mood swings, increased eye blink rate, or general lack of progress. It is vital that all such symptoms be recognized by the athlete and coach, since the popular practice of forcing oneself through these negative phases can lead to acute or chronic injury. Overtraining (as well as its acute form now known as 'overreaching') refers to or involves a specific type of physical and psychological stress, and an appreciation of the mechanisms underlying human stress is essential to understand overtraining. There are two types of overtraining: general and local. General overtraining affects the whole body and results in stagnation or a decrease in performance, whereas local overtraining affects a specific body part. Adaptation to physical, psychological or environmental stress depends on the inextricable links between the central nervous system (the fast control system of the body) and the endocrine system (the slow control system) (Fig. 5.12) Any changes in the central nervous and endocrine systems can affect performance in the muscular system.

For instance, the adrenal glands selectively prepare the skeletal muscle for physical activity in the face of stress. The hormone thyroxine, secreted by the thyroid gland, not only

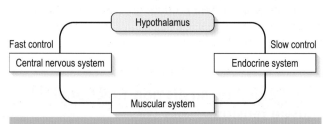

Figure 5.12.   Some of the physiological control systems involved with motor processes.

increases the rate at which cells burn their fuel (glucose) but it is involved in various anti-stress responses, including demands for extra energy. Human growth hormone (HGH), secreted by the pituitary gland in the brain, plays an essential role in general growth and in the elevation of blood glucose. Insulin, secreted by the pancreas, is concerned with the metabolism of glucose, and the sex hormones such as testosterone influence sexual behaviour and muscle growth, in the male.

This central role played by certain hormones in the occurrence and management of stress implies that it is logical to associate general overtraining, a stress-related phenomenon, with some disturbance of the endocrine system. Overtraining may also be associated with electrocardiographic changes, in particular a smaller T-wave. Local overtraining is simple to recognize, since it is often accompanied by stiffness or soreness of a particular muscle group, which does not subside with alternate days of rest. Moreover, the performance of that muscle group might be static or diminished and some of the symptoms of general overtraining, such as impaired coordination, might be present. In weight training, this situation may be revealed by outstanding performance in one supplementary exercise such as the squat, but diminished performance in another exercise such as the bench press. In the case of strength training, overtraining (or 'overreaching') injuries may be the result of too many repetitions or sets, regular training with near maximum loads, training the same muscle groups too frequently, inadequate recovery periods, insufficient rest or faulty execution of any movement.

Principles of safety in rehabilitation and physical conditioning

The design of any exercise programme would be incomplete without serious attention being paid to all aspects of safety, including safety of the means and methods of the individual exercises, the combination of exercises, the intensity, the volume of exercise, the timing of training loads, and the recovery periods (between repetitions, sets and sessions). An otherwise carefully devised training programme is of little value if it causes injury to the individual. Injuries may be caused by accident or overtraining. The former often depends on factors outside the direct control of the athlete and concern dangers arising unexpectedly in the environment.

With particular reference to injuries produced by inefficient patterns of movement, one must appreciate that deviations from normal patterns may be caused by:

- pain, soreness, stiffness or discomfort
- muscle weakness or imbalance between muscle groups
- any limitation in the range of joint range of movement in any direction
- inco-ordination of movement
- musculoskeletal changes

- fatigue
- changes in surface, footwear, equipment or environment
- neural changes
- visual or balance changes
- emotional disturbance.

Not all injuries are accompanied by pain. In many cases, such as disintegration of the menisci of the knee and intervertebral disc damage to the spine, the onset of pain may occur only once the injury has become extensive or serious. Micro-ruptures of soft tissue or similar minor injuries may be unheralded by pain signals until they have accumulated over a sufficiently long period to incapacitate the athlete. Overtraining or regular impact (e.g. caused by running on hard surfaces or by blows to the head in contact sports) are associated with this insidious type of injury process. However, it should be noted that the perception of pain by the CNS can reorganize the motor control system to minimize the pain, which can result in reflex inhibition of the muscles to exert maximal strength and thereby lead to muscle weakness. In fact, even if the injury is not accompanied by pain, this can also occur. This is very common with even relatively insubstantial injuries of the knee such as patellar tendinitis, peripatellar pain syndrome or chondromalacia patellae, which significantly reduce the ability of the quadriceps to produce powerful contraction. It is possible that the pain caused by muscle swelling or delayed onset muscle soreness (DOMS) may also provoke the CNS into responding with alternative motor programmes which distribute force production over a larger number of muscle fibres and diminish the efficiency and magnitude of strength output. The importance of dealing with even minor pain, soreness or injury then becomes obvious.

The models presented earlier also emphasize that strength training should focus not only on muscle development, but also on conditioning all the connective tissues associated with stability and mobility. This is further borne out by recent findings that increase in strength may not be related only to increase in density of the contractile protein elements of muscle, but also to improvement in the transmission of force from the muscle fibres to the skeletal system. In this respect, increase in connective tissue strength and improved rigidity of the muscle complex may decrease the dissipation of force generated by individual sarcomeres into the surrounding tissues.

REVIEW OF SOME IMPORTANT PRINCIPLES

Physical rehabilitation may be conveniently analysed if one notes the similarities between the production of motor output in human movement and the production of a musical symphony by an orchestra. In both cases the output is a complex pattern and perfection of this pattern in both cases is the ultimate objective. The central nervous system acts as the conductor which controls the different systems that contribute to the final pattern, just as the human conductor controls the players in an orchestra to produce the required musical pattern. Just as there are many different instruments played by different musicians in an orchestra, so there are many muscles, tendons and other physical units, which are controlled by different neural programmes in the human body. If the timing, intensities, duration and any other contributing factors are incorrect during any phase of the process in either case, the final result will be less than optimal.

The perfection of the output pattern depends on the ability to optimally use and integrate the contributions of every subsystem in space and time. This entails understanding how the nervous and neuromuscular systems interact to produce certain motor qualities that are necessary for successful performance in any given sport (Fig. 5.13). Essentially, the rehabilitation/training process simply involves compelling the body to adapt to a higher level of functioning via the imposition of appropriate physical and mental stresses. The existing levels of hormonal, neural and musculoskeletal integrity have to be raised at a rate which is optimal for the individual at a given stage. This means that a given intensity, volume and density of loading has to be used to alter both the actual and perceived thresholds of performance, a process that relies on feedforward and feedback mechanisms, as well as voluntary and involuntary methods of intervention to achieve the desired results. Rehabilitation is not simply a matter of strengthening the musculoskeletal system by altering the physical structure of all of its components and by increasing the ability of the neural system to orchestrate more powerful movements. In producing motor competence, the individual is strongly influenced by the psychological perception of the load involved,

not simply the actual load. If the load 'feels' insurmountable or technically too demanding, despite the fact that the body is well equipped to handle that given load, failure is highly likely. This is why the rehabilitation process must teach the individual to cope with both the perceived and actual load being handled.

In Figure 5.13 the arrow from Function to Structure is in bold to emphasize the well-known fact that function precedes structure. Humans operate in terms of a type of 'virtual reality' in which perceptions of effort and feedforward images of the forthcoming effort strongly determine the final outcome of the motor action. This is why the rehabilitative process is one which not only improves the structural and functional capabilities of the body, but also shows the individual how to manipulate 'virtual realities' for all of the actions involved in a given exercise. This 'virtual reality' training imparts to the individual great skill in minimizing the size of any detrimental differences between perceived and actual loading and technical skill. After all, the long-term goal of the rehabilitation process is to make the existing task feel easier and easier so that the existing level of performance may be raised. All physical demands and skills 'feel' progressively easier and this may be achieved by optimal implementation of principles such as that of fluctuating gradual overload (not simply progressive gradual overload) and SAID (specific adaptation to imposed demands).

The fundamental mechanical aspect of all resistance conditioning and musculoskeletal rehabilitation is the imposition of optimal progressive increases in loading so that muscle tension may be increased, thereby stimulating the neuromuscular and hormonal systems to adapt to higher levels of stress.

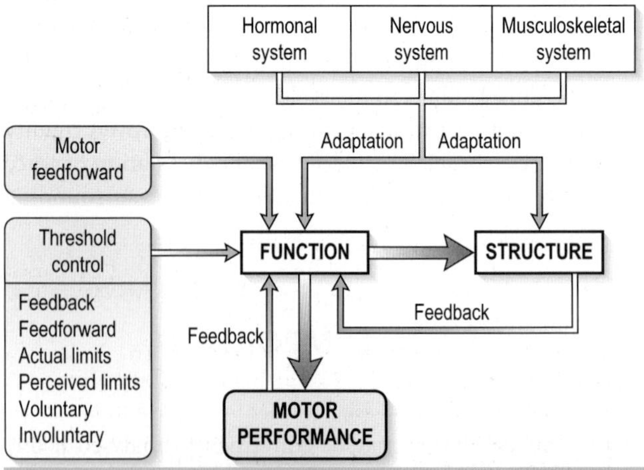

Figure 5.13.   The conditioning process summarized in the form of a systems model.

The following are some of the methods of increasing muscle tension which may be used in devising a rehabilitation programme:

1. Voluntary use of compensatory action to facilitate changes in movement characteristics.
2. Use of suddenly terminated eccentric actions.
3. Involuntary use of reflexive explosive rebound or plyometric actions.
4. Voluntary use of prestretch to facilitate stronger muscle contraction.
5. Use of free weights combined with elastic bands, chains or isokinetic loads.
6. Application of electrical stimulation (ES).
7. Concurrent combination of ES and voluntary movements.
8. Application of vibration to limbs.
9. Cognitive/Mental techniques (such as visualization and motivational strategies).

CONCLUSION

As we have seen, the various parts of the body can withstand only a certain level of physical stress, depending on many factors such as genetic background, level of training and adequacy of nutrition. Excessive stress may be caused by imposing too great a force for a short period, a smaller force for a prolonged period, or any type of force without adequate recovery periods. The results of such stress may range from the acute category of fractures, herniated spinal discs and torn ligaments to the chronic types of inflammation or tendinitis. In general, exercise safety is largely a consequence of skill development (neuromuscular efficiency) established upon a foundation of more than adequate physiological and anatomical soundness and may be enhanced by imposing activities which progress carefully with respect to factors such as complexity, intensity, volume, speed, range of movement, duration, variety, level of fatigue and mental state. In this respect, the engineering concept of designing any structure with a specific minimum 'safety factor' is highly relevant – thus, a safety factor of 2 means that a given structure is capable of handling stresses twice as great as those anticipated under the most severe operating conditions. This provides a solid rationale for the use of supplementary progressive strength training to enhance the ability of the body to perform not only efficiently, but also with a high degree of safety.

REFERENCES AND FURTHER READING

Structure and function of muscle

Davies A, Blakeley AGH, Kidd C (2001) Human Physiology. Edinburgh: Churchill Livingstone.

Komi P (1984) Physiological and biomechanical correlates of muscle function. Exerc Sport Sci Rev 14: 81–121.

Suzuki S, Sugi H (1983) Extensibility of the n-myofilaments in vertebrate skeletal muscle as revealed by stretching rigor muscle fibers. J Gen Physiol 81(4): 531–546.

Collagenous tissue

Minns R, Soden P, Jackson D (1973) The role of the fibrous components and ground substance in the mechanical properties of biological tissues. J Biomech 6: 153–165.

Loading of collagenous tissue

Tumanyan G, Dzhanyan S (1980) Strength exercises as a means of improving active flexibility of wrestlers. Teoriya i Praktika Fizischeskoi' Kullury 10: 10–11.

Viidik A (1973) Functional properties of collagenous tissues. Int Rev Connect Tissue Res 6: 127–215.

The role of stored elastic energy

Frankel V, Nordin M (1980) Basic Biomechanics of the Skeletal System. Philadelphia: Lea & Febiger, pp. 87–110.

Kovanen V, Suominen H, Heikkinen E (1984) Mechanical properties of fast and slow skeletal muscle with special reference to collagen and endurance training. J Biomech 17(10): 725–735.

Noyes F (1977) Functional properties of knee ligaments and alterations induced by immobilization: a correlative biomechanical and histological study in primates. Orthop Rel Res 123: 210–242.

Von der Mark K (1981) Localization of collagen types in tissues. Int Rev Connect Tissue Res 9: 265–305.

Woo S, Gomez M, Amiel D, et al. (1981) The effects of exercise on the biomechanical and biochemical properties of swine digital flexor tendons. J Biomech Eng 103: 51–56.

Fast and slow twitch muscle fibres

Abemethy PJ, Jurimae J, Logan P, Taylor A, Thayer R (1994) Acute and chronic response of skeletal muscle to resistance training. Sports Med 17(1): 22–38.

Andersen JL, Aagaard P (2000) Myosin heavy chain IIX overshoot in human skeletal muscle. Muscle Nerve 23(7): 1095–1104.

Andersen JL, Schjerling P, Saltin B (2000) Muscle, genes and athletic performance. Sci Am 283(3): 48–55.

Edstrom L, Grimby L (1986) Effect of exercise on the motor unit. Muscle Nerve 9: 104–126.

Enoka RM (1996) Commentary-Neural and neuromuscular aspects of muscle fatigue. Muscle Nerve Suppl 4: S31–S32.

Finer JT, Mehta A, Spudich J (1995) Characterization of single actin–myosin interactions. Biophys J 68(4 Suppl): 291S–297S

Grotmol S, Totland G, Kryvi H (1988) A general, computer-based method for the study of the spatial distribution of muscle fiber types in skeletal muscle. Anal Embryol 177: 421–426.

Jurimae J, Abernethy P, Quigley B, Blake K, McEniery M (1997) Differences in muscle contractile characteristics among bodybuilders, endurance trainers and control subjects. Eur J Appl Physiol 75: 357–362.

Kernell D (1998) Muscle regionalization. Can J Appl Physiol 23(1): 1–22.

Staron RS, Hikida RS (1992) Histochemical, biochemical and ultrastructural analyses of single human muscle fibers with special reference to the C fiber population. J Histochem Cytochem 40: 563–568.

Tesch PA (1988) Skeletal muscle adaptation consequent to long-term heavy resistance exercise. Med Sci Sports Exerc 20(5) Suppl: S132–S134.

Muscle proteins isoforms

Ennion S, Sant'ana Pereira J, Sargeant A, Young A, Goldspink G (1995) Characterization of human skeletal muscle fibres according to the myosin heavy chains they express. J Muscle Res Cell Motil 16(l): 35–43.

Goldspink G (1992) The brains behind the brawn. New Scientist 92 (1 Aug): 28–33.

Hamalainen N, Pette D (1995) Patterns of myosin isoforms in mammalian skeletal muscle fibres. Microsc Res Tech 30(5): 381–389.

Schiaffino S, Reggiani C (1994) Myosin isoforms in mammalian skeletal muscle. J Appl Physiol 77(2): 493–501.

Smerdu V, Karsch-Mizrachi I, Campione M, Leinwand L, Schiaffino S (1994) Type IIx myosin heavy chain transcripts are expressed in type Ib fibers of human skeletal muscle. Am J Physiol 267(6 Pt 1): C1723–1728.

Muscle fibres and exercise and muscle plasticity

Adams GR, Hather B, Baldwin K, Dudley G (1993) Skeletal muscle myosin heavy chain composition and resistance training. J Appl Physiol 74(2): 911–915.

Antonio J, Gonyea W (1994) Muscle fiber splitting in stretch-enlarged avian muscle. Med Sci Sports Exerc 26(8): 973–977.

Bacou F, Rouanet P, Barjot C, et al. (1996) Expression of myosin isoforms in denervated, cross-reinnervated and electrically stimulated rabbit muscles. Eur J Biochem 236: 539–547.

Banister EW, Calvert TW (1980) Planning for future performance: implications for long term training. Can J Appl Sport Sci 5(3): 170–176.

Banister EW, Morton R, Fitz-Clarke J (1992) Dose/response effects of exercise modeled from training: physical and biochemical measures. Ann Physiol Anthropol 11(3): 345–356.

Barjot C, Rouanet P, Vigneron P, et al. (1998) Transformation of slow- or fast-twitch rabbit muscles after cross-reinnervation or low frequency stimulation does not alter the in vitro properties of their satellite cells. J Muscle Res Cell Motil 19: 25–32.

Basmajian J (1978) Muscles Alive. Baltimore: Williams & Wilkins.

Bell DG, Jacobs I (1990) Muscle fibre area, fibre type and capillarization in male and female body builders. Can J Sport Sci 15(2): 115–119.

Caiozzo V, Haddad F (1996) Thyroid hormone: Modulation of muscle structure, function, and adaptive responses to mechanical loading. Exerc Sport Sci Rev 24: 321–361.

Caiozzo V, Herrick R, Baldwin K (1991) The influence of hyperthyroidism on the maximal shortening velocity and myosin isoform distribution in slow and fast skeletal muscle. Am J Physiol 261: C285–295.

Duchateau J (1995) Bed rest induces neural and contractile adaptations in triceps surae. Med Sci Sports Exerc 27(12): 1581–1589.

Eisenberg B, Brown J, Salmons S (1984) Restoration of fast muscle characteristics following cessation of chronic stimulation: the ultrastructure of slow-to-fast transformation. Cell Tissue Res 238: 221–230.

Hakkinen K (1985) Factors influencing trainability of muscular strength during short term and prolonged training. National Strength and Conditioning (NSCA) Journal 7(2): 32–36.

Hather BM, Tesch PA, Buchanan P, Dudley GA (1991) Influence of eccentric actions on skeletal muscle adaptations to resistance training. Acta Physiol Scand 143(2): 177–185.

Koh TJ, Herzog W (1998) Eccentric training does not increase sarcomere number in rabbit dorsiflexor muscles. J Biomech 31: 499–501.

Lynn R, Morgan DL (1994) Decline running produces more sarcomeres in rat vastus intermedius muscle fibers than does incline running. J Appl Physiol 11: 1439–1444.

MacDougall JD, Sale DG, Alway SE, Sutton J (1984) Muscle fiber number in biceps brachii in bodybuilders and control subjects. J Appl Physiol 57: 1399–1403.

Pette D, Vrbova G (1985) Neural control of phenotypic expression in mammalian muscle fibres. Muscle Nerve 8: 676–689.

Pipes TV (1994) Strength training and fiber types. Scholastic Coach 63 (March): 67–70.

Roy RR, Baldwin KM, Edgerton VR (1991) The plasticity of skeletal muscle: effects of neuromuscular activity. Exerc Sport Sci Rev 19: 269–312.

Vigneron P, Dainat J, Bacon F (1989) Properties of skeletal muscle fibers. II. Hormonal influences. Reprod Nutr Dev 29(1): 27–53.

Yamashita-Goto K, Okuyama R, Honda M, et al. (2001) Maximal and submaximal forces of slow fibers in human soleus after bed rest. Appl Physiol 91(1): 417–424.

High versus moderate intensity rehabilitation exercise

Noble EG, Pettigrew FP (1989) Appearance of 'transitional' motor units in overloaded rat skeletal muscle. J Appl Physiol 67(5): 2049–2054.

Tesch PA, Komi PV, Jacobs I, Karlsson J (1983) Influence of lactate accumulation of EMG frequency spectrum during repeated concentric contractions. Acta Physiol Scand 119: 61–67.

Timson BF, Bowlin BK, Dudenhoeffer GA, George JB (1985) Fiber number, area, and composition of mouse soleus muscle following enlargement. J Appl Physiol 58(2): 619–624.

The mechanism of muscle growth

Alway SE, Grumbt W, Gonyea WJ, Stray-Gundersen J (1989) Contrasts in muscle and myofibers of elite male and female bodybuilders. J Appl Physiol 67(1): 24–31.

Antonio J, Gonyea W (1993) Skeletal muscle fiber hyperplasia. Med Sci Sports Exerc 25(12): 1333–1345.

Gonyea W (1980) Role of exercise in inducing increases in skeletal muscle fiber number. J Appl Physiol: Respirat Environ Exerc Physiol 48: 421–426.

Heilig A, Pette D (1983) Changes in transcriptional activity of chronically stimulated fast twitch muscle. FEBS Lett 151(2): 211–214.

McDonagh M, Davies C (1984) Adaptive response of mammalian muscle to exercise with high loads. Eur J Appl Physiol 52: 139–155.

Nikituk B, Samoilov N (1990) The adaptive mechanisms of muscle fibres to exercise and possibilities for controlling them. Teoriya i Praktika Fizischeskoi Kultury 5: 11–14.

Tarnaki T, Uchiyama S, Nakano S (1992) A weight-lifting exercise model for inducing hypertrophy in the hindlimb muscles of rats. Med Sci Sports Exerc 24(8): 881–886.

Yamada S, Buffinger N, Dimario J, Strohman R (1989) Fibroblast growth factor is stored in fiber extracellular matrix and plays a role in regulating muscle hypertrophy. Med Sci Sports Exerc 21(5): S173–S180.

Neurophysiological aspects of muscle rehabilitation

Evarts E (1979) Brain mechanisms of movement. Sci Am 79 (July): 146.

Gao JH, Parsons LM, Bower JM, et al. (1996) Cerebellum implicated in sensory acquisition and discrimination rather than motor control. Science 272(5261): 545–547.

Kenyon GT (1997) A model of long-term memory storage in the cerebellar cortex: A possible role for plasticity at parallel fiber synapses onto stellate/basket interneurons. Proc Natl Acad Sci USA 94: 14200–14205.

Lotze M, Montoya P, Erb M, et al. (1999) Activation of cortical and cerebellar motor areas during executed and imagined hand movements: an MRI study. J Cognitive Neurosci 11: 491–501.

Nakazawa K, Yano H, Suzuki Y, Gunji A, Fukunaga T (1997) Effects of long term bed rest on stretch reflex responses of elbow flexor muscles. J Gravit Physiol 1997 4(1): S37–40.

Rapoport M, van Reekum R, Mayberg, H (2000) The role of the cerebellum in cognition and behavior: a selective review. J Neuropsychiatry Clin Neurosci 12: 193–198.

Ruegg DG, Kakebeeke TH, Gabriel JP, Bennefeld M (2003) Conduction velocity of nerve and muscle fiber action potentials after a space mission or a bed rest. Clin Neurophysiol 114(1): 86–93.

Yamanaka K, Yamamoto S, Nakazawa K, et al. (1999) The effects of long-term bed rest on H-reflex and motor evoked potential in the human soleus muscle during standing. Neurosci Lett 266(2): 101–104.

Soft tissue flexibility

Magnusson SP, Aagard P, Simonsen E, Bojsen-Moller F (1998) A biomechanical evaluation of cyclic and static stretch in human skeletal muscle. Int J Sports Med 19(5): 310–316.

Schutz R, et al. (1984) Mechanoreceptors in human cruciate ligaments. J Bone Jt Surg 64A(7): 171.

A model of physical fitness

Berger R (1982) Applied Exercise Physiology. Philadelphia: Lea & Febiger.

Booth F, Gould E (1975) Effects of training and disuse on connective tissue. Exerc Sports Sci Rev 3: 84–112.

Bosco C, Komi PV (1979a) Potentiation of mechanical behaviour of the human skeletal muscle through prestretching. Acta Physiol Scand 106: 467–472.

Bosco C, Komi PV (1979b) Mechanical characteristics and fiber composition of human leg extensor muscle. Eur J Appl Physiol 41: 275–284.

Muscle Disorders

Sue Madden

6

NON-ARTICULAR RHEUMATIC DISORDERS

Fibromyalgia syndrome

Fibromyalgia syndrome (FMS) is a chronic pain syndrome characterized by long-term widespread pain, tender points, generalized stiffness and fatigue. It has a long history within the medical fraternity and has been referred to by a number of names including fibrositis, primary fibromyalgia and secondary fibromyalgia. Despite being officially sanctioned as a distinct clinical syndrome by the American College of Rheumatology (ACR) and at the Myopain conference in Copenhagen in 1992, the issue of its existence remains a dominant discussion point for many members of the medical profession. The primary reason cited for this debate is the lack of pathophysiological abnormalities despite extensive research.

Classification criteria

FMS is currently classified using criteria identified by the ACR namely:

- Chronic widespread pain, which must be present above and below the waist, on both sides of the body and on the axial skeleton (cervical spine, anterior chest, thoracic spine or low back) and must be present for at least 3 months. Pain may be migratory or intermittent and may also occur as individual events in specific areas of the body, such as low back or neck pain.
- Tender points are identified with FMS, of which 18 potentially exist (Fig. 6.1). When palpated with a pressure of 4 kg/cm, 11 of the 18 points must produce pain.

A number of additional symptoms may be associated with FMS, including muscle tension, morning stiffness, chronic headaches, sensations of swelling around the joints, irritable bowel syndrome, premenstrual tension, jaw pain, sleep disturbances, microcirculatory disorders, post-exertion muscle pain, enhanced pain perception and cognitive dysfunction. These do not have to be present for a diagnosis to be made but may aid the clinician's diagnosis.

Pain and tender points

The use of chronic pain as a distinguishing symptom for FMS has many limitations; hence the ACR have argued that the most powerful discriminator between FMS and other similar syndromes such as myofascial pain syndrome and chronic fatigue syndrome are tender points. The ACR state that a tender point is positive if pain is produced in a specific point when a digital pressure of 4 kg/cm is applied to one of the 18 identified sites as seen in Figure 6.1. It should be noted that tender points in FMS are thought to be distinct to trigger points found in people with myofascial pain syndrome. Tender points in FMS reproduce pain in the specific area of

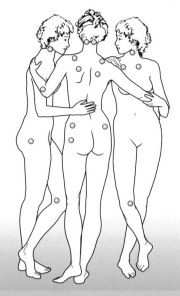

Figure 6.1.   The 18 tender points identified by the ACR (Wolfe et al., 1990).

the tender point only. However, trigger points exist within a taut band of muscle, which upon palpation reproduce the individual's pain and radiate in a specific pattern (see 'Myofascial pain syndrome' below for more information).

The use of tender points in FMS is controversial. Pain created by deep palpation can be produced in individuals who do not complain of chronic pain, albeit with lower degrees of subjective tenderness. It has also been discovered that people with FMS report increased sensitivity at almost every site examined, which has led to the theory that people with FMS have a decreased threshold to pressure. It has been concluded that people with FMS have the lowest threshold to pain pressure when compared with people who report no illnesses, as well as individuals who have various other rheumatological disorders. A further criticism of the tender point concept has been the number that must be present to characterize FMS. Individuals who complain of chronic widespread pain but fail to have 11 positive tender points risk being denied a diagnosis of FMS. Thus it has been argued that the tender point count is arbitrary.

Local muscle pathology

Numerous hypotheses have been proposed in an attempt to explain the clinical presentation of FMS. However, although each may explain certain symptoms, none have currently been able to account fully for the widespread chronic pain and tenderness identified by the ACR. The presence of tender points often leads clinicians and patients to assume that the cause of FMS must be due to localized pathology. For that reason a large number of biopsies have been taken from the tender areas. The results are unconvincing in demonstrating

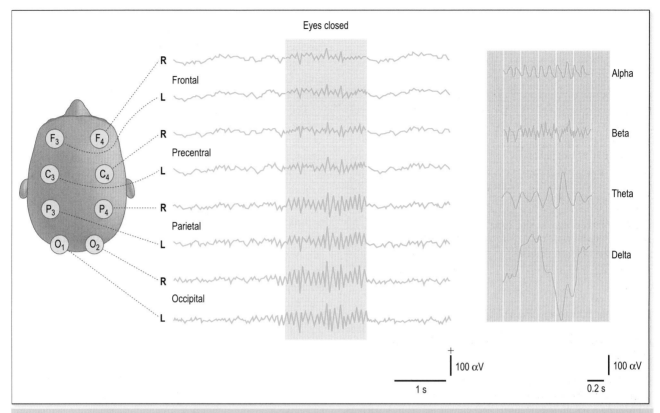

Figure 6.2. The electroencephalogram. The electrical activity of the cerebral cortex recorded on the surface of the skull has different amplitudes and rhythms depending on the recording site and mental activity. When a relaxed subject closes the eyes the activity 'synchronizes' into alpha waves. As the subject slips deeper into sleep, the waves become deeper and slower until rapid eye movement sleep intervenes. (Reproduced with permission from Davies et al., 2001.)

histological or biochemical changes which might seem sufficient to generate the pain. Studies of muscle biopsies have found that fibres may appear moth eaten, which may indicate the uneven distribution and proliferation of mitochondria. However, this finding is not unique to FMS and further studies are needed to demonstrate any link between FMS and muscle pathology.

Sleep pathogenesis

One of the most popular theories for the cause of FMS is the failure of patients to enter deep sleep. In order to measure what is occurring within the brain during sleep and wakefulness, an electroencephalogram (EEG) measures the electrical activity of the brain (Fig. 6.2). Waves can be divided into:

Alpha waves: These occur during periods of relaxation, but we are still awake. The brain becomes slower, and the amplitude of the wave is much larger.

Beta waves: These are associated with day-to-day wakefulness. These waves are the highest in frequency and lowest in amplitude. The waves are not very consistent in their pattern which is explained by various mental activity across the day.

Theta waves: These occur during the first stages of sleep, and have larger amplitudes than alpha waves. The difference between alpha and theta waves is often very subtle and the two can occur together.

Delta waves: These occur in deepest sleep, and are again much slower and have higher amplitudes than all other waves.

Sleep is traditionally divided into two phases: non-rapid eye movement (NREM) and rapid eye movement stages (REM). NREM, also known as slow wave sleep, can be divided into four phases and is believed to be affected by FMS. Stage one and two are lighter sleep stages, where alpha waves are interspersed with theta waves, and stages three and four represent deeper sleep, where delta waves are present. It is argued that patients with FMS do not enter the deeper sleep stages three and four.

The evidence supporting this theory is currently inconclusive. However, the neurotransmitters responsible for sleep and pain modulation are similar. One neurotransmitter of particular importance is serotonin, which is an inhibitory neurotransmitter. If levels of serotonin are insufficient, an increase in perceived pain will result (see 'Altered pain modulation' below for further details). Serotonin is also believed to

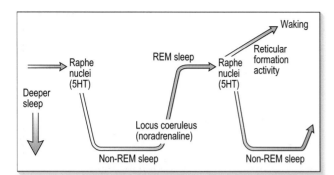

Figure 6.3.   Sleep–wakefulness. The rhythm between REM and non-REM sleep is established by release of serotonin (5HT) and noradrenaline in the brainstem. Activity in the ascending reticular activating system promotes wakefulness. (Reproduced with permission from Davies et al., 2001.)

trigger stage four sleep (Fig. 6.3), induce smooth muscle contraction and preserve the general well-being of the brain. It is generally believed that the lack of stage four sleep and the severity of pain mirror the degree of serotonin deficiency. Hence, it is generally believed that a deficiency in serotonin induces several biochemical abnormalities that best explain the symptoms of FMS. As a result, medications that elevate serotonin, such as serotonin selective reuptake inhibitors and tricyclic antidepressants, are commonly used for the treatment of FMS.

There are limitations to such theories. When patients' sleep patterns are treated and improved, a subsequent improvement in the symptoms of FMS does not occur. There also appears to be no association between patients attending a sleep disorder clinic and the prevalence of FMS symptoms. Of 108 consecutive patients attending a sleep disorder clinic, only 2.7% were considered to have FMS. At present, it is also unclear whether people get FMS as a result of the sleeping patterns or whether poor sleep results from the other symptoms of FMS, such as pain interrupting sleep. As a result, no conclusion can be made regarding sleep disorders and their relationship to FMS.

Altered pain modulation

Nociceptors are free nerve endings which normally have high stimulus thresholds. There are two types:

- *Mechano-nociceptors*. These are only activated by intense mechanical stimuli such as heavy pressure or pinching which respond with a slowly adapting discharge of action potentials. They do not respond to normal heating or cooling or to the application of *algogenic* (pain-producing) chemicals. However, they will respond to temperatures higher than 48°C.
- *Polymodalnociceptors*. Primarily located in the skin, these respond to a wide variety of stimuli.

If the nociceptors are stimulated, painful stimuli are transmitted through A delta and C fibres to the spinal cord. Nociceptors are not only stimulated via mechanical forces, but can also be stimulated by chemicals released within the body. One of these is serotonin, which is released from blood platelets.

The widespread nature of pain within FMS and associated tender points has focused attention towards hyperalgesia, which is where there is extreme sensitivity to a stimulant which results in the sensation of pain. Primary hyperalgesia is characterized by lowered pain threshold and increased pain sensitivity within the damaged tissue. Secondary hyperalgesia has increased pain sensitivity in the surrounding area without tissue damage, which is caused by central sensitization. Dorsal horn excitability is the mechanism that is primarily responsible. It is believed that FMS is due to secondary hyperalgesia, which is due to long-lasting input from deep nociceptors, thus resulting in long-term alteration of the central processing of pain. Peripheral nociceptors, which are involved with pain regulation, become sensitized by the release of substances from damaged tissue. This sensitization mechanism enables weak stimuli, such as local pressure, to elicit pain as in FMS. The nociceptors are also connected to the adjacent muscle by the dorsal horn neuron, which can lead to pain referring to other deeper tissues associated with hyperalgesia. As an inhibitory neurotransmitter, serotonin may prevent the firing of secondary neurons. Hence if levels of serotonin are low, there will be an increase in perceived pain.

Another neurotransmitter that has been associated with FMS is substance P. Substance P is an important mediator of the inflammatory process (Figs 6.4, 6.5 and 6.6) and it has been found that some patients with FMS have significantly higher levels than normal. The damaged tissue releases neurotransmitters that lower the mechanical threshold of the nociceptors (i.e. sensitization). The sensitization lowers the mechanical threshold of the nociceptive endings and weak stimuli are able to excite the nociceptors and elicit muscle pain; for example, local pressure elicits unpleasant sensation and pain, in the case of FMS local tenderness. Dorsal horn neurons, whose primary function is to conduct pain information, has afferents not only from nociceptors of a given muscle but also from neighbouring neurons that normally process information from other muscles and/or skin. Depending on the intensity of the stimulus, such a mechanism can lead to distal spread and/or referral to other deep tissues. This central sensitization might cause tenderness and hyperalgesia in patients through a general enhancement of neuronal excitability.

The relationship between neurotransmitters and pain is complex and as yet fails to explain why tenderness may occur in the absence of pain. In summary, long-lasting input from deep nociceptors is likely to increase the responsiveness of sensory dorsal horn neurons and peripheral painful lesions

Chapter 6 Muscle Disorders

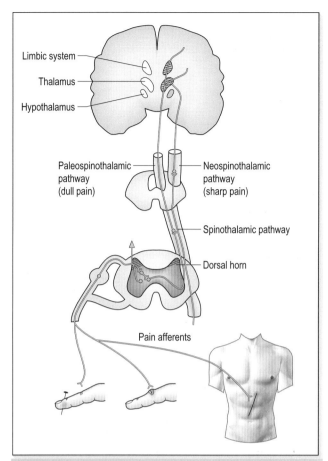

Figure 6.4.   Pathways of pain perception. Shaded areas are rich in opioid receptors. Opioid receptors are also found in medullary areas and the spinal cord. This shows in simplified form the pathways activated following stimulation of peripheral nociceptive nerve terminals. Many mediators are involved during afferent stimulation of the nociceptive pathway. Mediator release (bradykinin, 5-hydroxytryptamine, prostaglandins) stimulates the nerve terminals of pain fibres. Onward afferent transmission of ascending nerve impulses at the synapses in the dorsal horn involves neuropeptides such as substance P. Hyperexcitability of pain fibres can also be promoted by other mediators. The ascending pathways inner-vate areas of the midbrain and thalamus. (Reproduced with permission from Waller et al., 2001.)

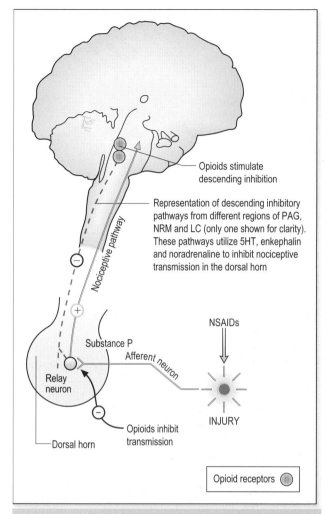

Figure 6.5.   Transmitters and receptors for pain perception. The nociceptive pathways use a variety of transmitter substances, and promoters of transmission in neurons, substance P, other neuropeptides and nitric oxide all appear to be involved. The afferent pathways are subject to inhibitory control. Opioids act at opioid receptor-rich sites in the periaqueductal grey matter (PAG), the raphe magnus nucleus (NMR) and other spinal sites to stimulate descending inhibitory fibres that inhibit nociceptive transmission in the dorsal horn. Descending pathways from the locus coeruleus (LC) that are noradrenergic are also involved. Opioids also act directly in the dorsal horn to inhibit transmission. The inhibitory pathways associated with 5-hydroxytryptamine (5HT) and noradrenergic neurons may also explain the analgesic properties of antidepressants and anticonvulsants in certain types of pain. NSAIDs, non-steroidal anti-inflammatory drugs. (Reproduced with permission from Waller et al., 2001.)

can result in long-term alteration of the central processing of pain.

Psychological factors

Psychological factors have been associated with FMS through-out the past 60 years of its history. In the 1950s and 1960s it was considered to be due to hysteria and acquired the name of psychogenic rheumatism. As a result, much research has been undertaken in an attempt to define possible psychologi-cal associations. However, these have produced conflicting results. Use of the Minnesota Multiphasic Personality Inventory (MMPI) has shown that people with FMS have higher scores relating to depression, hysteria and hypochon-driasis. These scores cannot be explained by degree of pain or

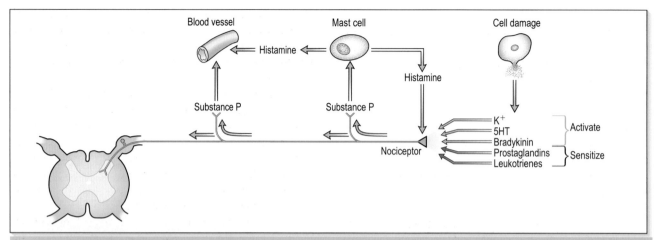

Figure 6.6.   The origins and effects of pain mediators. Activation of nociceptors is frequently brought about by damage but does not require the nociceptor itself to be damaged. For example, release of chemical mediators by damaged cells leads to the sensitization and activation of nociceptors, which in turn releases substance P by an axon reflex. Substance P then degranulates mast cells to release histamine, which stimulates nociceptors in a feedback loop. (Reproduced with permission from Davies et al., 2001.)

other associated symptoms of FMS, as patients with rheumatoid arthritis who report similar pain levels as patients with FMS do not have such scores on the MMPI. It is also suggested that patients with FMS have similar personality traits such as dependence and passivity, obsessive–compulsive personality and idealization of family relationships. As a result these manifest clinically in a depressive disorder which results in pain. However, it remains unclear how these factors relate to the clinical presentation of FMS and whether these psychological factors are present before the onset of FMS or whether they are as a result of the illness. Although individuals with FMS strongly reject the notion that FMS results from psychological problems it is acknowledged that these could result from the symptoms of FMS.

Other factors that have been proposed to cause FMS include various infections, overuse, trauma, stress and immunological factors. It is suggested that these in combination are the most likely triggers of FMS. However, at present there is no evidence to support any of these claims.

Treatment

Due to the symptom presentation many treatments have been developed in an attempt to resolve these problems.

Pharmacological approaches

Low doses of antidepressants are frequently prescribed. These are used to improve sleep patterns of patients rather than for an antidepressive effect. Analgesics, such as non-steroidal anti-inflammatory drugs (NSAID), have been advocated for treatment purposes although the results for their use remain inconclusive.

Non-pharmacological approaches

A number of non-pharmacological interventions have been identified as potential treatment modalities for FMS. These include exercise, electromyographic biofeedback training, electrotherapy, acupuncture and patient education and self-management programmes. Owing to the limited quality of studies to date, it is not possible to draw definite conclusions regarding these approaches.

Cognitive-behavioural therapy

Cognitive-behavioural therapy (CBT) allows a variety of components that may influence the nature of chronic pain to be addressed: namely the sensory, affective, cognitive and behavioural aspects. CBT is considered essential when treating FMS as many patients may suffer with depression or increased anxiety states. However, the true efficacy of these treatments is difficult to assess as they predominantly occur as part of a larger treatment programme, which uses a variety of other modalities such as aerobic exercise and stretching, pacing and enhancement of pain tolerance, family education and the use of tricyclic antidepressants.

Myofascial pain syndrome

Myofascial pain syndrome (MPS) is a regional pain syndrome. Although MPS has a long history, and is a well-known disorder, relatively little is understood about it. MPS is a controversial condition due to the lack of identifiable pathological abnormalities. However, there is increasing evidence to support the notion that trigger points exist in muscle and connective tissue.

Classification criteria

To date, there is still a lack of clarity about the classification criteria for MPS. Although not universally accepted, it has been proposed that there are major and minor criteria.

Major criteria include:

- trigger points
- regional pain
- pain in defined referral pattern of pain
- taut band at trigger point site
- focal tenderness at taut band and some restricted range of motion.

It is unclear whether all major criteria should be present for a diagnosis of MPS to be made, but it is accepted that the distinguishing feature of MPS are trigger points, which may be active or latent. Upon palpation, active trigger points give rise to local tenderness as well as a predictable pattern of referred pain in areas remote from the point of stimulation. This pattern does not correspond to segmental or dermatomal distribution. People with active trigger points complain of dull aching over the trigger point, which upon palpation produces dull aching or burning pain in the referred trigger zone. Latent trigger points are asymptomatic, but upon palpation produce the expected trigger point referred pain. Trigger points have three specific characteristics:

1. circumscribed deep tenderness
2. a localized twitch or fasciculation on pinching or pressing the muscle containing the trigger point
3. referred pain produced by pressure on the trigger point.

Trigger points are normally localized in taut bands of muscles, which can be as wide as a centimetre. These can be identified upon palpating the longitudinal axis of the muscle fibre, which may produce a 'twitch' response. Such a sign is classified as a minor criterion and it is uncertain how frequently people with MPS present with such signs. Additional minor criteria include:

- pain reproduced by pressure on the trigger point
- pain that is improved upon stretching, compressing or needling the trigger point.

Possible pathophysiology

The cause of MPS is unknown, but history of localized trauma, fatigue from muscle overuse, chronic posture imbalance and stress have all been proposed.

Histological findings in MPS are generally inconclusive. Early studies believed trigger points were caused by the release of mediators from locally degrading mast cells. It was hypothesized that this would lead to a release of histamine and 5-hydroxytryptamine (5HT) followed by sensitization of local C nerve fibres. However, all studies remain contradictory and inconclusive.

Trigger points may also lead to shortening and weakness of the muscles involved. Although sarcomere shortening does occur this is not present in the early stages of the illness. Therefore, this is believed to be secondary to, rather than the cause of, MPS.

At present, studies using electromyography (EMG) fail to identify any significant findings at trigger points. It has been suggested that the resting EMG level of a muscle with an active trigger point is higher than that of muscle with no trigger points, and that it subsequently decreased in response to trigger point injections. However, these findings have not been reproduced, and it is generally accepted that there is no abnormal activity at trigger point sites.

At present, the major limitation with much of the research in MPS is the lack of agreement as to the definition of the syndrome. Due to the lack of objective criteria, various interpretations are made regarding the classification criteria, and different studies have used different criteria; thus comparisons between studies are limited. A priority for MPS research is to agree a common definition which can be applied to all research studies.

Treatment of MPS: spray and stretch

The spray and stretch treatment was popularized by Travell and Simmons and is the most widely known and most controversial form of treatment for MPS. The skin overlying the trigger point is sprayed with ethyl chloride or dichlorodifluoromethane, which aims to cool the skin but not the underlying structures. After 10 seconds, the muscle is gently stretched. When successfully performed, it is reported that patients experience a feeling of looseness and diminished tension, with the effects lasting 12–36 hours, although it is reported that the more physically active the patient is the less time the results will last. In most patients spray and stretch will improve symptoms, but areas of pain tend to persist. To treat these remaining areas of pain, an injection into the trigger point is performed. Crucial to this form of therapy is being able to locate the trigger point precisely. Accurate localization of the trigger point is aided by the patient's account of intense pain as the needle enters the trigger point. Although it is often easy to find the trigger point over the skin, it is often more difficult to pierce the trigger point. The injecting solution used is 2–5 ml of 1% procaine containing a very small amount (0.1–0.3 ml) of an intermediate acting corticosteroid. The rationale of the corticosteroid is to minimize the irritant effect of the local anaesthesia. Following the injection, the whole muscle is stretched, followed by the spray and stretch technique described above. Ideally the patient should rest for 20–30 minutes after the injection, with the main relief reportedly lasting 2–4 days after the injection.

This form of treatment is controversial. Studies to date show varying degrees of efficacy, with many reporting the improvements occurring due to a placebo effect. A second major consideration is its cost effectiveness. It is highly time-consuming, particularly if a patient has several trigger points that need to be treated. As a result, many feel that the treatment is impractical and too costly for the results gained.

Differential diagnosis of FMS, MPS and other similar syndromes

A challenge facing healthcare professionals when considering FMS, MPS and other similar syndromes is the specificity and certainty of each diagnosis. For conditions such as FMS and MPS, which lack objective biomedical tests, this remains highly problematic as the clinical definition is very similar. For example, chronic fatigue syndrome (CFS), FMS and MPS are all classified in relation to subjective reporting of symptoms. Many of the symptoms used within these various criteria sets, such as myalgias, arthralgias and fatigue, are very similar and difficult to measure. MPS relies primarily on trigger points which are similar to tender points used within FMS, where even supposed experts in MPS have difficulty distinguishing between trigger points and tender points in clinical practice. It has also been suggested that the only difference between FMS and CFS is the level of reported pain and fatigue. Low back pain syndromes and cervical pain syndromes have been shown to result in clusters of local tender points. Similarly, knee joints affected by rheumatoid arthritis and osteoarthritis may have associated tender points. Local tenderness has been shown to exist in other rheumatological disorders but never to the extent or degree noted in FMS.

As a result, it has been argued that the diagnosis received is dependent on the clinical specialty to which the patient is referred rather than the uniqueness of the clinical picture. For example, a patient who is referred to a neurologist will in all likelihood be diagnosed with CFS, whereas if they were referred to a rheumatologist they would be diagnosed with FMS. It is also now proposed that rather than being distinct clinical syndromes, MPS, FMS and CFS represent one syndrome, which is represented by a spectrum of symptoms.

ABNORMALITIES OF ION CHANNELS

Myotonia

Myotonia is a term used to describe muscle stiffness caused by abnormalities of the muscle membrane, primarily hyperexcitability of the plasma membrane of skeletal muscle fibres. Myotonia may be present in a number of diseases, including myotonia muscular dystrophy, general myotonia congenita,

paramyotonia congenita, and some types of periodic paralysis (the key features of which are summarized in Table 6.1). Other symptoms associated with myotonia are muscle weakness, paralysis and muscle hypertrophy which may occur over a long period due to long-term muscle hyperactivity (see Table 6.2 for brief pathophysiology of each symptom). Myotonia can be present in myotonic dystrophy as well as non-dystrophic myotonia. However, myotonia in the former can affect skeletal, brain, eye and heart tissue rather than exclusively skeletal as in the latter. Myotonia also tends to be mild in myotonia dystrophy, with dystrophic changes being the primary symptom.

Myotonia can occur due to mutations in the genetic coding for the skeletal muscle sodium channel or the skeletal muscle chloride channel. Voltage-gated ion channels regulate membrane excitability, which is critical for muscle function. Excitability of skeletal muscle is needed to propagate action potentials from the neuromuscular junction along the fibre and into the transverse tubules, where depolarization triggers calcium release from the sarcoplasmic reticulum. Clinical myotonia is characterized by slowed muscle relaxation because of continuous spontaneous activity (electromyographic myotonia). Hence, the excitability is enhanced. A brief stimulus elicits a burst of myotonic discharges (known as myotonic runs on the EMG), lasting for several seconds.

Although myotonia can be caused by mutation in either the sodium or chloride channels, clinical myotonia occurs due to the same resultant effect. In both mutations, the after-discharges are dependent on the integrity of the transverse tubules. Transverse tubules are long, narrow invaginations of the sarcolemma that effectively propagate depolarization to the core of the fibre, as well as providing a barrier to potassium (Fig. 6.7). The accumulation of potassium in the transverse tubules depolarizes the fibre, which is normally prevented by chloride. The loss of chloride conductance and the accumulated potassium causes a larger depolarizing shift in the resting potential and triggers an after-discharge. With inactivation-deficient sodium channels, even a small potassium depolarization is sufficient to activate a substantial sodium current, which further depolarizes the fibre and triggers myotonic discharges.

Although the two resultant mutations may lead to myotonia, it is necessary to understand how each mutation can lead to such effects.

Chloride channel myotonia

Chloride channel myotonia may be inherited by dominant or recessive mechanisms. The overall effect is the same, with a reduction in skeletal muscle chloride conductance.

Chloride channel myotonia is caused by mutations in the CLCN1 gene coding. A reduction of the muscle chloride conductance electrically destabilizes the muscle fibre. This causes the repetitive action potential firing which results in the characteristic myotonic muscle stiffness. The channels are only

Table 6.1. An overview of the most common forms of myotonia

Na⁺ channel or Cl⁻ channel mutation	Disease	Family history	Age of onset	Clinical symptoms	Aggravating factors
Cl⁻ channel mutation	Dominant myotonia congenita (also known as Thomsen's disease)	Autosomal dominant inheritance	From birth to early childhood	Muscle stiffness which is worse after rest, and improves after exercise: the 'warm up phenomenon'. Myotonia fluctuates only slightly during lifetime, there is no progression and muscle hypertrophy is frequent	Patients may state that the cold increases myotonia. However, this is not substantiated with objective measurements of relaxation times
Cl⁻ channel mutation	Recessive generalized myotonia (Becker's disease)	Autosomal recessive inheritance	Occasionally in early childhood but usually occurs in teenagers	Muscle stiffness which is worse after rest, and improves after exercise: the 'warm up phenomenon'. Frequently transient weakness after rest which improves after several minutes of exercise. Weakness more pronounced in upper limbs, and stiffness worse in legs. Symptoms usually progress for first few years after onset and then stabilize	
Na⁺ channel mutation	Paramyotonia congenita (PMC)	Autosomal dominant inheritance	From birth	Muscle stiffness which may be accompanied by muscle weakness. Recovery from muscle weakness may last several hours but is not permanent	Stiffness increases with exercise: known as paradoxical myotonia. May also be increased in extreme cold
Na⁺ channel	Hyperkalaemic periodic paralysis (hyperPP)	Autosomal dominant inheritance	Early childhood to second decade in life	Attacks of weakness, usually in the morning, lasting 10 minutes to several hours and occasionally a couple of days. Severity can vary from patient to patient, with some experiencing a few attacks in a lifetime, with others having several attacks a week. Myotonic stiffness is not observed	Foods with high potassium content, rest after exercise, ethanol ingestion. Eating carbohydrates or mild exercise may diminish or stop an attack
Na⁺ channel	Potassium-aggravated myotonia (PAM). Also known as sodium channel myotonia (SCM). Includes a variety of distinct syndromes	Autosomal dominant inheritance		Muscle stiffness which may be provoked by exercise. Persistent generalized myotonia and muscle hypertrophy, particularly in the necks and shoulders. Muscle pain may be induced by exercise. Attacks of severe muscle stiffness in the thoracic muscles may be life-threatening in children due to impaired ventilation	Increases with ingestion of potassium. Also may be induced by exercise

Table 6.2.   Myotonia: pathophysiology of clinical symptoms

Clinical symptom	Pathophysiology
Stiff muscle	Several trains of action potentials of muscle fibres are triggered by single nerve stimulation. These present on EMG as 'myotonic runs'
Weak muscles	Unresponsiveness of the muscle fibre sodium channels that are inactivated by previous hyperstimulation. Also can occur due to high levels of potassium

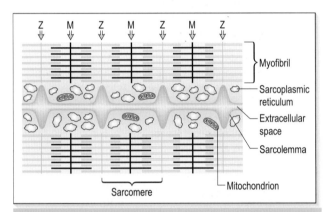

Figure 6.7.   Side view of the transverse tubular network in muscle cells. Transverse tubules are invaginations of the sarcolemma, which are in intimate contact with the sarcoplasmic reticulum (SR). The SR is a continuous, tubular compartment in close association with the myofibrils. The transverse tubules are extensions of the sarcolemma around the Z-line. They transmit the depolarizing nerve impulse to terminal regions of the SR, coordinating Ca^{2+} release and contraction of the myofibril. (Reproduced with permission from Baynes and Dominiczak, 1999.)

active at very large positive voltages, such that their contribution to the resting conductance at the physiological membrane potential is reduced, which affects the slow gate response of the channel.

Due to the genetic coding mutation of the chloride channel, treatment is very difficult. In general, most people manage the situation without any treatment, but if necessary, treatment is focused on reducing the excitability of muscle fibres by partially inhibiting the voltage-gated sodium channels with local anaesthetics.

Sodium channel myotonia/potassium-aggravated myotonia

To date, 23 different mutations have been identified which are associated with sodium channel diseases. As a result, several

different features of sodium channel behaviour have been identified. Hyperkalaemic periodic paralysis (HyperPP), paramyotonia congenita (PMC) and potassium-aggravated myotonia (PAM) are all associated with mutations in the adult isoform of the skeletal muscle sodium channel alpha subunit, SkM1. For all the mutant sodium channels studied to date, there is general agreement that the pore of the sodium channel is normal, and that the primary defect is an alteration in the voltage-dependent gating (opening and closing) of mutant channels.

A normal functioning sodium channel will activate quickly in response to depolarization and then close to a fast-inactivated state from which further openings are rare. The membrane must be hyperpolarized to induce recovery from inactivation and reprime sodium channels to become available to open with subsequent repolarization. However, in the mutations, there is disruption of fast inactivation which results in an increased tendency of the muscle fibres to depolarize. In addition, a subset of mutations produces a disruption in slow inactivation that occurs on a scale of seconds to minutes. Sodium influx at slight depolarization itself generates action potentials and myotonia, stronger depolarizations lead to general inactivation of both mutant and wild-type sodium channels and thus weakness. Such differences in gating behaviour may explain the differences in genotype–phenotype which are displayed.

Periodic paralyses

Periodic paralyses is a rare inherited disorder of skeletal muscle in which the primary defect is an alteration in the electrical excitability of the muscle fibre. Unlike myotonia, where excitability is enhanced, in periodic paralyses, excitability is reduced during attacks. Muscles are flaccid and electrically unexcitable. The resting membrane potential is depolarized at -50 to $-40\,mV$ from a normal value of $-95\,mV$. Such attacks only appear following defects in slow inactivation, where persistent sodium current induces prolonged episodes of depolarization-induced inexcitability.

Weakness is usually generalized and can last from a few minutes to several hours, with full strength not returning for days. People may have only a few attacks in a lifetime, or several a week if they are more severely affected having. During an attack a person may be unable to stand or move limbs against gravity. As only skeletal muscle is affected, this is not a life-threatening condition.

IDIOPATHIC INFLAMMATORY MYOPATHIES

Idiopathic inflammatory myopathies (IDM) are a group of muscle disorders of unknown cause that are characterized by muscle weakness and inflammatory infiltrates in the muscle.

Table 6.3.   An overview of idiopathic inflammatory myopathies

	Age at onset	Family history	Clinical features	Specific pathophysiology	Treatment
Polymyositis	Adult	No	Muscle weakness is progressive, proximal and symmetrical	Inflammatory infiltrates are mostly within the fascicles	Systemic corticosteroids with or without immunosuppressives
			Systemic	Necrotic fibres in polymyositis are scattered and not necessarily near the area of inflammation	
				Perifascicular atrophy is not usually found	
				CD8+ T-cells	
Dermatomyositis	All ages	No	Muscle weakness is progressive, proximal and symmetrical	Inflammatory infiltrates are perivascular or in the septa, and around rather than within the fascicles	Systemic corticosteroids with or without immunosuppressives
			Systemic	Necrosis and phagocytosis of muscle fibres and in advanced cases an increase of endomysial connective tissue	
				CD4+ and B-cells. More B-cells	
Body-inclusion myositis	>50 years	Rare	Muscle weakness is progressive, affecting both proximal and distal muscles. Most commonly affected muscle groups are finger flexors and quadriceps	Characterized by eosinophilic inclusions and vacuoles with basophilic granules at the rim of the vacuole	The disease is unresponsive to corticosteroids and immunosuppressives. Physiotherapy may be helpful to maintain mobility

Several conditions come under the umbrella term of inflammatory myopathies, including polymyositis, dermatomyositis and inclusion body myositis (see Table 6.3 for an overview of these conditions).

Although uncommon, IDMs are the most frequently encountered muscle disorders in clinical practice. There appear to be two peaks of onset, one in childhood, which present clinically as the most severe forms of the diseases, and one in the fifth decade of life. With the exception of inclusion body myositis, all are more common in females than males, although the precise incidence is unclear. The cause is unknown, but several hypotheses have been proposed including viral, environmental, drug related and hereditary.

The major clinical features of IDM are muscle weakness, tenderness and occasionally pain. Initial clinical symptoms may include myalgias, fatigue or weakness, with patients reporting difficulty in performing everyday functional tasks. IDMs are progressive disorders, with atrophy and fibrosis of skeletal muscle occurring. IDMs may also present systemically which may result in other diseases, the most common being arthritis and arthralgias. Other systems involved may include cardiac, pulmonary, gastrointestinal and endocrine, all of which contribute to the morbidity and mortality of the conditions. There is also an association between some myopathies and malignant cancers, although this is still open to debate.

Although referred to collectively, distinctions in the clinical course and pathophysiology are present in different IDMs, which need to be considered (see Table 6.3 for an overview).

Polymyositis/dermatomyositis

Traditionally polymyositis and dermatomyositis have frequently been considered to be the same disease with terms being used interchangeably, with the only additional clinical feature for dermatomyositis being skin disorders. Polymyositis is diagnosed using four key features: muscle disease which is progressive, proximal, with symmetrical weakness; an increased concentration of muscle enzymes; an abnormal EMG; and an abnormal muscle biopsy sample. Muscle pain and weakness may occur both during and after exertion. Dermatomyositis has the additional clinical features of a heliotrope rash, Gottron's papules, cuticular changes, a photo-erythema and a scaly alopecia. Polymyositis is rare in people under the age of 18, although dermatomyositis is common in children.

Traditionally, much of the research has focused upon understanding the relationship between inflammation and response to corticosteroids in polymyositis and dermatomyositis. It was originally hypothesized that the greater the inflammation upon muscle biopsy, the worse the muscle weakness would be. However, this does not reflect clinical findings where inflammation appears to be absent, but patients continue to respond slowly to the treatment, with some being left with decreased muscle function.

Although both conditions have similar inflammatory histological findings, abnormal pathophysiology differences exist. Dermatomyositis is thought to result from an antibody-mediated response, where the membrane of capillaries is attacked, leading to ischaemia. Although the antigen stimulus is unknown, it is assumed to be linked to the vascular endothelium. It has been proposed that involvement of the blood vessels could affect the perfusion of the muscle, which may lead to a disturbed muscle function. It has been shown that thickening of the endothelial cells is still present 3 months after corticosteroid treatment has commenced, despite the resolution of inflammatory infiltrates. Such changes to the endothelium could affect perfusion, causing hypoxia or other metabolic disturbances. This leads to muscle biopsy findings of necrosis, microinfarcts and perifascicular atrophy. Therefore, it is not a muscular disease per se, and explains, to a degree the involvement of other organs, particularly the skin. Further research has suggested that muscle bioenergetic metabolites such as phosphocreatine and ATP levels are reduced in dermatomyositis, with the ratio of inorganic phosphate to phosphocreatine increased, compared with controls, even at rest. Such findings give preliminary evidence to the cause of muscle weakness and pain. Further research is currently being done to explore this further.

Polymyositis, however, is believed to be an autoimmune response against muscle fibres which is mediated by CD8 T-cells. The inflammatory infiltrates tend to be within the muscle fascicles. CD8 T-cells cross the basal lamina, and through compression of normal muscle fibres appear to induce the release of necrosis substances, such as TNF-α, perforin (which forms tubular transmembrane complexes) and granzyme (granule content of T-cytotoxic cells). The antigen is assumed to be on the surface of the muscle fibre, but this is unclear. Typical muscle biopsy findings in polymyositis show evidence of endomysial inflammatory infiltrates, primarily CD8+ cytoxic T-cells and macrophages, which surround and invade non-necrotic muscle fibres. In polymyositis, muscle necrosis and regeneration may be present, although this varies depending on the severity and chronicity of the condition. In very severe cases connective tissues proliferation may also occur.

The mechanism for long-term decreased muscle function is less well studied but it is assumed to be a combination of atrophy from the disease itself, long-term corticosteroid treatment or disuse atrophy. Morbidity and mortality increases if systematic disease is present.

Body-inclusion myositis

Body-inclusion myositis is a slowly progressive form of IDM and only tends to develop when people are in their fifties. In the elderly, it is the most frequently seen myopathy. Due to the gradual onset of the disease, people may be symptomatic for 5 or 10 years before a diagnosis is made. Weakness can be distal and asymmetrical, with muscle groups such as wrist and long finger flexor muscles and knee extensors being affected, which is unlike other myopathies. However, proximal muscles can still be affected more than distal muscles. Muscle atrophy can also be prominent. Although body inclusion myopathy rarely responds to corticosteroid treatment, people with body-inclusion myopathy rarely die from the disease but do suffer from disability due to weak muscles.

Due to the onset being over 50 years, it is hypothesized that the pathophysiology changes are related to an ageing-based degenerative cascade. One theory is that the over-expression of amyloid beta-precursor protein occurs early in the pathological process, but this is still debated. Mitochondrial DNA depletion has also been found in IDM, leading to speculation as to whether this is the cause of the disease or as a result. A common pathological finding is rimmed vacuoles and 15–18 nm filamentous inclusions in the sarcoplasm and nucleus, containing many of the same protein components as are found in brain plaques in Alzheimer's disease.

MUSCULAR DYSTROPHIES

Muscular dystrophy (MD) is a general term referring to a group of heterogeneous genetic disorders which share clinical features of progressive muscle wasting and cardiac conduction

Table 6.4. Common forms of muscular dystrophies

Disease	Genetic abnormality	Age of clinical onset	Clinical presentation	Rate of progression
Duchenne MD	Almost complete absence of dystrophin	3	Weakness usually occurs initially in gluteal and lumbar regions. Eventually all areas involved. Complications include muscle contraction, kyphoscoliosis leading to impaired respiratory function and muscle wasting	Rapid, with wheelchair use by early teens and death by late teens early twenties. Usually due to respiratory or cardiac failure
Becker's MD	Abnormality of actin-binding domain of dystrophin	5 to 15	Similar to Duchenne MD, but less severe. Most remain ambulatory into their teens and early twenties	Less severe and rapid than Duchenne. Many live into middle age
Emery–Dreifuss MD	Emerin, which is localized on the nuclear membrane of muscle cells	Childhood or adolescence	Muscle contractures develop early in disease process, and primarily affect arms proximally and legs distally. Distribution referred to as 'scapulo-humero-peroneal' and cardiac arrhythmias leading to complete heart block in almost all patients	Slowly progressive. Usually live into middle age
Oculopharyngeal	Polyadenylation protein 2	Fifth decade in life	Ptosis (drooping of eyelids), dysphagia, weakness and atrophy of tongue, weakness of facial and proximal arm muscles	Progressive
Myotonic dystrophy	Myotonin protein kinase	Adult	Muscular weakness, muscular dystrophy, myotonia, cataracts, testicular atrophy, frontal balding, and cardiac conduction	Slowly progressive

defects. MD can be classified at a number of levels, whether by the mode of inheritance, age of onset or groups of muscles affected. The most commonly recognized MD is Duchenne muscular dystrophy, with other forms including various groups of limb girdle muscular dystrophy, myotonic dystrophy, Emery–Dreifuss muscular dystrophy and fascioscapulohumeral dystrophy (Table 6.4). It was originally hypothesized that the mutation resulted in a deficiency in dystrophin, a complex protein thought to be responsible for the mechanical reinforcement of the sarcolemma, thereby helping to protect muscle fibres from stresses which arise during muscle contraction. However, as the understanding of MD has developed, particularly in the last 10 years, other proteins have been identified which partly explain the clinical diversity in this group. As a result of such findings, MDs are currently being classified as dystrophinopathies or laminopathies, depending upon the protein identified as being the cause of the condition.

Dystrophinopathies

This group of MDs are the most common group of MDs and include Duchenne MD (DMD) and Becker's MD. In order to understand the phenotypical presentation of these conditions, it is necessary to consider the structure and wider function of dystrophin.

Dystrophin and dystrophin–glycoprotein complex

Dystrophin is an elongated cytoskeletal actin-binding protein structure with four important structural features: an

N-terminal actin binding domain; a long central rod domain; a cysteine-rich domain; and a C-terminal domain. Dystrophin is an integral part of a complex known as the dystrophin–glycoprotein (DGC) complex, which is believed to be essential in maintaining muscle function. A primary role of the DGC complex is to act as a link between the extracellular matrix and subsarcolemmal cytoskeleton. This would correlate with early research which found elevated serum creatine kinase levels in fetal blood before the development of the disease, which suggests an abnormality of the plasma membrane in DMD. Another function of the DGC complex is to protect muscle cells from contraction-induced damage. It is also thought to have a signalling role, although this is still being established.

The structure of the DGC comprises a number of membrane-associated proteins, all of which are essential for the integrity of skeletal fibres. These include dystrophin, the dystroglycans (alpha and beta), the sacroglycans (alpha, beta, delta and gamma), sarcospan, the dystrophins and alpha dystrobrevin (Fig. 6.8). The complex can be subdivided into three sections depending upon where they are localized: (1) an extracellular complex which includes alpha dystroglycan and laminin; (2) a transmembrane complex comprising the sarcoglycans, beta-dystroglycan and sarcospan; and (3) a subsarcolemmal complex comprising dystrophin, syntrophins and dystrobrevin.

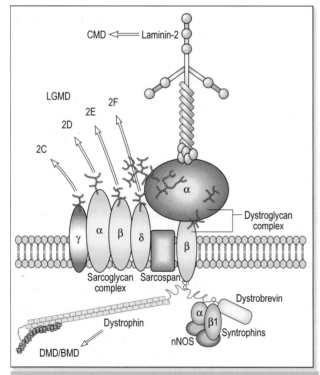

Figure 6.8.   The dystroglycan complex (DGC) in skeletal muscle. (Reproduced with permission from Durbeej and Campbell 2002.)

It is generally hypothesized that the type of muscular dystrophy will depend on where the mutation on the dystrophin complex is. It is established that DMD and Becker's MD both have mutations on the dystrophin protein itself. In the case of DMD it is completely absent, which explains, to a degree, the severity of the disease and its rapid progression. In the absence of dystrophin, muscle fibres are abnormally vulnerable to contraction-induced injury, which eventually leads to myofibre death and infiltration by connective tissue elements in DMD. The diaphragm and other respiratory muscles seem particularly susceptible to such effects due to the relatively continuous recruitment rate. In Becker's muscular dystrophy there is believed to be a malfunction in the actin-binding domain of dystrophin. The number of mutations found in the DGC can be explained, in part, by the fact that the dystrophin gene responsible for MD is a large gene, hence high numbers of mutations may occur.

Although it is now known that the DGC complex is involved in muscular dystrophy and can explain why there are wide variations in the clinical presentation of the diseases, it is still unclear exactly how these abnormalities result in skeletal muscle fibre destruction and connective tissue infiltration.

Laminopathies

Unlike the traditional belief that MD results from defects in proteins of the muscle membrane, laminopathies are due to deficiencies of nuclear proteins. The most commonly known laminopathies include Emery–Dreifuss muscular dystrophy (EDMD) and limb girdle muscular dystrophies (Table 6.5). Proteins found in the nuclear membrane, which is essential for maintaining the architecture of the nucleus, include emerin, LAP-1 and LAP-2 families and MAN1. In the case of EDMD, mutations have been found in emerin, but are also known to occur in lamin A and C, which bind to the inner nuclear membrane. Mutations of different sections of lamin

Table 6.5.   Common types of limb girdle muscular dystrophy (LGMD)

	Inheritance: autosomal dominant or recessive	Protein involved	Progressive nature
LGMD1A	Dominant	Myotilin	Difficult to assess as very rare
LGMD1B	Dominant	Lamin	
LGMD 2A	Recessive	Caplain 3	Gradual
LGMD 2B	Recessive	Dysferlin	Gradual
LGMD2C, 2D, 2E, 2F	Recessive	Sarcoglycan proteins	Variable

A and C have also been identified as being responsible for the limb girdle MD groups.

Although the mutations have now been identified, it is still unclear how nuclear deficiencies result in distinct forms of MD.

Exercise therapy

It is currently unclear whether exercise-induced therapy will be beneficial or harmful to those with dystrophin deficiency. Hence, the role of exercise in clinical management is controversial. The mechanical stress placed on the sarcolemma during muscle contraction may possibly increase the disease process. However, it is also possible to argue that exercise would include transformation of the muscle fibres towards a slower oxidative profile, which could also be beneficial. If exercise is used within the treatment process, it is advised that there should be sufficient muscle fibre to make a difference so the earlier the regime starts the more advantageous. It is possible to argue that exercise should involve low resistance training in which mechanical damage is avoided but which optimizes the metabolic and possibly contractile properties.

The role of botulinum toxin

Botulinum toxin has a number of serotypes, from A to G, although types A and B are the only ones to date that have been well studied. The most commonly used at present is botulinum toxin type A, which has become a popular and effective treatment for a number of disorders, such as cervical dystonia, juvenile cerebral palsy and adult spasticity. Botulinum toxin serotypes are made up of different neurotoxins, which are complex protein structures that act by binding to specific external high-affinity acceptors on the membranes of cholinergic neurons. As a result, the release of neurotransmitters is inhibited.

The primary mechanisms for how botulinum toxin type A works is by acting as an inhibitor of acetylcholine release from nerve terminals at the neuromuscular junction (Fig. 6.9). However, new research exploring the role of botulinum toxin type A suggests it may have wider effects and may be a useful treatment for chronic pain conditions such as myofascial pain syndrome and migraines. One reason for these effects may be that acetylcholine is released by gamma motor neurons that innervate intrafusal fibres of the muscle spindles; hence atrophy occurs both intra- and extrafusally, which may lead to changes in sensory input. Such sensory changes at an intrafusal level may have a subsequent effect in the central nervous system. Further recent research suggests that botulinum toxin type A may inhibit the release of other neurotransmitters, such as substance P.

Another effect of botulinum toxin type A is on the parasympathetic nervous system. Hence it is effective for treatment of hyperhidrosis and hypersalivation. The release of acetylcholine is inhibited in postganglionic fibres of the parasympathetic division of the autonomic nervous system.

The effects of botulinum toxin are temporary. As a result, clinically the injections need to be repeated to be therapeutically effective. The safety of botulinum toxin type A is currently unclear. It seems that whilst the safety of different serotypes is the same, the way in which the treatment is prepared in the laboratory will influence its safety. One of the most common side effects following treatment of cervical dystonia is dysphagia, which is likely to result from the diffusion of the drug to the pharyngeal muscles. Another side effect with the treatment of cervical dystonia is dry mouth, but appears more commonly associated with patients being treated with type B rather than type A.

RIPPLING MUSCLE DISEASE

Rippling muscle disease (RMD) is a very rare autosomal dominant disorder that may occur sporadically, and is mild and non-progressive. Little is known about the condition primarily because it is difficult to study as cases are rarely reported to doctors, due to their mild nature, and even if they are, are rarely identified by the clinician. Symptoms tend to appear in first or second decade of life and include muscle stiffness and slowness after rest, muscle cramps associated with stiffness which appear most pronounced in proximal muscles of the lower limbs, muscle hypertrophy and moderately elevated serum creatine kinase. Although it appears as a myotonia-like disorder, with signs of muscular hyperexcitability, it appears electrically silent on the EMG in as much as there are no motor unit action potentials or myotonia during the rippling effect. The electrically silent muscle contractions are frequently referred to as myxoedema, where tapping on a muscle may produce a mounding phenomenon. It seems that this effect is caused by calcium ions released from the sarcoplasmic reticulum. Such an effect can also be seen in people with malnutrition, cachexia and hypothyroidism.

RMD manifests itself in 'wave-like contractions' that seem to roll and spread across muscle. They are induced by stretch or percussion. Percussion-induced contractions release slowly and are clinically indistinguishable from myotonia. Biopsy findings are generally unimpressive and changes found are non-specific and clinically insignificant. The mechanism by which it works is not yet fully understood, but what appears to occur is that the muscle fibre action potential is 10 times slower than normal.

Treatment is difficult, but evidence exists to support the use of immunosuppressants. Further research is needed to fully understand the pathophysiology of the disease.

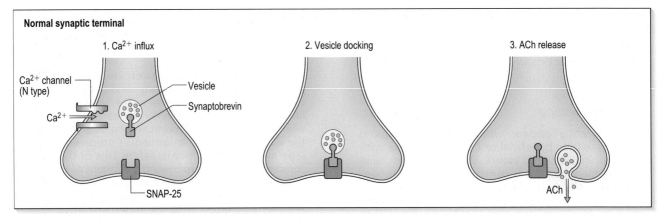

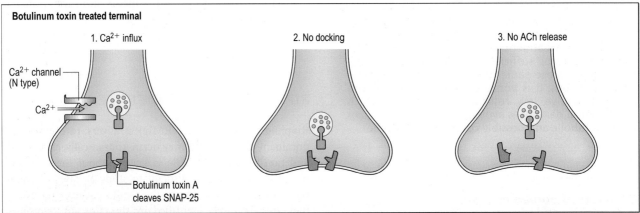

Figure 6.9.   The cellular mechanism of action of botulinum toxin. Botulinum toxin prevents vesicle docking and acetylcholine (ACh) release from motor nerves. It does this by cleaving synaptosomal-associated protein (SNAP-25), which is an important docking protein and has a molecular weight of 25 kDa. (Reproduced with permission from Page et al., 2002.)

MYASTHENIA GRAVIS

Myasthenia gravis (MG) is the most common disease affecting neuromuscular transmission. Its primary symptoms are skeletal muscle weakness and fatigue, but in more severe forms cardiac involvement and muscle myopathy may also occur. MG is believed to be an autoimmune disease where antibodies are directed to the muscle endplate postsynaptic nicotinic acetylcholine receptors (AChR) at the neuromuscular junction, thereby impairing neuromuscular transmission and muscle contraction. The severity of MG varies significantly, from very mild to life-threatening, and has traditionally been graded using Osserman's scale (Table 6.6). Diagnosis can be difficult and may take 2 years to reach, primarily due to the misinterpretation of symptoms and the severity of the symptoms when presented. Antibody testing is one of the most common ways, with elevated AChR antibodies being present in 85–90% of people with generalized MG and 50–60% of those with ocular MG. EMG results tend to be normal. The reason why people develop MG is unclear but it is believed to be linked to viral attacks, hereditary predisposing or abnormal thymus gland function.

Table 6.6.   Grading of myasthenia gravis – Osserman's scale (also referred to as Osserman and Genkin's scale)

Group I	Ocular muscle weakness. Characterized by ptosis and diplopia
Group IIA	Mild generalized weakness. Ocular signs present but respiratory muscles spared. Slow onset
Group IIB	Moderate generalized myasthenia gravis. Gradual onset. Usually includes dysarthria, dysphagia, and poor mastication
Group III	Acute fulminating MG. Severe and rapid onset of the bulbar and skeletal muscles, usually with early involvement of the respiratory muscles. The percentage of thymomas is highest in this group. Response to drug treatment is poor and mortality is high
Group IV	Late severe MG. This occurs when severe MG develops at least 2 years after the onset of type I or type II. Progression may be gradual or sudden. Response to drug therapy and prognosis is poor

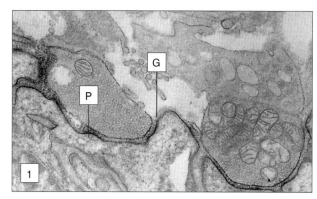

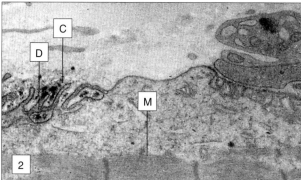

Figure 6.10.   Myasthenia gravis: motor endplate. (1) Electron micrograph showing IgG deposits (G) in discrete patches on the postsynaptic membrane (P). ×13 000. (2) Electron micrograph illustrating C9; (C) shows the postsynaptic region denuded of its nerve terminal: it consists of debris and degenerating folds (D). There is a strong reaction for C9 on this debris. M, muscle fibre. ×9000. (Courtesy of Dr A.G. Engel. Reproduced with permission from Roitt, 2001.)

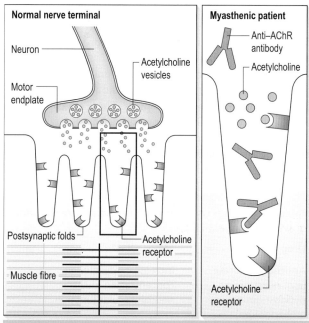

Figure 6.11.   Normally a nerve impulse passing down a neuron arrives at a motor endplate and causes the release of acetylcholine (ACh). This diffuses across the neuromuscular junction, binds ACh receptors on the muscle, and causes ion channels in the muscle membrane to open, which in turn triggers muscular contraction. In myasthenia gravis, antibodies to the receptor block binding of the ACh transmitter. The effect of the released vesicle is therefore reduced, and the muscle can become very weak. Antibody blocking receptors is only one of the factors operating in the disease. (Reproduced with permission from Roitt, 2001.)

Acetylcholine receptors and their relationship with myasthenia gravis

Acetylcholine receptors (AChR) or cholinoceptors are present in the post-junctional membrane of the motor endplate and are nicotinic in nature. AChR is a transmembrane protein composed of five subunits: two alpha units, one beta unit, one gamma unit and one delta unit, all of which are arranged to form a central pore which forms an ion channel. Acetylcholine release from the presynaptic cleft binds to nicotinic receptors on the motor endplate, which stimulates the AChR receptor, causing the opening of sodium channels (and some potassium channels); influx of sodium and potassium into the cell results in depolarization. In the case of MG, there are three main ways in which AChRs are lost.

1. Antigenic modulation. This is where there is accelerated endocytosis and degradation of the AChR. This results in the half-life of AChR being reduced from 7 to 2 days.
2. Destruction of the postsynaptic membrane. This results from a complement mediated focal lysis. The binding of antibodies to the AChR triggers a cascade effect that results in the focal destruction. The damage to the post-synaptic membrane is never fully restored, which results in the reduction in the number of postsynaptic folds (Fig. 6.10). This process facilitates antigenic modulation.
3. Blockage of the AChR ion channel by antibodies binding to the AChR on the postsynaptic cleft (Fig. 6.11).

As a result, muscular weakness and fatigue in MG is a consequence of a reduced number of functional receptors on the postsynaptic membrane.

Ryanodine receptor

AChR is widely accepted as causing major symptoms of MG, but not all symptoms, such as disorders of excitation–contraction coupling or myopathy in skeletal muscles which are found in most severe forms of MG, can be explained by AChR antibodies and decreased transmission at the neuromuscular junction.

The ryanodine receptor is a transmembrane protein which is the channel responsible for the release of calcium in the sarcoplasmic reticulum. As a result, it has a crucial role in the excitation–contraction coupling in skeletal muscle. Although primarily found in skeletal muscle, ryanodine receptors are also found in epithelial cells, neurons and smooth muscle.

Ryanodine receptor antibodies are found primarily in sera of MG patients with thymoma and bind to the skeletal and cardiac form of ryanodine receptors. There are correlations with patients with MG who die of sudden cardiac failure and ryanodine receptor antibodies. Such symptoms cannot be explained by the involvement of nicotinic AChR as these are not present in cardiac muscle. MG patients with ryanodine antibodies also have the more severe forms of MG, such as bulbar symptoms and respiratory failure which requires ventilation. The cause of the autoimmune response involving ryanodine receptor antibodies is still unknown.

Treatment and drugs

The main drugs used in the treatment of MG are listed in Table 6.7.

Table 6.7. Drugs used for the treatment of myasthenia gravis (Page et al., 2002)

Drug	Major effect
Anticholinesterase (e.g. neostigmine, pyridostigmine, ambenonium)	Increase acetylcholine concentration at the neuromuscular junction
Glucocorticoids (e.g. prednisolone, prednisone)	Inhibit the synthesis of nicotinic receptor antibody
Azathioprine	Inhibits the synthesis of nicotinic receptor antibody
Ciclosporin	Inhibits the synthesis of nicotinic receptor antibody

Thymoma and its links with myasthenia gravis

Thymoma is widely associated with the development of MG, and appears in patients with the more severe forms of MG. Although it is unclear why some patients with thymoma develop MG, it is believed that when fighting the thymoma, the immune system induces cross-reactive antibodies with AChR (Fig. 6.12). Patients with MG thymoma may develop ryanodine receptor antibodies, which is thought to explain why this group develop more severe forms of MG. However, only 30–50% of people with a thymoma actually develop MG. Treatment for this group usually consists of a thymectomy and although no large clinical trials exist, it is still widely used and is believed to be most effective in the treatment of MG.

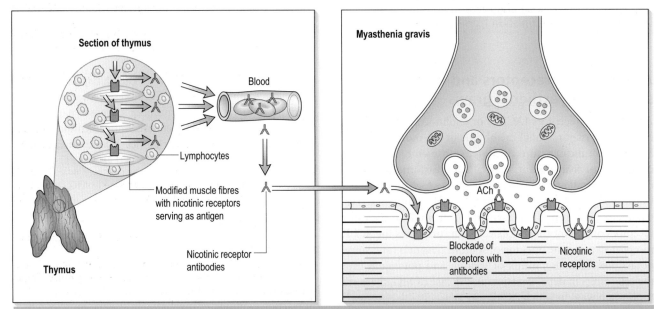

Figure 6.12. Postulated source of antigen and antibody production in myasthenia gravis. A diagrammatic representation of a section of the thymus gland containing modified muscle cells with nicotinic receptors on the surface. It is suggested that this gland may be the source of the antigen that serves as a template for the production of nicotinic antibodies in myasthenic patients. These antibodies block the nicotinic receptors at the neuromuscular junction and prevent interaction between the neurotransmitter and the nicotinic receptors. (ACh, acetylcholine). (Reproduced with permission from Page et al., 2002.)

REFERENCES AND FURTHER READING

Fibromyalgia syndrome

Ahles TA, Yunus MB, Riley SD, Bradley JM, Masi AT (1984) Psychological factors associated with primary fibromyalgia syndrome. Arthritis Rheum 27: 1101–1106.

Anch A, Lue F, Maclean A, Moldofsky H (1991) Sleep physiology and psychological aspects of the fibrositis (fibromyalgia) syndrome. Can J Psychol 45: 179–184.

Bengtsson A (2002) The muscle in fibromyalgia. Rheumatology 41: 721–724.

Buskila D, Langevitz P, Gladman DD, et al. (1992) Patients with rheumatoid arthritis are more tender than those with psoriatic arthritis. J Rheumatol 19: 1115–1119.

Consensus Document on fibromyalgia: the Copenhagen Declaration (1993) J Musculoskel Pain 1: 295–312.

Davies A, Blakeley AGH, Kidd C (2001) Human Physiology. Edinburgh: Churchill Livingstone.

Donald F, Esdaile JM, Kimoff JR, Fitzcharles MA (1996) Musculoskeletal complaints and fibromyalgia in patients attending a respiratory sleep disorders clinic. J Rheumatol 23: 1612–1616.

Gerdle B, Elert J (1995) Disability and impairment in fibromyalgia syndrome: possible pathogenesis and etiology. Crit Rev Phys Rehabilit Med 7: 189–232.

Henriksson KG (1994) Chronic muscular pain: aetiology and pathogenesis. Baillière's Clin Rheumatol 8: 703–719.

Leavitt F, Katz RS (1989) Is the MMPI invalid for assessing psychological disturbance in pain related organic conditions. J Rheumatol 16: 521–526.

McCain GA (1993) The clinical features of the fibromyalgia syndrome. In: Vaerøy H, Merskey H (eds) Progress in Fibromyalgia and Myofascial Pain. Amsterdam: Elsevier Science, pp. 195–215.

Moldofsky H, Scarisbrick P, England R, Smythe H (1975) Musculoskeletal symptoms and non-REM sleep disturbance in patients with 'fibrositis syndrome' and healthy subjects. Psychosom Med 4: 341–351.

Pillemer ST, Bradley LA, Crofford LJ, Moldofsky H, Chrousos GP (1997) The neuroscience and endocrinology of fibromyalgia. Arthritis Rheum 40: 1928–1939.

Schochat T, Croft P, Raspe H (1994) The epidemiology of fibromyalgia: workshop of the Standing Committee on Epidemiology European League Against Rheumatism (EULAR), Bad Säckingen, 19–21 November 1992. Br J Rheumatol 33: 783–786.

Scudds RA, Rollman GB, Harth M, McCain GA (1987) Pain perception and personality measures as discriminators in the classification of fibrositis. J Rheumatol 14: 563–569.

Scudds R, Trachsel L, Luchhurst B, Percy JS (1989) A comparative study of pain, sleep quality, and pain responsiveness in fibrositis and myofascial pain syndrome. J Rheumatol Suppl 19: 120–126.

Sim J, Adams N (1999) Physical and other non-pharmacological interventions for fibromyalgia. Baillière's Clin Rheumatol 13: 507–523.

Tamler MS, Meerschaert JR (1996) Pain management of fibromyalgia and other chronic pain syndromes. Phys Med Rehabil Clin N Am 7: 549–560.

Wall PD (1993) The mechanisms of fibromyalgia: a critical essay: In: Vaerøy H, Merskey H (eds) Pain research and clinical management. Progress in Fibromyalgia and Myofascial Pain. Amsterdam: Elsevier Science, pp. 53–59.

Waller DG, Renwick AG, Hillier K (2001) Medical Pharmacology and Therapeutics. Edinburgh: Saunders.

Wolfe F (1993) Fibromyalgia and problems of classification of musculoskeletal disorders. In: Vaerøy H, Merskey H (eds) Pain research and clinical management. Progress in Fibromyalgia and Myofascial Pain. Amsterdam: Elsevier Science, pp. 217–235.

Wolfe F, Smythe HA, Yunus MB, et al. (1990) The American College of Rheumatology 1990 criteria for the classification of fibromyalgia: report of the Multicenter Criteria Committee. Arthritis Rheum 33: 160–172.

Myofascial pain syndrome

Buskila D (2000) Fibromyalgia, chronic fatigue syndrome, and myofascial pain syndrome. Curr Opin Rheumatol 12: 113–123.

Carette S (1996) Chronic pain syndromes. Ann Rheum Dis 55(8): 497–501.

Fricton JR (1994) Myofascial pain. Baillière's Clin Rheumatol 8: 857–880.

Hudson JI, Pope HG (1994) The concept of affective spectrum disorder: relationship of fibromyalgia and other syndromes of chronic fatigue and chronic muscle pain. Baillière's Clin Rheumatol 8: 839–856.

McCain GA, Scudds RA (1988) The concept of primary fibromyalgia (fibrositis): clinical value, relation and significance to other chronic musculoskeletal pain syndromes. Pain 33(3): 273–287.

Travell JG, Simmons DG (1983) Myofascial pain and Dysfunction: The Trigger Point Manual. Baltimore, MD: Williams & Wilkins.

Wolens D (1998) The myofascial pain syndrome: a critical appraisal. Phys Med Rehabil 12: 299–316.

Myotonia and periodic paralysis

Baynes J, Dominiczak M (1999) Medical Biochemistry, St Louis: Mosby.

Cannon SC (1997) From mutation to myotonia in sodium channel disorders. Neuromuscul Disord 7: 241–249.

Cannon SC (2000) Spectrum of sodium channel disturbances in nondystrophic myotonias and periodic paralyses. Kidney Int 57: 772–779.

Fahlke C (2000) Molecular mechanisms of ion conduction in ClC-type chloride channels: Lessons from disease-causing mutations. Kidney Int 57: 780–786.

Finsterer J (2002) Myotonic dystrophy type 2. Eur J Neurol 9: 441–447.

Jurkat-Rott K, Lehmann-Horn F (2001) Human muscle voltage-gated ion channels and hereditary disease. Curr Opin Pharmacol 1: 280–287.

Pusch M (2002) Myotonia caused by mutation in the muscle chloride channel gene CLCN1. Hum Mutat 19: 423–434.

Idiopathic inflammatory myopathies

Askanas V, King Engel W (2002) Inclusion-body myositis and myopathies: different aetiologies, possibly similar pathogenic mechanisms. Curr Opin Neurol 15: 525–531.

Buchbinder R, Forbes A, Hall S, Dennett X, Giles G (2001) Incidence of malignant disease in biopsy-proven inflammatory myopathy. A population-based cohort study. Ann Intern Med 134: 1087–1095.

Callen JP (2000) Dermatomyositis. Lancet 355: 53–57.

Hilton-Jones D (2001) Inflammatory muscle diseases. Curr Opin Neurol 14: 591–596.

Kissel JT (2002) Misunderstandings, misperceptions, and mistakes in the management of the inflammatory myopathies. Semin Neurol 22: 41–51.

Lepidi H, Frances V, Figarella-Branger D, et al. (1998) Local expression of cytokines in idiopathic inflammatory myopathies, Neuropathol Appl Neurobiol 24: 73–79.

Lundberg IE (2001) The physiology of inflammatory myopathies: an overview. Acta Physiol Scand 171: 207–213.

Plotz PH, Dalakas M, Leff RL, et al. (1989) Current concepts in idiopathic inflammatory myopathies: polymyositis, dermatomyositis and related disorders. Ann Intern Med 111: 143–157.

Muscular dystrophy

Ansved T (2001) Muscle training in muscular dystrophies. Acta Physiol Scand 171: 359–366.

Aoki KR, Guyer B (2001) Botulinum toxin type A and other Botulinum toxin serotypes: a comparative review of biochemical and pharmacological actions. Eur J Neurol 9(Suppl.5): 21–29.

Arahata K (2000) Muscular dystrophy. Neuropathology 20: S34–S41.

Betto R, Biral D, Sandonà D (1999) Functional roles of dystrophin and of associated proteins. New insights for the sarcoglycans. Ital J Neurol Sci 20: 371–377.

Boyd RN, Hays RM (2001) Current evidence for the use of botulinum toxin type A in the management of children with cerebral palsy: a systematic review. Eur J Neurol 9(Suppl.5): 1–20.

Durbeej M, Campbell KP (2002) Muscular dystrophies involving the dystrophin–glycoprotein complex: an overview of current mouse models. Curr Opin Genet Devel 12: 349–361.

Gailly P (2002) New aspects of calcium signalling in skeletal muscle cells: implications in Duchenne muscular dystrophy. Biochim Biophys Acta 1600: 38–44.

Keep NH (2002) Structural comparison of actin binding in utrophin and dystrophin. Neurol Sci 21: S929–937.

Laing NG, Mastglia FL (1999) Inherited skeletal disorders. Ann Hum Biol 26(6): 507–525.

Maidment SL, Ellis JA (2002) Muscular dystrophies, dilated cardiomyopathy, lipodystrophy and neuropathy: the nuclear connection. Exp Rev Mol Med 30 July, http://www.expertreviews.org/02004842h.htm.

Petrof BJ (1998) The molecular basis of activity-induced muscle injury in Duchenne muscular dystrophy. Mol Cell Biochem 179: 111–123.

Sandri M, Carraro U (1999) Apoptosis of skeletal muscles during development and disease. Int J Biochem Cell Biol 31: 1373–1390.

Toniolo D, Minetti C (1999) Muscular dystrophies: alterations in a limited number of pathways? Curr Opin Genet Devel 9: 275–282.

Rippling muscle disease

Müller-Felber W, Ansevin CF, Ricker K, et al. (1999) Immunosuppressive treatment of rippling muscles in patients with myasthenia gravis. Neuromuscul Disord 9: 604–607.

Torbergsen T (2002) Rippling muscle disease: a review. Muscle Nerve Suppl 11: S103–107.

Myasthenia gravis

De Baets M, Stassen MHW (2002) The role of antibodies in myasthenia gravis. J Neurol Sci 202: 5–11.

Mortsensen Armstrong S, Schumann L (2003) Myasthenia gravis: diagnosis and treatment. J Am Acad Nurse Pract 15: 72–78.

Osserman K, Genkins G (1971) Studies in myasthenia gravis: review of twenty-year experience in over 1200 patients. Mount Sinai J Med 38: 497–537.

Page C, Curtis M, Sutter MC, et al. (2002) Integrated Pharmacology. Edinburgh: Mosby.

Roitt I (2001) Immunology. Edinburgh: Mosby.

Romi F, Gilhus NE, Varhaug JE, et al. (2002) Thymectomy and anti-muscle autoantibodies in late-onset myasthenia gravis. Eur J Neurol 9: 55–61.

Skeie GO, Lunde PK, Sejersted OM, et al. (2001) Autoimmunity against ryanodine receptor in myasthenia gravis. Acta Physiol Scand 171: 379–384.

Vincent A (2002) Unravelling the pathogenesis of myasthenia gravis. Nature Rev 2: 797–804.

Bone and Joint Disorders

Christine M. Schnitzler

Bone Disorders

Disorders of Joints

BONE DISORDERS

Structure of bone

The main function of the skeleton is to provide structural support. Bone also serves as a mineral reservoir. At the *macroscopic level*, bones are made up of a solid outer shell of cortical bone, and an inner 'spongy' component of trabecular (cancellous) bone (Fig. 7.1). Trabecular bone is found mainly in the central skeleton (spine, pelvis), the ends of the long bones, and in the small bones of the hands and feet. Cortical bone, on the other hand, predominates in the tubular bones, i.e. the long bones of the peripheral skeleton. Long bones are made up of structurally and functionally distinct zones (Fig. 7.1). The middle segment, also referred to as diaphysis,

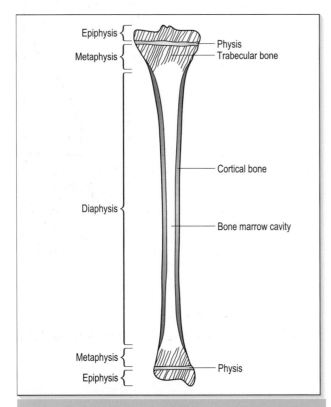

Figure 7.1. Anatomical subdivisions of a long bone. The diaphysis consists of a tube of solid cortical or compact bone. The metaphysis and epiphysis consist mainly of trabecular bone with a thin shell of cortical bone. In childhood the entire bone marrow cavity of the diaphysis and between trabeculae contains haematogenous (blood-forming) red bone marrow. In adults, on the other hand only a small portion of trabecular bone contains red marrow; and the diaphyseal bone marrow consists of yellow fatty tissue. The physis, or growth plate, is the site of longitudinal bone growth. It consists of cartilage during growth, but ossifies at the cessation of growth (age 14 years in girls, and 16 years in boys).

consists of a tube of solid cortical bone; the wider portions at the end of the bone are the metaphysis and the epiphysis which consist of trabecular bone with a thin cortical shell. In growing individuals, a plate of cartilage, the physis (growth plate; also sometimes referred to as 'epiphyseal plate'), lies between metaphysis and epiphysis. Bone growth in length takes place within the cartilage of the physis. The space between trabeculae is filled with red (haematogenous) bone marrow, but the cavity of the shafts of long bones contains yellow, i.e. fatty, marrow.

The skeleton is a surprisingly efficient construct designed to carry a maximum of load using a minimum of material. The beautiful trabecular architecture of the proximal femur resembling the gothic arches of cathedrals is an example (Fig. 7.2). This ingenious structure is the result of a highly coordinated collaboration among bone cells, namely osteoblasts (bone forming cells), osteocytes (bone maintaining cells), and osteoclasts (bone resorbing, i.e. destroying, cells).

At the *microscopic level* cortical and trabecular bone differ in the way osteons, the basic building blocks of bone, are constructed. *Cortical* bone is made up of closely packed, longitudinally arranged, branching and anastomosing osteons (Fig. 7.3). Cortical osteons are also referred to as Haversian systems. A *Haversian system* consists of a thick-walled tube of bone around a narrow canal, the Haversian canal (40 μm in diameter), which contains blood vessels, lymph vessels, and nerves (Fig. 7.4). The wall of the Haversian system is made up of concentrically arranged layers of lamellar bone (parallel collagen fibres), with embedded osteocytes. The wall thickness of the Haversian system reflects the efficiency of the team of osteoblasts that formed the system during bone renewal (turnover or remodelling, see below). The interstitial bone between the Haversian systems is the unremodelled part of old Haversian systems.

Trabecular bone, also referred to as cancellous bone, consists of an interconnected network of plates and rods that are aligned along lines of mechanical stress. Trabecular osteons are concavo-convex packets of bone that have formed on the trabecular bone surface (Fig. 7.5). Trabecular osteons correspond to cortical Haversian systems, opened up longitudinally (like a garden hose slit lengthwise and laid open). The surface facing the bone marrow cavity corresponds to the surface of the Haversian canal. The bone marrow cavity between the trabeculae also contains blood vessels, lymph vessels and nerves, similar to the Haversian canal. As in the cortex, osteons in trabecular bone consist of parallel layers of lamellar bone with embedded osteocytes. The wall thickness of the osteons reflects the efficiency of the team of osteoblasts that formed the osteon. If bone formation is impaired, wall thickness will decline and with it trabecular thickness. The haemopoietic marrow between the trabeculae is a rich source of cells, growth factors and cytokines that support bone remodelling and repair.

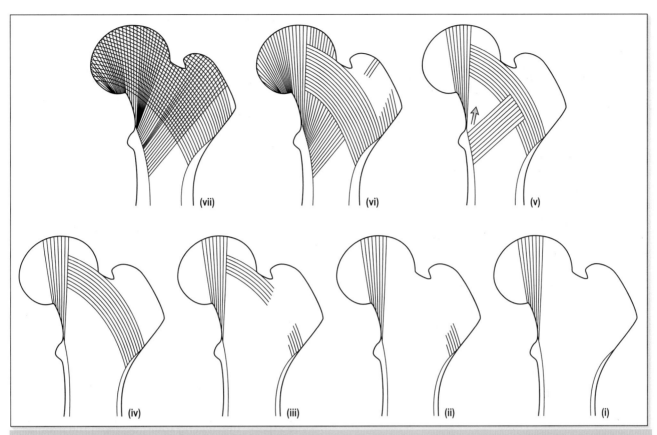

Figure 7.2.   Diagram of bone architecture of the proximal femur graded by the Singh index system. In the young adult (Singh index vii) the femoral head and greater trochanter are closely packed with compression and tension trabeculae, and the cortex of the femoral shaft is thick. With increasing age, and in osteoporosis, trabeculae are progressively resorbed, and cortices get thinner. Tension trabeculae disappear before compression trabeculae. Ward's triangle (arrow) loses bone early and is generally the region with the lowest bone density when examined by bone mineral densitometry. Before bone densitometry became widely available (1987) the seven trabecular patterns of progressive bone loss described by Singh (Singh index) were used in the assessment of the severity of bone loss. Singh indices iv and below were found to be associated with increasing vertebral fracture risk (Singh et al., 1973).

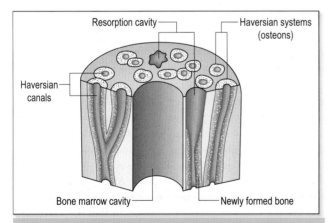

Figure 7.3.   Diagram of cortical bone microarchitecture. Osteons (Haversian systems; see Fig. 7.4) are aligned with the long axis of the bone, and their Haversian canals branch and anastomose. Bone is constantly being remodelled through resorption, followed by formation of a new osteon.

Composition of bone

Bone consists of cells, proteins, mineral and water (Table 7.1).

Bone cells

There are basically only two types of bone cells: osteoclasts and osteoblasts. *Osteoclasts* are multinucleate (containing many nuclei) bone-resorbing cells that are derived from blood monocyte/macrophage cell lines. The large number of nuclei enable an osteoclast to work with great speed, i.e. much faster than the bone-forming osteoblast, which has only one nucleus. The osteoclast attaches to bone by a sealing ring and thus closes off a sealed space ('sealing zone') (Fig. 7.6).The plasma membrane facing the sealed zone is laid in deep folds, referred to as 'ruffled border'. Across this ruffled border the osteoclast secretes into the sealing zone: (1) hydrogen ions to create a highly acidic environment in the sealing zone for the dissolution of bone mineral, and

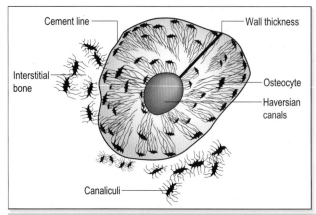

Figure 7.4. Diagram of a transverse section through a cortical osteon (Haversian system) and some interstitial bone (unremodelled part of an old osteon) as seen in the microscope. The Haversian system consists of a thick-walled tube of compact bone around a central canal that contains blood vessels, lymph vessels, and nerves. Osteocyte cell bodies are contained in small spaces referred to as lacunae, and their cell extensions project into the numerous canaliculi connecting the lacunae. The cement line is the boundary where a newly forming osteon is cemented to surrounding, older bone. The wall thickness of the osteon reflects the efficiency of the team of osteoblasts that formed the osteon.

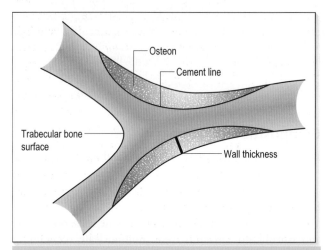

Figure 7.5. Diagram showing two trabecular osteons. In trabecular bone the osteon is a concavo-convex structure on the trabecular bone surface, facing bone marrow. The trabecular osteon may be thought of as a Haversian system slit lengthwise and laid open like a garden hose. The surface of the trabecular osteon facing the bone marrow cavity corresponds to the surface of the Haversian canal. Osteonal wall thickness is the distance between the trabecular bone surface and the cement line. Wall thickness determines trabecular thickness, and reflects the efficiency of the team of osteoblasts that formed it.

Table 7.1. Composition of bone

Component	% of bone
Protein	25–30
Type I collagen (90% of bone proteins)	
Non-collagenous proteins (10% of bone proteins)	
Mineral	60–70
Water	5–6

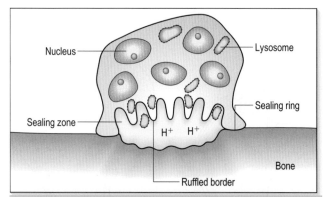

Figure 7.6. Diagram of an osteoclast in the process of resorbing bone. The osteoclast attaches to bone with the aid of its 'sealing ring' and thus creates a closed space, the 'sealing zone', between the plasma membrane of the osteoclast and bone. This sealed space permits the creation of a highly destructive acid milieu for the resorption of bone. The surface of the osteoclast's plasma membrane facing the sealing zone is vastly increased by a large number of deep folds ('ruffled border') across which the cell secretes (1) hydrogen ions for the dissolution of bone mineral, and (2) lysosomes that release destructive enzymes for the breakdown of organic bone matrix.

(2) lysosomes, which deliver lysosomal enzymes and collagenase for the breakdown of organic bone components.

Osteoblasts are bone-forming cells derived from marrow mesenchymal stem cells. They always work in teams of large numbers. They secrete proteins and enzymes, and induce the mineralization of the organic bone matrix they have produced (see 'Bone remodelling'). In the process of bone formation a proportion of the osteoblasts bury themselves as *osteocytes* in the bone they produce. At the completion of the formation phase the last osteoblasts become flat *lining cells* on the inner surfaces of bone, including the Haversian canals.

Osteocytes are the most numerous cells in bone. They are the mechanotransducers of bone that sense stimuli created by mechanical load, and transduce these stimuli into signal molecules which control the initiation of bone remodelling (see 'The lacunar–canalicular system', and 'Bone remodelling').

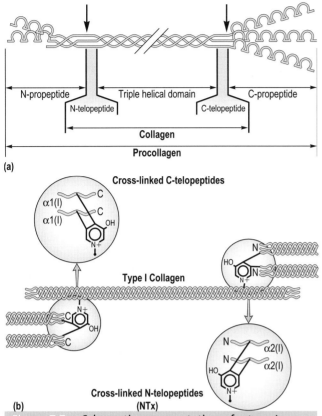

Figure 7.7. Schematic representation of a type I collagen molecule and cross-links. (a) The molecule consists of (1) a triple helix of three polypeptide chains wound around a common central axis, (2) a C- and an N-telopeptide (telos = end; C, carboxy terminal, N, nitrogen terminal of the molecule) for attachment of pyridinoline cross-links to other molecules, and (3) a C- and an N-propeptide. Osteoblasts secrete the molecule into the extracellular matrix as procollagen. Before the molecule can link up with neighbouring molecules (for increased tensile strength), the C-propeptide and the N-propeptide have to be split off at the cleavage sites (vertical arrows). This leaves the mature collagen molecule. The cleaved propeptides enter the bloodstream where they can be measured as bone formation markers. (b) Following propeptide cleavage, pyridinoline cross-links (the hexagonal ring structure in the circles) can now attach to the C- and N-telopeptides to link the collagen molecule to neighbouring collagen molecules, thus forming collagen fibrils of high tensile strength. Collagen fibrils then group together to form collagen fibres for even greater strength. During subsequent bone resorption, the cross-linked telopeptides (pyridinoline cross-link with attached telopeptides) become collagen breakdown products that enter blood and urine where they can be measured as bone resorption markers.

Bone proteins

The most abundant bone protein is *type I collagen* (Fig. 7.7a, b). It is made up of three polypeptide chains of approximately 1000 amino acids each (two alpha1 chains and one alpha 2 chain). The three polypeptide chains form a triple helix for stability, winding around a common axis. This stabilizing feature imparts great tensile strength and is present only in the fibrillar collagens that provide the structural framework of the body (types I, II, III, V and XI collagen).

In addition to bone, type I collagen is also present in ligaments, tendons, skin, dentin and sclerae. Type II collagen is found in cartilage, type III collagen in blood vessels and skin, and types IV to XIII in various sites. Type I bone collagen is secreted in immature form by osteoblasts as type I procollagen (Fig. 7.7a). Before neighbouring molecules can link up to form collagen fibrils, and these to collagen fibres for further stability, their C- and N-terminal propeptides (the 'curly tails' in Fig. 7.7a) have to be cleaved off. These C- and N-terminal propeptides spill over into the bloodstream where they can be measured as *bone formation markers* (other bone formation markers produced by osteoblasts are the peptides bone alkaline phosphatase and osteocalcin). Elevated levels of bone formation markers indicate high bone turnover. After propeptide cleavage, the collagen molecule can link up with neighbouring collagen molecules via pyridinoline cross-links that attach to the C- and N-telopeptide (telo = end) sites of the collagen molecules (Fig. 7.7a, b). During later bone resorption, bone collagen is broken down and the telopeptide cross-links enter the bloodstream and urine where they can be measured as *bone resorption markers*. Elevated levels reflect excessive bone resorption and likely rapid bone loss (high bone turnover).

Most bone collagen is deposited in closely packed parallel lamellae that give the microscopic image of bone under polarized light a striped appearance of alternating dark and light lines. Such bone is referred to as *lamellar bone*. In contrast, *woven bone* consists of a loosely woven network of collagen fibres with haphazard orientation. Lamellar bone is stronger than woven bone. Woven bone is deposited during very rapid bone formation as in the fetus and neonate, in fracture repair and in the new primary trabeculae formed at the growth plate. Most woven bone is subsequently resorbed and replaced with lamellar bone. Pathological conditions such as osteogenesis imperfecta, Paget's disease and bone tumours are also characterized by woven bone formation. Whereas collagen has largely a structural function, *non-collagenous proteins* have mainly regulatory functions (Table 7.2). The majority of non-collagenous proteins are also produced by osteoblasts.

Bone mineral

Bone mineral consists mainly of calcium and phosphorus in the form of hydroxyapatite $(Ca_{10}(PO_4)_6(HO)_2)$. It gives bone its rigidity. The hydroxyapatite crystals are attached to collagen fibrils.

The lacunar-canalicular system

Bone is a solid containing voids, namely the extensive network of lacunae and canaliculi (Fig. 7.4). From each lacuna

Table 7.2.   Non-collagenous proteins

Protein	Postulated function
Osteonectin	Calcium binding, HA binding, matrix protein binding
Fibronectin	Cell attachment
Thrombospondin	Cell attachment, growth factor binding
Osteopontin	Cell attachment, mineral proliferation
Bone sialoprotein	Cell attachment, calcium binding
Osteocalcin	Mineral maturation (used as bone turnover marker)
Alkaline phosphatase	Increase in local phosphate levels, destruction of HA inhibitors (used as bone turnover marker)

HA, hydroxyapatite (bone mineral).

numerous canaliculi extend to neighbouring lacunae, and to bone surfaces. The total internal surface area of the lacunae and canaliculi is 1000–5000 m^2 (about 20 times greater than that of lung capillaries). Each lacuna houses the cell body of an osteocyte. The long slender cell processes of the osteocyte reach into the canaliculi where they connect, by means of gap junctions, with the processes of neighbouring osteocytes (Fig. 7.8), and with the lining cells on bone surfaces, i.e. the Haversian canals, trabecular surfaces and endocortical surfaces. This permits rapid cell-to-cell communication, similar to that in a neuronal network. Within this warren of interconnected lacunae and canaliculi, the osteocytes and their cell processes are bathed in extracellular fluid which carries minerals, signal molecules, nutrients, waste and other substances. Importantly, extracellular fluid transmits pulsatile fluid flow through the lacunar–canalicular system, generated by loading. Here, osteocytes are ideally placed as the mechanotransducers of bone that control the initiation of bone remodelling (see 'Control of the remodelling cycle'). This function requires rapid cell-to-cell communication between osteocytes.

Bone remodelling

The remodelling cycle

Bone remodelling (bone turnover) controls bone mass and bone microarchitecture, in other words, bone strength. Bone remodelling is ongoing in the entire skeleton throughout life. It constantly replaces minute amounts of old bone with new in order to adapt the skeleton to ongoing mechanical demands, and to replace fatigue-damaged bone that would weaken the skeleton. Remodelling takes place on bone surfaces (also referred to as remodelling envelopes), namely the intracortical (Haversian), endocortical and trabecular surfaces (Fig. 7.9). The trabecular and endocortical surfaces

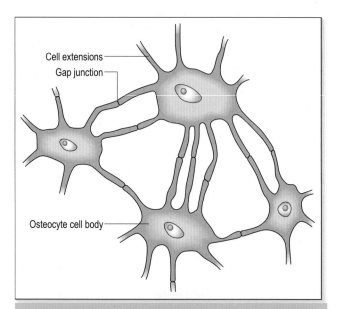

Figure 7.8.   Diagrammatic representation of isolated osteocytes cultured on a glass support. As in bone, each cell grew long thin extensions that linked up with similar extensions from neighbouring cells. This model demonstrates the inherent ability of the osteocyte to form a network of communicating cells, similar to neuronal networks.

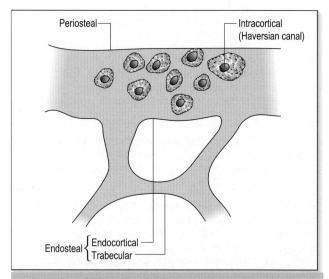

Figure 7.9.   Diagram showing bone remodelling surfaces. Bone remodelling and bone loss and gain take place on these surfaces.

combined constitute the endosteal surface. The extent of remodelling on the endosteal surface is greater than that on the intracortical surface because of the larger surface area available for such activities. On the *endosteal surface* remodelling takes place in a shallow resorption pit up to 60 μm in

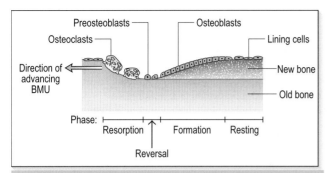

Figure 7.10.   Diagram of a basic multicellular unit (BMU) of bone remodelling on a trabecular bone surface. The first step is the resorption phase, lasting about 2 weeks. It starts with osteoclastic resorption, which advances at 10–20 μm a day, and is followed by slower resorption by mononuclear cells that 'mop up' the debris left behind by the osteoclasts. Thereafter preosteoblasts line the floor of the cavity (cement surface) during the reversal phase, lasting 1 week. Preosteoblasts then differentiate into osteoblasts that lay down new osteoid. About 3 weeks after osteoid deposition osteoblasts initiate mineralization of the osteoid. The formation phase lasts 4 to 8 months. In the course of bone formation about 15% of the osteoblasts become incorporated into new bone as osteocytes; other osteoblasts die by apoptosis (programmed cell death). On completion of the formation phase, the final group of osteoblasts become lining cells that cover the inner bone surfaces during the resting phase, which lasts a year or longer.

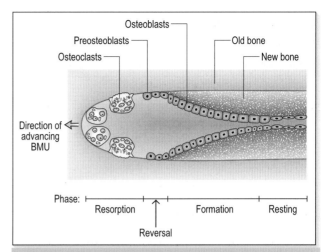

Figure 7.11.   Diagram of a basic multicellular unit (BMU) of bone remodelling in cortical bone. The sequence of events and the time frames are the same as in trabecular bone. First, osteoclasts cut a tunnel into solid bone, starting from within an existing Haversian canal that contains the necessary blood supply. Then mononuclear cells mop up the debris and preosteoblasts line the floor of the resorption cavity (cement surface) during the reversal phase. Preosteoblasts differentiate into osteoblasts that fill the tunnel with new bone, thus creating a new Haversian system (Fig. 7.9).

depth and 2–3 mm in greatest dimension (Fig. 7.10). In the *cortex* remodelling proceeds in a resorption tunnel, about 100–200 μm in diameter and up to 10 mm in length (Fig. 7.11). These tunnels are aligned parallel with the long axis of the bone (Fig. 7.3). Normal bone remodelling consists of a highly coordinated sequence of steps, namely (1) bone resorption, (2) matrix (osteoid) formation and (3) mineralization. The group of cells executing the remodelling process is referred to as the *basic multicellular unit (BMU)*. Each BMU consists of pre-osteoclasts, osteoclasts, mononuclear cells, pre-osteoblasts and osteoblasts, in that temporal order.

The first step in the *remodelling cycle* is excavation of a *resorption* cavity (Howship's lacuna) by osteoclasts. This process advances by 10–20 μm a day (Figs 7.10 and 7.11) and takes about 10 days at any one point of the BMU. Thereafter, mononuclear cells complete the resorption phase by 'mopping up' and smoothing the cavity. The floor of the cavity to which the new bone will be cemented is referred to as the cement surface (or cement line in histological sections). Next, *bone formation* commences. First, pre-osteoblasts line the cavity for about a week (reversal phase). They then differentiate (i.e. mature) into osteoblasts that secrete the osteoid. Osteoid consists of collagen, non-collagenous proteins, glycoproteins and proteoglycans (Table 7.2). Ten to 20 days later

the osteoblasts initiate *mineralization* of the osteoid by secreting calcification vesicles into it. These vesicles form the nucleus for bone crystal growth that is thereafter under the control of non-collagenous proteins – also products of the osteoblast. Mineralization proceeds in two phases. In the primary phase, lasting a few days, 70% of the bone mineral is deposited. The secondary phase extends over many years as more mineral continues to accumulate slowly. Because of this delay in full mineralization, bone with a high remodelling rate, as for example in children, has a large proportion of recently completed osteons and is therefore less highly mineralized than adult bone with lower bone turnover. As unremodelled bone accumulates with age, the skeleton becomes increasingly hypermineralized, and therefore more brittle.

In adults, the bone formation phase lasts 3 to 4 months at any one point of the BMU. The lifespan of the whole BMU, i.e. the remodelling period, is 4 to 8 months. The completed osteon is also referred to as bone structural unit (BSU). In adults, approximately one million remodelling cycles are active at any one time. In young adults the remodelling process is *balanced*, i.e. at the completion of each remodelling cycle as much new bone has been formed as was resorbed. However, with increasing age, and in bone-losing conditions, remodelling is in negative balance – or in *remodelling imbalance* – because less bone is formed than was resorbed (Fig. 7.12). Remodelling imbalance leads to a decline in

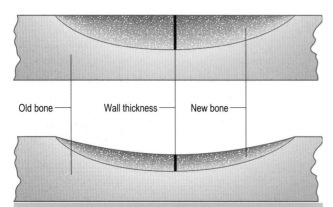

Figure 7.12.   Diagram representing normal osteonal wall thickness and trabecular thickness in a healthy young adult (top), and the effect of declining osteonal wall thickness on reduction of trabecular thickness in the elderly, or in osteoporosis (bottom).

osteonal wall thickness which results in loss of trabecular thickness and increased cortical porosity. This leads to *slow* but steady bone loss. If bone formation fails to follow resorption altogether, we speak of *uncoupling*. This leads to *rapid* bone loss. Rapid bone loss also results from an increase in the birth rate of new remodelling cycles (high bone turnover), particularly if combined with remodelling imbalance or uncoupling, as is the case at the menopause, in other forms of hypogonadism and in many bone-losing conditions. The sum of the voids created by bone remodelling is referred to as 'remodelling space'. The higher the bone turnover, the larger is the remodelling space and the greater the bone loss. If the high turnover is temporary, the remodelling space may 'close' again by filling in with new bone formation.

Control of the remodelling cycle

Osteocytes play a key role in the renewal of bone and in the optimization of bone mass and microarchitecture. The osteocyte is thought to be the *mechanotransducer* of bone that controls the activation of remodelling cycles. The osteocyte cell bodies in the lacunae, and their cell extensions in the canaliculi, are bathed in extracellular fluid that undergoes *pulsatile fluid flow*, generated by loading. Fluid flow over the cell surface subjects the cell to two kinds of stimuli: *fluid shear stress* and *streaming electrical potentials*. Furthermore, distortion of bone crystals caused by loading induces *piezo-electric potentials* (piezein = pressurize). The osteocyte is equipped to sense these various stimuli (mechanosensing), and to respond (transduction) by producing signal molecules (mechanotransduction) that serve to communicate messages to other cells within the lacunar–canalicular system and to lining cells on bone surfaces. On receipt of the appropriate signal, the lining cells retract, exposing mineralized bone for bone resorption, i.e. for a new remodelling cycle to start. The signal molecules involved in mechanotransduction

are thought to include *prostaglandins*, *nitric oxide (NO)*, and *insulin-like growth factor-1* (IGF-1). In addition, the *apoptosis* of osteocytes occurring in the vicinity of *fatigue-damaged bone* also stimulates activation of bone remodelling, presumably with the aim of removing damaged bone. Apoptosis is 'programmed cell death', a physiological process in which single cells 'shrivel up' without causing an inflammatory reaction; necrosis, on the other hand, is pathological cell death by rupture of many cells which incites inflammation.

Following arrival of an activation signal on the bone surface, haemopoietic pluripotent mononuclear cells proliferate and differentiate to *osteoclast precursors*. Under the influence of the cytokine interleukin-1 (IL-1) and the hormones PTH (parathyroid hormone) and 1,25-dihydroxyvitamin D, these cells fuse to form mature multinucleate (10–20 nuclei) *osteoclasts* that start resorbing bone. The spatial and temporal extent of resorption is limited by osteoclast apoptosis which is induced by oestrogen and transforming growth factor-beta (TGF-β). TGF-β is being released from degraded bone matrix during bone resorption, i.e. osteoclasts demise by the product of their labour. Oestrogen deficiency and the associated rise in IL-1, IL-6 and PTH levels, on the other hand, delay osteoclast apoptosis. As a consequence, osteoclasts work longer, resorption cavities get deeper, perforate trabecular plates and rods, and disconnect the trabecular network, further weakening bone. The direction of the resorption cavity is thought to be influenced by mechanical forces: low bone strain stimulates bone resorption, and high bone strain, formation. As the resorpton cavity deepens, bone strain increases, resorption ceases and formation starts. Mechanical forces thus belong to the 'coupling factors' that couple bone resorption to subsequent formation. Other coupling factors are transforming growth factor-beta (TGF-β), bone morphogenetic proteins (BMPs), insulin-like growth factor 1 and 2 (IGF-1, IGF-2), fibroblast growth factor (FGF) and platelet-derived growth factor (PDGF).

Bone formation is preceded by a series of intercations between growth factors and the cells of the osteoblast lineage. Coupling factors attract mesenchymal stem cells to the resorption cavity by means of chemotaxis (attraction by chemical means). These stem cells become *pre-osteoblasts* under the continued influence of the coupling factors. Final differentiation to mature *osteoblasts* occurs under the control of BMP-2 and IGF-1. Then osteoid formation can begin (see 'The remodelling cycle'). When osteoblasts have completed their task of osteoid deposition and its mineralization, their fate takes one of three forms: the majority of osteoblasts bury themselves as osteocytes in the bone they produce, the rest either become lining cells on the newly completed bone surface, or they die by apoptosis.

The regional acceleratory phenomenon

Bone responds to any disturbance (e.g. injury, infection, surgery, tumour) with activation of additional remodelling sites around the site of the disturbance, or in the entire limb in response to major disturbances (fracture, immobilization, tumour). This remodelling response is referred to as the 'regional accelerative phenomenon' (RAP). It is thought to be caused by the outpouring of local cytokines and growth factors that stimulate bone remodelling. A RAP can be identified on a bone scan as increased uptake of the radionuclide tracer technetium-99-methylene diphosphonate (^{99}Tc-MDP) in and around the affected region. The intravenously injected tracer attaches – by means of its diphosphonate component – to growing bone crystals at new bone formation sites. The radioactive component of the tracer, ^{99}Tc, emits gamma rays that can be photographed by a gamma camera, a specialized giant camera that photographs part or the whole of the patient. Clinical examples are the increased tracer uptake ('hot spots') around a new or loose arthroplasty endoprosthesis, a loose or infected implant, a tumour in bone, a healing fracture or a stress fracture. Indeed, a stress fracture can be identified in this way as soon as symptoms start, whereas the radiographic diagnosis depends on callus formation that appears only about 2 to 3 weeks later. The overgrowth of the leg in a child following a fractured femoral shaft is also the result of a RAP, here stimulating the growth plates. A RAP is expected to continue for at least one remodelling period (i.e. months) after the last disturbance.

Skeletal development and ageing

Bone mass increases during skeletal development, and peak bone mass is attained between 25 and 30 years of age. From age 40 years, bone mass slowly declines at the rate of 1% per annum in both men and women. Over and above this, women experience an acceleration of bone loss for several years around the menopause. The determinants of peak bone mass are mainly genetic, with contributions by calcium intake, physical activity and diet during childhood. The rate of later bone loss is influenced by a number of factors such as sex hormone deficiency, lifestyle and medical conditions. The transient bone loss of lactation is greater than that of pregnancy.

Skeletal development

During growth, bones change in size (length and width) and shape, but the proportions remain the same.

The growth plate

Growth in *bone length* takes place at the cartilaginous growth plate (physis; sometimes referred to as 'epiphyseal plate') (Fig. 7.1) by endochondral ossification, i.e. by bone formation from cartilage. During growth the end of the bone (epiphysis and physis) moves further away from its mid-length (Fig. 7.13). The *physis* consists of four distinct zones: (1) *resting* or reserve chondrocytes, (2) *proliferating* chondrocytes, (3) *hypertrophic* chondrocytes, and (4) zone of *provisional*

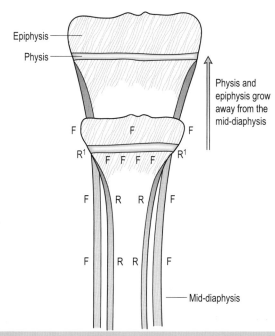

Figure 7.13. Modelling of growing bone. During growth, bone increases in length and changes in width. Longitudinal growth occurs within the cartilaginous physis. This new cartilage is converted to bone by resorption of cartilage and new bone formation (FFFF) at the physeal-metaphyseal junction (endochondral bone formation). In this way, physis and epiphysis move further away from the mid-diaphysis as the bone elongates. Growth in width is achieved by bone formation (F) on the periosteal surface (intramembranous bone formation). At the same time, the marrow cavity is widened by bone resorption (R) on the endocortical surface. The cortex thus moves outwards, increasing the width of the bone. An increase in cortical thickness is achieved as slightly more bone is formed on the periosteal surface than is resorbed on the endocortical surface. To maintain the normal proportions of the bone, the metaphysis has to slim down to diaphyseal width by bone resorption (R^1) on the outside. The epiphysis enlarges circumferentially by bone formation (F) on the outside, and cortical thickness is controlled by endocortical resorption as in the diaphysis.

calcification (Fig. 7.14). The proliferating chondrocytes of zone 2 multiply rapidly and produce abundant cartilaginous matrix. These cells are responsible for the rate of longitudinal growth and final body height. They are arranged in columns. The intervening vertical cartilage columns form the template for bone trabeculae. Next, the proliferating chondrocytes mature and enlarge to become the hypertrophic chondrocytes of zone 3. These cells then initiate calcification of the surrounding matrix, a process that induces their apoptosis, i.e. the chondrocytes die. The older part of the zone of provisional calcification therefore has empty cell columns. Chondroclasts open up these empty cell columns by resorbing the horizontal calcified cartilaginous septae. This allows

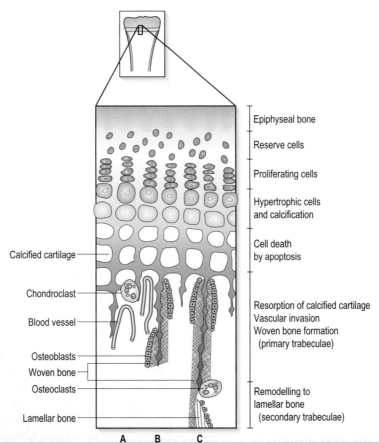

Epiphyseal bone

Reserve cells

Proliferating cells

Hypertrophic cells and calcification

Cell death by apoptosis

Calcified cartilage

Chondroclast

Blood vessel

Resorption of calcified cartilage
Vascular invasion
Woven bone formation
   (primary trabeculae)

Osteoblasts
Woven bone

Osteoclasts

Remodelling to lamellar bone
   (secondary trabeculae)

Lamellar bone

A   B   C

Figure 7.14.   Schematic representation of a physis (growth plate). The cartilaginous part of the growth plate consists of several layers of cartilage cells with different metabolic profiles. These layers are: (1) reserve cells, (2) proliferating cells, and (3) hypertrophic cells. The rate of longitudinal growth depends on the rate of cell division of the proliferating cells. These cells then become the hypertrophic cells that prepare the cartilage matrix for calcification, and finally calcify it. Once enclosed in calcified cartilage, the hypertrophic cells die by apoptosis. The vertical bars of calcified cartilage form the templates for trabecula formation. Subsequent steps are depicted in temporal order from left to right as A–C. A, Chondroclasts advance from the metaphysis and resorb the horizontal septae of calcified cartilage, opening up the empty cell columns for vascular invasion and bone formation. Chondroclasts also resorb two-thirds of all vertical septae so that only about 30% of vertical septae remain as templates for trabecula formation. B, Blood vessels import the necessary stem cells that will differentiate into osteoblasts which settle on the surface of the remaining vertical septae. Here they rapidly form woven bone, encasing the calcified cartilage septae. The vertical septae of calcified cartilage thus become the core of pillars of woven bone. These pillars are the primary trabeculae which are soon remodelled to lamellar bone, i.e. to secondary trabeculae (C).

hairpin-shaped sinusoidal blood vessels to grow into the 'empty' columns. These blood vessels import osteoblasts that populate the inside of the empty cell columns, i.e. the outer surface of the vertical calcified cartilage septae, on which they lay down woven bone. These then are the primary trabeculae which consist of woven bone around a calcified cartilage core. Primary trabeculae are rapidly remodelled to lamellar bone. Only about one-third of the vertical cartilage columns results in trabecula formation, the rest are resorbed. The number of trabeculae in an individual is thus determined at the growth plate, i.e. in childhood. Trabeculae do, however increase in thickness until peak bone mass is reached at age 30. Trabeculae thicken as a result of a positive remodelling balance, i.e. under age 30 more bone is formed during the remodelling cycle than is resorbed.

Increase in *bone width* is by intramembranous ossification, i.e. bone formation from periosteal soft tissue (Fig. 7.13). At the same time, the bone marrow cavity gets wider through endocortical bone resorption. Since slightly more bone is being added to the outside of the cortex than is removed on the inside, cortical thickness gradually increases until peak bone mass is reached.

For a child's bone to attain adult size and maintain its proportions, a change in bone shape is required (Fig. 7.13). This change in bone shape is referred to as *modelling*. Bone modelling occurs only during growth. *Remodelling* of the entire

Table 7.3. Systemic and local factors enhancing (+) or retarding (−) longitudinal bone growth

Factor	Effect
Systemic factors	
Growth hormone	+
Thyroid hormone	+
Vitamin D metabolites	+
Sex steroids	−
High dose glucocorticoids	−
Local factors	
Insulin-like growth factor-1 (IGF-1)	+
Transforming growth factor-beta (TGF-β)	+
Bone morphogenetic proteins (BMP)	+
Fibroblast growth factor (FGF)	+
Platelet-derived growth factor (PDGF)	+

skeleton, on the other hand, continues throughout life, i.e. during growth and in adulthood. The two processes differ in several other respects. In remodelling, resorption and formation take place sequentially and in the same place, with coupling of resorption to formation. In contrast, in modelling, resorption and formation occur simultaneously and on different surfaces, without coupling of resorption to formation.

Factors influencing bone growth are numerous (Table 7.3). Hormones with a positive effect on bone growth are growth hormone, thyroid hormone and vitamin D metabolites. Hormones with a negative effect on longitudinal bone growth are the sex steroids and high doses of glucocorticoids. While sex steroids slow longitudinal growth through physeal closure at 14 years in girls and 16 years in boys, they are necessary for the continued rise in bone mass through increases in cortical and trabecular thickness until attainment of peak bone mass between ages 25 and 30. Growth-promoting local factors are insulin-like growth factor-1 (IGF-1), transforming growth factor-beta (TGF-β), bone morphogenetic protein (BMP), fibroblast growth factor (FGF), epidermal growth factor (EGF), platelet-derived growth factor (PDGF), and others. A hormone is an endocrine substance that is produced elsewhere in the body and is carried by the bloodstream to its point of action; local factors may be paracrine (produced by other cells in the neighbourhood), or autocrine (produced by the cell to act upon itself). Other factors beneficial for normal growth are physical activity, vitamins and an adequate diet.

Disorders of the growth plate

The junction of physis and metaphysis, i.e. the region of calcified cartilage and primary trabeculae, is weak and therefore vulnerable to trauma.

Fracture-separation of the epiphysis is a common childhood injury. The epiphysis separates from the metaphysis through the weak region of calcified cartilage and primary

trabeculae. After fracture healing, growth continues because the cartilage cells of the physis have not been damaged.

Compression injuries of the physis, however, may damage the growing chondrocytes and lead to growth arrest. Since compression forces usually damage only part of the full width of the physis, only a portion of the physis will cease to grow and an angular deformity such as a varus, valgus, flexion or hyperextension deformity may result because the rest of the physis will continue to grow.

Slipped upper femoral epiphysis (SUFE) typically affects overweight, sexually immature teenagers aged 11 to 16 years. The pubertal growth spurt is associated with rapid formation of new primary trabeculae. This immature bone is unable to withstand the load of a by now adult-sized body, particularly at the proximal femoral growth plate with its high shear stresses. This combination of adverse factors, together with minor trauma, may lead to separation of the proximal femoral epiphysis through the weak region of calcified cartilage and primary trabeculae. SUFE is, in a way, a pathological fracture-separation of the epiphysis.

Acute *haematogenous osteomyelitis* in children starts in and around the new hairpin-shaped sinusoidal blood vessels of the primary trabeculae where blood flow is sluggish (Fig. 7.14). Bacteria carried in the bloodstream (bacteraemia) as a result of a minor skin or other infection settle here and form an abscess. Furthermore, these thin-walled sinusoids are easily traumatized and bacteria may settle in the haematoma and lead to abscess formation. As the abscess enlarges and the pressure within the confined spaces of bone rises, pus eventually tracks into the marrow cavity, and under the periosteum, stripping it from bone. The affected portion of the cortex is thus devitalized, bathed in pus, and becomes a sequestrum (loose piece of dead, infected bone; sequester = isolate). The periosteum produces new bone (involucrum = covering) around the sequestrum. At this stage, the condition has become chronic osteomyelitis.

Achondroplasia, a form of short-limbed dwarfism, is due to a genetic mutation (single amino-acid substitution in fibroblast growth factor receptor-3). This mutation prevents the proliferative chondrocytes of the physis (zone 2) from multiplying. Bones depending on endochondral bone formation for longitudinal growth, especially limb bones, therefore fail to attain full length.

Gigantism is characterized by exceptionally tall, but normally proportioned stature that results from continued production of excessive amounts of growth hormone by the pituitary gland and failure of physeal closure after puberty.

Skeletal ageing

Skeletal ageing commences in the fourth or fifth decade, and is characterized by a decline in bone mass and deterioration in bone quality (microarchitectural deterioration, hypermineralization, micropetrosis, see below). If these changes are exaggerated, fragility fractures (fractures due to non-violent trauma) may result. Bone loss is always associated with microarchitectural deterioration. Both bone loss and microarchitectural deterioration are due to derangements of bone remodelling, such as a negative remodelling balance, uncoupling of resorption from formation in favour of resorption, increased resorption depth, and/or high bone turnover. Eighty per cent of bone strength is accounted for by bone mass, and 20% by bone quality. The predominant *mechanism of the bone loss* of ageing is remodelling imbalance (Fig. 7.12), either due to excessive bone resorption or impaired formation, or both. Around the menopause excessive resorption predominates through an increase in resorption depth and an excessive number of resorption sites. Still later in life, remodelling imbalance is mainly due to impaired formation. Decreased bone formation is the result of impaired osteoblast recruitment contributed to by stem cell depletion, deficient microcirculation, premature osteoblast apoptosis, and stem cell differentiation to fat cells rather than to osteoblasts (adipogenesis instead of osteoblastogenesis).

Trabecular bone loss

Bone loss and microarchitectural deterioration in trabecular bone are more severe and occur more rapidly than in cortical bone because of the larger bone surface area available in trabecular bone on which deranged bone remodelling can wreak havoc. The derangements of bone remodelling in trabecular bone lead to (1) thinning of trabeculae, (2) perforation of trabeculae and loss of connectivity of the trabecular network, (3) fatigue damage, and (4) trabecular lattice irregularity.

Thinning of trabeculae results from declining wall thickness of trabecular osteons with age (Figs 7.5 and 7.12). Reduction in trabecular thickness leads to a disproportionate decline in bone strength since reducing the cross-sectional area of a rod leads to an exponential loss of its buckling strength (Fig. 7.15). Trabecular bone strength is also reduced in individuals with high remodelling rates because trabecular thickness is reduced at every resorption site, and a trabecula is only as strong as its thinnest part.

Perforation of trabeculae and loss of trabecular connectivity will eventually occur when thin plates and rods are perforated by resorption sites, especially when resorption depth increases. Trabecular perforations constitute a critical phase in bone loss because they cannot be repaired. When resorption switches to formation, new bone is deposited only on the edge of the perforation but the centre of the gap remains unrepaired and fills with bone marrow (Fig. 7.16). In this way, trabecular plates are gradually transformed to rods. When rods are eventually also perforated, the disconnected portions no longer transmit load and will therefore also be resorbed. In this way, the trabecular network becomes progressively disconnected, and weaker. In the vertebral body, horizontal trabeculae are perforated before vertical ones. This results in longer free-standing segments of vertical

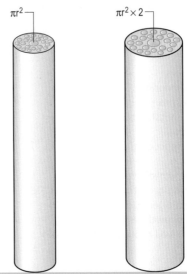

Figure 7.15. Diagram to show the relationship between trabecular cross-sectional area and bone strength. Reducing the cross-sectional area of the rod on the right by half to that of the rod on the left (41% thinner) decreases its buckling strength b not to half, but to a quarter i.e. exponentially. A small change in trabecular thickness thus causes a disproportionately greater change in bone strength.

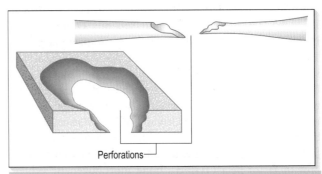

Figure 7.16. Diagram showing perforations of a trabecular plate and a trabecular rod by bone resorption. When resorption switches to formation, only the margins of the perforations will be covered with new bone. The remainder of the perforation remains unrepaired and fills with bone marrow. This constitutes irreversible bone loss. Repeated plate perforations gradually convert trabecular plates to rods. A rod, once perforated, no longer transmits load and will therefore be resorbed in its entirety.

trabeculae. This elongation is associated with an exponential loss of bone strength (Fig. 7.17). If removal of a supporting horizontal beam increases the length of the now unsupported vertical rod by a factor of 2, the vertical rod's resistance to buckling is reduced, not by a factor of 2, but by a factor of $2^2 = 4$, i.e. exponentially. Derangements of remodelling

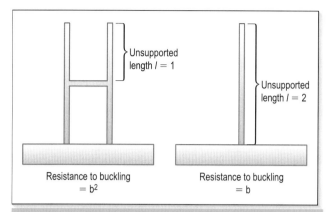

Figure 7.17. Schematic representation of the effect of the loss of horizontal trabeculae on the strength of the remaining vertical trabeculae. Removal of the horizontal trabecula (left image) doubles the length of the free-standing portion of the vertical trabecula (right image). This decreases the resistance to buckling b of the vertical trabecula not to half, but to one quarter, i.e. exponentially. A small loss in bone mass thus leads to a disproportionately greater loss in bone strength.

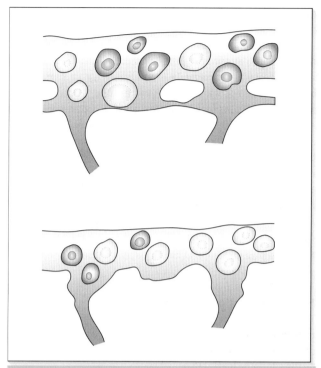

Figure 7.18. Diagrammatic representation of reduction in cortical thickness with ageing and in osteoporosis. Top: Impaired bone formation leads to decreasing wall thickness of Haversian systems so that Haversian canals remain wide and the cortex becomes increasingly porous, especially in the inner portion of the cortex next to bone marrow. The larger intracortical cavities fill with bone marrow so that this portion of the cortex begins to resemble cancellous bone. This process is referred to as 'cancellization' of the cortex. Bottom: Resorption of the thin bony septae separating intracortical cavities from bone marrow joins these cavities to the marrow cavity. In this way the cortex gets progressively thinner, and the marrow cavity wider.

thus pose a triple threat to trabecular bone: trabeculae get thinner, longer and fewer. According to our current state of knowledge, no remedy exists that will repair perforations, or build new trabeculae within bone marrow. Bone gain is only possible through bone deposition on existing bone scaffolding. Hence the importance of early prevention of bone loss.

Fatigue damage develops in bone weakened by bone loss and microarchitectural deterioration. Fatigue failure takes the form of microcracks in cortical bone and microfractures in trabecular bone. As a result of microdamage, bone gets weakened further (see below, 'Fatigue failure of bone').

Lattice irregularity of the trabecular network stems from perforations and microfractures. Even though bone mass may be little changed initially, trabecular lattice irregularity by itself is associated with loss of bone strength as a result of the conversion of simple compression forces to a mixture of compression and bending forces.

Cortical bone loss

Cortical bone is lost on the endocortical and intracortical (Haversian canals) surfaces (Fig. 7.9). Remodelling on the *endocortical* envelope takes place on a flat surface as in trabecular bone (Fig. 7.10). As a result of decreasing osteonal wall thickness, the cortex gets a little thinner and the marrow cavity a little wider with every remodelling cycle (Fig. 7.12). In *intracortical* remodelling (Fig. 7.11), on the other hand, reduction in osteonal wall thickness leads to an increase in *cortical porosity* because new Haversian canals remain wider as less new bone is formed than was resorbed (Fig. 7.18). The widest Haversian canals are situated near the bone marrow

cavity. The canals eventually coalesce to form large intracortical spaces that fill with bone marrow. Since this portion of the cortex now resembles cancellous bone, this change is referred to as 'cancellization' of the cortex. This change may be evident on radiographs as loss of distinction of the cortico-cancellous junction. Eventually, the thin plates of bone separating the intracortical spaces from the marrow cavity are also perforated, and the intracortical space is added to the marrow cavity. Thus, the cortex gets thinner and the marrow cavity wider (Fig. 7.18).

The *periosteal* surface shows little remodelling activity and no age-related bone loss. Indeed, a small but measurable amount of bone is added to the periosteal surface throughout life. Maximal strength is derived from this small amount of bone because it is advantageously placed biomechanically, namely furthest away from the centre of the bone. This change makes up, to some extent, for the loss of bone strength from bone loss and microarchitectural deterioration on other bone surfaces.

Osteocytes have a maximal lifespan of 20–25 years and then undergo apoptosis (programmed cell death). *Osteocyte apoptosis* may also take place prematurely, e.g. in patients on high dose glucocorticoid therapy, around microfractures, and in the vicinity of resorption sites. If bone containing apoptotic osteocytes is not remodelled, its lacunae and canaliculi calcify, a change referred to as *micropetrosis*. This adds to the hypermineralization of old unremodelled bone. More importantly, the absence of osteocytes as mechanotransducers of bone leads to a failure of bone to sense strain, detect microdamage, and initiate repair.

Fatigue failure of bone

Microfractures, microcracks and stress fractures are fatigue phenomena of bone.

Microfractures and microcracks

The term *microfracture* is used to describe fatigue damage in trabecular bone, presumably because the globular mass of callus surrounding the fracture of a trabecula resembles a healing long bone fracture.

Fatigue damage in cortical bone, on the other hand, takes the form of *microcracks*. These develop mostly in interstitial bone, i.e. in the oldest (unremodelled) bone which is the most highly mineralized, and therefore the most brittle bone. Since healing of microcracks by callus formation is obviously not possible within solid bone, the bone containing the microcrack has to be remodelled, i.e. resorbed and replaced with new bone.

Stress fractures

At what stage microfractures and microcracks become stress fractures is probably a matter of degree. Trabecular stress fractures consist of multiple microfractures, and cortical stress fractures of multiple or propagated microcracks. Whereas small numbers of microfractures and microcracks are mostly asymptomatic, stress fractures cause pain and swelling.

The development of a stress fracture is determined by a number of factors, namely (1) load, (2) number of loading cycles per unit time, (3) bone mass and deterioration of microarchitecture, (4) remodelling disorders. These factors are interdependent. Stress fractures develop predominantly in the lower limbs because of the *load* of body weight. Non-ambulant osteoporotic patients (e.g. with rheumatoid arthritis) rendered ambulant by a total hip or knee arthroplasty may develop stress fractures in the lower limbs and pelvis because of a sudden increase in the number of *loading cycles* (gait). With declining *bone mass* and *deteriorating microarchitecture* the stress fracture risk increases; for this reason microfractures and microcracks increase exponentially with age. Whereas normal bone *remodelling* removes incipient

microdamage, low remodelling rates may not keep up with the development of new lesions, and high remodelling rates weaken bone, thus increasing the stress fracture risk. The *healing* of stress fractures is the healing of their component microfractures, or microcracks. Trabecular stress fractures heal by callus formation around each individual microfracture (Fig. 7.19), and cortical stress fractures heal by remodelling of the cracked portion of bone. Some periosteal new bone formation accompanies the healing of most stress fractures.

Stress fractures can be divided into insufficiency stress fractures and fatigue stress fractures. *Insufficiency stress fractures* typically occur in trabecular bone of osteoporotic individuals, and affect the proximal and distal metaphyses of femur and tibia, the pelvis, sacrum, and the posterior half of the calcaneum. These insufficiency stress fractures develop *in abnormal bone under normal load*. The term 'insufficiency' refers to osteoporosis. *Fatigue stress fractures*, on the other hand, are thought to develop *in normal bone under abnormal load* mostly in healthy young individuals. Unaccustomed, strenuous and repetitive activity causes material fatigue in cortical bone because cortical bone with its small surface area is unable to respond sufficiently rapidly with additional new

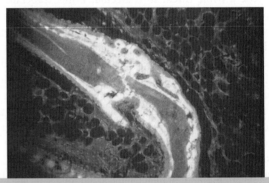

Figure 7.19.   Photomicrograph of an unstained section of undecalcified bone, photographed under ultraviolet light, showing a healing trabecular microfracture (biopsy of a calcaneal stress fracture similar to that shown in Fig. 7.21). The trabecula (dark) shows an oblique fracture line (light) and is surrounded at this site by a spindle-shaped mass of callus (light). The very dark background is bone marrow. The light colour is produced by fluorescence of the antibiotic tetracycline under ultraviolet light. Tetracycline attaches to enlarging bone crystals at bone formation sites and so allows identification of newly forming bone on microscopic examination. The patient in question had been given the tetracycline for routine bone labelling twice, namely for 2 days, and again for 4 days after a 10-day interval. The biopsy of the stress fracture was taken 5 days later. Such timed labelling and measurement of the interlabel distance permits the calculation of bone formation rates. The tetracycline-labelled new callus in this case was formed between days 21 and 5 before the biopsy.

bone formation to meet the new physical demand, nor can it rapidly increase bone remodelling to replace damaged bone. Fatigue stress fractures typically present in the shafts of lower limb bones and in the cortex of the femoral neck of athletes and military recruits, and in the pars interarticularis of lumbar vertebrae in young ballet dancers. Some athletes suffering from 'shin splints' may in fact have an incipient fatigue stress fracture of the tibial shaft that is not yet evident on radiographs. Fatigue stress fractures in the 17- to 26-year age group are partly due to the physiological high bone turnover of a skeleton that has not yet reached peak bone mass (which occurs at age 25–30 years). High turnover bone has a large remodelling space, i.e. the remodelling space (the sum of all resorption cavities) is large. In other words, bone in a high turnover state is more porous than bone with lower turnover. Furthermore, high-turnover bone also has lower stiffness than lower-turnover bone because recently formed bone is not yet fully mineralized since the secondary phase of mineralization takes years to complete. Both factors, namely increased porosity and low stiffness, result in a combination of (1) increased bone strain (deformation within bone), and (2) increased strain rates in bone when external stresses are applied. These features are thought to be the reasons for the higher stress fracture rates in young than in older adults. Between ages 17 and 26 years, stress fracture risk in military recruits was found to decline by 28% for every year of age. In other words, with time affected individuals will grow out of the stress fracture phase.

The *diagnosis* of a stress fracture frequently has to be delayed by 2–3 weeks because callus formation on which the radiologic diagnosis depends takes this long to develop. However, a radionuclide bone scan using the bone-seeking isotope compound ^{99}Tc-MDP will show increased uptake in and around the fracture site from the onset of symptoms (see 'The regional acceleratory phenomenon'). Magnetic resonance imaging (MRI), too, shows early changes, namely the bone marrow oedema accompanying the stress fracture. MRI may identify the marrow oedema accompanying even a small number of microfractures, referred to as *bone bruise*.

Bone mineral metabolism

Bone is a mineral reservoir for calcium, sodium, phosphate and other substances. The minute-to-minute supply of *calcium* for calcium homeostasis comes from bone crystals and is provided by osteocytes across the walls of their lacunae and canaliculi, which have a vast surface area. Calcium supply for homeostasis could not rely on osteoclastic resorption alone because osteoclast activation responds too slowly (hours, days) for homeostatic metabolic needs. *Magnesium* is thought to enhance bone quality by influencing hydroxyapatite crystal growth. It may also improve parathyroid hormone (PTH) secretion and intestinal calcium absorption. Magnesium deficiency is seen in alcoholics in whom it is associated with hypocalcaemia, reduced PTH secretion and impaired 1,25-dihydroxyvitamin D response to PTH. Magnesium deficiency is thought to possibly also contribute to the development of postmenopausal osteoporosis.

Calcium homeostasis

The three calcitropic hormones parathyroid hormone, 1,25-dihydroxyvitamin D and calcitonin fine-tune the extracellular concentration of calcium to safeguard an optimum supply of calcium for cellular function of all body tissues (Fig. 7.20). When serum calcium levels drop even minimally, they will be restored immediately by supply of calcium from bone. So important is calcium to cellular function, that provision of sufficient calcium from bone gets preference over skeletal structural integrity. Highly efficient feedback loops guard against hypo- and hypercalcaemia.

Vitamin D is derived from the diet and from photosynthesis in skin. Ultraviolet rays of sunlight convert 7-dehydrocholesterol to vitamin D (cholecalciferol) in skin exposed to direct sunlight. Exposure of a small area of skin to direct sunlight for 15 minutes a day suffices to provide sufficient vitamin D. However, UV light does not penetrate clothes or window glass. Vitamin D is converted in the liver to *25-hydroxyvitamin D* (calcidiol), and passes via the bloodstream to the kidneys, where it is converted to *1,25-dihydroxyvitamin D* (calcitriol) by the enzyme 1-alphahydroxylase. 1,25-Dihydroxyvitamin D behaves as a hormone. It stimulates intestinal absorption of calcium and phosphorus, and thus

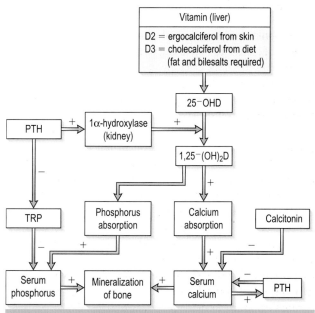

Figure 7.20.   Schematic representation of the control of calcium homeostasis by vitamin D metabolites, parathyroid hormone (PTH) and calcitonin. TRP, tubular reabsorption of phosphate by the kidney.

raises serum calcium and phosphorus levels; it also releases calcium from bone. *Vitamin D deficiency* leads to inadequate intestinal absorption of calcium and phosphorus with a resultant drop in serum levels so that newly forming bone cannot mineralize adequately and *rickets* and *osteomalacia* may develop. However, before full-blown rickets and osteomalacia develop, the drop in serum calcium levels causes secondary hyperparathyroidism. This increases bone turnover, which raises the demand for calcium for newly formed bone, and thus hastens the development of rickets and osteomalacia. The mineralization defect of bone in rickets and osteomalacia is a result of low calcium and/or phosphorus concentrations in extracellular fluid, and not of low levels of vitamin D; as far as is known, vitamin D itself plays no direct role in the deposition of bone mineral into osteoid. Vitamin D status is assessed by measuring serum levels of 25-hydroxyvitamin D rather than those of 1,25-dihydroxyvitamin D because only 25-hydroxyvitamin D has vitamin qualities (depending on extraneous source) whereas 1,25-dihydroxyvitamin D behaves like a hormone (produced and controlled within the body). Rickets and/or osteomalacia can also be caused by dietary calcium deficiency and renal loss of phosphorus (see 'Osteomalacia and rickets').

Parathyroid hormone is produced by four minuscule (2 grams each) parathyroid glands situated behind the upper and lower poles of the thyroid gland. PTH production is increased in response to a drop in serum calcium levels or a rise in serum phosphorus. PTH enhances the renal conversion of 25-hydroxyvitamin D to 1,25-dihydroxyvitamin D. This then increases intestinal absorption of calcium so that serum calcium levels are restored to normal. PTH also increases renal tubular reabsorption of calcium, and decreases renal tubular reabsorption of phosphate (TRP), thus conserving calcium and increasing renal phosphate excretion. In calcium homeostasis, calcium and phosphorus always move in opposite directions. PTH also causes calcium release from bone. There exist thus a number of mechanisms that guard against hypocalcaemia. Hypercalcaemia is, however, counteracted only by the hormone *calcitonin*, which is produced by the C-cells of the thyroid gland; calcitonin is not associated with any known disease state. High PTH levels, on the other hand, cause hyperparathyroidism, which may lead to osteoporosis over a period of years if left untreated (see 'Hyperparathyroid bone disease').

Pathophysiology of bone disorders

Most bone diseases are caused by derangements of bone remodelling.

Osteoporosis

Osteoporosis is the commonest bone disease. It is the final common end-stage of all bone-losing conditions and may therefore be due to any of many different causes. Osteoporosis

without an identifiable cause is referred to as idiopathic or primary osteoporosis, and that due to a known cause as secondary osteoporosis. *Risk factors for osteoporosis* are given in Table 7.4. Osteoporosis can present at any age and in both sexes, but the commonest form is postmenopausal osteoporosis. The current *definition* of osteoporosis, adopted by the World Health Organization, is: 'Osteoporosis is a systemic skeletal disorder characterised by low bone mass and microarchitectural deterioration of bone tissue, leading to enhanced bone fragility and a consequent increase in fracture risk'.

Pathogenesis

Both low bone mass and microarchitectural deterioration are the result of deranged bone remodelling. During each remodelling cycle less bone is formed than was resorbed (see 'Skeletal ageing'). This results in gradual thinning of trabeculae and their eventual perforation (Figs 7.12 and 7.16). The result is a disconnected trabecular network and loss of bone strength. Cortical thickness decreases as a result of a negative remodelling balance on the endocortical surface, and cortical porosity increases as the remodelling imbalance leaves wider new Haversian canals (Fig. 7.18). Although the skeleton is made up of more cortical (80%) than trabecular (20%) bone, the clinical manifestations of osteoporosis are first evident in trabecular bone because of the larger surface area available on which deranged bone remodelling can cause rapid bone

---

Table 7.4.   Risk factors for osteoporosis

Genetic factors
  Female sex (white, Asian)
  Family history of osteoporosis
Lifestyle factors
  Alcohol abuse
  Sedentary lifestyle, immobilization
  Excessive exercise with low energy intake
  Heavy smoking
Diseases/Drugs
  Endocrinopathies (e.g. hyperparathyroidism, hyperthyroidism, Cushing's disease, hyperprolactinaemia)
  Gut disorders (inflammatory bowel disease, gluten enteropathy, gastrectomy)
  Rheumatic disorders
  Anorexia nervosa, malnutrition
  Malignant disease (myeloma, metastases)
  Chronic organ failure (lung, liver, kidney)
  Bone toxic drugs (corticosteroids, excessive thyroxine replacement, chemotherapy, immunosuppressive therapy, anticonvulsants)
Ageing
  Sex hormone deficiency (male and female)
  Calcium and vitamin D deficiency (causing secondary hyperparathyroidism)

destruction. For this reason, sites containing a high proportion of trabecular bone are typical sites for fragility fractures (fractures caused by non-violent trauma), namely vertebral bodies, proximal femur and distal radius.

Assessment of osteoporosis

Risk factor analysis (Table 7.4) is the first step in the assessment of a patient with suspected osteoporosis. A diagnosis of osteoporosis can be made in the presence of a *fragility fracture*, or on the basis of *low bone mineral density (BMD)*. *Dual X-ray absorptiometry* (DXA) is the current 'gold standard' for the measurement of BMD (Fig. 7.21a, b). It is used to (1) diagnose osteoporosis, (2) assess future fracture risk, (3) monitor BMD response to therapy, and (4) guide therapeutic decision-making. Standard measurement sites are the lumbar spine and hip (proximal femur). The *diagnosis* of osteoporosis is based on so-called T-scores. A T-score is one standard deviation (SD) from the young normal mean BMD (age 30 years) (Fig. 7.21b). In other words, every patient's BMD result is expressed in the number of T-scores that this value differs from the young normal mean. In this way all individuals are compared with a single norm (age 30), and

thus also become mutually comparable. The World Health Organization has defined the following diagnostic categories of bone loss, based on the T-score system:

Normal bone: T-score above −1
Osteopenia: T-score between −1 and −2.5
Osteoporosis: T-score below −2.5
Severe osteoporosis: T-score below −2.5 plus existing fragility fractures.

Comparison with age-related normal values is expressed in so-called Z-scores. One Z-score is one SD of the age-specific (same age group) mean BMD. A Z-score within the age-specific normal range, i.e. less than 2 SD below the age-specific mean (Z-score above −2), suggests that the bone loss is age-related. However, a Z-score below the normal range for age, i.e. below −2, indicates the possible existence of an underlying disorder in addition to age-related bone loss.

The *future fracture risk* doubles with every SD (T-score) below the young normal mean: at T-score = −1 the fracture risk is double that of young normals, at −2 it is 4-fold, at −3 it is 8-fold, etc. At a T-score of −3 many individuals already have fragility fractures. *Therapeutic decision-making*

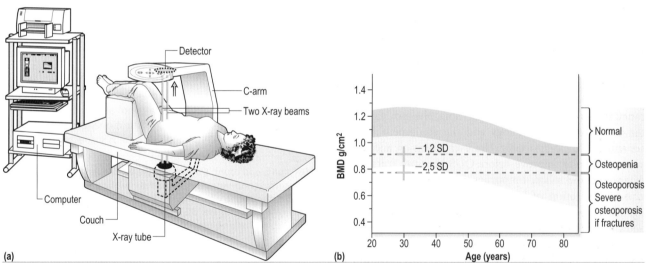

Figure 7.21.   Diagnosis of osteoporosis by measurement of bone mineral density (BMD) using dual X-ray absorptiometry (DXA). (a) Diagram depicting a densitometer. Two X-ray beams (hence 'dual') of different energy pass through the patient. One beam measures the density of bone plus soft tissue, and the other that of soft tissue only; the difference gives the bone value (subtraction radiography). The intensity of the emerging beam is inversely related to the patient's bone mineral content. The attenuation (weakening) of the X-ray beams is measured by the detector, located above the patient. The result is expressed as bone mineral density (BMD) = bone mineral content (BMC)/bone area in g/cm². (b) The two bands on the graph reflect the normal range of BMD for women (mean ± 2 SD). The patient's BMD value is expressed as a T- and a Z-score. A T-score is one SD of the young normal mean (age 30). The upper of the two red crosses in the graph represents a T-score of −1.2, and the lower a T-score of −2.5. The World Health Organization (WHO) has defined diagnostic categories of bone loss based on T-scores. Normal bone: T-score above −1; osteopenia: T-score between −1 and −2.5; osteoporosis: T-score below −2.5; severe osteoporosis: T-score below −2.5 plus fragility fracture(s). The Z-score compares the patient's result with age-related normal values. One Z-score is one SD of the age-related mean. A Z-score result below the normal range for age (i.e. below −2) suggests that the patient's bone loss is greater than can be accounted for by age-related bone loss and that an underlying disorder should be looked for.

may also be guided by BMD measurements: normal bone density requires no intervention other than lifestyle counselling, osteopenia calls for prevention, and osteoporosis requires treatment.

Limitations of DXA are falsely high readings caused by degenerative changes in spine and hip (osteophyte formation in osteoarthritis), vascular calcifications, and fractured lumbar vertebrae. Previous surgery also renders the measurement invalid. Even in the absence of such confounding factors, the methodology has inherent limitations, namely an accuracy error of 3–10% and a precision error of 1–3%. Accuracy states to what extent a BMD value reflects true bone mineral density. An accuracy error of 3–10% means that 3–10% of the measured BMD value may be due to technical error. Precision refers to the ability to obtain the identical reading on repeat measurement. A precision error of 1–3% states that 1–3% of a repeat BMD measurement may be due to technical error. A follow-up BMD measurement during osteoporosis therapy should not be carried out in less than 1 year because the expected changes are within the range of the precision error of the equipment. If the measurement were to be repeated in less than one year, it would be unclear whether a change is due to a true BMD change in the patient, or to the precision error of the equipment.

Single energy X-ray absorptiometry (SXA) of peripheral sites (e.g. forearm) is less costly than DXA and is also used to diagnose osteoporosis. Its precision and accuracy are similar to those of DXA. However, this technology is not used for monitoring therapy because BMD changes at peripheral sites (mainly cortical bone) are too small.

Ultrasonometry (quantitative ultrasound, QUS) of the calcaneum and other peripheral sites (tibia, phalanx, patella) is the least costly methodology and the equipment has the advantage of being portable. However, precision and accuracy will have to improve before QUS becomes suitable for diagnostic, and follow-up purposes. Currently it can at best give an indication of hip fracture risk. Ultrasonometry is thought to reflect changes in bone microarchitecture, in addition to those of bone mass.

Bone turnover markers, i.e. formation markers and resorption markers (see 'Bone proteins' under 'Composition of bone', Fig. 7.7a, b), are physiological chemical compounds that are produced during bone turnover. They can be measured in blood or urine (Table 7.5). Whereas bone formation markers are products of osteoblastic activity, bone resorption markers are breakdown products of bone collagen. The rationale for their use in clinical practice and research is the fact that high bone turnover in adults leads to bone loss as a result of a negative remodelling balance and uncoupling of resorption from formation. High bone turnover markers may therefore predict rapid bone loss, but they are not a diagnostic test for existing osteoporosis – this would require BMD measurement. Bone resorption markers can also be used for advance assessment of response to antiresorptive

Table 7.5.   Biochemical markers of bone turnover

Bone formation markers
  Bone-specific alkaline phosphatase (produced by osteoblasts)
  Osteocalcin (bone GLA protein, BGP) (produced by osteoblasts)
  Propeptides of type I collagen
    C-propeptide (PICP)
    N-propeptide (PINP)
Bone resorption markers (collagen cross-links)
  Deoxypyridinoline (DPD)
  Cross-linked N-telopeptides (NTX)
  Cross-linked C-telopeptides (CTX)

Table 7.6.   Biochemical investigations in osteoporosis

Investigations	Over 50 years	Under 50 years
Routine		
Serum calcium (ionized)	+	+
Urine calcium (24 hour)	+	+
Alkaline phosphatase (total)	+	+
FBC and ESR	+	+
PTH	+	
TSH	+	
Serum protein electrophoresis	+	
Bone turnover marker(s)	+	+
Serum creatinine	+	
Optional		
FSH, LH, oestrogen/testosterone (women under 50 y/men)		
AST, GGT, MCV, uric acid (if alcohol abuse suspected)		
Serum 25-hydroxyvitamin D (institutionalized individuals)		
Serum cortisol (if Cushing's disease is suspected)		

FBC, full blood count; ESR erythrocyte sedimentation rate; PTH, parathyroid hormone; TSH, thyroid-stimulating hormone; FSH, follicle-stimulating hormone; LH, luteinizing hormone; AST aspartate transaminase; GGT, gamma glutamyltransferase; MCV, mean corpuscular volume of red cells.

therapy of osteoporosis since a decline in levels in the case of a good response will already be evident after 2 to 3 months of treatment, whereas repeat BMD measurement by DXA has to be delayed to 1 year. It must be emphasized that bone turnover markers are no substitute for BMD measurements because the two methodologies reflect different time frames in the life of the skeleton. Whereas BMD is the historical static result of past gains and losses of bone, bone turnover markers reflect the dynamics of current, and likely future bone loss or gain.

Other *biochemical investigations* (Table 7.6) yield normal results in most cases of primary osteoporosis but are carried out to exclude underlying causes. *Primary hyperparathyroidism* is characterized by elevated levels of serum ionized calcium, PTH and alkaline phosphatase. *Secondary hyperparathyroidism* due to dietary calcium deficiency, calcium malabsorption, and/or vitamin D deficiency also presents with raised values of PTH and alkaline phophatase, but serum ionized calcium and urinary calcium excretion are low. This condition is common in the elderly, particularly in patients presenting with femoral neck fractures. If untreated, secondary hyperparathyroidism due to calcium and/or vitamin D deficiency does not only cause osteoporosis but also leads to *osteomalacia*, which further increases bone fragility. *Myeloma* can present as osteoporosis but is characterized by abnormal serum electrophoresis (monoclonal gammopathy), an elevated ESR, and in advanced cases with hypercalcaemia. Osteoporosis is also a known complication of *thyrotoxicosis*, or too high a dose of thyroxine replacement therapy (suggested by low thyroid-stimulating hormone levels in serum).

All conditions of high bone turnover (e.g. hyperparathyroidism, thyrotoxicosis and many other forms of osteoporosis) are associated with increased levels of bone turnover markers; these decline with successful therapy. *Hypogonadism* in both males and females presents with elevated levels of follicle-stimulating hormone and luteinizing hormone, and low levels of gonadal (sex) hormones. A suspicion of *alcohol abuse* as the cause of osteoporosis may be confirmed if two or more of the markers of alcohol abuse, i.e. aspartate aminotransferase, gamma-glutamyltransferase, uric acid and MCV (mean corpuscular volume of red blood cells), are elevated (Table 7.6).

Clinical features

Bone loss develops silently. Osteoporosis is not a chronic pain syndrome until fragility fractures occur. Typical fracture sites are the vertebral column (below T5), the distal radius, the proximal femur (neck and greater trochanteric region) and the proximal humerus. When a fracture has healed, osteoporosis is once again painless in most patients.

Vertebral compression fractures develop spontaneously, or with minimal trauma, and usually occur in phases of several fractures in close succession. The most commonly affected vertebrae are T6 to L3. A vertebral fracture due to osteoporosis causes sudden and severe midline back pain that is relieved by rest, and gradually decreases over a period of 4 weeks. Osteoporotic vertebral fractures are not associated with nerve root symptoms or a neurological deficit, in contrast to intervertebral disc prolapse, or malignant vertebral lesions. Vertebral compression fractures may also be diagnosed radiologically at an asymptomatic stage. Such fractures may date back to an undiagnosed past episode of back pain, or they may have developed without causing major symptoms, presumably as a result of multiple microfractures. A vertebral fracture is diagnosed when there is a 20% or greater reduction in anterior and/or central vertebral height relative to the posterior height of the same or the

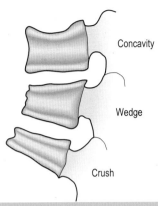

Figure 7.22.   Diagram showing the three most common forms of vertebral body compression fractures due to osteoporosis. A vertebral body compression fracture is considered present when there is a 20% or greater reduction in anterior and/or central height relative to its own, or the nearest intact posterior height. A reduction in central height constitutes a concavity fracture, a reduction in anterior height (with or without reduction in central height) a wedge fracture, and reduction in all three heights a crush fracture. Crush fractures are indicative of severe osteoporosis.

nearest intact vertebra. Reduction in central height constitutes a *concavity fracture*, reduction in anterior height, a *wedge fracture*, and reduction in all three heights, a *crush fracture* (Fig. 7.22). The crush fracture signifies a more severe form of osteoporosis than the other two fracture types. Complete collapse of all three heights (vertebra plana) should arouse suspicion of malignancy; other features of malignancy are spinal pain not relieved by rest, spontaneous vertebral fractures above T6, and non-traumatic long bone shaft fractures. Since a collapsed vertebra does not spontaneously regain normal height, the height loss and spinal flexion deformity (kyphosis) remain. As a result of the kyphosis, the sagging rib cage causes painful impingement on the iliac crest, and the abdominal muscles become slack so that the abdomen protrudes. Furthermore, the stooped patient has to hyperextend the low lumbar and the cervical spine to compensate for the kyphosis. This causes intermittent lumbar and cervical pain, and muscle fatigue. Indeed, lumbar back pain in most elderly women is caused by degenerative changes rather than by osteoporosis.

Vertebroplasty and *kyphoplasty* are surgical procedures that involve percutaneous injection of bone cement (methylmethacrylate as used in joint replacements) into collapsed vertebrae for the treatment of osteoporotic patients who have severe prolonged pain following vertebral fracture. Whereas vertebroplasty aims to stabilize the collapsed vertebra without correcting the deformity, kyphoplasty expands the collapsed vertebra with a bone tamp (balloon) before injecting cement. The technique is at an investigative stage.

Table 7.7.   Optimum daily calcium intake

Age	Elemental calcium (mg)
Infant	
0–6 months	400
6–12 months	600
Children	
1–5 years	800
6–10 years	800–1200
Adolescents/Young adults	
11–24 years	1200–1500
Women	
25–50 years	1000
50+ years (postmenopausal)	
On oestrogen	1000
Not on oestrogens	1500
65 + years	1500
Pregnancy and lactation	1500
Men	
25–65 years	1000
65+ years	1500

Source: NIH Consensus Development Panel on Optimum Calcium Intake (1994). JAMA 272:1942–1948.

Hip fractures are mostly caused by a fall from standing height as a result of motor incoordination or a giddy spell. However, spontaneous fractures do occur. In this event the patient may have groin pain for several days before the complete fracture occurs without trauma. In such cases a stress fracture may have weakened the bone and led to the hip fracture. Stress fractures of the femoral neck may only be demonstrable on a ^{99}Tc-MDP bone scan or by MRI. Such fractures should be pinned before they become complete in order to reduce morbidity.

Prevention of osteoporosis

The prevention of osteoporosis begins in childhood. Adequate dietary intake of *calcium* and regular *physical exercise* (weight bearing) during childhood have been shown to be beneficial for bone mass accumulation. In adults, however, exercise at best slows bone loss because the adult skeleton is less responsive than the young skeleton. Optimum daily intake of calcium is listed in Table 7.7. In adults, calcium slows bone loss but does not prevent it altogether. Calcium supplementation in adulthood is most effective in the presence of calcium deficiency, and least effective in a state of calcium sufficiency. An adequate supply of *vitamin D* ensures optimal intestinal calcium absorption. The adequate intake (AI) per day of vitamin D is 200 IU (International Units) (5 μg) from birth to age 50 years, 400 IU from age 51–70, and 800 IU from age 71 years. Since photosynthesis is less efficient in individuals with dark skin, particularly those living in northern climates (e.g. Asians in Britain), the daily AI may well be higher for these individuals. Although

adequate *dietary protein* is necessary for optimal skeletal development (bone mass, skeletal size) and maintenance of muscle mass in the elderly, a high protein diet increases dietary calcium requirements. Every additional gram of protein metabolized by an adult causes an additional urinary excretion of 1 mg of calcium. This increased calcium excretion is thought to be needed in the excretion of sulphates from metabolized sulphur-containing amino acids in protein. Similarly, for every additional 100 mg of sodium excreted by the kidney, 1 mg of calcium is co-excreted. Thus a high protein and salt content of the diet calls for increased calcium intake.

Treatment of osteoporosis

The drug treatment of osteoporosis falls into two major categories: inhibition of resorption by antiresorptives, and stimulation of bone formation by anabolic agents. *Antiresorptive agents* inhibit osteoclast differentiation and/or function. This results in a lower birth rate of new remodelling cycles, i.e. resorption sites. At the same time, previously created resorption sites fill in with new bone (closure of the remodelling space). For this reason bone mass tends to increase slightly during the first 2–3 years of antiresorptive therapy. Antiresorptive agents are currently the most commonly used drugs in the treatment of osteoporosis. Available in clinical practice are HRT (hormone replacement therapy), bisphosphonates (e.g. alendronate, risedronate, pamidronate), calcitonin, calcium and SERMs (selective (o)estrogen receptor modulators, e.g. raloxifen, tamoxifen), calcitonin and calcium. SERMs have oestrogen-like bone-sparing and serum lipid-lowering actions, but have anti-oestrogenic effects on breast and uterus. A large 3-year clinical trial of antiresorptive therapy has shown that subjects with the greatest decline in bone turnover markers had the lowest number of new vertebral fractures, irrespective of BMD changes. This effect is attributed to inhibition of trabecular plate perforations, and therefore to preservation of trabecular connectivity and strength. Moreover, trabeculae are no longer weakened by an excessive number of resorption sites. The associated increase in bone mass was presumably too small to be detectable by BMD measurement. *Anabolic agents* capable of stimulating bone formation, namely pulsed PTH therapy, fluoride, growth hormone, and insulin-like growth factor-1 (IGF-1) and other substances await introduction into clinical practice.

Two to 5% of all *falls* and 25% of sideways falls in the elderly result in hip fractures. Risk factors for falling that need attention are environmental hazards (e.g. rugs, furniture, poor lighting), gait and balance disorders, muscle weakness, mental impairment (e.g. due to medication), and visual impairment. External *hip protectors*, worn in underwear, cushion the greater trochanter during a sideways fall, and so reduce hip fracture risk. *Exercise programmes* are aimed at fall prevention by improving muscle strength and coordination, rather than at increasing bone mass.

Hyperparathyroid bone disease

Hyperparathyroidism (HPT) may be primary or secondary. *Primary HPT* is due to a secreting adenoma of one of the four parathyroid glands (over 90% of adenomas are benign) and is characterized by hypercalcaemia. *Secondary HPT*, most commonly found in renal failure, is caused by hyperplasia of all four glands and is associated with normal or low serum calcium and high serum phosphorus levels. Secondary HPT may also be caused by low dietary calcium intake and vitamin D deficiency as is seen in the elderly, particularly those with femoral neck fractures. HPT causes high bone turnover that may result in osteoporosis characterized by cortical thinning. In advanced cases of primary HPT, vigorous bone resorption may cause localized bone destruction in the form of intraosseous cysts that contain old blood which is brown, hence 'brown tumour'. The treatment of hyperparathyroid bone disease is by parathyroidectomy of the tumour-bearing gland. This will normalize bone turnover, and some of the bone loss may be reversed. In over 90% of cases hypercalcaemia is caused by primary HPT or by malignancy unrelated to the parathyroid glands. *Hypercalcaemia of malignancy* is due to secretion of *parathyroid-hormone-related protein* (*PTHrP*) by a tumour (e.g. carcinomas of the lung, kidney, ovary, bladder, breast, oesophagus, head and neck). Although PTHrP is a member of the PTH family, PTHrP cannot be measured by the test for PTH. PTH is in fact suppressed in hypercalcaemia of malignancy. Commercial assays for PTHrP are now available. PTHrP is also a physiological substance with vital functions in development and normal cell biology and is expressed in small quantities in many fetal and adult tissues.

Osteomalacia and rickets

Osteomalacia (OM) means 'soft bones'. New bone formed during the remodelling process fails to mineralize, i.e. the soft unmineralized new osteoid does not harden because no hydroxyapatite crystals are deposited on the collagen fibres. In all cases of OM, the failure of mineral deposition is due to low serum concentrations of either calcium or phosphorus, or both. Vitamin D plays no direct role in the mineralization process; its role is merely the provision of sufficient calcium and phosphorus through intestinal absorption. Bone mass in osteomalacia is usually normal, but it may be increased or decreased. If bone mass is low, the patient suffers from both osteomalacia and osteoporosis (Fig. 7.23). Bone densitometry cannot distinguish between OM and osteoporosis because it only measures bone mineral density and merely shows 'low bone density' in both conditions. Osteomalacia and rickets may be inherited or acquired.

The term *osteomalacia* refers to failed mineralization of bone in the skeleton as a whole, and in both adults and children. The term *rickets* refers to the condition in children who in addition to having osteomalacia show features of failed mineralization at the growth plate. The disorder has typical

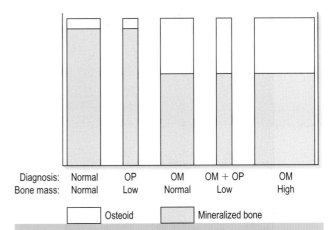

Diagnosis:	Normal	OP	OM	OM + OP	OM
Bone mass:	Normal	Low	Normal	Low	High

☐ Osteoid   ▦ Mineralized bone

Figure 7.23. Schematic representation of proportions of mineralized and unmineralized bone in normal, osteoporotic (OP) and osteomalacic (OM) bone. The width of the columns represents bone mass. Approximately 5% of normal and of osteoporotic bone consists of osteoid (unmineralized bone), irrespective of bone mass. A marked increase in the proportion of unmineralized bone constitutes osteomalacia, irrespective of bone mass.

histological, clinical, radiological and biochemical features. The *histological* picture of bone is characterized by an excessive proportion of unmineralized bone matrix, i.e. osteoid (Plate III; see plate section p. xi). *Clinical features of osteomalacia* in adults are bone pain and occasionally deformities. Because of rapid growth and high bone turnover in children the *clinical features of rickets* are usually more severe than those of OM in adults. These include painful enlargement of the growth plate regions at the ends of the long bones, and the costo-chondral junctions ('ricketty rosary' on the anterior chest wall), bowing and rotational deformities of long bones, bossing of the frontal bones, flat parietal bones, indentation of the lower rib cage due to pull by the diaphragm (Harrison's groove), and retardation of growth. *Radiological features of osteomalacia* in adults are *Looser's zones*. These are broad, radiolucent transverse bands in ribs, pubic rami (see Fig. 7.26), femoral neck and shaft, ulna, metatarsal bones and the axillary border of the scapula. These sites are areas of high biomechanical stress where bone turnover is high. Because of low concentrations of phosphorus or calcium the newly deposited osteoid cannot mineralize. Histologically Looser's zones consist of osteoid that has failed to mineralize. Although Looser's zones are considered by some to be insufficiency stress fractures, they differ from stress fractures in that they are symmetrically distributed and do not form callus (see Fig. 7.26). The distinction between Looser's zones and stress fractures is of clinical importance because true Looser's zones point to an underlying severe osteomalacia that will require special attention. Furthermore, stress fractures heal

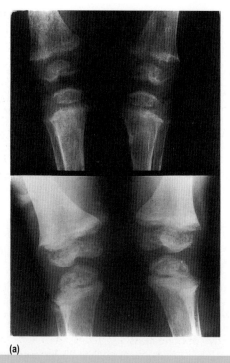

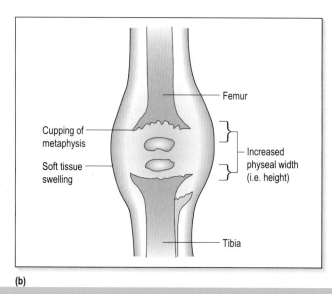

(a) (b)

Figure 7.24.   Radiographs of the knees (a) of a patient with rickets at baseline and on treatment, and (b) explanatory diagram (for baseline radiograph). The radiograph taken at baseline (top) shows (1) increased physeal width due to a mineralization failure in cartilage and new bone, (2) cupping and sideways spread of the metaphysis due to anatomical disorganization of physeal microstructure, and (3) low radiographic bone density. A radiograph taken after 6 months of therapy for rickets (bottom) shows evidence of healing: the physes are less wide because mineral is now being deposited at the physis. Radiographic bone density appears to be increasing.

with rest and Looser's zones do not. Looser's zones only heal with medical intervention. Radiological features of rickets are wide growth plates, cupped metaphyses (Fig. 7.24), and angular and rotary deformities of long bones (Fig. 7.25). *Biochemical features* are similar in osteomalacia and rickets and depend on the underlying metabolic abnormality. Phosphorus and/or calcium levels are low or normal. Vitamin D metabolites and PTH are variously affected, but alkaline phosphatase is always elevated. A number of different metabolic abnormalities may cause rickets. The following are the commonest forms.

Privational rickets and osteomalacia
Privational rickets or osteomalacia may be caused by deficiency of vitamin D or calcium, or both. *Vitamin D deficiency* results from lack of exposure of skin to direct sunlight in the absence of dietary supplementation of vitamin D. Vitamin D deficiency is seen for example in institutionalized elderly individuals, and in Asian immigrants in Britain. In the general population serum 25-hydroxyvitamin D levels are lower in winter than in summer. However, vitamin D may be stored in the body for several months. British children who enjoyed a seaside summer holiday still had higher serum 25-hydroxyvitamin D levels at the end of the following winter than controls.

Dietary *calcium deficiency* due to insufficient intake of dairy products in African countries has been shown to lead to rickets and osteomalacia. The calcium deficiency is aggravated by the high phytate content of the corn-based diet because phytates bind calcium. Dietary calcium deficiency at first causes nutritional secondary HPT with bone loss, and later OM. *Phosphate deficiency* is rare because phosphate is readily available in food. However, premature infants fed unsupplemented breast milk develop a deficiency of both phosphorus and calcium.

X-linked hypophosphataemic rickets
Hypophosphataemic rickets is due to low serum phosphate levels as a result of a proximal renal tubular phosphate leak that may be caused by a circulating hypophosphataemic factor. The condition is inherited as an X-linked dominant trait with the mutant gene in the distal part of the short arm of the X-chromosome. This led to the condition being referred to as 'X-linked hypophosphataemic rickets'. It is characterized by three features:

- hypophosphataemia
- lower limb deformities
- and stunted growth.

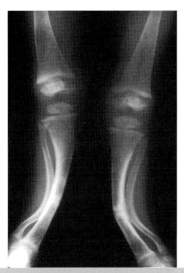

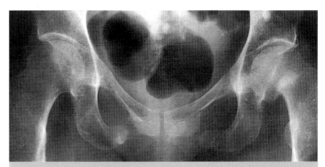

Figure 7.26. Radiograph of the pelvis of an elderly woman who complained of discomfort when walking. There was no history of injury. The radiograph shows a spontaneous fracture of the left femoral neck, and Looser's zones in the inferior and superior pubic rami. She was found to have both osteoporosis and osteomalacia as a result of intestinal malabsorption following extensive small bowel resection for intestinal obstruction earlier in life.

Figure 7.25. Radiograph showing leg deformities in a patient with rickets. The patient had recently started treatment to correct the metabolic abnormality. As a result the bone disease had begun to heal: the excessive width of the growth plates has begun to decline, the radiodensity of the metaphyses has increased, and the Looser's zone (resembling a fracture) in the shaft of the left tibia is healing. The bowing of the tibiae will, however, not correct spontaneously, but will require surgical correction by osteotomy. This will have to be deferred until the bone disease (osteomalacia) has healed completely, to ensure that the new bone uniting the osteotomies mineralizes.

In the presence of low levels of serum phosphorus, newly deposited bone throughout the skeleton cannot mineralize, and as a result bones gradually deform. The hypertrophic cell layer of the growth plate (Fig. 7.14) also fails to calcify, and primary trabeculae are not formed because they require calcified cartilage as scaffolding. Since the proliferative layer of the growth plate continues to grow, the cartilaginous growth plate gets wider (i.e. it gains in height). These disturbances at the growth plate lead to reduced longitudinal growth. Bone mass is usually normal because there is no hypocalcaemia to cause HPT and bone loss (as is the case in calcium deficiency rickets). However, bone mineral density is low because of the mineralization failure. The condition is treated with oral phosphate supplements with the aim of raising serum phosphorus levels. A side effect of high oral phosphate intake is a drop in serum calcium levels and the development of secondary HPT. To counteract this effect, vitamin D is added to oral phosphate with the aim of increasing intestinal absorption of both calcium and phosphorus.

Vitamin D resistant rickets

Vitamin D resistant rickets is due to an inborn end-organ resistance to 1,25-dihydroxyvitamin D. This type of rickets can be improved only with high doses of 1,25-dihydroxyvitamin D, in an attempt at overcoming the block.

Vitamin D dependent rickets

Vitamin D dependent rickets is due to an inborn deficiency of renal 1-alphahydroxylase so that 25-hydroxyvitamin D cannot be converted to the active metabolite 1,25-dihydroxyvitamin D. As a result, intestinal calcium and phosphorus absorption are impaired, serum calcium and phosphorus levels are low and bone cannot mineralize normally. In this instance measurement of 1,25-dihydroxyvitamin D is the test of choice to establish vitamin D status, and not 25-hydroxyvitamin D. This condition is treatable with physiological doses of 1,25-dihydroxyvitamin D.

Tumour-induced rickets and osteomalacia

Tumour-induced rickets and osteomalacia is a rare, acquired condition and may present at any age. It is caused by a small and usually benign mesenchymal tumour that produces a phosphate transport inhibitor (a peptide). This inhibitor prevents renal tubular reabsorption of phosphate from the glomerular filtrate, and also inhibits intestinal phosphorus absorption of phosphate. Thus, phosphorus is lost in the urine and not replaced by intestinal absorption. The resulting osteomalacia and rickets are usually severe, but can be cured by surgical removal of the secreting tumour, if its location can be identified. Failing this, medical therapy with large doses of phosphorus and vitamin D may improve the mineralization defect.

Metabolic bone disease in chronic gastrointestinal, hepatobiliary and pancreatic disorders

These disorders are caused by impaired absorption of calcium and vitamin D, or by failure of hepatic hydroxylation of vitamin D (in the case of liver disease). Other deficiencies, e.g. of protein, also contribute. Gastrectomy, gastric stapling and intestinal bypass for obesity, extensive small bowel resection (aetiology of osteomalacia shown in Fig. 7.26), gluten enteropathy (synonyms: gluten sensitivity, coeliac disease, sprue), inflammatory bowel disease (e.g. Crohn's disease), cystic fibrosis, liver cirrhosis, and obstructive biliary disorders have been documented to be associated with metabolic bone disease. Indeed, the first presenting feature of gluten enteropathy may be osteoporosis or osteomalacia. The bone diseases in gastrointestinal (GI) disorders fall into three categories: *osteoporosis, secondary hyperparathyroidism* and *osteomalacia,* in this order of frequency. Combinations of these disorders also occur. Treatment of the underlying GI disorder with corticosteroid or immunosuppressive agents aggravates the bone disease, as do alcohol abuse, hypogonadism and smoking. Treatment of the bone disease consists of provision of adequate amounts of calcium and vitamin D.

Renal osteodystrophy (ROD)

The kidneys play a key role in the control of mineral metabolism. As a result, renal failure leads to ROD. Derangements of mineral metabolism in renal failure are: (1) hyperphosphataemia as a result of impaired renal phosphorus excretion, (2) impaired 1,25-dihydroxyvitamin D production as a result of 1-alpha-hydroxylase deficiency in the failing kidneys, (3) hypocalcaemia due to hyperphosphataemia and impaired intestinal absorption (low 1,25-dihydroxyvitamin D), and (4) high levels of PTH as a result of hypocalcaemia, hyperphosphataemia, low levels of 1,25-dihydroxyvitamin D, and diminished renal degradation of PTH. These derangements give rise to ROD, which may present as one of three types of bone disease: (1) secondary hyperparathyroidism (high bone turnover), (2) adynamic bone disease (low bone turnover), or (3) osteomalacia.

Secondary hyperparathyroidism

Secondary hyperparathyroidism is characterized by extremely high levels of bone turnover as a result of extremely high concentrations of PTH (up to 40 times normal). The condition causes unexplained severe bone pain. Bone mass declines, subperiosteal erosions appear and fractures may develop. The condition can be improved medically with calcium, 1,25-dihydroxyvitamin D and phosphate binders. Parathyroidectomy may alleviate bone pain.

Adynamic bone disease

Adynamic bone disease is characterized by low bone turnover that may result from overzealous vitamin D and calcium therapy of secondary HPT.

Osteomalacia

Osteomalacia may accompany secondary HPT in 'mixed ROD' as a result of persistent hypocalcaemia. Osteomalacia as a result of aluminium toxicity is no longer seen since aluminium has been eliminated from dialysate solutions used in haemodialysis.

Clinical features of ROD

The clinical features are bone pain, muscle weakness, skeletal deformities, fractures and extraskeletal calcifications. Children develop angular (varus, valgus) and rotational deformities of upper and lower limbs, growth retardation and slipped epiphyses (separation from the metaphysis).

Treatment of ROD

Treatment of ROD aims at maintenance of normal serum calcium and phosphorus levels by administration of calcium, 1,25-dihydroxyvitamin D and phosphate binders. These measures improve the severity of the bone disease. Parathyroidectomy may become necessary to control secondary HPT. Osteotomies of lower limb deformities in children may be required. Renal transplantation heals the bone disease but has its own skeletal complications: glucocorticoid therapy necessary to counteract graft rejection causes bone loss and osteonecrosis of convex joint surfaces (e.g. femoral head, femoral condyles, humeral head) may develop. The use of non-glucocorticoid immunosuppressants has reduced the incidence of osteonecrosis.

Osteogenesis imperfecta

Osteogenesis imperfecta (OI) is a heritable (mostly autosomal dominant) disorder of type I collagen which is normally found in bone, skin, ligaments, sclerae and dentin. The skeletal effects of OI are low bone mass, recurrent fractures and bone deformities resulting from malunions of fractures (Fig. 7.27).

Pathogenesis

The abnormality of the condition is a gene defect in osteoblasts and fibroblasts which produce abnormal type I collagen that contains amino acid substitutions in the alpha-1 and/or alpha-2 chains of the triple helical domain of the collagen molecule (see 'Structure of bone'). Osteoblasts are normal or increased in numbers, but as a result of the gene defect produce too little collagen, and the collagen fibres are thin and irregularly arranged. Such bone is weak.

Clinical features

The clinical features of OI vary from a lethal form to no more than adult-onset osteoporosis. Affected individuals have normal intelligence. The classification by Sillence into clinical types 1–4 is widely used.

- *Type 1 OI* (mild form) presents with mild osteopenia, infrequent fractures, blue sclerae, normal height, adult-onset deafness in 50% of individuals and rarely dentinogenesis imperfecta. This mild form may be mistaken for

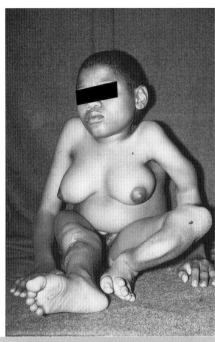

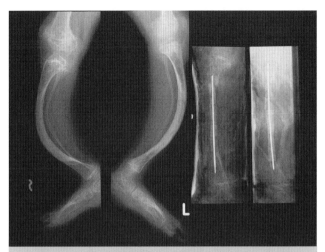

Figure 7.28.   Radiographs of lower limb deformities in osteogenesis imperfecta before and after surgical correction by intramedullary rodding.

Figure 7.27.   Clinical photograph of a young woman with gross bone deformities and short stature due to osteogenesis imperfecta, Sillence type 3. The skull shows bulging of the temporal bones. The patient is wheelchair-bound.

postmenopausal osteoporosis. Radiographic features of type I OI do not differ from those of osteoporosis.

- *Type 2 OI* (lethal form) is the most severe form that leads to perinatal death from respiratory complications. Affected neonates are small, have short, bowed limbs and numerous fractures. Respiration is impossible because of multiple rib fractures.
- *Type 3 OI* (severe from) is characterized by frequent fractures, progressive bone deformity, and short stature (Fig. 7.27), partly from fragmentation of growth plates. There may be temporal bulging of the skull, and the weight of the head may lead to basilar impression (base of the skull invaginates into the skull) that can cause brainstem compression and hydrocephalus (obstruction of cerebrospinal fluid flow from ventricles to lumbosacral region). Cases coming to clinical attention are usually type 3 OI.
- *Type 4 OI* has variable pathology that does not clearly fit into types 1 and 3.

Treatment of OI

Treatment of OI would ideally consist of molecular correction of the gene defect. However, In our current state of knowledge this is not yet possible. The use of *bisphosphonates* in children with OI leads to increase in bone density and body height, a decrease in pain and fracture rates and in

improved mobility. *Rodding* of the long bones corrects deformity and prevents fractures (Fig. 7.28). In this procedure the bony deformity is corrected by osteotomies and an intramedullary rod is inserted into the full length of the bone. The use of extensile rods that elongate with growth obviates the need for frequent rod changes. Fractures in OI heal normally.

Paget's disease of bone

Paget's disease of bone is an acquired localized disorder of bone remodelling that causes pain and deformity. It is found in 0.5–6% of Caucasian adults over the age of 50 years, but is rare in Asians and Africans.

Aetiology and pathophysiology

Paget's disease may affect one (monostotic) or more bones (polyostotic). The most commonly affected sites are the pelvis, femur, tibia, spine and skull and humerus. The aetiology of Paget's disease is thought to be an infection of osteoclast nuclei with a paramyxovirus, probably of the measles variety. Despite lack of conclusive proof of a viral aetiology, most investigators believe that a viral infection earlier in the life of a genetically predisposed individual reactivates, infects osteoclasts and re-programmes their behaviour. Affected osteoclasts proliferate, have an excessive number of nuclei and show greatly increased activity. They resorb bone haphazardly, rather than by the dictates of biomechanical or metabolic needs. Although bone resorption and bone formation remain coupled, the 'crazy' osteoclasts resorb new bone as soon as it is formed. This deranged bone remodelling results not only in disorganized microarchitecture and therefore

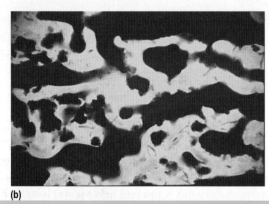

(a)

(b)

Figure 7.29.   Microradiographs of iliac crest cortical bone biopsies of normal (a) and pagetic (b) bone. Mineralized bone appears in a light colour and soft tissue in black, as in a clinical radiograph. (a) Normal cortical bone consists of numerous osteons (Haversian systems) most of which are in the resting phase (the Haversian canal is small and smooth) (see Fig. 7.11). This appearance is the result of normal bone remodelling. (b) Pagetic bone lacks ordered remodeling and therefore no Haversian systems form. Instead, numerous haphazardly placed resorption tunnels (dark spaces with irregular outline) have rendered the cortex excessively porous. Pagetic bone is weaker than normal bone.

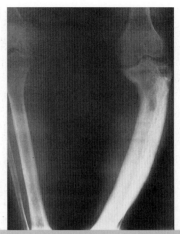

Figure 7.30.   Radiograph of a normal right tibia and a pagetic left tibia. The pagetic bone is bowed, enlarged, and sclerotic (more radiodense, i.e. a lighter colour; scleros = hard). Other features typical of Paget's disease are the thickened cortex, and coarse trabeculae.

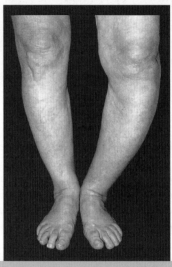

Figure 7.31.   Clinical photograph of both legs of the same patient with Paget's disease of the left tibia as in Figure 7.30. Bowing of the left tibia led to varus deformity of the leg. The skin over the left tibia felt unusually warm because of hypervascularity of underlying pagetic bone.

weak bone (Fig. 7.29a, b) but also in a change in bone size, density and shape (bowing) (Fig. 7.30). The affected bone seems to have lost its memory of its own shape and size. Pagetic bone is hypervascular so that the skin over subcutaneous bones feels unusually warm, and extensive pagetic involvement of the skeleton may be complicated by high output cardiac failure.

Although pagetic lesions tend to spread within an affected bone, Paget's disease, once established, does not spread to other bones, presumably because the sites of involvement are determined earlier in life. The extent of pagetic involvement of any patient's skeleton can be readily assessed by a total body radionuclide (^{99}Tc-MDP) bone scan (see 'The regional acceleratory phenomenon' under 'Bone remodelling'). The disease process goes through a lytic, i.e. predominantly resorptive phase in the initial years, and later on changes to a sclerotic, i.e. predominantly formative phase.

Clinical features

Clinical features include pain, deformity, neurological deficit, fractures and rarely malignant change. Most pagetic lesions are painful. *Pain* may be caused by secondary osteoarthritis due to subchondral pagetic bone, by short transverse stress fractures on the convex side of a bowed femur, or by a rapidly advancing pagetic lesion. Bowing *deformity* is most noticeable in the femur and tibia (Fig. 7.31). Enlarging pagetic bone

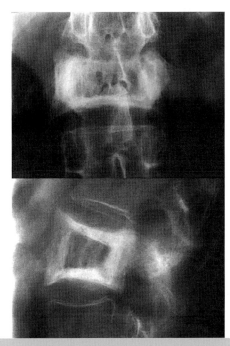

Figure 7.32. Radiographs (anteroposterior and lateral views) of a pagetic vertebra. Paget's disease has led to enlargement of the vertebral body, thickening and sclerosis of the cortex ('picture frame' vertebra), and a coarse trabecular pattern. A spinal cord neurological deficit may be caused by bony expansion, but more likely results from a vascular 'steal syndrome' (diversion of local blood flow from the spinal cord to hypervascular pagetic bone).

in spine (Fig. 7.32) and skull may cause compression of neural structures and result in a *neurological deficit* such as hearing loss or spinal stenosis (narrowing of the spinal canal). Neurological deficits reminiscent of cord compression may be caused the vascular 'steal syndrome', whereby hypervascular pagetic bone of a vertebra 'steals' blood from the neighbouring spinal cord. *Fractures* of pagetic bone tend to occur in long bones at sites of maximum stress, e.g. in the subtrochanteric region of the femur. The fractures are usually transverse and require open reduction and internal fixation. Regular intramedullary rods may be impossible to introduce into deformed bone so that plates and screws have to be used. This is a less than ideal choice for this highly stressed skeletal site because the last screw hole is a stress raiser predisposing to a new fracture. Fracture healing of pagetic bone tends to be slower than normal. Rarely, pagetic bone may undergo *neoplastic* change (osteosarcoma, chondrosarcoma or fibrosarcoma).

Treatment of Paget's disease

Treatment of Paget's disease aims to suppress osteoclastic activity by the use of antiresorptives (bisphosphonates, calcitonin). Treatment response is monitored by decline in bone turnover markers (usually total alkaline phosphatase). Following a 6-month course of bisphosphonate therapy, remission may last up to 1 year. When turnover markers rise again, treatment is repeated. In our current state of knowledge no cure is available. Neurological deficits may recover more rapidly than could be explained by relief of bony compression. The rapid response is attributed to reversal of the steal syndrome as vascularity decreases. Pain, too, diminishes with reduction in vascularity. In preparation for a surgical procedure on pagetic bone, patients should receive antiresorptive therapy (preferably for some weeks) in order to reduce the vascularity of bone and prevent disastrous blood loss at surgery. Surgical procedures necessary may be open reduction and internal fixation of a fracture, joint replacement, or a corrective osteotomy to straighten a deformed bone.

Fibrous dysplasia

Fibrous dysplasia is a rare, sporadic developmental, i.e. not heritable, disorder. Monostotic (one bone affected) or polyostotic (more than one bone affected) expanding fibrous lesions of bone give rise to deformity, pain and fractures. The condition is referred to as McCune–Albright syndrome if it is associated with patches of hyperpigmented skin (café-au-lait spots) and hyperfunction of one or more endocrine glands (usually premature ovarian activity and precocious puberty). Widespread skeletal involvement may be associated with renal phosphate wasting that causes rickets and osteomalacia. It is thought that the abnormal skeletal tissue produces a phosphaturic factor (increases loss of phosphate in urine).

Diagnosis

The diagnosis can be made by radiological examination. The affected part of a bone appears ballooned with a thin cortex, and has a ground-glass texture on radiographs. The skeletal distribution of the disease can be ascertained by increased uptake in affected areas on a ^{99}Tc-MDP total body bone scan (see 'Bone remodelling').

Clinical features

Clinical features include deformities and fractures of affected bones. Commonly involved sites are femur, tibia and ribs, but any bone may be affected. Facial involvement can lead to grotesque disfigurement and consequent social isolation. Whereas monostotic fibrous dysplasia tends to present in young adults and is rarely progressive, polyostotic disease manifests under the age of 10 years and tends to progress. Lesions do not spontaneously regress. If a lesion becomes painful, an impending fracture must be suspected. Nerve compression by an expanding lesion may also be a cause of pain. Fractures heal normally. Malignant degeneration is rare.

Pathogenesis of fibrous dysplasia

The pathogenesis of fibrous dysplasia lies in an activating mutation in the Gs-alpha subunit of the receptor/adenylate cyclase-coupling G protein. This gene defect is a somatic rather than germ-line mutation, i.e. it occurred at some cell division after fertilization. The abnormal gene is only found in fibrous dysplasia tissue and not in the rest of the skeleton, a condition referred to as *somatic mosaicism*. The gene mutation causes marrow stem cells to differentiate into fibroblasts rather than into osteoblasts.

Pathology

Histological examination of fibrous dysplasia lesions show masses of spindle-shaped fibroblasts, arranged in twists and swirls, instead of bone. Some cells produce small spicules of woven bone that give the lesion the radiographic ground-glass appearance. This abnormal bone is rapidly resorbed again. There is no specific *treatment* for fibrous dysplasia. Antiresorptive therapy with bisphosphonates is said to improve bone pain and radiological appearances, presumably by reducing resorption of bone spicules. Fractures are treated along conventional lines. Deformities may require corrective osteotomy. Curettage and bone grafting of lesions is frequently followed by recurrence.

Sclerosing bone disorders

Sclerosing bone disorders (scleros = hard) are a group of rare, mostly heritable disorders characterized by hard, dense and often brittle bone. The disorders may be due either to impaired resorption, or to excessive formation of bone.

Disorders due to impaired resorption (bone fragility increased)

Osteopetrosis (petra = rock) or *marble bone disease* (Albers–Schönberg disease) is characterized by impaired haematopoiesis and dense, fragile bones. The severity of the disorder varies from being incompatible with life to asymptomatic presentation and normal life expectancy. The failure of normal bone resorption is most evident at the growth plate. The primary trabeculae (woven bone with a calcified cartilage core; see 'Skeletal development') persist because they cannot be remodelled to normal lamellar bone as a result of the absence of osteoclastic resorption (resorption is the necessary first step of bone remodelling). There is also failure of removal by resorption of about 75% of the primary trabeculae (see 'Skeletal development') so that an unusually large number of primary trabeculae persist. These are responsible for the uniformly high bone density. There is neither a cortex nor a marrow cavity but only a homogeneous, chalk-like substance. The small spaces between the trabeculae are taken up by fibrous tissue instead of by blood-forming tissue. This results in life-threatening anaemia. Although high in bone density, osteopetrotic bone is brittle because it lacks normal

bone microarchitecture as a result of absent bone remodelling. Fractures heal slowly and require internal fixation. The absence of osteoclastic resorption also manifests in absent bone modelling, i.e. shaping of bone with growth (Fig. 7.13). As a result the metaphysis does not slim down when it converts to the diaphysis, and cranial nerve palsies develop as a result of failure of cranial foramina to widen by resorption. There is no effective *treatment* for osteopetrosis. Bone marrow transplantation with the aim of importing osteoclast progenitors may help some children.

Pyknodysostosis (pyknos = stocky, short) is another rare heritable sclerosing bone disorder caused by diminished rates of bone resorption and remodelling. Although cortices are thick and microarchitecture is normal, bones fracture easily (Fig. 7.33). Patients are short in stature and all affected individuals resemble one another because of characteristic facial features, namely a small face with prominent eyes, a beaked nose and a large cranium. The painter Henri Toulouse-Lautrec (1864–1901) is believed to have had pyknodysostosis. There is no medical therapy. Fractures require internal fixation.

Disorders due to excessive bone formation (bone fragility not increased)

Progressive diaphyseal dysplasia (Engelmann's disease) is transmitted as an autosomal dominant trait. It presents during childhood with progressive painful enlargement of the

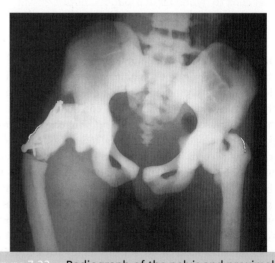

Figure 7.33.   Radiograph of the pelvis and proximal femora of a patient with a sclerosing bone disorder (pyknodysostosis). The femoral cortex is abnormally thick, and the marrow cavity extremely narrow. Internal fixation of a subtrochanteric fracture of the femur with an intramedullary rod, the method of choice, was therefore not possible. Following internal fixation with a plate and screws the femoral shaft fractured through the last screw hole. This event might have been foreseen since a screw hole is a stress raiser, especially in brittle bone as in this case.

diaphyses of tubular bones, and muscle wasting. New bone apposition takes place on the periosteal and endosteal surfaces of the cortex. Bone histology is normal. It has been suggested that Engelmann's disease may be an inflammatory connective tissue disorder in view of an elevated erythrocyte sedimentation rate in some patients, and responsiveness to glucocorticoids.

Endosteal hyperostosis (van Buchem's disease) is a rare, heritable (autosomal recessive) condition of excessive bone formation on the endocortical and trabecular bone surfaces of children and adults. Bones become dense but rarely enlarge in size. There is no specific medical treatment.

Melorheostosis (melos = limb; rheo = flow) is characterized by localized and excentric excessive bone formation on one or more bones that resembles flowing wax on a candle. It is non-heritable, and thought to be an embryonic defect. The condition presents with pain and deformity during childhood. Progression of the lesions slows in adulthood. There is no medical treatment.

Osteopoikilosis (spotted bones) and *osteopathia striata* (longitudinally striped bones) are radiologic curiosities that have no clinical significance. The radiologic appearance is caused by islands of cortical bone within trabecular bone.

Fracture healing

A fracture results from a mismatch between bone strength and load. Either the load is excessive or the bone is weak, or both. The configuration of a fracture is determined by the direction of force. As a general rule, bending forces cause transverse fractures, compression forces compression fractures, and a combination of forces, more complex patterns.

Cellular and molecular events

Fracture healing is a specialized form of wound healing that, instead of leaving a scar, restores the original tissue. Fracture repair goes through a number of phases, namely (1) haematoma formation, (2) inflammatory reaction, (3) angiogenesis (ingrowth of blood vessels), (4) differentiation of mesenchymal stem cells to chondrocytes and cartilage formation, (5) calcification of cartilage, (6) resorption of cartilage, (7) ingrowth of blood vessels into the resorption spaces, (8) differentiation of stem cells into osteoblasts, and formation of woven bone where there was cartilage, (9) remodelling of woven to lamellar bone. These steps describe fracture healing by endochondral ossification in the presence of micromovement due to non-rigid fixation. Following rigid fixation, the interim stage of cartilage formation is omitted (steps 4 to 7), and bone formation occurs directly (intramembranous ossification).

The fracture haematoma is a rich source of signalling molecules that initiate the many cascades of cellular events and control fracture healing. Platelets release important growth factors, i.e. TGF-β (transforming growth factor beta) and PDGF (platelet-derived growth factor) that are necessary for cell proliferation and differentiation. Cytokines and other molecules produced in the inflammatory reaction aid angiogenesis and chemotaxis (attraction of cells by chemical means). Both formation and composition of bone and cartilage at the fracture site are the same as at other skeletal sites (see 'Composition of bone', 'The remodelling cycle', 'Synovial joints'). The speed and adequacy of fracture repair are influenced by a number of local and systemic factors.

Local factors in fracture repair

Local factors influencing fracture repair are (1) cancellous versus cortical bone, (2) fracture configuration and number of fragments, (3) loss of the fracture haematoma, (4) soft tissue disruption and infection, (5) vascularity of bone, (6) accuracy of reduction and (7) rigidity of immobilization.

Fractures of *cortical bone* take at least twice as long to unite as those in cancellous bone because less bone surface area is available on which callus can be laid down. *Transverse fractures* take longer to unite than spiral fractures because the contact area between the fragments is smaller. The greater the *comminution* of the fracture the greater is the likelihood of avascularity of the fragments and the slower is the healing process. Loss of the *fracture haematoma* in an open fracture or through surgical intervention is detrimental to fracture healing because of the loss of important growth factors and other signalling molecules that initiate the cellular events of the healing process. *Soft tissue disruption*, especially in open fractures, slows fracture healing because of loss of the fracture haematoma, deficient soft tissue cover of bone, poor blood supply and the likelihood of infection. An *avascular fragment* of bone cannot contribute to fracture healing because it cannot provide the blood supply essential for fracture repair. Small avascular fragments can be bridged by callus, or may be remodelled (resorbed and replaced with new bone). Inaccurate *fracture reduction* leaves large gaps that have to be filled in with callus. The greater the direct contact area between the fragments, the stronger will be the fracture union.

The *rigidity of immobilization* of a fracture determines the type of tissue that will form to join the fragments. In the absence of movement, mesenchymal stem cells differentiate into osteoblasts (primary fracture union), but in the presence of micromovement they differentiate into chondrocytes (callus formation, i.e. secondary fracture union), and in the presence of excessive movement they differentiate into fibroblasts (fibrous non-union). *Rigid internal fixation*, e.g. by compression plating, ensures the largest direct contact area between fragments. At points of intimate contact, union is established by Haversian remodelling (see 'Bone remodelling'). Osteoclasts cut a longitudinally aligned resorption tunnel into both fragments, straddling the fracture site. Blood vessels enter the tunnel and import osteoblasts which form a new Haversian system that acts as a dowel, joining the two fragments. Small gaps between fragments are filled with woven bone before Haversian remodelling of the gaps can start. *Non-rigid stabilization*, on the other hand, e.g. by intramedullary nailing, external skeletal fixation or plaster cast, allows controlled micromovement that causes callus formation around the fracture. The strain generated by micromovement in the fracture gap makes mesenchymal stem cells differentiate into chondrocytes. These will become hypertrophic chondrocytes (as in the growth plate; see 'Skeletal development') that induce calcification of their cartilage matrix. Chondroclasts then resorb the calcified cartilage, and blood vessels grow into the resorption cavities and supply mesenchymal stem cells. These are now able to differentiate into osteoblasts since stability has been established by cartilaginous callus. The osteoblasts then lay down woven bone that is later remodelled to lamellar bone.

Systemic factors in fracture repair

Systemic factors with adverse effects on fracture healing are smoking, diabetes, corticosteroid therapy, and some non-steroidal anti-inflammatory drugs (NSAIDs) such as indomethacin. Although time to fracture union increases with age, osteoporotic fractures heal normally.

Treatment of fracture non-unions and bone gaps

A number of different methods are available for the treatment of non-unions and bone gaps.

1. Bone grafting with autografts, allografts, or rarely xenografts. Grafts can consist of cancellous or cortical bone, and may be non-vascularized or vascularized.
2. Osteoconductive methods make use of ceramics and bioactive glasses.
3. Osteoinductive methods use bone growth factors to produce bone in soft tissue.
4. Physical methods such as electromagnetic fields and low-intensity ultrasound aim to stimulate bone formation.

Bone grafting

A graft taken from another site and implanted in the same individual is an autogenous graft or *autograft*, one from another human being is an allogeneic graft or *allograft*, and one from another species a *xenograft* (auto = self, allo = other, xeno = foreign). A *non-vascularized bone graft* (no blood supply) first dies and has to be gradually resorbed and replaced with new bone from the host bed. The *stages of graft incorporation* of a *non-vascularized cancellous autograft* are: bone death, inflammatory reaction around the graft, ingrowth of blood vessels into graft marrow spaces, population of the trabecular surfaces by osteoblasts differentiated from host mesenchymal stem cells imported by the new blood vessels. The osteoblasts use the dead trabeculae of the graft as scaffolding

on which they lay down new bone. At other sites osteoclasts start resorbing dead graft bone in preparation for replacement with new bone.

This remodelling continues for up to 2 years, depending on the size of the graft, the vascularity of the host tissues and the mechanical forces acting on the graft. Incorporation of a *non-vascularized cortical autograft* takes longer than that of a non-vascularized cancellous autograft. Because of its solid structure the cortical graft can be vascularized only on the outside, or after osteoclasts have cut tunnels for vascular ingrowth and new bone formation. In this way the graft will be slowly replaced by live bone, although small amounts of dead bone may persist. The incorporation of cortical or cancellous *allografts* follows similar steps to those described for autografts, but the process takes substantially longer and remains incomplete. Bone banks provide a large selection of cortical and cancellous allografts in many shapes and sizes. *Xenografts* have performed disappointingly.

Osteoconductive methods

Osteoconduction is the propagation of bone formation from host bone onto an implanted three-dimensional porous non-bone structure with a suitable surface. Examples of osteoconductive materials are some ceramics, bioactive glasses and synthetic polymers. *Ceramics* are made up of hydroxyapatite and tricalcium phosphate which act as structural support and as template for bone formation. They compare favourably with autogenous bone grafts. With time they are resorbed and remodelled to host bone. *Bioactive glasses* consist of silicophosphatic chains that are implanted for structural support and can be used as carriers of bone growth factors. Synthetic polymers such as polyglycolic acid (also used as absorbable suture material) can be used as biodegradable plates and screws that can at the same time act as carriers of bone growth factors.

Osteoinductive methods

Osteoinduction is the process of heterotopic (heteros = other, topos = site) new bone formation in soft tissue. An osteoinductive substance induces proliferation and differentiation of mesenchymal stem cells derived from soft tissue into osteoblasts. Bone morphogenetic proteins (BMPs, see 'Control of the remodelling cycle') are the most powerful of the osteoinductive substances. When added to a carrier, e.g. collagen, they can be introduced into bone gaps where they will induce new bone formation that will re-establish continuity between the disconnected bone ends.

Other bone growth enhancing substances

When introduced into fracture sites these substances can enhance callus formation. Such substances are transforming growth factor-beta (TGF-β), fibroblast growth factor-2 (FGF-2) and platelet-derived growth factor (PDGF).

Physical enhancement of fracture repair

Electromagnetic fields. Two types of small physiological electrical currents are generated in bone by loading, namely (1) streaming electrical potentials, produced by pulsatile fluid flow of extracellular fluid over the osteocyte cell surface in the lacunar-canalicular system, and (2) piezoelectric currents induced by deformation of bone crystals. Osteocytes sense these electrical signals and transduce them into chemical messages that regulate bone remodelling (see 'Control of the remodelling cycle'). It was hoped that externally applied currents might stimulate bone cells in the absence of loading. A number of different currents have been examined for this purpose. Pulsed electromagnetic fields (PEMF) have reached clinical use (e.g. the Bassett coil) for the treatment of slowly healing fractures. Delayed unions treated with PEMF showed significantly increased union rates, and osteotomies united more rapidly when treated with PEMF. Nevertheless, controversy continues to surround the use of the method because of inconsistent scientific evidence in support of proposed mechanisms of action.

Low intensity ultrasound. Ultrasound (US) is mechanical energy that can be transmitted in the body as high frequency acoustic pressure waves. It has found wide application in the medical field. *Diagnostic US* devices employ low magnitudes of 1 to $50\,mW/cm^2$ in the examination of organs, fetuses, peripheral blood flow and osteoporosis. These low intensities cause neither heating of the tissues nor destruction. *Therapeutic US*, on the other hand, uses higher intensities, namely 1 to $3\,W/cm^2$ which can cause considerable heating of tissues. Much higher intensities of 5 to $300\,W/cm^2$ are used *surgically* to ablate diseased tissues, fragment calculi and to remove methylmethacrylate bone cement during arthroplasty revisions. The effect of low intensity US of $30\,mW/cm^2$ on *bone healing* has been examined in experimental fractures which were found to achieve union more rapidly, and fracture callus was stronger in US treated animals than in controls. Investigation of the possible mechanism of action revealed that US increases intracellular adenylate cyclase activity and TGF-β synthesis in osteoblasts (see 'Control of bone remodelling'), and stimulates upregulation of aggrecan (see 'Structure of joints') gene expression in chondrocyte cultures. Clinical fractures treated with US at $30\,mW/cm^2$ also showed reduced time to union, and prevented delayed union in double-blind placebo-controlled multicentre trials.

DISORDERS OF JOINTS

Structure of joints

There are three categories of joints (Fig. 7.34):

1. synovial joints
2. cartilaginous joints
   - primary cartilaginous joints
   - secondary cartilaginous joints
3. Fibrous joints.

Most of the joints in the human body are synovial joints.

Synovial joints, also referred to as diarthrodial (freely mobile) joints, have a joint space, two or more cartilage-covered bone ends, a capsule lined by a synovial membrane, synovial fluid for lubrication and ligaments and muscles to control stability and mobility. Synovial joints have a greater range of movement than cartilaginous or fibrous joints.

Primary cartilaginous joints are the costo-chondral junctions of the ribs. The bone ends are joined by hyaline cartilage. Such joints are quite immobile.

Secondary cartilaginous joints are the intervertebral discs, the sternomanubrial joint and the symphysis pubis. The bone ends are covered with hyaline cartilage, and dense fibrous tissue joins these cartilage covers. There is no joint space. These joints have a limited range of movement.

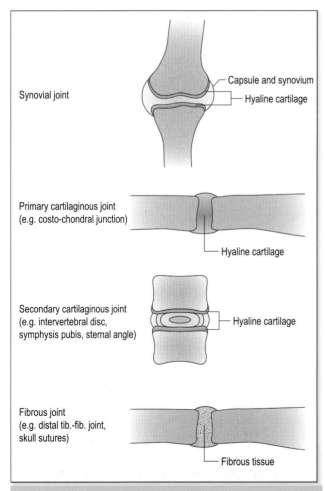

Figure 7.34. Categories of joints.

Fibrous joints are the distal tibio-fibular joints and the skull sutures. The bone ends are simply joined by fibrous tissue, and movement is minimal. Synovial joints warrant more detailed description because a large number of pathological conditions may affect these joints.

Synovial joints
Articular cartilage
Articular cartilage is hyaline cartilage and has two functions: it acts as gliding surface and as shock absorber. It is made up of extracellular matrix and a sparse number of chondrocytes. The extracellular matrix consists of water (65–80%), collagen fibres and proteoglycans. Articular cartilage can be divided into four zones that differ in collagen fibre arrangement: the superficial tangential zone, the intermediate zone, the deep zone and the zone of calcified cartilage next to subchondral bone (Fig. 7.35). The water content is highest in the superficial zone, whereas the proteoglycan content is highest in the deep zone. Chondrocytes are dispersed throughout the four zones.

Chondrocytes are secretory cells that produce the extracellular matrix consisting of proteoglycans, collagen and other proteins. Chondrocytes also control cartilage maintenance, i.e. degradation and repair of the extracellular matrix. To this end, they secrete degrading enzymes (the metalloproteinases collagenase, gelatinase, cathepsin), their inhibitors, and growth factors for repair (TGF-β, IGF-1, FGF, PDGF and others). In arthritis, chondrocytes also contribute to the production of pro-inflammatory cytokines that promote cartilage degradation, namely interleukin-1 beta (IL-1β), tumour necrosis factor-alpha (TNF-α), and others. The chondrocyte is therefore a surprisingly versatile cell. In normal cartilage a chondrocyte lasts a lifetime.

Extracellular matrix has two major components that are structurally intricately interwoven, namely collagen fibres and proteoglycans (Fig. 7.36). Cartilaginous *collagen* is predominantly type II collagen, which resembles type I collagen of bone except that it does not support mineral deposition (see 'Composition of bone'). The collagen fibres of the superficial tangential zone of articular cartilage run parallel to the joint surface, those in the intermediate zone arch downwards towards the deep zone and those in the deep zone are arranged vertically (Fig. 7.35). The spaces between collagen fibres are distended by proteoglycans and water. This arrangement holds the collagen fibres taut and prevents them from fracturing. *Proteoglycans* are macromolecules (Fig. 7.37) that are responsible for the shock-absorbing quality of articular cartilage. They consist of a protein core which carries about 150 side chains of glycosaminoglycans (100 long side chains of chondroitin sulphate, and 50 shorter side chains of keratan sulphate) like the bristles on a brush. The protein core with its 150 side chains is also referred to as aggrecan because many molecules are aggregated. About 300 aggrecans are assembled along a very long hyaluronate chain (an unsulphated

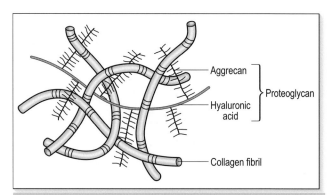

Figure 7.36.   Schematic representation of molecular architecture of articular cartilage. Collagen and proteoglycans are intricately interwoven for stability.

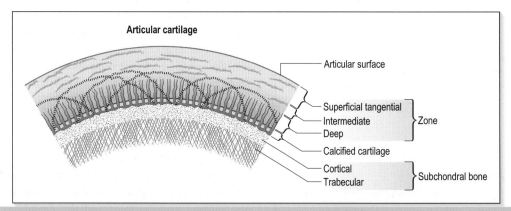

Figure 7.35.   Schematic representation of zones of collagen fibre arrangement in articular cartilage. In the superficial tangential zone collagen fibres run parallel to the joint surface, in the intermediate zone fibres arch downwards towards the deep zone and in the deep zone fibres are arranged perpendicular to subchondral bone.

proteoglycan) to form a truly huge proteoglycan macromolecular complex. Proteoglycans trap water by two mechanisms: (1) chondroitin and keratan sulphate side chains carry negative charges (COO^- and SO_3^-) that create a strong mutually repulsive force between the molecules and open up the space between them for water to distend this 'molecular sponge'; (2) the negative charges attract the counter-ions sodium (Na^+) and calcium (Ca^{2+}) that increase the osmotic pressure, and likewise attract water. These two phenomena are so effective that they put the trapped water under about five times the pressure of a motor vehicle tyre. This explains the shock-absorbing quality of articular cartilage. As the chondroitin and keratan sulphate side chains get shorter with age and in osteoarthritis, the repulsive negative charges decline, the water content and tissue turgor decrease, collagen fibres become distorted and fracture. These changes soften cartilage and may lead to its break-up.

Synovial membrane

Paracelsus (early sixteenth century) described joint fluid as 'synovia' (like egg) because it is slippery like egg white. The synovial membrane lines the entire interior of the joint, except cartilage and menisci. It consists of two layers, the

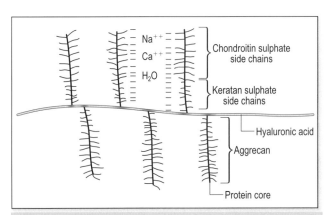

Figure 7.37. Schematic representation of a cartilage proteoglycan macromolecular complex. About 100 chondroitin sulphate and 50 keratan sulphate side chains are mounted on a protein core like the bristles on a brush. The protein core with its 150 side chains is called an aggrecan. Up to 300 aggrecans are assembled along a hyaluronic acid molecule, thus forming a huge proteoglycan macromolecular complex, also referred to as proteoglycan aggregate. The chondroitin sulphate and keratan sulphate side chains carry negative electrical charges that attract positively charged counter ions, namely Na^+ and Ca^{2+}. These create a high osmotic pressure that attracts water into the molecule. Furthermore, the mutually repulsive force of the negative charges helps to open up the intermolecular space, to be distended with water. The water content of articular cartilage determines its tissue turgor and its ability to absorb shocks.

synovial lining cell layer and the sublining. The lining cell layer, 1–3 cells deep, contains macrophages (so-called type A cells) and secretory fibroblast-like cells (so-called type B-cells); the latter produce synovial fluid. The sublining consists of fibrous tissue, capillaries, arterioles, venules and lymphatics. Synovial lining cells lack a basement membrane. This permits a rapid exchange of plasma dialysate, nutrients and waste products and the migration of leucocytes from blood vessels into the joint cavity. These features also facilitate the development of arthritis.

Lubrication of joints

The lubrication of synovial joints by *synovial fluid* ensures low friction gliding between articular surfaces and reduces articular cartilage wear during motion. Synovial fluid is produced by the synovial membrane as a plasma dialysate. Synovial cells also secrete hyaluronate, a large glycosaminoglycan, as lubricating agent. The amount of synovial fluid in a normal joint is small, amounting to no more than 1–5 ml, even in large joints. A synovial fluid film covers the whole of the joint interior, namely cartilage, synovial membrane and menisci at all times. As joint motion commences, movement takes place within this fluid film by so-called *fluid film lubrication*, and the articular cartilage surfaces do not come into direct contact (Fig. 7.38, top). As the load increases, the fluid film is slowly squeezed out from between the loaded regions of the cartilage surfaces. This is, though, not the end of lubrication. A boundary of a thin layer of glycoprotein molecules called lubricin remains adsorbed onto articular cartilage surfaces like the pile of a carpet (Fig. 7.38, bottom). This boundary layer provides cushioning, low friction gliding and protection against abrasions. It remains in place to provide so-called *boundary lubrication*, and the cartilage surfaces do still not come into direct contact, even under high load. When load decreases, the fluid film returns to the joint space and fluid film lubrication resumes. Both, fluid-film and boundary lubrication usually are present side by side (mixed lubrication) in the same joint, depending on the congruity of the joint surfaces: prominent regions move by boundary lubrication and receding areas by fluid lubrication. Moreover, joint surfaces themselves may slightly alter their shape temporarily during loading. Under load the collagen–proteoglycan network undergoes elastic deformation, and a small amount of water is displaced, but returns on unloading. The viscosity, and therefore the lubricating quality of synovial fluid, is reduced in inflammatory arthritis.

Joint capsule and ligaments

The *joint capsule* is like a cuff around the joint. It consists of interlacing bundles of white connective tissue fibres, strengthened in places by ligaments. In the embryo, the joint capsule is attached to the growth plate. With growth the attachment may move onto the epiphysis or the metaphysis. With migration onto the metaphysis, part or the whole of the

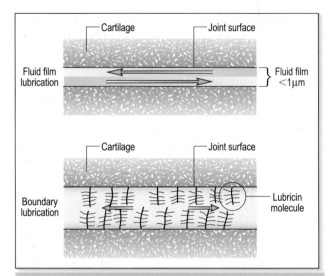

Figure 7.38.   Schematic representation of joint lubrication by fluid film lubrication and boundary lubrication. Fluid film lubrication (top): joint movement takes place within the fluid film of the synovial fluid (arrows). The articular surfaces do not come into direct contact. With increased loading the fluid film is squeezed out from between the articular surfaces so that fluid film lubrication is no longer possible and boundary lubrication (bottom) takes over. A boundary of a thin layer of glycoprotein molecules (lubricin) remains attached to cartilage to coat each articular surface. Joint movement now takes place between the two lubricin layers (arrows) and cartilage surfaces still do not come into direct contact. When the load is reduced, the fluid film and fluid film lubrication return.

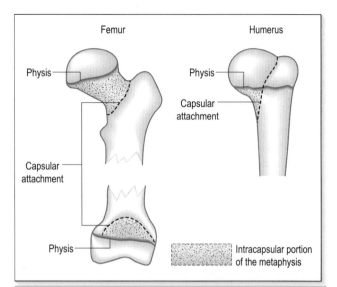

Figure 7.39.   Diagram to show the attachment of joint capsules to the proximal and distal femur, and proximal humerus in children. The metaphysis of the proximal femur is entirely intracapsular, and those of the distal femur and proximal humerus are partially intracapsular. Acute osteomyelitis in children arises in the metaphysis and pus may track to the surface. In the case of an intracapsular metaphysis this leads to septic arthritis.

metaphysis becomes an intracapsular structure (e.g. at the proximal and distal ends of femur, and the proximal humerus, Fig. 7.39). The significance of this migration lies in the pathogenesis of septic arthritis complicating acute haematogenous osteomyelitis in children. Acute osteomyelitis starts in the metaphysis. When pus from the metaphyseal marrow cavity breaks through the cortex at an intracapsular site, septic arthritis and joint destruction ensue.

Ligaments (ligare = to bind) are tough, glistening white bands of connective tissue that connect the bones across a joint. They are flexible, allowing normal joint movement, but they do not stretch, and so provide joint stability. The nerve supply of joints and ligaments is by the nerve supply of the muscles acting on the joint.

Menisci

Menisci are found in a number of joints, e.g. knee, sternoclavicular and temporomandibular joints. They are peripherally attached mobile rings or discs of fibrocartilage that are interposed between the joint surfaces like washers. Menisci serve as shock absorbers, increase the contact area between incongruous joint surfaces and improve lubrication and proprioception. Of greatest clinical significance are the menisci of the knee because they tear when trapped between femur and tibia during loading, despite their mobility. The medial meniscus is particularly vulnerable because it is restrained at its attachment to the medial collateral ligament and may fail to move out of the way. Meniscal fibrocartilage consists of type I and type II collagen and proteoglycan aggregates (see 'Articular cartilage'). The collagen fibres are predominantly circumferentially aligned. This explains why traumatic bucket handle tears and degenerative in-substance horizontal cleavage tears in the elderly occur in a circumferential direction. The meniscal blood supply is confined to the peripheral 10–25% of meniscal width. For this reason, peripheral tears or detachments of menisci will heal when repaired, but tears in the inner, non-vascularized portion cannot heal because healing requires a blood supply.

Bursae, fat pads, plicae

Bursae are sac-like cavities that facilitate gliding between tissue planes in the vicinity of joints. The outer surface of a bursa is attached to the two gliding structures, e.g. to the deep surface of the fascia lata and the greater trochanter. The movement between fascia lata and greater trochanter now takes place within the bursa, and not between fascia lata and greater trochanter (Fig. 7.40). There are about 20 bursae around the knee joint alone. Some bursae communicate with the joint cavity and may therefore become distended with

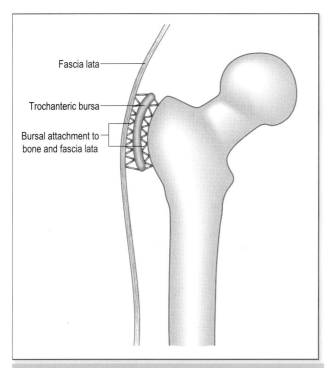

Figure 7.40.   Diagram to show attachments of the trochanteric bursa. The external surfaces of the bursal sac are attached to the greater trochanter and to the undersurface of the fascia lata. Movement between fascia lata and greater trochanter takes place within the bursa.

synovial fluid when there is a synovial effusion in arthritis. Bursae are lined by a synovium-like membrane that secretes a small amount of lubricating fluid. Overuse may cause friction within a bursa and result in inflammation, a condition referred to as bursitis. *Fat pads* are space fillers within joints where the articulating parts are not in direct contact. They are covered in synovium and thus aid in joint lubrication. *Plicae* are synovial folds extending into the joint cavity. They are thought to result from incomplete tissue resorption during embryonic joint cavity formation. If thickened, they may cause symptoms.

Osteoarthritis

Osteoarthritis (OA) causes pain, stiffness and deformity. It is the commonest cause of pain after age 50 years. Degenerative joint disease and osteoarthrosis are synonyms for osteoarthritis. The term osteoarthritis emphasizes the inflammatory component of the disorder, and osteoarthrosis the degenerative aspect. OA is characterized by deterioration of articular cartilage, formation of new bone at joint surfaces (subchondral sclerosis and osteophytes), cyst formation and capsular fibrosis. Although the prevalence of OA increases with age, ageing by itself does not cause OA. OA is not a single entity, but rather the final common end-stage of a cluster of different disorders. OA is considered to be 'primary' or idiopathic when no cause can be identified, and 'secondary' when a known cause exists, such as trauma, joint instability, congenital dislocation of the hip, infection, osteonecrosis, Paget's disease, multiple epiphyseal dysplasia, previous Perthes' disease, previous slipped upper femoral epiphysis (SUFE), bleeding disorders, 'burnt out' rheumatoid arthritis, crystal deposition disease, hypermobility of joints and neuropathic disorders as seen in diabetics. The features of primary OA may be indistinguishable from secondary OA.

Pathogenesis and pathology of OA

Pathogenetic factors can be grouped into (1) faulty cartilage (e.g. in crystal deposition disease), (2) faulty subchondral bone (e.g. in Paget's disease), and (3) faulty loading (e.g. irregular joint surfaces after intra-articular fractures). The disease process consists of cartilage degradation, new bone formation and chronic synovitis.

Cartilage degradation and synovitis

Destruction and repair of articular cartilage normally go on side by side, controlled by cytokines (destruction) and growth factors (repair). Whereas in healthy cartilage, destruction and repair are well balanced, in OA destruction predominates. What tips this balance in primary OA remains uncertain. There is some evidence of an autoimmune response to circulating articular cartilage molecules, but it is not clear whether this is the cause or the result of OA. The evolution of cartilage degradation in OA can be divided into three stages: stage I, proteolytic degradation of cartilage matrix; stage II, fibrillation of the cartilage surface; stage III, chronic synovitis in resonse to cartilage breakdown products in the synovial cavity.

Stage I.   The production by synovial cells of *metalloproteinases* (collagenase, stromelysin, gelatinase) is increased and *cartilage matrix destruction* commences. Chondrocytes also show enhanced expression of metalloproteinases, cathepsins, aggrecanase and other degradative enzymes as a result of increased sensitivity of their receptors to cytokines (IL-1, TNF-α) (Fig. 7.41). Aggrecans (see 'Articular cartilage') are the first cartilage matrix component to be broken up. This is done by aggrecanase, stromelysin, plasmin and other enzymes. As chondroitin sulphate and keratan sulphate chains become shorter, the negative repulsive electrical charges diminish and the osmotic pressure drops. This results in reduced water content, lower tissue turgor and softening of cartilage. Next, collagen fibres are cleaved by collagenase, gelatinase and other enzymes. These changes loosen the tightly woven network of the cartilage matrix so that it becomes increasingly softer and allows easy deformation. This leads to fracture of collagen fibres, and the cartilage surface begins to split.

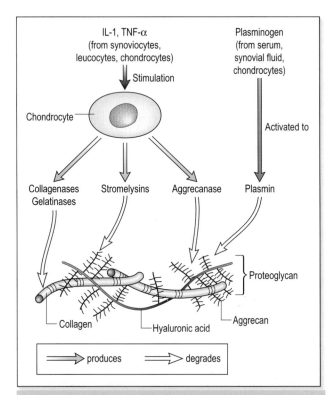

Figure 7.41. Schematic representation of the main degradative enzymes involved in cartilage destruction in OA. Proteoglycans are degraded by aggrecanase, stromelysins and plasmin. Collagen is broken up by collagenase and gelatinase. The activators and inhibitors that fine-tune the activities of these enzymes are not shown.

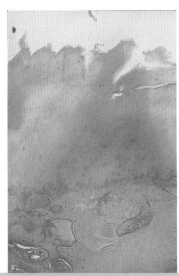

Figure 7.42. Photomicrograph of a histological section of articular cartilage (upper two-thirds of image) and subchondral bone (lower one-third) from an osteoarthritic femoral head. The cartilage surface shows fibrillation and early vertical clefts extending deeper into the cartilage substance. Haematoxylin and eosin stain.

Stage II. The initial small surface splits run parallel to the surface, between the superficial collagen fibres. This change is referred to as *fibrillation* (Fig. 7.42). As cartilage degradation progresses, fibrillations propagate along the deeper vertical collagen fibres and become deep vertical fissures that may reach all the way to subchondral bone. Chondrocytes initially increase their output of new matrix to repair the damage, but their capacity is soon overwhelmed by rapid destruction, and they eventually succumb by apoptosis (programmed cell death). Areas of now acellular cartilage disintegrate even more rapidly, leading to full thickness cartilage loss (cartilage ulcer).

Stage III. Synovial phagocytes engulf particles from cartilage breakdown, rupture and release degradative enzymes that elicit a *chronic synovitis.* Synovitis is associated with increased production of destructive cytokines, further cartilage degradation and more synovitis, thus establishing a vicious cycle of destruction. Keratan sulphate particles escape into the bloodstream where they can be measured as indicators of ongoing cartilage destruction. Synovitis leads to thickening and fibrosis of the capsule that contribute to joint deformity. Cartilage breakdown with accompanying synovitis

initially progresses in bouts. This explains the fluctuating severity of symptoms of OA.

Periarticular bone

New bone formation in the form of subchondral sclerosis (scleros = hard) and marginal osteophytes (osteon = bone, phyton = growth) is a cardinal feature of OA (Fig. 7.43a, b). The stimulus for new bone formation is variously thought to be mechanical or chemical. *Subchondral sclerosis* develops as articular cartilage is destroyed and its shock-absorbing quality is lost. The impact of *loading* is therefore transmitted directly to bone where it stimulates bone formation. This would explain the thickening of trabeculae and the increase in bone density beneath the joint surface at points of maximal joint loading. Because of its increased stiffness such sclerotic bone does not absorb load well so that what little cartilage is left is subjected to still greater impact loading and destruction. *Chemical substances,* such as growth factors produced by osteoarthritic cartilage and synovium, are also implicated as stimulators of subchondral bone formation and marginal osteophyte growth. There is histomorphometric and molecular evidence that bone remodelling (see 'Bone remodelling') in osteoarthritic individuals is unbalanced in favour of formation, and that this may be a systemic rather than a purely local phenomenon. Indeed, bone of patients with OA contains larger amounts of the growth factors IGF-1 and IGF-2, and TGF-β than bone of non-arthritic controls, even at sites other than joints. This would explain why

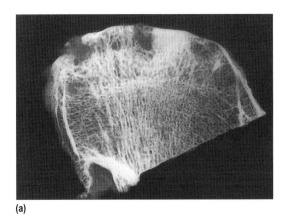

(a)

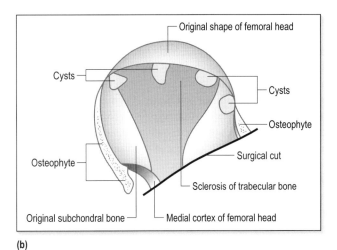

- Original shape of femoral head

Cysts

Cysts

Osteophyte

Surgical cut

Osteophyte

Sclerosis of trabecular bone

Original subchondral bone

Medial cortex of femoral head

(b)

F6/79

(c)

Figure 7.43.   Radiograph (a) with explanatory diagram (b) of a coronal slab (c) of a femoral head removed at total hip arthroplasty for osteoarthritis. The radiograph shows three of the four radiographic features of osteoarthritis, namely subchondral sclerosis, osteophytes and subchondral cysts. The earliest radiological change, i.e. narrowing of the joint space, is obviously not seen because the acetabulum is not shown. The femoral head is flattened superiorly where subchondral bone has been worn away following cartilage destruction. The increased radiodensity (light grey) in subchondral bone is due to increased bone sclerosis (new bone formation) under the weight-bearing surface. Cysts have developed in subchondral bone. Osteophytes have begun to form on the medial and lateral aspects of the femoral head. (Parts (a) and (c) by courtesy of Professor L. Solomon, University of Bristol, UK.)

patients with OA, especially those with hypertrophic OA (abundant osteophyte formation), tend to have good bone density and are less likely to develop osteoporosis than normal controls. Controversy persists as to whether OA is initiated by stiff subchondral bone that leads to mechanical cartilage damage, or whether cartilage degradation is the initiating factor that leads to stiff subchondral bone. It is assumed that both processes go on side by side.

When full thickness cartilage loss is established, sclerotic subchondral bone is exposed. Its surface appears polished and resembles ivory, hence the term 'eburnation' (ebur = ivory) for this appearance. Here and there, pinhead-size crops of

fibrocartilage appear on this surface, representing a futile attempt at cartilage repair.

Subchondral cysts, filled with fibrous or gelatinous material, form in the depth of subchondral bone, or just beneath the joint surface. These cysts may have a connection to the joint surface. It remains unclear how these cysts form. Once bared of cartilage, the eburnated joint surface gradually wears away, and bony deformity results (Fig. 7.43a–c). In this process cysts are broken into, and rapid collapse of the joint surface may occur, e.g. destruction of half or more of the femoral head.

Different changes take place at the periphery of the joint surfaces where osteophytes form. What causes marginal *osteophyte formation* (Fig. 7.43a–c) remains unclear. Growth factors and cytokines from surrounding arthritic tissues are thought to contribute. Osteophytes grow by endochondral ossification. First, hyaline cartilage thickens at the joint margins. When this new cartilage is about 2 mm thick, blood vessels penetrate its substance and bone is formed from within out. The cartilage cover continues to grow, to be followed by further ossification. Osteophytes may stabilize a disintegrating joint, but they limit the range of motion.

Abnormal loading

Joint incongruity as for example in acetabular dysplasia and congenital deformity of the hip, or from intra-articular fractures, leads to point loading that concentrates abnormally high forces over a small joint surface area. Such high load initiates cartilage damage and OA.

Clinical features of OA

The predominant features of OA are pain, stiffness and deformity. *Primary OA* comprises a cluster of diseases with different presentations and genetic backgrounds. *Large joint OA* most commonly affects hips and knees. It may present as hypertrophic OA with marked subchondral sclerosis and osteophyte formation, or as atrophic OA with scant new bone formation. In atrophic OA, joint destruction may progress rapidly as bone is eroded and collapses. In hypertrophic OA, on the other hand, progression is much slower because new bone formation stabilizes the joint. *Generalized OA* (GOA) predominantly affects the small joints of the hand, namely distal (DIP) and proximal interphalangeal (PIP) joints, and the first carpometacarpal joints (1st CMC) in postmenopausal women (Fig. 7.44). The condition is inherited as an autosomal dominant trait. Mutations of the collagen 2A1 gene are thought to be responsible. Large joints may be affected as well. GOA has both erosive and hypertrophic features. It manifests as painful inflammatory swelling of the DIP and/or PIP joints, lasting several months. After this acute phase, inflammation and pain abate, but unsightly knobbly swellings (osteophytes) remain. These swellings are referred to as Heberden's (DIP joints) and Bouchard's nodes (PIP joints), hence the term 'nodal OA'. Subcutaneous mucus cysts may appear over the joints. These cysts are herniations of synovium, contain synovial fluid and communicate with the joint cavity. Mucus cysts should be excised to prevent rupture and subsequent septic arthritis, should the overlying skin break down. OA of the first CMC joint runs a more protracted course of pain, stiffness, instability and eventually subluxation or dislocation. This leads to first web space contracture.

DIP swelling in a male should arouse suspicion of gout. The distribution of affected joints in GOA differs from that in rheumatoid arthritis (RA) and may aid in the differential diagnosis. Whereas in GOA, DIP and PIP joints are involved, in RA, PIP joints and metacarpophalangeal (MCP) joints are

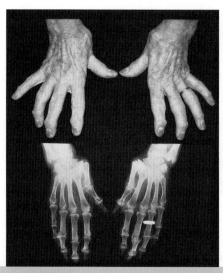

Figure 7.44.   Clinical photograph and radiograph of the hands of an elderly woman with general osteoarthritis (GOA). The clinical photograph shows Heberden's (DIP joints) and Bouchard's (PIP joints) nodes. The back of the hand appears square because of the prominence of the osteoarthritic first carpometacarpal joint and the adducted first metacarpal (first web space contracture caused by first CMC joint instability). (By courtesy of Professor L. Solomon, University of Bristol, UK.)

affected. Moreover, RA affects the wrist and elbow, whereas GOA does not. Clinical features of *secondary OA* do not differ from primary OA except that the anatomical distribution of affected joints is determined by the underlying cause.

Diagnosis of OA

The diagnosis of OA is made on clinical and radiological grounds. Routine laboratory examinations are normal. The clinical features are pain, post-inactivity stiffness, deformity and swelling (synovitis, synovial effusion, osteophytes). Radiological features are (1) narrowing of the joint space, (2) subchondral sclerosis, (3) osteophytes and (4) subchondral bone cysts (Fig. 7.49a–c). Chondrocalcinosis (calcification of cartilage) may be a manifestation of calcium pyrophosphate crystal deposition disease (CPPD), referred to as 'pseudogout' (see 'Other crystal arthropathies'). This is a rare systemic disorder that predisposes to polyarticular OA, mainly of large joints. However, up to 10% of normal elderly individuals have chondrocalcinosis but are asymptomatic and do not have OA.

Treatment of OA

Treatment of OA is mainly symptomatic. There is no medical treatment that will prevent or arrest OA because the causative agent is still unknown. Non-steroidal anti-inflammatory drugs (NSAIDs) may diminish pain and stiffness but do not affect the outcome. *Intra-articular cortocosteroid injections* may temporarily diminish inflammation, but if given too frequently, may lead to analgesic arthropathy. This means that freedom from pain encourages increased joint usage that will damage the joint further. Moreover, intra-articular steroids are absorbed and have systemic effects. *Weight reduction* may retard progression of joint destruction. *Physiotherapy* can improve the range of movement, increase muscle power and possibly prevent deformity. *Surgical treatment* may have to be resorted to, such as arthroscopic debridement, joint lavage, osteotomy to redistribute loading and replacement arthroplasty. The indications for the latter are pain and/or bone destruction.

Rheumatoid arthritis

Rheumatoid arthritis (RA) should more correctly be called 'rheumatoid disease' because it is a chronic systemic disorder. Although RA affects mainly synovial joints and tendon sheaths, multiple other tissues may be involved. The term 'rheumatoid' is derived from the Greek word 'rheo', meaning 'flow'. It is based on the old concept of the disease 'flowing' through the body. The disorder affects about 1% of the general population, is commoner in women than in men, and mostly develops between ages 40 and 50 years, but children may also be affected.

Aetiology of RA

The aetiology of RA remains 'one of the great unsolved mysteries of modern medicine' (D.A. Fox). The currently accepted view is that RA is a multifactorial disease that may develop when genetic, environmental and immune-mediated factors coincide. Individuals with certain genetic markers, e.g. HLA-DR4 (HLA, human leucocyte antigen), are at increased risk of developing RA. These markers are thought to bind to foreign antigenic agents such as viruses, or the body's own (self) type II collagen from cartilage, and then present these for processing to T-lymphocytes which direct other cells in this immune-mediated inflammatory disorder (see Ch. 2).

Pathogenesis and pathology of RA

If unchecked, joint pathology progresses through three incremental stages: stage I – synovitis, stage II – cartilage destruction and periarticular bone erosions, stage III – joint disintegration and tendon ruptures leading to deformities.

Stage I – synovitis

The synovium of joints and tendon sheaths increases in thickness by: (1) an increase in the number of layers of synovial lining cells from 2 to around 10 or more, (2) an increase in the number of blood vessels, (3) accumulation of leucocytes, (4) deposition of fibrin, (5) oedema. These inflammatory changes are mediated through the actions of cytokines, free radical donors (nitric oxide (NO) and oxygen free radicals), arachidonic acid metabolites (prostaglandins, leukotrienes), and other substances. *Cytokines* are produced by leucocytes, macrophages, synovial fibroblasts and chondrocytes. Cytokines are peptides that regulate inflammatory and immune responses. Most cytokines act in a paracrine (affecting surrounding tissues) manner, but autocrine (affecting the producing cells themselves) and endocrine (general effect via the bloodstream) actions are involved as well. More than a dozen pro-inflammatory cytokines have been identified in RA. The most destructive pro-inflammatory cytokines are tumour necrosis factor-alpha (TNF-α) and interleukin-1 beta (IL-1β). In addition to many other actions, IL-1β is thought to be responsible mainly for activation of matrix metalloproteinases that destroy cartilage (see 'Osteoarthritis'), and TNF-α for induction of adhesion molecule production. Adhesion molecules cause circulating leucocytes to stick to other cells such as the lining cells of capillaries (endothelium). This enables leucocytes to slip through the capillary wall into synovial tissue. From here they are attracted by chemokines (chemotactic cytokines) to sites of inflammatory action. Chemokines achieve this by locking onto leucocyte cell surface receptors to direct the cell. Subtypes of leucocytes respond to different chemokines.

Leucocyte types migrating from blood vessels into synovium are: macrophages (mainly producing inflammatory cytokines), T-lymphocytes (directing other inflammatory cells), B-lymphocytes and plasma cells (producing antibodies), and small numbers of polymorphonuclear cells. B-lymphocytes produce the rheumatoid arthritis factor, an autoantibody (IgG immunoglobulin) directed against the body's own IgG immunoglobulin which now becomes an antigen. The resultant antigen–antibody complexes aggravate the inflammatory reaction. The RA factor is also used as a laboratory test in the diagnosis of RA. False positive tests may be present in 5% of normal subjects, in chronic infections (tuberculosis), and in other connective tissue diseases. Plasma cells also produce autoantibodies, e.g. against type II collagen of cartilage.

Stage II – cartilage destruction and periarticular bone erosion

Cartilage destruction begins at its junction with the synovium. Here the inflammatory process gives rise to a large number of aggressive synovial fibroblasts that grow like a tongue (Fig. 7.45) onto the cartilage surface which they invade and destroy by means of proteolytic enzymes. This invading tumour-like tissue is referred to as 'pannus' (=rag). The bone underlying the cartilage–synovial junction is also eroded. These small marginal bone erosions in RA joints have a rat-eaten appearance on radiographs.

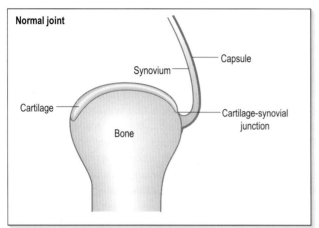

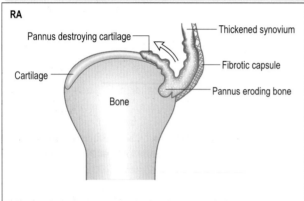

Figure 7.45.   Diagram to show cartilage–synovial junction in a normal joint (left), and in RA (right). In RA the inflamed synovium at its junction with articular cartilage gives rise to a large number of aggressive fibroblasts that invade the articular cartilage as a tongue-shaped pannus and destroy it. The same inflammatory tissue erodes subchondral bone, starting at the cartilage–synovial junction.

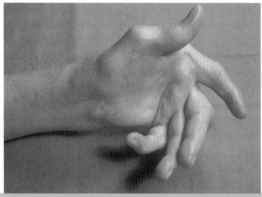

Figure 7.46.   Clinical photograph of severe hand deformities in a patient suffering from long-standing rheumatoid arthritis (RA). The metacarpophalangeal joints (MCP) are dislocated and in marked ulnar deviation. The first carpometacarpal joint is subluxated and the wrist is swollen by synovitis. (By courtesy of Dr J. Fleming, University of the Witwatersrand, Johannesburg, South Africa.)

Stage III – joint disintegration and tendon ruptures

Pannus will eventually cover and destroy the entire joint cartilage and erode the underlying bone. The capsule and ligaments contract, or are also invaded and destroyed. Tendons are invaded by pannus from their synovial sheaths and may rupture, particularly where they glide over eroded sharp bony edges. Subluxation and dislocation of joints constitutes the end-stage of joint destruction (Fig. 7.46). After a variable number of years, the inflammatory nature of the disease tends to cease, but osteoarthritis secondary to rheumatoid destruction continues.

Extra-articular manifestations of rheumatoid disease

The commonest extra-articular manifestations of rheumatoid disease are *rheumatoid nodules* in subcutaneous tissue of regions exposed to pressure and trauma. They may, however, be found in all tissues: heart, lungs, meninges, eyes, spinal cord etc. A rheumatoid nodule in the sclera can cause rupture of the eyeball and blindness. Rheumatoid nodules consist of an acellular necrotic centre, surrounded by macrophages and inflammatory tissue. *Vasculitis* is a serious complication of RA because it may block blood vessels and cause life-threatening infarctions. Blood vessels of all sizes may be affected. All layers of the vessel wall may be infiltrated by an inflammatory infiltrate consisting mainly of lymphocytes and plasma cells. Intimal (endothelium and underlying connective tissue) proliferation may lead to thrombosis. Recanalization is possible. Clinical features include digital gangrene, gastrointestinal bleeding and infarction, peripheral neuropathy and cutaneous ulcers. RA patients with vasculitis have high levels of rheumatoid factor, cryoglobulins (abnormal proteins), and decreased levels of circulating complement. Such patients also have higher levels of circulating TNF-α and IL-6 than RA patients without vasculitis. Rheumatoid disease may also cause *diffuse inflammatory changes* in muscles, myocardium, lungs and other tissues.

Bone in RA

Juxta-articular osteoporosis (juxta = next to) is an early feature of RA. It is radiographically evident even before joint destruction or marginal bone erosions appear. Juxta-articular bone loss occurs as a result of excessive bone resorption induced in a paracrine fashion by inflammatory cytokines from the neighbouring joint. Furthermore, circulating cytokines and other catabolic substances which cause cachexia also cause generalized bone loss. Juxta-articular

Table 7.8.   Criteria for the classification of rheumatoid arthritis[a]

Criterion	Definition
1. Morning stiffness	Morning stiffness in and around joints, lasting at least one hour before maximal improvement
2. Arthritis of three or more joint areas	At least three joint areas simultaneously have had soft tissue swelling or fluid (not bony overgrowth alone) observed by a physician. The 14 possible areas are right or left PIP, MCP, wrist, elbow, knee, ankle and MTP joints
3. Arthritis of hand joints	At least one area swollen (as defined above) in wrist, MCPs or PIPs
4. Symmetric arthritis	Simultaneous involvement of the same joint areas (as defined in 2) on both sides of the body (bilateral involvement of PIPs, MCPs or MTPs is acceptable without absolute symmetry)
5. Rheumatoid nodules	Subcutaneous nodules, over bony prominences, or extensor surfaces, or in juxta-articular regions, observed by a physician
6. Serum rheumatoid factor	Demonstration of abnormal amounts of serum rheumatoid factor by any method for which the result has been positive in <5% of normal control subjects
7. Radiographic changes	Radiographic changes typical of RA on PA hand and wrist radiographs, which must include erosions or unequivocal bony decalcification localized in or most marked adjacent to the involved joints (OA changes alone do not qualify)

[a] For classification purposes, a patient shall be said to have RA if he/she has satisfied at least four of these seven criteria. Criteria 1 through 4 must have been present for at least 6 weeks. Patients with two clinical diagnoses are not excluded. Designation of classic, definite, or probable RA is *not* to be made.
Adapted from Arnett FC, Edworthy SM, Bloch DA, et al. (1988) The American Rheumatism Association 1987 revised criteria for the classification of rheumatoid arthritis. Arthritis Rheum 31: 315–324. (Reprinted by permission of Wiley-Liss, Inc., a subsidiary of John Wiley & Sons, Inc.)

bone destruction is accelerated in the presence of osteoporosis. Disuse of inflamed joints further aggravates bone loss.

Diagnosis of RA

The diagnosis of RA may be based on the Criteria for the Classification of RA, as defined by the American College of Rheumatologists (Table 7.8).

Clinical features of RA

The initial presentation of RA most frequently takes the form of symmetrical chronic (more than 6 weeks) polyarthritis of the small joints of the hands (Fig. 7.46) and feet. Large joints soon also become involved. Tenosynovitis, especially on the dorsum of the wrist and of the flexor tendon sheaths of the fingers, is usually present from the outset, whereas other extra-articular features tend to present later. The anatomical distribution of affected joints differs from that of OA (Fig. 7.47). A positive RA factor test is not a necessary prerequisite for a diagnosis of RA (seronegative RA has a negative RA factor test). Symptoms and signs reflect the three stages of progression of joint pathology (see 'Pathogenesis and pathology of RA'). In stage I (synovitis) patients complain of painful swelling of joints, morning stiffness and weight loss. In stage II (cartilage and bone destruction) joint function is increasingly impaired, deformities begin to develop and muscles waste. In stage III (joint disintegration and tendon rupture) deformities are marked. The hands show ulnar deviation of the fingers at the MCP joints that

may progress to volar dislocation. Hips and elbows may develop flexion deformities, and the knees flexion/valgus deformities. At the subtalar joint, valgus deformity is common, and at the metatarsophalangeal (MTP) joints of the lesser toes, dorsal dislocation (claw toes). This latter deformity causes painful callosities under the metatarsal heads; if the skin ulcerates, the metatarsal heads are exposed in the sole of the foot and the patient walks on bare bones. When a large popliteal cyst (herniations of synovium) ruptures, the contents of the knee joint cavity (effusion, fibrin clots) spread into the calf, mimicking deep vein thrombosis. The synovial joint between the transverse ligament of the atlas and the dens of the axis (C2) is frequently affected by synovitis and erosions on the posterior surface of the dens. The posterior half and more of the dens may disappear with the result that the atlas slides forward on the axis and may compress the spinal cord. Forceful neck flexion, e.g. during anaesthesia, may prove fatal in such a case. Destruction of the temporomandibular joints may lead to an inability to open the mouth wide enough for oral intubation on induction of anaesthesia. RA progresses in repeated acute exacerbations ('flare-ups'), but after many years tends to 'burn itself out', leaving secondary OA to contend with. In about 15% of patients the disease goes into remission at an earlier stage in the disease.

Radiographs show soft tissue swelling and juxta-articular osteoporosis in stage I; to these come joint space narrowing and marginal bone erosions in stage II, and joint destruction and widespread osteoporosis in stage III.

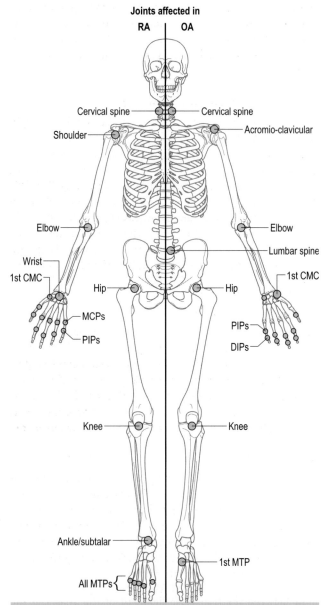

Joints affected in

RA   OA

Cervical spine — — Cervical spine

Shoulder — — Acromio-clavicular

Elbow — — Elbow

— Lumbar spine

Wrist
1st CMC — — 1st CMC

Hip — — Hip

MCPs — — PIPs

PIPs — — DIPs

Knee — — Knee

Ankle/subtalar —
— 1st MTP

All MTPs {

Figure 7.47.   Diagram of the anatomical distribution of joints affected by rheumatoid arthritis and osteoarthritis. CMC, carpometacarpal joint; MCPs, metacarpophalangeal joints; PIPs, proximal interphalangeal joints; DIPs, distal interphalangeal joints; MTPs, metatarsophalangeal joints.

Treatment of RA

Since the aetiology of RA remains unknown, no treatment of the underlying cause exists. Treatment therefore aims to (1) slow disease progression, (2) provide symptomatic relief of pain, (3) prevent deformity, (4) surgically reconstruct, and (5) rehabilitate. Disease progression may be slowed by *disease-modifying antirheumatic drugs (DMARDs)* such as immunosuppressive drugs (methotrexate, azathioprine,

cyclophosphamide, cyclosporin), chloroquine, sulphasalazine, gold, minocycline and TNF-α blockers (e.g. entanercept). *Symptomatic relief* can be provided by controlling inflammation with the use of non-steroidal anti-inflammatory drugs (NSAIDs), physiotherapy, splinting and possibly low dose corticosteroids. Analgesics are also used. Despite achieving symptomatic relief, most treatment modalities fail to arrest progression of the disease. *Deformity may be diminished* by physiotherapy, splinting, synovectomy (surgical, or by intra-articular radiocolloid injection) and stabilization (tendon transfer, arthrodesis). *Reconstructive surgery* may consist of osteotomy, excision arthroplasty, arthrodesis or replacement arthroplasty. Rehabilitation has to address physical, social and psychological aspects.

Seronegative spondyloarthropathies

This group of chronic inflammatory rheumatic disorders includes ankylosing spondylitis, reactive arthritides (e.g. Reiter's syndrome), psoriatic arthritis and the enteropathic arthropathies associated with chronic inflammatory bowel disease. Common features of these conditions are (1) negative rheumatoid factor, (2) chronic inflammation of spinal and sacroiliac joints, (3) oligoarticular (four joints or less affected; oligos = few) asymmetrical arthritis, (4) inflammation of tendon and ligament insertions (enthesis = attachment of ligament or tendon to bone; enthesopathy or enthesitis gives the bony attachment a frayed appearance on X-ray), (5) presentation under age 40 years, (6) familial clustering and (7) strong association with the major histocompatibility complex HLA-B27.

Ankylosing spondylitis

Ankylosing spondylitis (AS) (ankylos = bent; spondylos = spine) is a chronic inflammatory disorder of the spinal joints, sacroiliac (SI) joints and costovertebral joints that results in ascending ankylosis (spontaneous fusion) of the spine in a flexed position. Large peripheral joints and extraskeletal sites (heart, eyes) may also be affected. Over 90% of patients with AS have the major histocompatibility marker HLA-B27 (8–14% of the general population are HLA-B27 positive).

Pathology and radiographic appearance of AS

The inflammatory changes commence in the SI joint and gradually ascend to involve the lumbar, dorsal and cervical spine over a period of months or years. Rarely does progress cease at a lower spinal level. The *SI joints* show both erosions and sclerosis (new bone formation), and eventually go on to bony ankylosis. In the spine several distinct changes are seen: (1) bone erosions appear on the vertebral body margins at the attachments (entheses) of the *outer layers of the annulus fibrosus*, and bone forms in these outer layers and in the

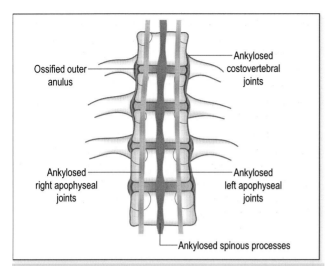

Figure 7.48.   Diagram of the radiological features of a 'bamboo spine' in ankylosing spondylitis. The prominent soft tissue ossifications around the intervertebral discs are thought to resemble the wider, and the receding waist of the vertebral bodies, the narrower sections of a bamboo rod. The three vertical lines of radiodensity resembling a rail track are ossification bars of the right and left apophyseal joints and of the spinous processes.

anterior longitudinal ligament leading to ankylosis; (2) the *apophyseal joints* are destroyed by inflammation and go on to bony ankylosis; (3) the *spinous processes* fuse by ossification of the interspinous and supraspinous ligaments. Over a period of many years the entire spine may gradually ankylose from the lumbar region upwards, including the costovertebral joints, and become a single rigid structure from sacrum to skull.

The anteroposterior *radiographic* appearance of ankylosing spondylitis is reminiscent of a bamboo stick with its alternating wider (ossified disc) and narrower (vertebral body) sections. Hence the term '*bamboo spine*'. Overlying this 'bamboo stick' are three longitudinal parallel lines, resembling a rail track (Fig. 7.48). The two outer lines are the fused apophyseal joint, and the central line the fused spinous processes. Vertebral osteoporosis is common in AS, possibly as a result of stress-shielding at ankylosed levels, and inflammatory cytokine production in nearby joints.

Some large joints (hips, knees, shoulders) may also undergo destruction but tend to ankylose only in patients with juvenile onset. Enthesopathies are also seen at non-spinal tendon and ligament insertions, e.g. that of the Achilles tendon and the plantar fascia to the calcaneum. *Non-skeletal soft tissue inflammation* can have serious consequences: iritis may lead to blurred vision, and aortic incompetence can lead to heart failure. The pathological changes of *synovitis and cartilage destruction* resemble those in RA, except that synovial thickening is less pronounced, fewer lymphocytes and plasma cells are present, and pannus does not always develop.

Bone erosions show T-lymphocytes, macrophages and high concentrations of tumour necrosis factor-alpha (TNF-α) and transforming growth factor-beta (TGF-β). The latter is probably responsible for new bone formation (sclerosis) at these sites.

Aetiology and pathogenesis of AS

Although the aetiology of AS remains unknown, it is thought that *Klebsiella pneumoniae*, a common colonizer of the gut, may constitute one factor in disease causation. Another factor is the genetic marker HLA-B27, which shares sequence homologies with some enteric bacteria, including *Klebsiella pneumoniae* (molecular mimicry). This fact could result in an increased immunological reaction against self in HLA-B27 positive individuals when they develop antibodies against enteric bacteria. The antibodies cannot distinguish between HLA-B27 and enteric bacteria. AS may be caused by such a reaction against self.

Clinical features of AS

Pain and stiffness as a result of the inflammatory process start in the low back, and over the years progressively involve higher spinal levels. The pain is worst at rest. Once the spine is ankylosed, the pain disappears. Reappearance of pain in a fused spine must arouse suspicion of a vertebral fracture. Chest expansion diminishes as the costovertebral joints ankylose. Iritis and valvular heart lesions must be looked for.

Treatment of AS

Treatment aims at (1) *control of inflammation and pain* by NSAIDs and analgesics, and (2) *preservation of mobility* through physical exercise, and (3) prevention of spinal flexion deformity by physical means. Sulphasalazine may be a disease-modifying agent through its antibiotic effect on intestinal bacteria, in addition to its anti-inflammatory effect.

Reiter's syndrome

Reiter's syndrome is a chronic inflammatory disease characterized by asymmetrical oligoarticular synovitis, sacroiliitis, enthesopathy and mucocutaneous lesions. The *synovitis* resembles that in RA but without pannus formation or erosions. The inflammatory infiltrate by macrophages and lymphocytes at entheses and around the *SI joints* results in small erosions of bone. The *mucocutaneous* lesions on hands and feet resemble those of psoriasis. They consist of infiltrates of lymphocytes and plasma cells, thickening of the keratin layer and epidermal vesicles filled with epithelial and inflammatory cells. Most patients also have subclinical inflammation of the *terminal ileum and colon*.

Aetiology and pathogenesis of Reiter's syndrome

In a large proportion of cases of Reiter's syndrome a triggering infectious agent, either an enteric (e.g. *Shigella, Salmonella,*

Yersinia) or urogenital organism (e.g. *Chlamydia*), can be identified. It is postulated that the disorder is brought about either by an immune reaction against the causative organism, or by the presence of non-viable antigenic microbial material (i.e. fragments of the causative organism) at sites of inflammation.

Clinical features of Reiter's syndrome

Symptoms of Reiter's disease appear up to one month after a diarrhoeal or genitourinary infection. Initially only a few, usually lower limb joints are affected by *chronic arthritis*. This may progress in an additive fashion to involve the SI joints, the spine and upper limb joints. Sites of *enthesopathy* become painful, namely the heel (attachment of the Achilles tendon and plantar fascia), fingers, toes, ischium, symphysis pubis, greater trochanter and ribs. *Mucocutaneous lesions* appear on hands and feet, in the mouth and as conjunctivitis. Radiographs may show joint space narrowing, small erosions and new bone formation (frayed appearance of bone) at sites of enthesopathy.

Treatment of Reiter's syndrome

Treatment aims at *reducing inflammation* by NSAIDs and *eradication of infection* by antimicrobials. Immune suppression with azathioprine, methotrexate or anticytokine therapy (TNF-α blocker) may have to be used in unresponsive cases. Intervention aimed at *preservation of function*, and prevention of reinfection are also needed. Many cases follow a relapsing–remitting course over years.

Psoriatic arthritis

Psoriasis is a chronic autoimmune and heritable skin disorder found in 2% of Caucasians. Up to 40% of affected individuals develop a chronic inflammatory arthritis referred to as *psoriatic arthritis* (PSA), and *enthesopathy*. In some cases the skeletal manifestations may precede the onset of skin lesions.

Pathogenesis and pathology of psoriatic arthritis

The pathogenetic basis of PSA appears to be an interplay between genetic, immunological and environmental factors. PSA is thought to be triggered by bowel or psoriatic plaque flora. It is postulated that skin keratinocytes process exogenous (bacterial or viral) or endogenous antigens and activate T-lymphocytes that then direct the inflammatory response. The exact relationship between skin, joint and bone changes remains unclear. The synovitis in PSA resembles that in RA. There are, however, greater concentrations of collagenase in synovial fluid in PSA than in RA. This feature may be responsible for the severe joint and bone destruction in some PSA patients. Moreover, there is a preponderance of CD8 lymphocytes in PSA, whereas CD4 lymphocytes predominate in RA. This reversal of the CD4/CD8 ratio is thought to underlie the different response of the two disorders to concomitant HIV

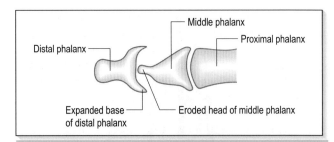

Figure 7.49.   Diagram of the radiographic appearance of the 'pencil-in-cup' deformity of DIP joint destruction in psoriatic arthritis. The head and part of the shaft of the middle phalanx have been destroyed by erosions (arthritis mutilans).

infection, namely RA improves and PSA worsens in HIV-infected individuals.

Clinical features of PSA

PSA may have a juvenile or adult onset, and may be either symmetrical and polyarticular, or asymmetrical and oligoarticular. The *polyarticular PSA* affects predominantly DIP (unlike RA) and other small joints of hands and feet. In about 5% of patients the digits may turn into grotesquely deformed, shortened appendages as a result of bone destruction (arthritis mutilans). *Oligoarticular PSA* affects scattered DIP, PIP, MCP and MTP joints, and some large joints. Joints may go on to ankylosis or destruction. The spine and SI joints may also be involved in PSA. Although PSA runs a protracted course, the outcome in most patients is less disabling than that of RA. *Radiographic features* of PSA are joint narrowing, erosions, marginal osteophytes, ankylosis of small joints, and osteolysis of the distal ends of phalanges ('pencil-in cup' deformity, Fig. 7.49).

Treatment of PSA

Medical and surgical management of PSA are the same as for rheumatoid arthritis. The skin lesions of psoriasis tend to respond favourably to 1,25-dihydroxyvitamin D which effects a downregulation of keratinocyte responsiveness to growth factors. It remains to be shown whether PSA also responds to such treatment.

Gout

Gout is caused by urate crystal formation in tissues. Uric acid and monosodium urate crystallize from supersaturated extracellular fluid. Clinical features are *gouty arthritis, tophus formation* (collections of crystal deposits) and *renal* disease (uric acid calculi and interstitial nephropathy). Phagocytosis of urate crystals by leucocytes and their subsequent rupture generates a severe inflammatory reaction.

Pathogenesis of gout

Uric acid is derived from purines in the diet (proteins) and from the body's own purine nucleotides (components of

DNA from dead cells). Purines are metabolized to xanthine which is then converted to uric acid by xanthine oxidase, and uric acid is excreted by the kidneys. Overproduction and/or underexcretion of uric acid may lead to hyperuricaemia. Over 90% of patients with hyperuricaemia or gout are *under-excreters*, either on a hereditary basis, or as a result of acidosis (e.g. alcohol abuse, diabetic ketoacidosis) or drug therapy (e.g. diuretics, low dose salicylates). *Overproduction* of uric acid may be due to high cell turnover (e.g. in malignancy), or more rarely due to an inborn enzyme defect.

Whereas in men serum uric acid levels tend to rise during adulthood, aided by overweight, alcohol excess and a diet rich in purines, in women a rise commences only after the menopause (oestrogens appear to enhance renal excretion of uric acid). A *low pH* of tissues due to diminished perfusion as a result of *low ambient temperatures*, or *local pressure* (e.g. first MTP joints, olecranon bursae, ears) favours precipitation of urate in the form of microscopic needle-shaped crystals. These crystals cause an intense acute inflammatory reaction known as an acute attack of gout. An attack may also be precipitated by a *rapid fall or rise in serum uric acid levels*. Even the disappearance overnight of oedema in the legs that has accumulated during the day changes the local uric acid concentration. This may explain why gouty attacks commonly start at night. Urate crystals activate synovial cells and macrophages to produce inflammatory cytokines (IL-1, IL-6, TNF-α). Among other actions, the cytokines initiate the production of adhesion molecules that cause leucocytes to adhere to endothelial cells and to transmigrate from the blood vessel into extravascular tissue. Here, and in synovial fluid the polymorphonuclear cells phagocytize the crystals, subsequently rupture and release their destructive enzymes that then damage soft tissues, cartilage and bone. The cytokines also enter the circulation and cause fever, malaise, leucocytosis and elevation of acute phase reactants (ESR, C-reactive protein). These systemic features accompanying an attack of acute gouty synovitis, together with turbid synovial fluid containing polymorphonuclear leucocytes, may lead to the wrong diagnosis of septic arthritis. Only the microscopic demonstration of uric acid crystals in the synovial fluid, and a negative culture of synovial fluid, will clinch the diagnosis of gout.

Pathology of gout

In gouty *synovitis* the synovium and synovial fluid contain large numbers of polymorphonuclear leucocytes which may show intracellular needle-shaped crystals that they have engulfed. Small clusters of needle-shaped crystals are also found in the synovium, capsule and surrounding soft tissues. The crystal clusters are surrounded by mononuclear cells and multinuclear giant cells. Larger masses of urate crystals referred to as *tophi* develop at capsular attachments to bone where they cause bone erosions. *Gouty bone erosions* are therefore situated a little further way from the articular

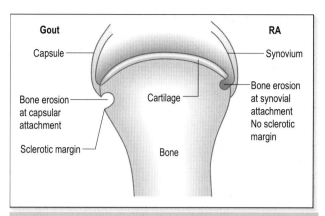

Figure 7.50.   Diagram to show the differences in bone erosions at joints in gout and in rheumatoid arthritis. In gout erosions occur at capsular, and in RA at synovial attachments. Erosions in gout are therefore further away from the joint surface than in RA. Moreover, gouty erosions have a sclerotic margin, whereas RA erosions blend into surrounding osteoporotic bone.

cartilage than rheumatoid erosions which develop at synovial attachments to bone, i.e. at the junction of synovium and cartilage (Fig. 7.50). Moreover, gouty erosions have a sclerotic margin whereas RA erosions are surrounded by osteoporotic bone. These features may be helpful in differential diagnosis. There is no periarticular osteoporosis in gout until late in the disease when tophi lead to bone destruction. Macroscopically, tophi contain a white material resembling toothpaste.

Clinical features of gout

If untreated, gout progresses in three phases: (1) asymptomatic hyperuricaemia (lasting decades), (2) acute intermittent gout (lasting years), (3) chronic tophaceous gout (probably continuing indefinitely). Acute intermittent gout starts with the first acute attack of nonarticular synovitis which comes on rapidly, usually during the night, lasts several days and is self-limiting. The first joint affected is usually the first MTP joint, or an ankle or a knee. Initially, attacks occur infrequently (e.g. once a year) but with time the frequency increases and any joint may be affected, including intervertebral discs. More and more joints are involved, tophi appear, and joint destruction sets in (Fig. 7.51). Other organs may become involved such as heart and kidneys.

Treatment of gout

The goals of treatment are (a) rapid control of the acute inflammation, and (b) prevention of further attacks and complications, such as renal stones and tophi. Treatment is thus tailored to the stage of the disease. *Asymptomatic hyperuricaemia* generally requires no more than lifestyle adjustments: weight reduction, purine (i.e. protein) restriction, and

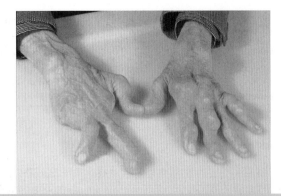

Figure 7.51.   Clinical photograph of the hands of a patient with neglected long-standing gout. Large cumbersome tophi have formed on the digits. The patient had requested amputation of one, and then another of the deformed digits of his right hand because they got in the way of the remaining functional digits. (By courtesy of Professor L. Solomon, University of Bristol, UK.)

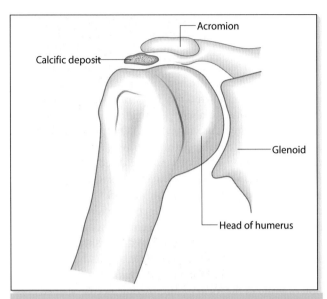

Figure 7.52.   Diagram of a radiographic image of calcific tendinitis of the supraspinatus tendon of the right shoulder. The calcific deposit in the degenerating tendon presents as a disc-shaped opacity between the humeral head and the acromion.

avoidance of alcohol excess. *Acute intermittent gouty attacks* are treated with NSAIDs or colchicine, and rarely with corticosteroids. Antihyperuricaemic drugs such as a xanthine oxidase inhibitor (allopurinol) or a uricosuric agent (enhancing renal excretion of uric acid, e.g. probenecid) may be indicated to prevent frequent attacks. It should be remembered that antihyperuricaemic drug therapy should only be commenced under cover of an NSAID or colchicine in order to prevent precipitation of an acute attack of gout when serum uric acid concentrations change, i.e. decline rapidly. *Tophaceous gout* and/or severe hyperuricaemia require long-term therapy with antihyperuricaemic drugs. Since it is extremely difficult to 'melt' tophi with such therapy, prevention of tophus formation is a more realistic goal.

Other crystal arthropathies

Crystalline particles other than monosodium urate can cause acute attacks of crystal-induced arthritis resembling gout. Examples are hydroxyapatite (HA, $Ca_{10}(PO_4)_6OH_2$) crystal deposition disease and calcium pyrophosphate dihydrate (CPPD) crystal deposition disease (pseudogout).

Hydroxyapatite crystal deposition disease

This is a non-heritable disorder of HA deposition in periarticular tendons (e.g. supraspinatus tendon), intervertebral discs and in cartilage. The cause is unknown. Identification of HA crystals is beyond the scope of most clinical laboratories because the crystal size is below the power of resolution of the light microscope, although large crystal aggregates may be identifiable by staining. The diagnosis rests mostly on clinical and radiographic evidence.

Pathogenesis of HA crystal deposition disease

There are no known underlying systemic metabolic abnormalities of calcium and phosphorus metabolism. Although body fluids are normally close to supersaturation for calcium and phosphorus, these substances stay in solution because of natural inhibitors of crystal formation in body fluids. When these inhibitors are overwhelmed by a rise in calcium or phosphorus concentrations, or when they are absent, e.g. in avascular or damaged tissue, crystal deposition may commence, as for example in the damaged and avascular portion of the supraspinatus tendon of the shoulder. A *supraspinatus calcific deposit* remains asymptomatic as long as it remains localized. At this stage radiographs show a well-defined disc-shaped opacity between the humeral head and the acromion (Fig. 7.52). However, when the deposit breaks up, crystals disperse into the subacromial bursa and the surrounding tissues where they elicit an outpouring of inflammatory cytokines (IL-1, TNF-α). These initiate an intense acute inflammatory reaction. At this stage the radiographic opacity becomes fluffy and may disappear. In *cartilage*, HA deposition may occur around chondrocytes which are thought to produce calcification vesicles that act as nucleation centres for crystal formation. These crystal aggregates within cartilage generally cause no problems, but when they shower into the joint cavity they elicit inflammation. Most cases of OA have HA crystals in the synovial fluid, but it is not known whether the crystals caused the OA, or whether they are shed into the joint as a result of the OA.

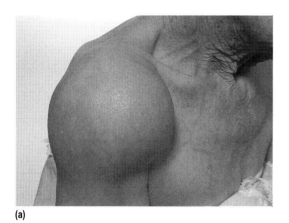

(a)

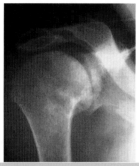

(b)

Figure 7.53. Hydroxyapatite crystal deposition disease ('Milwaukee shoulder' or 'cuff-tear arthropathy'). (a) Clinical photograph of the right shoulder showing a chronic massive effusion. (b) Radiograph of the same shoulder shows: (1) narrowing of the subacromial space indicating a rotator cuff tear, (2) narrowing of the glenohumeral joint, (3) subchondral bone erosions indicating cartilage and bone destruction. (By courtesy of Professor L. Solomon, University of Bristol, UK.)

Clinical features of HA crystal deposition disease

The majority of radiographically demonstrable periarticular calcific deposits are asymptomatic. In a small proportion of cases an acute inflammation develops as crystals are shed into the surrounding tissues. The most commonly calcified structure is the supraspinatus tendon, but lesions may also be found in the hand, feet and spine. In the case of an attack, the pain is intense, of sudden onset, and incapacitating. The affected part may be red, hot and swollen. The episode is self-limiting within days or weeks but can be shortened by the use of NSAIDs. Rapid resolution can be brought about by surgical removal of the HA deposit. The material removed resembles toothpaste.

An apatite-associated destructive arthritis of the shoulder ('Milwaukee shoulder' or 'cuff tear arthropathy') is seen in the elderly (Fig. 7.53a, b). The patient presents with a chronic massive cool effusion, pain and stiffness. There is progressive destruction of bone, joint and soft tissues, and large amounts of HA crystals are present in the synovial fluid. The condition is thought to start as rotator cuff degeneration, followed by HA crystal deposition, rotator cuff tear and shedding of crystals into the joint cavity. The condition cannot be cured, but is improved by NSAIDs, joint aspiration and arthroscopic joint lavage.

Calcium pyrophosphate dihydrate crystal deposition disease

CPPD arthropathy is a disorder of crystal deposition in articular cartilage (chondrocalcinosis), and less frequently in periarticular soft tissues. The condition may be heritable, sporadic or associated with metabolic disorders of calcium and phosphorus metabolism (e.g. hyperparathyroidism). The prevalence of the sporadic form increases with age.

Pathogenesis of CPPD deposition disease

There are no systemic biochemical abnormalities. The disorder is thought to originate locally. Articular chondrocytes may produce an enzyme that causes crystal nucleation and growth of pyrophosphate crystals formed from physiological phosphate compounds. In this way, clusters of pyrophosphate crystals develop in articular cartilage. In the course of cartilage wear, crystal clusters are broken into, and crystals disperse into the joint cavity. Here they elicit the production of inflammatory cytokines, and are phagocytized by leucocytes which in turn rupture and release destructive proteases. Thus full-blown synovitis, and later joint damage result.

Radiographic features of CPPD disease

Calcification of hyaline and fibrocartilage is most commonly seen in one or more of the following sites: articular cartilage (Fig. 7.54) and menisci of the knee joint, articular cartilage and labrum if the hip joint, triangular fibrocartilage of the wrist, intervertebral discs and symphysis pubis.

Clinical features of CPPD disease

The condition is referred to as 'pseudogout' because it presents with episodes of acute synovitis indistinguishable from those in gout. The diagnosis can be confirmed microscopically by the demonstration of rod-shaped crystals that are birefringent under polarized light. CPPD may strike in any joint, and one or more joints may be affected at a time. An untreated attack of 'pseudogout' is self-limiting within days or weeks. With repeated attacks, cartilage destruction and secondary OA will supervene. The pattern of distribution of affected joints of this form of OA differs from that of primary OA in that wrists, MCP joints, elbows and ankles may be involved, in addition to hips and knees. Another feature is severe patellofemoral OA (Fig. 7.54). Although attacks are self-limiting, they can be shortened with the help of NSAIDs, colchicine or corticosteroids. There is no treatment that will reduce the crystal burden, as is possible in gout.

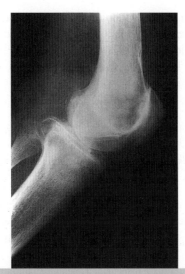

Figure 7.54.   Lateral radiograph of the knee of a patient suffering from severe patellofemoral arthritis due to calcium pyrophosphate crystal deposition disease (CPPD). Calcification is seen in the articular cartilage of the femoral condyles. The patellofemoral joint space has been obliterated as a result of cartilage destruction.

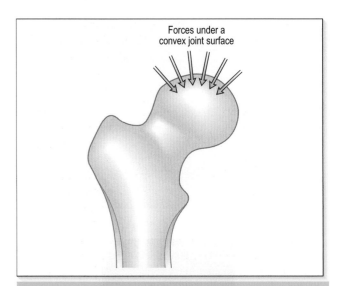

Figure 7.55.   Schematic representation of convergent forces of joint loading on convex articular surfaces.

Osteonecrosis

The term osteonecrosis, i.e. dead bone, refers to dead bone cells. The synonym 'avascular necrosis' emphasizes the most common pathogenetic mechanism, namely lack of blood circulation. Osteonecrosis may occur as a consequence of a bone infarct deep in the substance of a bone where its existence may go unnoticed. In contrast, osteonecrosis in subchondral bone may become disabling when the overlying joint surface collapses and OA develops. Sites most commonly affected are convex joint surfaces, namely those of the femoral head, the femoral condyles, the head and the capitellum of the humerus, the dome of the talus, the capitellum, and the proximal pole of the scaphoid. Convex joint surfaces are thought to be predisposed to osteonecrosis on account of the endarterial arrangement of the blood supply (few collateral vascular connections) under these joint surfaces. Blockage of endarteries can therefore not be compensated for by collateral circulation. Moreover, in convex joints the forces of joint loading converge in subchondral bone where they are thought to contribute to fragmentation of the osteonecrotic bone segment (Fig. 7.55).

Aetiology and pathogenesis

Impaired circulation of bone may come about through (1) mechanical disruption of blood vessels, (2) occlusion of blood vessels from within the blood vessel, (3) pressure on blood vessels from without, and (4) damage to blood vessel walls from within.

Mechanical disruption of blood vessels may be due to a fracture involving the joint, or a dislocation. The commonest examples are subcapital fractures of the femoral neck, traumatic dislocation of the hip and fracture of the scaphoid.

Occlusion of blood vessels from within may result from embolism, arterial thrombosis and circulation of fat globules. Circulating nitrogen bubbles may block small blood vessels when blood gases come out of solution during too rapid an ascent by deep-sea divers from work at great underwater depths. The condition is referred to as decompression sickness or caisson disease, and is popularly known as 'the bends'. Blood vessels may also be occluded by intravascular sludging of red blood cells as in for example sickle cell disease.

Pressure on blood vessels from without will interrupt blood flow. In a closed compartment such as the femoral head the pressure rises when marrow oedema develops or fat cells enlarge as for example in hypercortisolism, or alcohol abuse. Intraosseous pressure rises gradually, first above venous pressure obstructing venous outflow, and then above arterial pressure preventing inflow of arterial blood. Occlusion of blood vessels may also occur in Gaucher's disease, a storage disorder of the lipid cerebroside in bone marrow macrophages. As these cells enlarge, pressure in the femoral head rises and blood vessels are compressed.

Damage to the blood vessel wall from within occurs for example in vasculitis and in radiation damage (see Ch. 3.2).

High dose glucocorticoid therapy has been shown to induce *osteocyte apoptosis*, even in the presence of an intact blood supply. This is thought to constitute an alternative pathogenetic mechanism of steroid-induced osteonecrosis. In fact, the term 'avascular necrosis' for steroid-induced osteonecrosis is considered to be a misnomer because the process is based on apoptosis (see 'Control of the remodelling cycle') and the blood supply is frequently intact.

Pathology of osteonecrosis

The pathological features of osteonecrosis will be described for the femoral head since this is the most frequently affected site. Interruption of blood supply leads to cell death in bone marrow and in bone (osteocytes, osteoblasts, osteoclasts) within a number of hours. The anterolateral portion of the femoral head is most commonly affected, but half or more of the femoral head may be involved. Osteonecrotic bone stimulates neighbouring live bone to revitalize the dead segment as if the dead bone were a bone graft by (1) ingrowth of blood vessels, (2) deposition of new bone on dead trabeculae, and (3) remodelling of dead bone (i.e. resorption followed by formation). However, such repair manages to revitalize only the periphery of the osteonecrotic lesion, the rest remains dead bone.

Despite cell death, the dead bone continues to function structurally in a normal way for months, and occasionally for up to 2 years. However, fatigue damage within the devitalized bone gradually sets in. In the absence of both a blood supply and viable osteocytes (the mechanotransducers of bone) bone remodelling and repair cannot take place (see 'Control of the remodelling cycle'). As a result, damaged bone is not repaired, microfractures and microcracks accumulate, and finally a macroscopic fracture supervenes. In the femoral head the fracture plane traverses subchondral bone, parallel to the joint surface. The fracture gap is evident radiographically as the 'crescent sign'. A thin sliver of subchondral bone usually remains attached to the undersurface of articular cartilage. The articular cartilage overlying the fractured dead bone, however, remains viable, presumably being nourished by synovial fluid. With time the overlying cartilage subsides into the fragmenting dead bone. At this stage the superior surface of the femoral head begins to flatten. Eventually, the cartilage tears at the edge of the bony defect and lifts like a lid from the underlying dead bone (Fig. 7.56a–c). This allows fragments of necrotic bone to escape into the joint cavity where they cause synovitis and articular cartilage damage. This is the beginning of secondary OA.

Clinical features of osteonecrosis of the femoral head

The clinical and radiological staging system described by Arlet and Ficat (modified by Cruess) is widely used in clinical practice because it has therapeutic implications.

Stage 1 is a pre-radiologic stage. However, magnetic resonance imaging (MRI) may demonstrate marrow oedema, and scintigraphy with a ^{99}Tc-MDP radionuclide bone scan may show decreased uptake in the avascular segment, and increased uptake in the surrounding repair zone. Some pain

and restriction of movement may be experienced intermittently at this stage.

Stage 2 is characterized by increased bone density in the osteonecrotic segment, and osteopenia in the remainder of the femoral head. The higher bone density in the dead segment is variously thought to be due to (1) new bone apposition on dead trabeculae (repair) at the periphery of the necrotic segment, or (2) inability of dead bone to develop osteopenia (this requires a blood supply) in contrast to surrounding viable bone. The femoral head still has a normal shape at this stage. Pain and stiffness remain mild and intermittent.

Stage 3 is characterized by the classical radiological 'crescent sign' of a subchondral fracture. There may be slight flattening of the femoral head in the region of the osteonecrotic segment. Increasing pain, especially on weight bearing, and stiffness are experienced.

Stage 4 is characterized by marked collapse of the osteonecrotic segment and flattening of the femoral head. Pain and stiffness have now become incapacitating.

Stage 5 is established OA with arthritic changes also in the acetabulum. Symptoms remain incapacitating.

Treatment of osteonecrosis of the femoral head

Whether an asymptomatic hip in *stage 1* should be treated remains a matter of controversy. Some proponents of intervention would measure intraosseous pressure in the proximal femur, and if this were elevated, would carry out a *core decompression*. In this procedure, a core of bone measuring up to 1 cm in diameter is removed from the femoral neck and head with the aim of lowering the intraosseous pressure. This may improve blood flow and thus aid repair of dead bone. Such repair takes place by new bone apposition on dead trabeculae, and by remodelling (formerly called 'creeping substitution'). In *stage 2* a patient with a small lesion may derive some benefit from an *intertrochanteric osteotomy* that realigns the femoral head in such a way that the necrotic segment is subjected to less mechanical loading.

Most patients present in *stage 3*. The appropriate treatment for stages 3–5 lesions is *total hip arthroplasty*.

Diffuse idiopathic skeletal hyperostosis

Diffuse idiopathic skeletal hyperostosis (DISH) is a disorder of excessive periosteal new bone formation on vertebral bodies, around peripheral joints, and at tendon and ligament attachments to bone. Synonyms are ankylosing hyperostosis and Forestier's disease. DISH is a vertebral ankylosing disorder that may be confused with AS. However, the radiographic shape of the spinal osteophytes differs between the two conditions and should serve to distinguish DISH from AS. Whereas osteophytes in DISH are large beak-like excrescences projecting horizontally from the disc margins

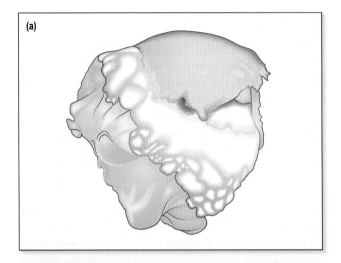

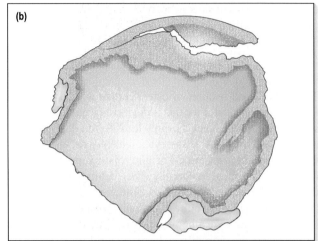

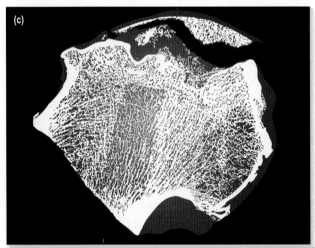

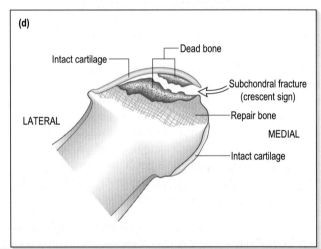

Figure 7.56.   Illustration of a whole femoral head (a), a coronal slab (b) and a slab radiograph (c), together with an explanatory diagram (d) for (b). The right femoral head had been removed at total hip arthroplasty for steroid-induced osteonecrosis in a renal transplant patient. (a) The articular cartilage overlying the osteonecrotic segment of the femoral head flipped up like a lid. On lifting the lid, fragmenting dead bone was exposed. (b and c) The coronal slab and corresponding slab radiograph show the subchondral fracture ('crescent sign') through osteonecrotic bone, and the covering cartilage 'lid'. The subchondral fracture appeared as a crescent sign also on a clinical radiograph of the hip.

(Fig. 7.57), those in AS are more vertically oriented and less prominent because they are confined to within the longitudinal ligament and the outer anulus fibrosus. DISH is not classified among the spondyloarthropathies. It is neither an inflammatory nor a degenerative disorder, although the radiographic appearance of the spinal osteophytes is similar to that in spondylosis. Although hyperglycaemia is a common clinical finding, the cause of DISH remains unknown. The *spinal lesions* of DISH are characterized by the large beak-shaped anterolateral osteophytes that project from the disc margins and unite with similar osteophytes a level above and below, thus bridging the discs and ankylosing the spine. Disc height is mostly preserved. *Peripheral joints* may show para-articular (next to the joint) osteophyte formation, but OA

may be present in large joints. Periosteal new bone formation appears on the shafts of tubular bones, and numerous tendon and ligament attachments to bone ossify, e.g. at the olecranon, the patella, the pelvis and the calcaneum. These enthesophytes show neither erosions nor sclerosis in underlying bone, unlike those in spondyloarthropathies. Considering the impressive radiological features of DISH, affected individuals experience remarkably few symptoms other than some restriction of movement.

Patients with DISH have a tendency to develop extensive heterotopic ossification in soft tissues around the hip following total hip arthroplasty. This complication causes permanent restriction of joint movement. Surgical removal of established heterotopic ossification tends to be followed by

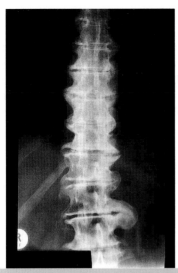

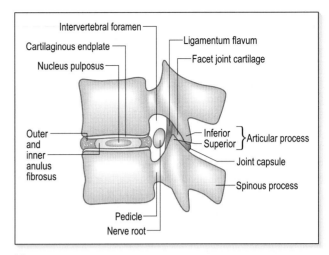

(a)

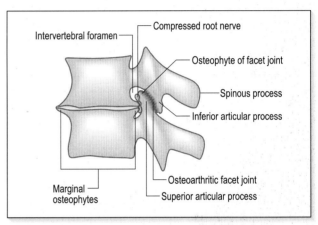

(b)

Figure 7.57.   Anteroposterior radiograph of the thoracolumbar spine of a patient with idiopathic skeletal hyperostosis (DISH). Large beak-like osteophytes project horizontally from the vertebral bodies at multiple disc levels. Neighbouring osteophytes tend to fuse, leading to spinal ankylosis.

Figure 7.58.   Diagrams of a lateral view of a normal (a) and a degenerating (b) lumbar motion segment. (a) Adequate space is available in the intervertebral foramen to accommodate the nerve root. (b) Disc degeneration has led to loss of disc height and circumferential marginal osteophyte formation (spondylosis). Loss of disc height has also resulted in malalignment and OA of the facet joint with osteophyte formation. This chain of events results in narrowing of the intervertebral foramen by a number of structures: the bulging disc, marginal disc osteophytes, osteophytes on facet joints, thickening of the ligamentum flavum (as a result of shortening), and possibly spondylolisthesis. The nerve root may become compressed to a thin ribbon, and neurological symptoms and signs may develop in its distribution.

recurrence. Awareness of the presence of DISH in patients coming to total hip arthroplasty should lead to preventive measures pre- and postoperatively that will suppress osteoblast differentiation (indomethacin, radiotherapy).

Degenerative spinal disorders

The vertebral column has 23 intervertebral discs and at least 100 synovial joints; this includes the costo-vertebral joints. It is therefore not surprising that arthritic disorders and degenerative changes affect the spine. The commonest spinal disorders are intervertebral disc degeneration and degenerative OA of the facet joints, especially at levels of greatest mobility, i.e. at C5–6 an L4–S1. The structures affected in a lumbar motion segment are shown in Figures 7.58a and b.

Structure of the intervertebral disc

Intervertebral discs connect the vertebrae, allow spinal movement and act as shock absorbers. The intervertebral disc has four distinct regions: (1) nucleus pulposus, (2) inner anulus fibrosus, (3) outer anulus fibrosus, and (4) cartilaginous end plates (Fig. 7.58a). The intervertebral disc has few cells. A blood and nerve supply are present only in the peripheral layers of the outer anulus. Nutrition of disc cells and dispersal of their waste products occurs by diffusion through the cartilage end plates and the anulus. In early life the *nucleus pulposus* is a gel-like substance, but in adulthood it firms up through loss of water. The nucleus pulposus derives its consistency from macromolecules (aggrecans bound to hyaluronan) that hold water in a way similar to that of articular cartilage (see 'Synovial joints'). The macromolecules are trapped in a sparse network of randomly oriented type II collagen fibres. High intradiscal pressures are created by a combination of osmotic and hydraulic pressures. The cells responsible for matrix production in the nucleus pulposus are chondrocyte-like cells. The *inner anulus fibrosus* consists of fibrocartilage with more or less concentrically arranged type II collagen fibres and embedded chondrocytes. The *outer anulus* fibrosus is made up almost entirely of tightly packed, circumferentially oriented type I collagen fibres. The embedded cells are fibroblasts. The anulus is thinnest posteriorly, the site of nucleus pulposus prolapse. The proteoglycan content of the intervertebral disc decreases and the collagen content increases from the nucleus pulposus outwards. The *cartilaginous end plates* cover the bony vertebral end plates and consist of hyaline cartilage. The cartilage is traversed by collagen fibres that bind the anulus fibrosus firmly to vertebral bone.

Function of the intervertebral disc

The structure and composition of the intervertebral disc makes it ideally suited to withstand high compressive loads and bending forces. During loading, the nucleus pulposus undergoes particularly high compressive stresses that amount to many times superincumbent body weight because of added muscle action and lever arm effects. In contrast, the anulus fibrosus develops high tensile stresses that hold the nucleus pulposus in place. Under load, water is extruded from the nucleus pulposus through the cartilaginous end plates, and the disc loses height as a result. This loss of nucleus pulposus volume increases the circumferential bulge of the anulus fibrosus. On unloading, the high osmotic pressure within the nucleus pulposus ensures the return of water, and restoration of disc height. These changes explain the slight loss in body height during the day, and its restoration during the night.

Prolapse of the intervertebral disc

Degenerative fissures and clefts in the anulus fibrosus may allow material from the nucleus pulposus to herniate. Since the anulus fibrosus is thinnest posterolaterally and posteriorly, disc herniations occur here where they protrude into the nerve root canal and the spinal canal. This leads to compression of the nerve root in the nerve root canal and of the cauda equina in the spinal canal. Pain and neurological deficits are experienced in the distribution of the compressed neural structures. Disc herniations tend to occur on rising in the morning because the hydrostatic pressure in the nucleus pulposus has risen during the night's recumbency as a result of the return of water into the nucleus. The sudden resumption of upright posture generates additional hydrostatic pressure within the nucleus pulposus that may cause the fissured anulus to tear, and the nucleus pulposus to prolapse. Furthermore, spinal posture affects intradiscal pressure. Lumbar intradiscal pressure is lowest in supine recumbency, and increases, in ascending order, in lateral recumbency, upright posture, sitting, upright posture carrying a load beside the body, bending forward and bending forward carrying a load

in front of the body. Thus, loaded forward bending is the posture most likely to result in disc prolapse. A soft nucleus pulposus in young adulthood is more likely to prolapse than a firm fibrotic nucleus in an older person. What starts as age-related disc changes may go on to complete degeneration of all disc tissue until the disc consists of no more than a thin fibrotic layer between the bony end plates of the vertebrae.

Ageing and degeneration of disc and facet joints

Age-related changes commence after age 20 years and at first affect the nucleus pulposus. As a result of an age-related decline in blood supply and cell numbers in the disc, the matrix of the nucleus pulposus cannot be replaced when the large proteoglycan molecules fragment. This has the following far-reaching consequences over the years. The nucleus pulposus holds less water, the disc loses height, the anulus becomes slack and bulges, and abnormal movements forwards, backwards and sideways occur between vertebrae. This *instability* creates abnormal traction forces on the periosteum and spinal ligaments, leading to traction osteophytes at the disc margins. The condition is referred to as *spondylosis* (Fig. 7.58a, b). Loss of disc height also causes incongruity of the facet joints as the inferior facet of the upper vertebra slides down on the superior facet of the vertebra below (Fig. 7.58a, b). This leads to articular cartilage wear and marginal facet joint osteophytes. Episodes of acute facet joint synovitis develop in response to cartilaginous and bony detritus being shed into the joint cavity. The clinical picture is referred to as *facet joint syndrome* (see below). Facet joint osteophytes may compress nerve roots in the lateral recess of the spinal canal, particularly in individuals with a small triangular spinal canal with an already narrow lateral recess. Destruction of facet joint cartilage and subchondral bone allows the upper vertebral body to slip forward on the one below, a condition referred to as degenerative *spondylolisthesis* (spondylos = vertebra, olisthesis = slip). The sum of the structures encroaching on the spinal canal, namely marginal disc osteophytes, bulging disc, facet joint osteophytes, shortened and therefore thickened ligamentum flavum, and spondylolisthesis, may severely compress neural structures and cause *spinal stenosis*. A vertebra may also slip backwards as a result of disc degeneration. This is referred to as *retrolisthesis*.

Spinal stenosis

As osteophytes, bulging disc, spondylolisthesis and thickened ligamentum flavum encroach on the spinal canal (Fig. 7.59a, b), insufficient space remains for the dilatation of nerve root blood vessels necessary for increased metabolic activity during walking. This causes nerve root ischaemia which manifests as 'spinal claudication', a pain and limp indistinguishable from intermittent claudication due to peripheral vascular disease. Initially, relief of pain is obtained by standing still

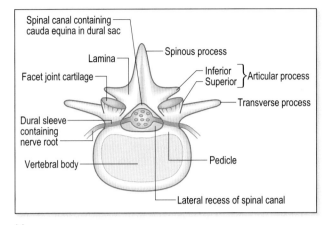

(a)

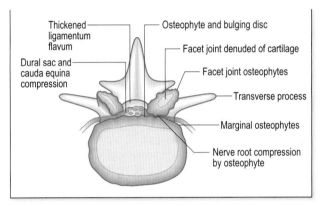

(b)

Figure 7.59. Cross-sectional diagrams of a normal (a) and a degenerating (b) lumbar motion segment with spinal stenosis. (a) In the normal spinal canal there is ample space to accommodate the dural sac containing the cauda equina and the emerging nerve roots. As the nerve root leaves the dural sac, the nerve root takes with it a dural root sleeve that enwraps it within the lateral recess of the spinal canal and in the intervertebral foramen. (b) In spinal stenosis due to degenerative changes the spinal canal is narrowed anteriorly by marginal disc osteophytes and the bulging disc (not shown), laterally by facet joint osteophytes, and posteriorly by the shortened and therefore thickened ligamentum flavum. The spinal canal cross-sectional area may be reduced to a small fraction of normal, and the cauda equina may be severely compressed as a result. The lateral recess of the spinal canal may be obliterated by osteophytes, thus strangulating the exiting nerve root to a thin ribbon. At this advanced stage neurological symptoms and signs are inevitable.

and bending forward (spinal flexion widens the spinal canal). As constriction of the spinal canal increases over months or years, spinal flexion is no longer able to widen the spinal canal, and neurological deficits may develop. Surgical decompression consisting of removal of the constricting structures relieves the condition.

Low back pain

Spinal pain is most commonly experienced in the lumbosacral and cervical regions, i.e. at sites of greatest mobility and therefore most advanced degeneration. Low back pain (LBP) may arise in different anatomical structures and have different causes. The following sites are known sources of LBP.

Disc degeneration may give rise to low back, buttock, posterior thigh and even calf pain at an early stage of the disease, i.e. long before there is evidence of disc prolapse, loss of disc height or nerve compression. This early pain is thought to be due to chemical irritation caused by acidic breakdown products of proteoglycans from the nucleus pulposus that seep through fissures in the anulus fibrosus and irritate the nerve endings in the dura and the dural root sleeve of the nerve root. The pain in the buttock and lower limb is a referred pain from dural root sleeve irritation. Neurological symptoms and signs are absent at this stage. When the nucleus pulposus prolapses, mechanical irritation of the dural root sleeve causes severe pain in the distribution of its nerve root. Stretching of the sciatic nerve, as in the straight leg raising test ('sciatic stretch test'), aggravates this pain because the nerve root and its dural sleeve are pinned down by the prolapse, and stretching tugs on the irritated structures. Under normal conditions the nerve root and its dural sleeve move freely into and out of the intervertebral foramen over a range of 8–10 mm during straight leg raising. Neurological symptoms and signs in the leg develop when the nerve root itself becomes compressed.

Advanced disc degeneration is associated with ingrowth of nerves and blood vessels into what is left of previously avascular disc material. These nerves are thought to become a source of LBP.

Facet joint OA is associated with episodes of synovitis caused by the shedding of cartilaginous or bony detritus into the joint cavity. These episodes are referred to as *facet joint syndrome*. The onset is usually sudden following an unaccustomed movement, and the back pain is sharp and immobilizing. Protective muscle spasm is a prominent feature. The attack may last days or weeks. Although the pain may be referred distally in the distribution of the sclerotome of the affected facet joint, neurological deficits are not a feature. However, in advanced facet joint OA with large osteophytes and nerve root compression, a neurological deficit may be present and the pain may be continuous.

The LBP of *spinal stenosis* comes on while standing or walking because during these activities the spine is in extension which further narrows the spinal canal. The pain is deep-seated and dull, extends into the legs and causes limping (spinal claudication). An overwhelming sensation of 'lameness' makes further steps impossible. These symptoms are relieved by spinal flexion such as standing still with one leg flexed, or by sitting (spinal flexion widens the spinal canal). Neurological deficits are absent in the early stages of the condition but may develop if surgical decompression is not carried out.

Low back pain relieved by sitting or lying down is generally considered to be a 'mechanical back pain', i.e. due to degenerative or traumatic changes. In contrast, an unrelenting rest pain and night pain should arouse suspicion of malignancy or infection.

Location of the pain may suggest the site of pathology. 'Hip pain' behind the hip and pain in the posterior thigh most commonly originate in the low lumbar spine, and pain in front of the hip and anterior thigh in the hip joint itself, or less frequently at a high lumbar level. 'Meralgia paraesthetica' is a syndrome of localized pain and paraesthesia in the anterolateral thigh. It is caused by compression of the lateral cutaneous nerve of the thigh as it passes through the inguinal ligament just medial to the anterior superior iliac spine; local pressure at this point will aggravate symptoms. Surgical release may be required. Pain located over the SI joint is sometimes assumed to be caused by 'sacroiliac joint arthritis' or sacroiliitis, but is more likely referred pain from the much commoner low lumbar spinal derangements. A ^{99}Tc-MDP bone scan can be used to exclude sacroiliac pathology. The clinical features of many low back derangements overlap. In many cases of LBP it is impossible to accurately pinpoint the site of origin of the pain and to arrive at a pathological diagnosis without elaborate investigations. The attending doctor may therefore be unable to put an accurate diagnostic label to the condition, and may instead choose simply to call it 'low back pain' until further clarification. Many patients get better anyway.

REFERENCES AND FURTHER READING

Bone disorders
Structure of bone
Baron RE (1996) Anatomy and ultrastructure of bone. In: Favus MJ (ed.) Primer on the Metabolic Bone Diseases and Disorders of Mineral Metabolism, 3rd edn. Philadelphia: Lippincott-Raven, pp. 3–10.

Bostrom MPG, Boskey A, Kaufman JK, Einhorn TA (2000) Form and function of bone. In: Buckwalter JA, Einhorn TA, Simon SR (eds) Orthopaedic Basic Science, 2nd edn. Rosemont, IL: American Academy of Orthopaedic Surgeons, pp. 320–369.

Parfitt AM, Villanueva AR, Foldes J, Rao S (1995) Relations between histologic indices of bone formation: implications for the pathogenesis of spinal osteoporosis. J Bone Miner Res 10: 466–473.

Singh M, et al. (1973) Mayo Clin Proc 48: 184–189.

Composition of bone
Burger EH, Klein-Nulend J (1999) Mechanotransduction in bone – role of the lacuno–canalicular network. FASEB J 13: S101–S112.

Eyre DR (1996) Biochemical basis of collagen metabolites as bone turnover markers. In: Bilezikian JP, Raisz LG, Rodan GA (eds) Principles of Bone Biology. San Diego: Academic Press, pp. 143–153.

Mundy GR (1996) Bone-resorbing cells. In: Favus MJ (ed.) Primer on the Metabolic Bone Diseases and Disorders of Mineral Metabolism, 3rd edn. Philadelphia: Lippincott-Raven, pp. 16–24.

Puzas JE (1996) Osteoblast cell biology: Lineage and functions. In: Favus MJ (ed.) Primer on the Metabolic Bone Diseases and Disorders of Mineral Metabolism, 3rd edn. Philadelphia: Lipincott-Raven, pp. 11–16.

Rossert J, de Crombrugghe B (1996) Type I collagen: structure, synthesis, and regulation. In: Bilezikian JP, Raisz LG, Rodan GA (eds) Principles of Bone Biology. San Diego: Academic Press, pp. 127–142.

Termine J, Robey PG (1996) Bone matrix proteins and the mineralization process. In: Favus MJ (ed.) Primer on the Metabolic Bone Diseases and Disorders of Mineral Metabolism, 3rd edn. Philadelpia; Lippincott-Raven, pp. 24–28.

Bone remodelling
Eriksen EF (1986) Normal and pathological remodeling of human trabecular bone: Three dimensional reconstruction of the remodeling sequence in normals and in metabolic bone disease. Endocr Rev 7: 379–408.

Frost HM (1963) Bone Remodeling Dynamics. Springfield, IL: Charles C. Thomas.

Jilka RL, Weinstein RS, Bellido T, Parfitt AM, Manolagas SC (1998) Osteoblast programmed cell death (apoptosis): modulation by growth factors and cytokines. J Bone Miner Res 13: 793–802.

Mundy GR (1995) Bone Remodelling and its Disorders. London: Martin Dunitz, chap. 1.

Parfitt AM (1983) The physiological and clinical significance of bone histomorphometric data. In: Recker RR (ed.) Bone Histomorphometry: Techniques and Interpretation. Boca Raton, FL: CRC Press, pp. 143–223.

Parfitt AM (1994) Osteonal and hemiosteonal remodelling: the spatial and temporal framework for signal traffic in adult human bone. J Cell Biochem 55: 273–286.

Smit TH, Burger EH (2000) Is BMU-coupling a strain-regulated phenomenon? A finite element analysis. J Bone Miner Res 15: 301–307.

Verborgt O, Gibson GJ, Shaffler MB (2000) Loss of osteocyte integrity in association with microdamage and bone remodeling after fatigue in vivo. J Bone Miner Res 15: 60–67.

Skeletal development and ageing
Bell GH, Dunbar O, Beck JS, Gibb A (1967) Variations in strength of vertebrae with age and their relations to osteoporosis. Calcif Tissue Int 1: 75–86.

Frost HM (1960) Micropetrosis. J Bone Joint Surg 42A: 144–153.

Heaney RP, Abrams S, Dawson-Hughes B, et al. (2000) Peak bone mass. Osteoporosis Int 11: 985–1009.

Iannotti JP, Goldstein S, Kuhn J, et al. (2000) The formation and growth of skeletal tissues. In: Buckwalter JA, Einhorn TA, Simon SR (eds) Orthopaedic Basic Science, 2nd edn. Rosemont, IL: American Academy of Orthopaedic Surgeons, pp. 77–109.

Jensen KS, Mosekilde Li, Mosekilde Le (1990) Model of vertebral trabecular bone architecture and its mechanical properties. Bone 11: 417–423.

Manolagas SC, Weinstein RS (1999) New development in the pathogenesis and treatment of steroid–induced osteoporosis. J Bone Miner Res 14: 1061–1066.

Parfitt AM (1987) Trabecular bone architecture in the pathogenesis and prevention of fracture. Am J Med 82 (Suppl 1B): 68–72.

Parfitt AM, Travers R, Rauch F, Glorieux FH (2000) Structural and cellular changes during bone growth in healthy children. Bone 27: 487–494.

Section II: Calcium, Magnesium, Phosphorus Homeostasis and Physiology, and Biochemistry of Calcium Regulating Hormones (1996). In: Favus MJ (ed.) Primer on the Metabolic Bone

Diseases and Disorders of Mineral Metabolism, 3rd edn. Philadelphia: Lippincott-Raven, pp. 41–87.

Stress fractures

Burr DB, Milgrom C (eds) (2001) Musculoskeletal Fatigue and Stress Fractures. Boca Raton, FL: CRC Press.

Milgrom C, Finestone A, Shlamkovitch M, et al. (1994) Youth is a risk factor for stress fracture. A study of 783 military recruits. J Bone Joint Surg 76B: 20–22.

Resnick D, Goergen TG, Niwayama G (1995) Physical injury: concepts and terminology. In: Resnick D (ed.) Diagnosis of Bone and Joint Disorders, 3rd edn. Philadelphia: WB Saunders, pp. 2561–2693.

Osteoporosis

Delmas PD (2000) How does antiresorptive therapy decrease the risk of fracture in women with osteoporosis? Bone 27: 1–3.

Looker AC, Bauer DC, Chesnut III CH, et al. (2000) Clinical use of biochemical markers of bone remodeling: Current status and future directions. Osteoporosis Int 11: 467–480.

Marcus R, Feldman D, Kelsey J (eds) (2001) Osteoporosis. San Diego: Academic Press.

Osteomalacia

McKenna MJ, Kleerekoper M, Ellis BI, et al. (1987) Atypical insufficiency fractures confused with Looser zones of osteomalacia. Bone 8: 71–78.

Pettifor JM, Daniels ED (1997) Vitamin D deficiency and nutritional rickets in children. In: Feldman D, Glorieux FH, Pike JW (eds) Vitamin D. San Diego: Academic Press, pp. 663–678.

Section V: Metabolic bone diseases (1996). In: Favus MJ (ed.) Primer on the Metabolic Bone Diseases and Disorders of Mineral Metabolism, 3rd edn. Philadelphia: Lippincott-Raven, pp. 301–360.

Paget's disease of bone

Siris ES (1996) Paget's disease of bone. In: Favus MJ (ed.) Primer on the Metabolic Bone Diseases and Disorders of Mineral Metabolism, 3rd edn. Philadelphia: Lippincott-Raven, pp. 409–419.

Other skeletal disorders

Glorieux FH, Bishop NJ, Plotkin H, et al. (1998) Cyclic administration of pamidronate in children with severe osteogenesis imperfecta. N Engl J Med 339: 947–952.

Section VI: Genetic, developmental, and dysplastic skeletal disorders (1996) In: Favus MJ (ed.) Primer on the Metabolic Bone Diseases and Disorders of Mineral Metabolism, 3rd edn. Philadelphia: Lippincott-Raven, pp. 362–387.

Fracture healing and osteonecrosis

Day SM, Ostrum RF, Chao EYS, et al. (2000) Bone injury, regeneration, and repair. In: Buckwalter JA, Einhorn TA, Simon SR (eds) Orthopaedic Basic Science, 2nd edn. Rosemont, IL: American Academy of Orthopaedic Surgeons, pp. 371–399.

Joint disorders
Structure of joints

Mankin HJ, Mow VC, Buckwalter JA, Iannotti JP, Ratcliffe A (2000) Articular cartilage structure, composition, and function. In: Buckwalter JA, Einhorn TA, Simon SR (eds) Orthopaedic Basic Science, 2nd edn. Rosemont, IL: American Academy of Orthopaedic Surgeons, pp. 443–470.

Mow VC, Flatow EL, Ateshian EA (2000) Biomechanics. In: Buckwalter JA, Einhorn TA, Simon SR (eds) Orthopaedic Basic Science, 2nd edn. Rosemont, IL: American Academy of Orthopaedic Surgeons, pp. 133–180.

Recklies AD, Poole RA, Banerjee S, et al. (2000) Pathophysiologic aspects of inflammation in diarthrodial joints. In: Buckwalter JA, Einhorn TA, Simon SR (eds) Orthopaedic Basic Science, 2nd edn. Rosemont, IL, USA: American Academy of Orthopaedic Surgeons, pp. 489–530.

Arthritides, spondyloarthropathies, gout, crystal arthropathies

Koopman WJ (ed.) (2001) Arthritis and Allied Conditions, 14th edn. Philadelphia: Lippincott Williams & Wilkins.

Diffuse idiopathic skeletal hyperostosis

Resnick D, Niwayama G (1995) Diffuse idiopathic hyperostosis. In: Resnick D (ed.) Diagnosis of Bone and Joint Disorders, 3rd edn. Philadelphia: WB Saunders, pp. 1463–1495.

Osteonecrosis

Cruess RL (1986) Osteonecrosis of bone. Clin Orthop 208: 30–39.

Day SM, Ostrum RF, Chao EYS, et al. (2000) Bone injury, regeneration, and repair. In: Buckwalter JA, Einhorn TA, Simon SR (eds) Orthopaedic Basic Science, 2nd edn. Rosemont, IL: American Academy of Orthopaedic Surgeons, pp. 371–399.

Manolagas SC (2000) Corticosteroids and fractures: A close encounter of the third cell kind. J Bone Miner Res 15: 1001–1005.

Degenerative spinal disorders

Buckwalter JA, Mow VC, Boden SD, Eyre DR, Weidenbaum M (2000) Intervertebral disc structure, composition, and mechanical function. In: Buckwalter JA, Einhorn TA, Simon SR (eds) Orthopaedic Basic Science, 2nd edn. Rosemont, IL: American Academy of Orthopaedic Surgeons, pp. 547–556.

Buckwalter JA, Boden SD, Eyre DR, Mow VC, Weidenbaum M (2000) Intervertebral disc ageing, degeneration, and herniation. In: Buckwalter JA, Einhorn TA, Simon SR (eds) Orthopaedic Basic Science, 2nd edn. Rosemont, IL: American Academy of Orthopaedic Surgeons, pp. 557–566.

Movement and Immobility

Karen Barker

8

INTRODUCTION

The concepts of motion and rest are the basic building blocks underpinning all treatment of the musculoskeletal system since the time of Hippocrates. Over time the emphasis has shifted away from the early tenet that 'rest was best' towards a greater understanding of the effect that rest, activity and inactivity has on the different tissues of the musculoskeletal system.

For many years the view of physicians was the time-honoured tradition that rest allowed diseased and injured tissues to heal. More recently the effect of rest on the physiology of the body's tissues has been extensively investigated and a better understanding gained of the relative benefits and dangers of rest and immobilization on musculoskeletal tissues. Similarly, there have been extensive studies of the effect of mobilization, stretch and exercise on the tissues of the body.

This chapter reviews the effect of immobility, mobilization and exercise on the musculoskeletal tissues and suggests the clinical impact of changes to a normal balance of motion and rest on the body's ability to function normally.

BONE

Introduction

Bone is made up of two types of tissue: compact bone, which is dense in texture, and cancellous bone, which is composed of a meshwork of trabeculae.

Both types are a mixture of collagen and hydroxyapatite. Bone mineral is embedded in variously orientated collagen fibres forming an extracellular matrix. The collagen matrix composes approximately 95% of the bone and between 35 and 30% of its dry weight. The collagen fibres have a low modulus of elasticity and thus respond with good tensile strength but with poor resistance to compression. The calcium phosphate portion of bone provides a stiff, brittle component that is resistant to compressive load.

This results in tissue that can resist tension, compression and shear forces. Bone is able to resist the most load under compression and the least under shear. Cancellous bone is 5–10% stiffer and five times more deformable than compact bone. It is a dynamic tissue able to constantly change and remodel itself to withstand the stresses placed upon it (Wolff's law).

Mature bone demonstrates a curvilinear response to loading, with a stress/strain curve that shows both elastic and plastic properties.

Mature bone demonstrates the usual elastic response to loading, but some yielding is possible during loading within this elastic region. The stiffness of a bone is dependent on its shape, density and the forces applied to it. If a bone is subject to fast loading, it behaves with more stiffness, meaning that it may sustain a greater overall stress and store more energy before failure. Thus a high-energy fracture tends to be comminuted because of the added energy stored in the bone before failure.

If the frequency of loading is excessive, there will not be sufficient time for repair to occur and the bone may fail due to fatigue.

Effect of increased activity on bone

There is a direct relationship between the mechanical property of bone and the intensity of exercise.

If bone is subjected to levels of physical stress that are higher than normal, it becomes more tolerant to subsequent stresses and more resistant to injury, provided that the tissues are given time and are able to recover and adapt to previous bouts of physical stress. Higher than normal levels of physical stress will cause bone to remodel. Wolff's law evolved from observations by Julius Wolff, a medical student in Berlin in the 1860s. He proposed that tissues adapt to physical stress. His law states that bone will alter its size, shape and trabecular pattern in both the subchondral and cortical bone according to the distribution of mechanical stresses placed upon the bone. Thus the strength of the bone is greatest in the direction in which loads are most commonly placed.

Increases in cyclic loading of bone cause bone formation to exceed bone removal and can result in significant increases in bone density, strength and size.

Animal studies have shown that newly weaned rats subjected to low level exercise intensities showed no effect on either bone weight or length in relation to body weight over a 7-week period, although the absolute weight of the bone increased. Bone weight and length decreased after high intensity exercise training compared with normal controls. Low intensity exercise training appears to either stimulate bone growth or to have no effect. High intensity exercise training inhibits bone growth in immature animals.

In an experiment in pigs the ulnar diaphysis was resected. This increased the compressive strain on the radius by a factor of 2–2.5 times its normal value. The radius responded by a rapid increase in its diameter so that within 3 months the cross-sectional area of the radius was equivalent to the area of the combined radius and ulna on the contralateral side, and the compressive strain on the radius had decreased to the normal value.

Bone density has been shown to be unchanged following low intensity exercise programmes, but to increase under high intensity exercise conditions. Runners demonstrate a marked increase in their bone mineral density in the lower limbs, but not in the upper limbs as a result of mechanically induced adaptations in the bone. Similarly, professional racquet sport players demonstrate contralateral differences in the bone mineral density, cross-sectional area and diaphyseal diameter in the humerus of the dominant arm compared with the non-dominant side, as a result of the stresses placed upon the limb.

Effect of inactivity on bone

Disuse results in loss of both bone mass and size. Patients with conditions that result in disuse such as spinal injury or poliomyelitis demonstrate bone loss over time. Similarly, immobilizing a limb in a cast or by traction results in bone loss. The cause of the decrease in bone mass appears to be increased bone resorption rather than decreased bone formation. Osteoclasts resorb trabecular and cortical bone and osteoblasts fail to replace enough bone to maintain the mass and strength of the tissue. Whilst decreased activity will not result in observable changes in the shape or strength of the bone radiographic changes will be evident. These include decreased bone mineral density of cancellous bone and loss of trabeculae with thinning and increased porosity of cortical bone. The changes seen in humans with age are very similar to those seen from disuse. Decreased activity leads to decreased osteoclast stimulation.

The change in bone mass resulting from inactivity or immobilization affects the bone's mechanical strength. The stress that a bone can withstand is proportional to its mass. A decrease in bone mass results in a decrease in the stress that it can withstand before failure and in less elasticity. Thus the fractures suffered by elderly patients, or those who have been immobile, are usually low energy non-comminuted fractures as the bone has less ability to dissipate the strain energy.

In animal studies primates were immobilized in full body casts for 60 days. After 60 days the vertebrae were tested in vitro and compared with a control group who had not had any restrictions to their mobility. The immobilized primate vertebrae showed a threefold decrease in the load it could withstand before failure, decreased energy storage capacity and decreased stiffness.

In the absence of weight bearing, bone mass decreases to half its normal value after 12 weeks, decreasing bone strength and increasing the likelihood of fracture. Following a period of immobilization it takes several months of weight-bearing exercise to regain the bone mineral density, even in young patients. In elderly patients the bone mineral density may never recover to its previous level.

Effects of motion on bone tissue healing

Conventionally, fractured limbs have been held in a rigidly immobilized, non-weight-bearing position to facilitate healing. More recently the beneficial effects of some cyclical loading on tissue repair has been recognized. Early loading and movement by micro-motion promotes fracture healing of long bones. Clinical studies have demonstrated that early or immediate controlled loading of long bone fractures promotes fracture repair. However, excessive movement at a fracture site or uncontrolled loading results in delayed or failed fracture healing.

Effect of imposed stretch stimulus to bone

Under certain biological and mechanical conditions bone can be carefully divided and the two bone ends separated in a controlled manner to allow new bone to be generated in the gap that is created, a process known as *distraction osteogenesis*. This occurs naturally under certain conditions; for example, the bone growth at the perimeter of the growth plate is the result of traction forces from the surrounding attached periosteum. Surgeons can use mechanical distraction to reproduce and accelerate this natural phenomenon and exploit it to address a range of clinical problems including limb length discrepancy.

The Russian surgeon Ilizarov was the first to describe and exploit this process for limb-lengthening surgery. He states that certain mechanical and biological factors are essential for osteogenesis:

- maximum preservation of extraosseous and medullary blood supply
- stable external fixation
- a delay period prior to distraction of between 5 and 10 days, to allow the initial inflammation to settle
- a distraction rate of 1 mm per day in small frequent steps
- a period of stable fixation after the correction is completed (consolidation)
- physiological use of the elongating limb.

New bone is stimulated to grow, the regenerate bone matures and neocorticalization occurs as the bone is remodelled. By 4 weeks after distraction new bone is laid down in the central growth zone. The content of the new bone includes water 15%, lipid 5%, calcium 25%, phosphate 12% and collagen 24%. These are found in approximately the same ratios as in normal bone. The cortices of the bone form 4–6 months after distraction, and remodelling of the bone continues for up to a year or more.

Once matured the regenerate bone formed by distraction osteogenesis is indistinguishable from host bone, unlike the new bone seen in fracture healing, in which there is a disorganized collagen network of bone and where the bone often does not recover its normal contour.

Summary of clinical implications

Bone demonstrates a viscoelastic response to imposed load. Increases in cyclic loading of bone cause bone formation to exceed bone removal and can result in significant increases in bone density, strength and size. In conditions of non-weight-bearing, bone mass decreases to half its normal value after 12 weeks, with a corresponding decrease in bone strength and increase in the likelihood of fracture. Following a period of immobilization it takes several months of weight-bearing exercise to regain the bone mineral density, even in young patients. The viscoelastic properties of bone may be exploited to facilitate fracture repair. Clinical studies have demonstrated that early or immediate controlled loading of long bone fractures promotes fracture healing. These properties may be exploited by applying a tension force to bone ends separated by an osteotomy to promote distraction osteogenesis. This may be used to facilitate procedures such as leg-lengthening surgery.

CARTILAGE

Introduction

Articular cartilage is a viscoelastic tissue that is a mixture of a viscous fluid and elastic solid. It consists of 60% water and a solid matrix that is composed of 60% collagen and 40% proteoglycan gel. Structurally, cartilage consists of sparsely scattered chondrocytes in a vast extracellular matrix composed of a highly organized molecular framework filled with water. Chondrocytes synthesize this molecular framework from three classes of molecule: collagens, proteoglycans and noncollagenous proteins. It is the proteoglycans that give the cartilage its resistance to compression, through their binding interaction with water. The collagen provides a fibrous ultrastructure with bundles of collagenous fibres forming arcades, similar to the ribs of an open umbrella. This arrangement gives the collagen a layered characteristic and accounts for the tensile strength of cartilage.

Biomechanically, a stress/strain curve for cartilage will demonstrate an exponential function, with an initial low slope thought to be the result of the alignment of the collagen fibres and the linear steep section of the curve representing the tensile stiffness of the collagen. Whilst its tensile strength is only 5% of bone, it has high viscoelastic properties, making it well suited to compressive loading. Initial loading is characterized by large amounts of deformation as water is extruded. Once the water is expelled, the gel portion of the cartilage carries the load and the response is stiffer than in the initial phase. The rate of loading will influence the mechanical properties that cartilage exhibits: rapid loading gives a relatively elastic appearance, while low rates of loading result in the cartilage indenting with very slow resolution.

Normal articular cartilage provides a low-friction, self-lubricating bearing surface with load distribution properties that minimize the peak stresses on subchondral bone; i.e. they have a shock-absorbing effect. It is resilient, durable, has tensile strength and is resistant to wear. However, the disadvantage that it has little capacity for repair has been recognized for many years, together with knowledge of its lack of blood supply. Whilst healthy cartilage can resist normal or even strenuous loading, injury to articular cartilage may be a precursor to pain and eventually osteoarthritic changes.

Degeneration of cartilage may be a consequence of an imbalance between the remodelling and maintenance processes of the chondrocytes that are embedded in the dense extracellular matrix of the articular cartilage. There is poor understanding of the mechanisms responsible for controlling the balance between the degradation and synthesis of cartilage, but it is thought that local changes in the biomechanical loading of chondrocytes are important.

Effect of immobilization on cartilage

Numerous experimental models have demonstrated that immobilized joints develop cartilage changes. Even simple immobilization in a plaster of Paris cast may result in hyaline cartilage changes, fibrillation, flaking, fissuring and thinning of the cartilage. When immobilized, chondrocytes degenerate and die within a short period of just weeks or a few months. This would suggest that they need mechanical stimulation to exist. If a normally weight-bearing joint is subjected to a period of immobilization combined with non-weight-bearing or non-loading, there is a substantial loss of matrix proteoglycans of the articular cartilage. The reason for this is likely to be a combination of lack of weight-bearing and lack of movement, although there is little consensus about the relative importance of each of these factors.

Salter and co-workers investigated the effect of immobilization of synovial joints by holding a rabbit knee joint in fixed flexion for periods of between 3 and 10 weeks. They found that after even a short period of immobilization, the synovial membrane became adherent to the surface of the articular cartilage that was not in contact with the opposing joint surface. This obliterated the fluid space between the cartilage and synovial membrane, preventing the normal synovial fluid nutrition of the cartilage and causing it to become necrotic or degenerate. Similarly, it has been demonstrated that if a joint is immobilized in an extreme position, for even a short period of time, necrosis of the cartilage will occur in the contact area, similar to a pressure sore.

Basic science experiments on animal models have demonstrated that a combination of immobilization and non-weight-bearing results in approximately a 20% decrease in the glycosaminoglycan content of articular cartilage and a 41–47% decrease in the synthesis of cartilage. In ovine models the relative importance of weight-bearing and immobilization has been investigated in an experimental model in which sheep legs were subjected to varying combinations of immobilization and weight-bearing status. After 4 weeks under each test condition, full thickness samples of articular cartilage from the radiocarpal joints were taken and examined. It was found that joints that were immobilized and subject to non-weight-bearing conditions suffered the greatest decrease in glycosaminoglycans.

However, in other animal studies, investigators have found that joints that were subject to non-weight-bearing conditions, but allowed to move, maintained their glycosaminoglycan content. The experimental design of this study placed the animals under an experimental condition analogous with patients following a regime of non-weight-bearing status but with the joints free to move.

Effect of mobilization on cartilage

In the early 1900s Retterer observed that increased functional stress resulted in increased cartilage thickness from $300\,\mu m$ to $400\,\mu m$ and caused hypertrophy of the superficial cartilage cells. Studies by Saaf on the effects of exercise on the articular cartilage of the shoulder joints of adult guinea pigs demonstrated that exercise stimulated a temporary increase in the number of chondrocytes per unit volume of matrix. Other investigators have demonstrated that a period of immobilization of the knee applied to animals with a full thickness defect of the knee articular cartilage will result in the formation of adhesions. Conversely, the same injury treated by normal active motion, i.e. intermittent mobilization, resulted in strikingly better healing and an absence of adhesions.

Effect on cartilage of stretch stimulus/traction of the lower limb

Cartilage damage might be induced during such orthopaedic procedures as limb-lengthening surgery. When the limb is lengthened, the soft tissues are stretched and put under tension. When a muscle crosses a joint this tension results in high joint compression forces, which increase the pressure on the articular cartilage and may lead to cartilage breakdown. In canine studies a 30% lengthening of the femur resulted in reproducible cartilage injury ranging from fibrillation to frank loss of substance. However, other researchers have shown that articular surfaces could be preserved during lengthening of 30% magnitude by preventing large compressive forces during lengthening. This was achieved by techniques such as extending the external fixation mechanism over the knee joint and allowing motion of the knee. In rabbit studies it was found that increasing the frequency of distraction, so that the bone was lengthened in more frequent, smaller stages, resulted in less damage to the cartilage of adjacent joints.

Effect of reduced weight bearing, but retaining joint movement

Clinically this kind of presentation would occur by amputation of a distal extremity. In animal studies it has been demonstrated that chondrocytes survived prolonged non-weight-bearing situations, but that the cells could not form solid bands of intercellular matrix substance that would enable the cartilage to resist heavy loading. Loss of loading leads to marked decreases in the glycosaminoglycan content of the articular cartilage. Further animal studies using sheep

have shown that joints that were subject to no weight-bearing but allowed to move maintained their glycosaminoglycan content.

In a study of patients with amputated lower limbs over half were reported to have reduced thickness of the articular cartilage on the amputated side. This loss of cartilage correlated with the length of the remaining limb, as 11 of 13 patients with an upper third amputation had decreased thickness cartilage, but none of the lower third amputees.

Thus it is clear that joint unloading by immobilization has a deleterious effect on the articular cartilage with atrophy, indicated by the reduced content of proteoglycans in superficial zones and in alterations to their interaction with other matrix constituents. The decrease in articular cartilage glycosaminoglycans found after reduced weight-bearing in animal models appears to be reversible in some cases.

Clinically, this basic science research would suggest that there is a need to carefully consider the benefits of unloading a joint by rest or cast, compared with the possible atrophy that might develop with long-term treatment.

Effects on cartilage of remobilization after a period of immobilization

The level of matrix proteoglycans is key to the ability of the articular cartilage to withstand compressive forces. This is obviously important in the clinical setting as decreased proteoglycans will predispose the cartilage to damage, particularly if it is subsequently subjected to loads, for example the loads imposed in the early rehabilitation of a patient after immobilization in a cast.

In an experiment by Sood rabbits were subjected to immobilization of the knee in flexion for 7–12 weeks before remobilization. After a remobilization period of 12 weeks the stainability of the intercellular matrix was only slightly decreased and the articulate surface appeared intact on histological sections. These observations suggested that after immobilization in flexion, regressive changes in cartilage were completely reversible. Other investigators offer a different opinion with reports that articular lesions became coated with fibrous lesions on remobilization. Palmoski reported that dogs showed immobilization-induced defects of proteoglycans that were reversible after 2 weeks of mobilization following an immobilization period of 6 weeks. However, when the dogs were immobilized for 11 weeks, only partial restoration of the proteoglycans and physical properties of the articular cartilage was observed after 15 weeks' remobilization.

It is suggested that when unloading has occurred for long periods, care should be taken, using a phased introduction of weight-bearing status on recommencing weight-bearing, to avoid irreversible damage to the cartilage. There is a delicate balance of the relative times of immobilization versus mobilization that affects the ability of the cartilage to regenerate.

Summary of clinical implications

Sustained decreases in either the motion of a synovial joint or the loading through the joint cause articular cartilage changes. Chondrocytes change their synthesis activity, proteoglycan concentrations decrease, matrix organization decreases and the mechanical properties of cartilage deteriorate. The results of the studies on the effect of immobilization on articular cartilage would support the practice used in rehabilitation of encouraging exercise, including passive movements to limbs, in the absence of weight-bearing to maintain the articular cartilage matrix. Loading of an immobilized joint by repeated isometric muscle contractions may help preserve cartilage. The studies of the effect of weight bearing on cartilage support the importance of rehabilitation efforts to encourage weight-bearing through immobilized joints where clinically applicable. For short periods of immobilization or unloading changes will be temporary. However, the longer-term maintenance of normal, healthy cartilage requires a combination of both loading and motion.

SYNOVIAL JOINTS

Introduction

Synovial joints have to achieve a balance between mobility and stability to achieve a state of effective functional ability. The deleterious effects of immobility on joints remain the main risk factor for joint contractures. These present a frequent problem, impeding the performance of everyday tasks and limiting independence. Much of the focus of musculoskeletal physiotherapy is directed at either preventing or treating joint stiffness.

Joints will be affected by mobilization and immobility through the interactions of bone, cartilage, muscle and the collagenous or dense fibrous tissues such as ligaments and tendons. There is natural variation in the amount of stiffness in a joint, determined by the physical properties of the soft tissues that cross the joint. As the joint is moved the soft tissues are lengthened, developing tension that resists further lengthening and further movement of the joint, in the same way that a spring responds to tension. The main restraint to the movement of joints comes from the periarticular, dense fibrous connective tissues (ligament and capsule) and from muscle. A normal joint will experience a large amount of movement in response to a given torque, whereas a stiff joint will experience relatively little movement in response to the same torque.

It is still not clearly established which tissues have the greatest influence on joint immobility. In contractures uncomplicated by skin or neural changes the articular structures and muscles are deemed responsible. Some studies implicate myogenic restrictions as the primary cause of joint restrictions whereas others favour arthrogenic restrictions. A third suggestion is that during the first 90 days of immobility, the limitation was predominantly myogenic but after 90 days the limitation is mainly arthrogenic.

The dense fibrous periarticular tissues are only effective at resisting tensile deformation. The structure of the different types of tissues reflects their function. Tendon fibres are arranged almost completely parallel to each other, so that the fibres are aligned parallel to the load and are thus able to resist tensile load. Ligaments, including joint capsule, have a fibre arrangement that varies between two extremes. If it is required to resist major joint stresses then its fibres will be more parallel, if it is not required to resist forces from any particular direction then its fibre orientation will be more random. The mechanical properties of tendon and ligament vary with loading. Under high rates of loading collagenous tissue stores more energy, fails at higher maximum load and has increased elongation. It is very resistant to slow loading; thus with this form of loading the mode of failure is at the bone–ligament complex and results in osseous avulsion. In fast loading the ligament is the weakest component and is the site of the majority of failures.

Effect of immobilization on synovial joints

Total immobilization of a joint will result in a series of changes to the structures of the joint. These may primarily have an effect on the intra-articular environment of the joint or affect the periarticular connective tissues.

Studies on both animal models and humans have demonstrated that when a joint is immobilized fibro-fatty connective tissue proliferates in the synovial joint space, forming pannus. This pannus proliferates over the surface of the articular cartilage, together with proliferation of the synovial cells, and the joint space can be filled with fibro-fatty tissue. With continued immobilization, the fibro-fatty tissue becomes more fibrous and forms strong bands of dense connective tissues that form adhesions to the surrounding joint surfaces and restrict the mobility of the joint.

The adhesions are very strong, such that if forced manipulation is attempted tears may occur at the sites of attachment of the synovium, capsule and cartilage and there will be enzymatic degradation of the surrounding connective tissues in response to an inflammatory reaction to the trauma.

These damaging changes occur very quickly and the repair is extremely slow and unpredictable.

The ligaments and joint capsule form dense fibrous tissue that has the function of resisting tension. This responds to decreased loading and prolonged immobilization by a decrease in the glycosaminoglycan and water content of the matrix collagen fibres. There is an increase in collagen cross-linking and decreased collagen mass. These changes can occur after just 6 weeks of immobilization.

In the ligaments around the joint there is an increased rate of collagen synthesis. The collagen fibres cease to be aligned in a parallel fashion and the pattern of deposition of collagen becomes increasingly random. At the ligament bone attachment there will be marked osteoclastic resorption. The increase in the synthesis of collagen and proteoglycans by the fibroblasts that occurs in the ligaments during total immobilization is unexpected. However, the collagen fails to aggregate in a parallel array, instead forming in a random fashion resulting in a disorganized tissue matrix that does not have the high tensile strength necessary for the ligament to function. Thus immobilization results in the formation of a new, poorly functioning substitute for normal ligament tissue.

In animal studies the bone–ligament complex of knees in primates were immobilized for 8 weeks. The anterior cruciate ligaments were collected and tested to failure. The ligaments from the immobilized primates demonstrated a 39% decrease in the load they could withstand before failing, and a 32% decrease in the energy storage capacity compared with a control group. Similarly experiments in rabbits demonstrated that if the medial collateral ligament of rabbits was immobilized for 9 weeks there was a decline in the mechanical properties of the ligament. Stiffness, ultimate load before failure, and the energy-absorbing capacity of the ligament–bone complex were approximately one-third of those of the control, contralateral non-immobilized limb.

Akeson and co-workers demonstrated that immobilization of rabbit knees resulted in an increase in the joint stiffness that was associated with changes in the biochemical composition of the periarticular connective tissues. There was a decrease in the concentration of the glycosaminoglycans, which produced a substantial loss of water from the tissues. Normally, the high water content of the tissues acts as a spacer keeping the collagen fibres apart. It is hypothesized that the loss of water from the connective tissues allows the collagen fibres to become sufficiently close to form additional interfibre cross-links. These additional cross-links cause the tissues to become inextensible and the joints to become stiffer. It has not been established whether these changes are dependent on the position of the tissues when immobilized, i.e. do the periarticular connective tissues become inextensible only if immobilized in a shortened position, or after immobilization in any position? Limited clinical observations have suggested that the stiffness induced by the periarticular connective tissues is position dependent. When the metacarpophalangeal joints of the hands are immobilized in extension, the collateral ligaments are held immobilized in a shortened position and become stiff, yet when the metacarpophalangeal joints are immobilized in a flexed position, this stiffness does not occur.

Decreased loading also alters the insertion of the ligaments and tendons into the bone. In some insertions the collagen fibres pass directly into the bone matrix through a series of zones of tendon or ligament, then a zone of fibrocartilage, a zone of calcified cartilage then bone. This is termed *direct insertion* and responds to decreased loading by resorption around the insertion, but relatively little resorption activity around the insertion itself, e.g. cruciate ligament of the knee. For other insertions the insert is *indirect or periosteal* and the collagen fibres join the periosteum with relatively few passing into the bone matrix, e.g. tibial insertion of the medial collateral ligament. Decreased ligament loading produces subperiosteal osteoclast resorption of the bony insertion of the ligaments. This leaves the ligament attached primarily to periosteum and there is significant weakening of the bone–ligament junction within 6–8 weeks. These changes are reversible once normal joint use is resumed with cells in the insertion site forming new bone and restoring the structure and mechanical properties of the tendon insertion. A prolonged period of active loading is required to reverse the changes that occur after just 6–8 weeks of immobilization. It takes up to one year for there to be complete restoration of the ligament insertion structure and for full mechanical properties to be restored.

Effect of reduced weight bearing, but retaining joint movement

Clinically, when a joint has been subject to non-weight-bearing status, e.g. after a fracture, physical methods have traditionally been employed to prevent the development of stiff joints, usually by passive cyclical movements or joint mobilization.

The dense fibrous tissues appear to be less sensitive to decreased load and motion than the surrounding bone. In dogs that were prevented from weight-bearing for 8 weeks but allowed active motion of the joints, there was decreased bone density but no resorption or weakness of the knee ligaments. This suggests that the loading provided by active joint motion might be sufficient to maintain the composition and mechanical properties of the periarticular dense fibrous tissues, at least for a few months.

Studies investigating the effect of passive movements on the paws of dogs immobilized after flexor tendon repair showed that dogs who received 5 minutes of daily passive movements had significantly greater joint range of motion after 6 weeks of immobilization than dogs who were immobilized without receiving passive movements. The dogs that received passive movements did not develop adhesions between the tendon and sheath, whereas those completely immobilized did.

A large number of studies have investigated the efficacy of using continuous passive motion (CPM) to prevent joint stiffness. When CPM is used after knee arthroplasty there is evidence that it is beneficial at reducing joint stiffness. However, under controlled experimental conditions the same benefits could be attained by active exercises and stretching. In a recent randomized controlled trial CPM was compared with stand and exercises and with use of a sliding board after total knee arthroplasty. No benefit was found to have occurred by using adjunct continuous passive motion.

Effect of increased use/loading

If a stretch stimulus is applied to dense fibrous tissues such as tendon or ligament they will respond with a characteristic stress/elongation curve as shown in Figure 8.1. Initially the curve will be concave (zone 1), reflecting changes in the alignment of the collagen fibres; with a small stretch load the wavy collagen fibres straighten. This change may also reflect interfibrillar sliding and shear of the interfibrillar gel. Only a small amount of load is required to make these initial changes. As stretching continues, the stiffness of the tissues progressively increases and greater force is needed to produce elongation of the tissues (zone 2). The tissue then follows a linear curve when the collagen fibres become more parallel. Towards the end of zone 2 there will be some deformation with sequential failure of stretched fibre bundles. At the end of the linear zone the curve levels off and major failure of the fibre bundles occurs.

Repetitive loading of the dense fibrous tissues of the joint (tendons, ligaments, capsule) will increase the strength, size and matrix organization of the tissues. Increased loading can cause adaptation of dense fibrous tissue in animal studies. In studies using rabbit models the load on the medial collateral ligament was increased by 200–350% by the insertion of a pin underneath the ligament to alter the mechanical axis and angle of pull. This resulted in a significant increase in the strength of the bone–ligament complex over a 12-week period. The dense fibrous tissues respond to changes in the intensity and frequency of loading. Tendon regions subjected to tension demonstrate linearly arranged dense collagen fibrils, elongated cells, a lower proteoglycan content and higher rate of collagen synthesis than tendon subjected to more variable forces. Tendon subject primarily to compression consists of a network of collagen fibrils separated by a proteoglycan matrix and more rounded cells. Subjecting tendons to compression increases the hyaluronic acid and chondroitin sulphate content, whereas applying tension decreases the glycosaminoglycan content. These differences result from adaptation to differences in loading.

Effect of stretch on joints

Stretching stiff joints by forced manipulation may result in improvement by tearing the intra-articular adhesions that develop after immobilization. However, this may result in tearing of tissues, promoting further scar formation and joint stiffness. Physiotherapists tend to use less forceful techniques to try to improve decreased joint range of motion. Techniques tend to focus on the effect of sustained stretch on the length of the tissues around the joint: the joint is positioned at the limit of its range of motion and overpressure applied and sustained. Immediately after a period of slow, sustained stretching the soft tissues exhibit less resistance to lengthening than prior to stretching and consequently the joint has greater mobility. Stretching can be applied for a few minutes or for prolonged periods of up to 24 hours a day using splints, casts or orthoses. Stretching increases the extensibility of the soft tissues by both viscous deformation and structural adaptation of the soft tissues. Viscous deformation is a temporary effect that is reversed once the stretch stimulus has been removed. In human studies recovery from viscous deformation occurs at a similar rate to the effects of the initial stretch stimulus. In contrast, structural adaptations are less easily reversible. In experimental models it took over 50 minutes of sustained stretching before changes to the connective tissues were effected. This suggests that stretching needs to be applied for far longer than is the norm in clinical practice, if maximum benefit is to be gained.

There is some evidence to suggest that low load is sufficient to achieve increases in range of motion. The effect of a high load, brief stretch or a low load prolonged stretch on elderly patients with bilateral knee flexion contractures has been studied. High load stretching was applied by ten passive movements and one minute of forced passive stretching each day. Low load stretching was applied by traction applied for an hour a day. Over the 4-week experimental period the legs stretched using a low load prolonged stretch demonstrated significantly greater increases in joint range of motion.

In a further study on the effect of low-load prolonged stretch on knee flexion contractures in the elderly, passive range of motion exercises were compared with low load stretching provided by a splint applied over a 6-month period. It was found that there was no statistically significant difference between the patients treated by passive exercises alone and those who also received the low-load prolonged stretching.

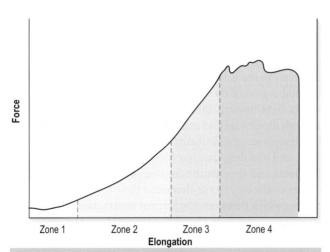

Figure 8.1.   Stress/elongation curve for tendon/ligament. Zone 1, tissue elongates with little increase in force as collagen fibres straighten. Zone 2, fibres straighten and stiffness increases. Deformation of tissue is nearly linear with increased force. 3, End of zone 2. Progressive failure of collagen fibres produces irregular dips. 4, Maximum load = tensile strength of tissue; complete failure.

There is considerable debate about whether stretching really does induce lasting increases in joint mobility. A recent systematic review concluded that stretching produces increases in joint range of motion that are still evident one or more days after cessation of treatment.

Effect of mobilization to joints

Specifically applied movement may be applied to joints for therapeutic benefit in treating joint stiffness, for example in such techniques as Maitland mobilizations. Exercise of the joint increases the penetration of cartilage to nutrients from the synovial fluid. Compression and decompression of the fluid film on the cartilage surface results in an increased flow of nutrients from the synovial fluid into the cartilage. Patients with intra-articular joint pain present with either marked restriction due to pain felt within the joint, or with intermittent, mild pain felt when the joint is placed under conditions of load, or compressive force. Where there is a severe restriction in the range of motion with an irritable joint that easily becomes painful and takes a long time to settle, Maitland advocates the application of gentle, large amplitude passive mobilizations of the joint. These may be applied as either accessory joint movements or utilizing the pain-free portion of the physiological range. The techniques effectively produce the agitation or stirring of the fluid film on the joint surfaces that is necessary to improve the nutrition of the cartilage. Patients who present with minor intermittent pain aggravated by joint compression or loading also benefit from passive mobilization techniques applied to the joints, but with smaller amplitude movements applied with the joint surfaces compressed adjacent to each other.

Summary of clinical implications

Joint mobility is essential for normal locomotor activity. Joints will become stiff if deprived of the normal forces and movement that they are used to experiencing. Joint stiffness is a response to a combination of changes in the soft tissues, particularly the muscles and periarticular soft tissues. Periarticular connective tissue responds to immobilization by becoming inextensible.

The joint also responds to immobilization by developing fibro-fatty tissue that forms fibrous adhesions, limiting the movement between adjacent joint surfaces or the joint surfaces and soft tissues. Once the soft tissues have adapted, they may cause permanent restrictions in joint mobility affecting the completion of activities of daily living.

In cases where a joint needs to be unloaded, but some motion is allowed, studies have demonstrated that passive movements can ameliorate some of the effects of immobility.

Many common rehabilitation modalities are directed at either preventing or treating joint stiffness. Techniques such as stretching, orthotics to maintain joint position and joint mobilizations have all been advocated and have various degrees of success at treating and/or preventing joint contractures developing. The research evidence from clinical trials would tend to support low-load prolonged stretches over high-load brief stretches and would support the use of serial splinting in established joint contractures of neurological origin. As yet there is no consensus about the most effective regimen for maintaining joint range of motion in the immobilized patient, nor for treating joint contractures once they have developed.

MUSCLE

Introduction

Muscles are complex structures consisting of both contractile and connective tissues. The basic contractile unit of a muscle is the sarcomere. This consists of a rod-like structure, the myofibril. Within the myofibril proteins are arranged with thick filaments (myosin) interdigitating with thinner filaments (actin). The myofibril is divided into short sections by z-bands. The area between one z-band and the next forms a sarcomere. Units of this contractile unit in series form myofibrils. The myofibrils group together to form a multinucleate muscle fibre enclosed in a layer of connective tissue, the endomysium. Bundles of muscle fibres are grouped together to form fasciculi, and these are enclosed in another connective tissue sleeve, the perimysium. A large number of fasciculi are grouped together enclosed in a connective tissue sheath, the epimysium, to form a muscle.

The intermuscular connective tissue sleeves provide physical structure to the muscle and assist in muscle shortening by providing a lubricated surface for the fibres to slide over.

The working mechanism of the contractile tissue consists of sliding together of the actin and myosin filaments. During contraction the thick myosin filaments remain stationary in the mid-region of the sarcomere, whilst the thinner actin filaments slide inwards interdigitating with them drawing the z-bands closer together and shortening the sarcomere. Cross-bridges between the filaments are made and broken, generating force and enabling the thin filaments to slide over the thick filaments and shorten the muscle. Skeletal muscle has three elements: the contractile element, a passive series elastic component which transmits the force of contraction, and a parallel elastic component which distributes the forces associated with passive stretch and maintains the relative positions of the fibres.

The connective tissue component of muscle is predominantly made up of collagen fibres. At rest the collagen fibres of the perimysium have a wavy appearance. As the muscle lengthens, the angle between these collagen fibres and the muscle fibres becomes more acute and they become less wavy. As collagen straightens, it becomes stiffer, suggesting that intramuscular connective tissue has a role in maintaining the

Table 8.1.   Characteristics of muscle fibres

Type	Structural properties	Characteristics
Type I – slow twitch, slow oxidative	Aerobic metabolism High number of mitochondria Wide z-bands	Slow contraction speed Resistant to fatigue
Type IIA – fast twitch, oxidative, glycolytic	Contain both oxidative and glycolytic enzymes Anaerobic and aerobic metabolism	Fast contraction speed Intermediate tension-generating capacity Resistant to fatigue
Type IIB – fast twitch, glycolytic	High supply of glycolytic enzymes, poor supply oxidative enzymes Anaerobic metabolism Few mitochondria Narrow z-bands	Fast contraction speed Generate large amount of muscle tension Fatigue rapidly

stiffness of relaxed muscle. Further stiffness is provided by intracellular structure. The amount and structure of the intramuscular collagen is thought to be related to differences in elastic compliance between the different types of muscle. Slow, tonic muscle has a higher concentration of collagen than fast twitch muscle.

Whilst muscle has the same basic units there are different types of muscle based upon differing proportions of contractile and connective tissue components. They have been placed into a classification system based upon contraction times and enzyme capacities (Table 8.1).

Effect of immobilization on muscle

Effect of immobilization on contractile tissue component of muscle

In normal muscle the number of sarcomeres in series determines the distance through which the muscle can shorten and the sarcomere length at which it has to develop force. The number of sarcomeres can increase or decrease in adult muscle depending upon the demands placed upon it. However, the length of the sarcomere is constant. The addition or subtraction of sarcomeres is an adaptation to changes in the functional length of a muscle (Fig. 8.2).

When muscle is immobilized, for example, in a plaster cast, the sarcomere numbers rapidly adapt to a change in length by adding or removing sarcomeres. These changes result in the optimum sarcomere length being attained, irrespective of the position of immobilization.

If a muscle is immobilized in a shortened position there will be a decrease in the number of sarcomeres so that the remaining sarcomeres are pulled to a length which enables the muscle to develop its maximum tension in the immobilized position. If muscles are immobilized in a lengthened position sarcomeres will be added and this will result in sarcomere length being reduced compared with before adaptation to the new length. This will again allow the muscle to

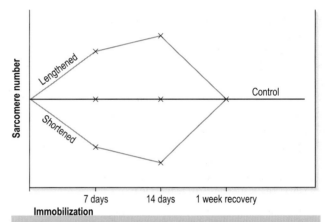

Figure 8.2.   Change in sarcomere numbers with immobilization position. (Adapted from Goldspink and Williams, 1990.)

generate maximum tension in the immobilized position. The addition/subtraction of sarcomeres will result in changes in the length/tension curve of the muscle; the curve of muscles immobilized in the shortened position being to the left of normal becomes steeper, i.e. the muscle becomes stiffer and shorten. The length/tension curve for lengthened muscle shifts to the right of normal (Fig. 8.3). Thus the muscle adapts to the imposed changes of length during immobilization.

If a muscle is immobilized in a shortened position it can lose up to 40% of its sarcomeres. This decrease will be proportional to the decrease in muscle length. The adaptations to muscle length and serial sarcomere number are readily reversible. Once the cast is removed, the number of sarcomeres returns to its original 'normal' number and the original length–tension relationship is restored. Return to normal functional activity alone appears to provide sufficient stimulus to return to normal stiffness and length after immobilization, irrespective of the position in which the muscle was immobilized.

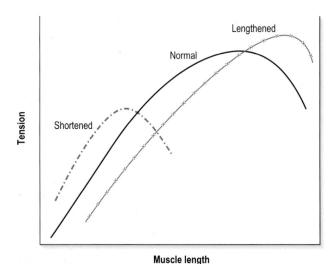

Figure 8.3.   Changes in length/tension curve of muscle with position of immobilization.

The trigger for the muscle to either add or subtract sarcomeres is thought to be related to the muscle tension along the myofibril and/or the fibre attachment. High tension leads to addition of sarcomeres and low tension to sarcomeres being subtracted. Sarcomere number is regulated so as to achieve optimum sarcomere length at the position where most force is exerted on the fibre attachment. However, the exact nature of the control mechanism is not clear.

In animal studies a difference in the behaviour of animals of different ages has been observed. All animals initially respond to a period of immobilization in a lengthened position by increasing the number of serial sarcomeres. After 5 days the muscle of adult rabbits continues to show an increase in the numbers of sarcomeres, whilst in the young animals there is a rapid decrease in sarcomere number and a corresponding lengthening of the tendon.

With complete immobilization muscle will atrophy with a decrease in fibre diameter and myofibril loss. Despite being in a state of atrophy and decreasing fibre diameter, the longitudinal length of the myofibril can grow if subject to an imposed functional length, e.g. by application of a cast. This would imply that there are different stimuli that trigger transverse muscle fibre growth/atrophy than those for longitudinal growth.

Effect of immobilization on connective tissue component of muscle

In muscle that has been immobilized the connective tissue component will also show characteristic changes. If the collagen of a muscle is selectively stained with Sirius red, immobilization of a muscle in a shortened position will result in an increase in the proportions of the endomysium and the perimysium, making the muscle stiffer. The increase in perimysium was

observed after only 2 days of mobilization, i.e. before there was evidence of loss of serial sarcomere numbers. This implies that the effect on the connective tissue is directly caused by the immobilization, rather than the increase being due to redistribution of connective tissue after shortening of the fibres. If a muscle is immobilized in a lengthened position the same changes are not seen and the proportions of connective tissue to contractile muscle tissue remains unchanged. Thus it would seem that although the muscle can adapt to changes in position of immobilization by adapting the number of serial sarcomeres, the position of immobilization is more critical for the connective tissue component and will have an influence on muscle stiffness. It is suggested that lack of activity, rather than lack of stretch, is the determining factor in connective tissue remodelling. If a muscle is immobilized in a neutral position, i.e. it is deprived of movement but without any imposed change in length, it does not demonstrate any changes in length or stiffness.

Effect of immobilization on fibre type

Cast immobilization of normal adult muscle results in preferential atrophy of slow twitch fibres. They decrease in size and lose some of their capacity for oxidative metabolism. There is a decreased rate of protein synthesis in all types of muscle fibre, but greatest in type I fibres. Type I fibres also increase their rate of tension development after immobilization. In animal studies using rats, where the soleus muscle (predominantly slow twitch) is immobilized, there is a loss in the number of slow twitch fibres resulting in an increase in the contraction time of the muscle. There is some debate about whether this decrease in slow twitch fibres is due to preferential degeneration or whether some slow twitch fibres convert to fast twitch fibres. Fibre type changes in humans have also been studied.

The influence of the position of immobilization may be important (Table 8.2). In rabbit studies immobilization produces increases in the resting stiffness of the muscle-tendon unit, but this effect was not influenced by the position in which the muscle was immobilized. However, the muscle alone is subject to position-dependent increases in muscle stiffness. The position of immobilization does influence the effect on muscle weight, muscles immobilized in a shortened position demonstrating a marked decrease in weight compared with those immobilized in a lengthened position. The relationship between the position of immobilization and loss of muscle weight is non-linear, suggesting a threshold position of immobilization. Booth suggests that the threshold position beyond which an immobilized muscle does not atrophy rapidly is the position that corresponds to the pre-immobilization resting length of the muscle. The results from studies on human subjects are less conclusive. Sargeant and co-workers studied young adults who had their lower limb immobilized in a plaster cast for between 53 and 213 days (mean 131 days) following fractures. Needle biopsy specimens of the lateral part

Table 8.2.   Effect of position of immobilization

Effect of immobilization in shortened position	Effect of immobilization in lengthened position
Decreased number of sarcomeres	Increased number of sarcomeres
Shorter muscle	Longer muscle
Increase in muscle stiffness	No change in muscle stiffness
Increase in proportion of connective tissue	No change to connective tissue
Connective tissue becomes more longitudinally orientated	
Marked atrophy	Less atrophy
Marked decrease in muscle weight	No marked change in muscle weight

of quadriceps femoris were obtained and the fibre type calculated. They found that the numbers of type I and type II fibres remained unchanged. There was a greater decrease in the cross-sectional area of the type I fibres than the type II, with a mean decrease of 46% in type I fibres and an average 37% decrease in type II fibres. These results would suggest that there is not selective degeneration of fibres, but that there is preferential atrophy of type I fibres. These changes occurred after a lengthy period of immobilization and using the contralateral limb as a control, so the differences may partly be due to hypertrophy of the contralateral limb. Haggmark and co-workers also studied fibre type after immobilization. They studied pre- and post-immobilization changes in patients undergoing anterior cruciate ligament reconstruction. The limbs were immobilized in a cast for 5 weeks and patients were actively encouraged to perform a regime of isometric muscle contraction throughout the period of immobilization. Following immobilization there was a decrease in overall muscle bulk. The type I fibres were found to have atrophied selectively.

There are several possible explanations for the difference in findings of selective fibre atrophy between the two studies. Sargeant found mixed fibre atrophy, but compared the immobilized limb to the contralateral limb. Haggmark demonstrated selective type I fibre atrophy, but immobilized patients for a shorter period of time and had a regime of isometric muscle contractions that patients found very painful to perform. Thus the pain may have had an inhibitory influence on the type I fibres and the atrophy may have been due to pain and not immobilization.

Effect of immobilization on muscle strength

Immobilization is associated with a progressive decrease in muscle strength. Various authors report that the knee extensors show a decrease of around 25–30% in dynamic muscle strength after 14 days of immobilization, but decreases of 40–75% after immobilization up to 49 days. Similarly isometric strength decreases with immobilization. Reports of a decrease of 12–30% in isometric strength are made after 14 days of immobilization and of 45–80% decreases after 49 days of immobilization. These decreases in muscle strength are largely a function of the atrophy that occurs with immobilization.

Effect of disuse

Disuse may arise from immobilization following injury, after cerebral or spinal cord damage, through illness or through decreased postural activity such as bed rest. Irrespective of the cause, the highly active anti-gravity muscles will be most profoundly affected by disuse. These slow twitch muscles will rapidly exhibit extensive atrophy, if deprived of their normal stimulus from everyday activity. Disuse results in both muscle atrophy and decreases in muscle strength. Disuse or decreased use is easily detected by changes in the shape, volume and functional capacity of skeletal muscle. Within 14 days there is a decrease in both the number of myofibres and in the volumes of the myofibres. There is a decrease in the intensity of activity and a reduction in the oxidative capacity of the muscle. These changes cause a decrease in both muscle mass and muscle strength.

In the myofibres there is an increase in the intramuscular connective tissue volume relative to the overall volume of the myofibril and a decrease in the intramuscular capillary density. These changes are less severe than those seen where complete immobilization and disuse are combined.

The effect of muscle disuse will have greater impact than just on the muscle tissue itself. Normal muscle function is necessary for normal functioning and growth of other musculoskeletal tissues. For example, without the stresses placed upon it by the musculature, bone will decrease both its cortical thickness and mineral density; thus disuse and inactivity has the impact of inducing atrophy of both the muscles and the skeleton.

Many years of experimental studies have been conducted to investigate the effect of space travel using a suspended rat model. In these experiments rats are suspended in a body harness from a metal bar placed above the cage. The forelimbs are placed on a shelf for access to food and water, but the hind limbs are completely suspended and deprived of all weight-bearing stimuli. Within a few hours the rats cease to move their hind limbs, leaving them to hang in space. Scientists have demonstrated that there is a hierarchy in the order in which the muscles waste dependent on the proportion of slow postural muscles that each muscle comprises. Thus the soleus wastes faster than gastrocnemius, followed by plantaris, extensor digitorum longus and tibialis anterior. This wasting of the anti-gravity muscles is explained by a decrease in the fraction of the protein mass of the muscle synthesized each day, and an increase in the rate of protein breakdown after 3–5 days of suspension and unloading of the limbs. The degree of atrophy in disused muscle is affected by the amount of stretch that is applied to the muscle. Passive stretching applied to the muscle for 5 days can counteract some of the changes induced by disuse. In rats studied under experimental conditions, passive stretching of the soleus muscle for 3 days produced marked changes in protein turnover in both suspended and walking animals. These changes can be detected after as short a period of 6 hours after the imposition of stretch. Clinically, stretching one muscle group in a disused limb is unlikely to be helpful, as reducing the atrophy of an individual muscle is likely to be accompanied by an adverse effect on the antagonist muscles. It is more beneficial therefore to provide intermittent stretch to prevent atrophy in patients. The optimum duration and degree of stretch and the cycles it needs to be applied in to prevent disuse atrophy are not known.

Disuse results in both muscle atrophy and decreases in muscle strength. Animal studies demonstrate that when subject to conditions of disuse, muscle responds after a short, threshold period of no atrophy, with an initial rapid decrease in cross-sectional area and then slower progressive atrophy. In humans this response is more variable. The effect of 5 weeks' immobilization in a cast has been reported as producing decreases in cross-sectional area that range from nil to 25–30%. It has been suggested that when disuse is the result of injury, and not just immobilization, the atrophy response that follows is accelerated.

Effect of stretch on muscle

When a muscle is stretched the stretch reflex mechanism is initiated. Stretching a muscle lengthens both the muscle fibres (extrafusal fibres) and the muscle spindles (intrafusal fibres). Deformation in the muscle spindles results in the initiation of the stretch reflex, which contracts the muscle. This stretch effect has a tonic and a phasic component. A tonic reflex is such as those found when trying to initiate a knee jerk response by hitting the patellar tendon. The tapping of the patellar tendon stretched muscle spindles located in parallel to the fibres being stretched within the tendon. Firing of the primary muscle afferents is increased, sent to the spinal cord and brain and an efferent response sent to the quadriceps causing them to contract and take the tension off the muscle spindles.

The tonic stretch component initiates a reflex in response to stretch of secondary afferents, causing the contraction of anti-gravity muscles in response to such stimuli as a shift in centre of gravity.

Applied stretch to a muscle can be effective at counteracting the changes in muscle connective tissue and sarcomere number that occur after immobilization. Normally, a reduction in muscle compliance is found after both immobilization or a period of prolonged bed rest in the presence of joint disease. The problem of the deleterious effect on the antagonist muscle

group prevents the use of immobilization in a lengthened position as a strategy for preventing the muscle tightness that occurs after immobilization. Williams studied the effect of intermittent stretch on immobilized muscle. In an animal model the soleus muscle of a mouse was immobilized in a cast in a shortened position for a period of 10 days. Every 2 days the cast was removed and the muscle passively stretched for a period of 15 minutes. This prevented the connective changes normally seen when muscle is immobilized in a shortened position, but did not prevent reduction in muscle fibre length, resulting in considerable loss of range of motion at the foot. Changes to the experimental design so that daily sessions of 30 minutes stretching were applied prevented both loss of serial sarcomeres and connective tissue remodelling and enabled a normal range of motion to be retained.

Stretching may be used to try and prevent injury occurring during activity. Repeated stretching to a specific length results in small increases in muscle length and corresponding decreases in tension. At the wrist the increase in the length of extensor digitorum longus increased by approximately 3% between the first two stretches. This has the effect of reducing the load on the muscle-tendon units, i.e. the muscle-tendon unit would have to be stretched to a greater length in order to achieve the tension necessary to cause damage.

When a tissue is exposed to a passive force (stretch) it will deform according to its material properties and in the presence of sustained stretch can be expected to deform in a time-dependent manner. This behaviour is called 'creep' and reflects the viscoelastic properties of the tissue. When the force is no longer applied the tissue will return to its original length in a time-dependent manner (relaxation). Increased range of motion following passive stretching can be explained by the viscoelastic behaviour of muscle and by short-term changes in muscle extensibility. Clinical tests of passive stretching have demonstrated that mobility gained with stretch-based rehabilitation protocols are maintained after the stretch is removed, suggesting that a permanent adaptive response is possible. Other authors disagree and argue that any changes are only temporary and that permanent effects can only be achieved by prolonged stretching such as by specific orthoses or serial casts.

Effect of distraction on muscle

Orthopaedic techniques such as leg lengthening using distraction osteogenesis subject the muscle to gradual incremental imposed increases in length. Although different tissues react to distraction in different ways, they all involve two predominant mechanisms: reorganization of collagen in response to stretch and neohistogenesis. Ilizarov demonstrated that muscle would proliferate in response to a sustained distraction force. Using metal clips to mark the length change in different parts of the distracted muscle and fascia in a canine limb, he found that with up to 20% lengthening of the bone, the new tissue was distributed along the total length of the muscle and fascia. Ilizarov stated that under experimental conditions parts of the distracted muscle developed an identical appearance ultrastructurally as embryonic muscle tissue. He postulated that, like bone, soft tissues responded to tension–stress distraction by forming new tissue, not by simply stretching.

Simpson and co-workers lengthened the tibias of New Zealand white rabbits in twice daily increments. They found that new contractile tissue formed during lengthening but that damage to muscle fibres occurred at rates of distraction as low as 1 mm/day. There was proliferation of fibrous tissue between the muscle fibres at distraction rates of over 1 mm/day. Schumacher and co-workers lengthened the tibia of New Zealand white rabbits and compared them to a control group. The nuclei of the tibialis anterior muscle in the proliferative phase were evaluated and found to demonstrate a significant increase in the weight of the lengthened muscle and in the number of proliferating cell nuclei compared with a control group. This response was observed only during the lengthening period and ceased when the lengthening was stopped. The authors concluded that muscle cell proliferation occurred only during the distraction phase of limb lengthening and agreed with Ilizarov that stretch was the major stimulus for longitudinal muscle growth. However, there is a limit to the amount of distraction that muscle tissue can tolerate. Kyberd and co-workers distracted rabbit tibiae by 20%. They found evidence of muscle damage including the presence of internal nuclei, necrosis, thickening of the perimysial connective tissue and enlargement of muscle fibres. Other researchers have also reported histopathological changes such as endomysial fibrosis and internalization of nuclei after 20% lengthenings, which may suggest irreversible muscle damage.

Effect of strength training/exercise on muscle

Muscle fibres respond to exercise by hypertrophy. Fast twitch muscle fibres are recruited relatively infrequently for short-lasting power movements. If they are selectively trained by recruitment and overloading, for example in weight lifting, they readily hypertrophy. Slow fibres may also increase in size as a result of training, but to a lesser extent than fast fibres.

When muscle tissue is repetitively loaded or trained it responds by producing an increased number of mitochondria and oxidative enzymes. There will also be an increase in the number of capillaries per muscle fibre. These responses give the muscle increased resistance to fatigue and an increased aerobic power output. McDonagh reports that a threshold of 66% of the maximum that a person can lift exists, below this level dynamic strength training will not induce increases in isometric strength. Rapid responses can be made with progressive high resistance strength training. Increases of up to 3% per day have been documented. Training results in increases in muscle fibre size, rather than an increase in the number of muscle fibres during normal training loads. There is a parallel addition of myofilaments to myofibrils, causing the muscle fibres to become larger in cross-sectional area. As the intrinsic tension-generating capacity of the muscle is directly related to the muscle cross-sectional area, hypertrophy will result in gains in both muscle size and muscle strength. Increases in muscle cross-sectional area are usually smaller than the accompanying gains in muscle strength. In a study on older men a 117% increase in dynamic strength was accompanied by a 10% increase in cross-sectional muscle area. This would indicate that training-induced strength increases are not only due to adaptations to the muscle itself. Some of the increase in strength may be accounted for by a motor learning effect, or neural adaptation as subjects learn to recruit motor units more effectively or more completely.

Use of isometric muscle training to prevent disuse atrophy

Isometric muscle training has been advocated to try to counteract the effect of immobilization in a cast during fracture repair/tissue healing. A number of clinical trials have been conducted investigating the effect on muscle strength post-immobilization. One study reported that the decrease in muscle strength after immobilization was 30% less in a group of patients that performed isometric muscle contractions compared with those who did no exercises. Patients were allocated to no exercise or to perform ten repetitions of a 10 second isometric contraction of the quadriceps throughout the day. On testing of the patients 10 RM (the maximum load a patient could lift 10 times), the isometric exercise group demonstrated a significantly greater mean strength and greater isometric strength.

In studies of subjects on bed rest who followed specific exercise protocols, high resistance training was effective at preventing muscle wasting. The frequency of exercise is an important factor. In one study five sets of 6–10 repetitions to failure of constant resistance concentric and eccentric plantarflexion performed alternate days for 14 days of bed rest was effective at preventing any decline in torque or power when plantarflexion was tested using an isokinetic dynamometer. However, the training has to be specific to the muscle that is to be tested. During 14 days of bed rest subjects performed 5 sets of leg press exercises to fatigue every other day. Before and after the period of bed rest, an isokinetic concentric–eccentric knee extension protocol was used to test extensor strength. Over the period of bed rest angle-specific power values dropped by 20%, and no differences were seen between the group of subjects who exercised whilst on bed rest and a control group who followed a regime of bed rest alone.

Summary of clinical implications

Decreased use of skeletal muscle whether induced by immobilization or disease results in decreases in muscle mass, structure and strength. Immobilization by a cast induces decreases in muscle protein synthesis within 6 hours of the cast application. After as little as 10 days of immobilization muscle fibres will show a decrease in size and myofibrils will be lost. As the myofibrils degenerate, fibrous tissue and fat become a progressively larger proportion of the tissue. If muscles are immobilized in a shortened or lengthened position, they will adapt to a position at which they can achieve the optimum tension-generating properties by either increasing or decreasing the number of sarcomeres in series in the muscle fibre.

Increases in use, or training will result in changes to the structure, size and functional capacity of a muscle. Different patterns of muscle training induce different responses. Low tension, high repetition use primarily increases muscle endurance, whilst high tension, low repetition training increases muscle strength. There is limited evidence that stretching programmes can counteract the effect of muscle shortening after immobilization if the stretch is sustained for a sufficient period. Stretching may also be used to accelerate muscle protein turnover, causing hypertrophy and increases in strength.

REFERENCES AND FURTHER READING

Bone

Aronson J (1997) Limb lengthening, skeletal reconstruction and bone transport with the Ilizarov method. J Bone Joint Surg [Am]. 79-A: 1243–1258.

Bamman MM, Caruso JE (2000) Resistance exercise counter measures for space flight: implications of training specificity. J Strength Cond Res 14: 45–49.

Bamman MM, Hunter GR, Stevens BR, Guilliams ME, Greenisen MC (1997) Resistance exercise prevents plantar flexor deconditioning during bed rest. Med Sci Sports Exerc 29: 1462–1468.

Calbert JA, Moysi JS, Dorado C, Rodriguez LP (1998) Bone mineral content and density in professional tennis players. Calcif Tissue Int 62: 491–496.

Cornwall MW (1984) Biomechanics of noncontractile tissue: A review. Phys Ther 64: 1869–1873.

Goodship AE, Lanyon LE, McFie H (1979) Functional adaptation of bone to increased stress. J Bone Joint Surg 61-A: 539–546.

Ilizarov GA (1990) Clinical application of the tension-stress effect on the genesis and growth for limb lengthening. Clin Orthop. 250: 8–26.

Kazarian LE, Von Gierke HE (1967) Bone loss as a result of immobilisation and chelation. Preliminary results in *Macaca mulatta*. Clin Orthop 65: 67–75.

Kenwright J, Goodship AE (1989) Controlled mechanical stimulation in the treatment of tibial fractures. Clin Orthop 241: 36–47.

Kenwright J, Richardson JB, Goodship AE, et al. (1986) Effect of controlled axial micromovement on healing of tibial fractures. Lancet ii: 1185–1187.

Nordin M, Frankel VH (1989) Basic Biomechanics of the Skeletal System, 2nd edn. Philadelphia, PA: Lea and Febiger.

Sarmiento A (1967) A functional below-the-knee cast for tibial fractures. J Bone Joint Surg 49-A: 855–875.

Tetsworth K, Paley D (1995) Basic science of distraction histogenesis. Curr Opin Orthop 6: 61–68.

Turner CH (1998) Three rules for bone adaptation to mechanical stimuli. Bone 23: 399–407.

Uhthoff HK, Jaworski ZFG (1978) Bone loss in response to long term immobilisation. J Bone Joint Surg 60-B: 420–429.

Cartilage

Bell DF (1994) The effect of limb lengthening on articular cartilage: an experimental study. Clin Orthop 301: 68.

Buckwater JA, Rosenberg LC, Hunziker E (1990) Articular cartilage: composition, structure, response to injury and methods of facilitating repair. In: Ewing JW (ed.) The Science of Arthroscopy. New York: Raven Press, pp. 19–56.

Cornwall MW (1984) Biomechanics of noncontractile tissue: A review. Phys Ther 64:1869–1873.

Culaw EM, Clark CH, Merrilees MJ (1999) Connective tissues. Matrix composition and its relevance to physical therapy. Phys Ther 79: 308–319.

Helminen HJ, Kirviranta I, Tammi M, et al. (eds) (1987) Joint Loading – Biology and Health of Articular Structures. Bristol: John Wright.

Houlbrooke K, Vause K, Merrilees MJ (1990) Effects of movement and weightbearing on the glycosaminoglycan content of sheep articular cartilage. Aust J Physiother 36: 88–91.

McPherson JM, Tubo R (2000) Articular cartilage injury. In: Lanza RP, Langer R, Vacanti J (eds) Principles of Tissue Engineering. San Diego: Academic Press.

Palmoski M, Perricone E, Brandt KD (1979) Development and reversal of a proteoglycan aggregation defect in normal canine knee cartilage after immobilisation. Arthritis Rheum 22: 508–517.

Palmoski MJ, Colyer RA, Brandt KD (1980) Joint motion in the absence of loading does not maintain normal articular cartilage. Arthritis Rheum 23: 325–334.

Salter RB (1993) Continuous Passive Motion. Baltimore: Williams & Wilkins.

Sood SC (1971) A study of the effects of experimental immobilisation on rabbit articular cartilage. J Anat 108: 497–507.

Stanitski DF, Rossman K, Torosian M (1996) The effect of femoral lengthening on knee articular cartilage: The role of apparatus extension across the joint. J Paediatr Orthop 16: 151–154.

Vanwanseele B, Lucchinetti E, Stussi E (2002) The effects of immobilization on the characteristics of articular cartilage: current concepts and future directions. Osteoarthritis Cartilage 10: 408–419.

Joints

Akeson WH, Woo SL-Y, Amiel D, Matthews JV (1974) Biomechanical and biochemical changes in the periarticular connective tissue during contracture development in the immobilised rabbit knee. Connect Tissue Res 2: 315–323.

Akeson WH, Amiel D, Woo SL (1980) Immobility effects on synovial joints. The pathomechanics of joint contracture. Biorheology 17: 95–110.

Beaupre LA, Davies DM, Jones CA, Cinats JG (2001) Exercise combined with continuous passive motion or slider board therapy compared with exercise only: a randomised controlled trial of patients following total knee arthroplasty. Phys Ther 81: 1029–1037.

Buckwalter JA (1996) Effects of early motion on healing of musculoskeletal tissues. Hand Clin North Am 12: 13–24.

Davies DM, Johnston DW, Beaupre LA, Lier DA (2003) Effect of adjunctive range of motion therapy after primary total knee arthroplasty on the use of health services after hospital discharge. Can J Surg 46: 30–36.

Duong B, Low M, Moseley AM, Lee RY, Herbert RD (2001) Time course of stress relaxation and recovery in human ankles. Clin Biomech 16: 601–607.

Enneking WF, Horowitz M (1972) The intra-articular effects of immobilization on the human knee. J Bone Joint Surg 54-A: 973.

Farmer S, James M (2001) Contractures in orthopaedic and neurological conditions: a review of causes and treatment. Disabil Rehabil 23: 549–558.

Gelberman RH, Botte MJ, Spriegelman JJ, Akeson WH (1986) The excursion and deformation of repaired flexor tendons treated with protected early motion. J Hand Surg (Am). 11-A: 106–110.

Harburn KL, Potter PJ (1993) Spasticity and contractures. Phys Med Rehabil State of the Art Rev 7: 113–132.

Harvey L, Herbert R, Crosbie J (2002) Does stretching induce lasting increases in joint ROM? A systematic review. Physiother Res Int 7: 1–13.

Herbert R (1993) Preventing and treating stiff joints. In: Crosbie J, McConnell J (eds) Key Issues in Musculoskeletal Physiotherapy. Oxford: Butterworth Heinemann, pp. 120–122.

Lau SK, Chiu KY (2001) Use of continuous passive motion after total knee arthroplasty. J Arthroplasty 16: 336–339.

Light KE, Nuzik S, Personius W, Barstrom A (1984) Low-load prolonged stretch vs high-load brief stretch in treating knee contractures. Phys Ther 64: 330–333.

MacDonald SJ, Bourne RB, Rorabeck CH, et al. (2000) Prospective randomised clinical trial of continuous passive motion after total knee arthroplasty. Clin Orthop 380: 30–35.

Maitland GD (1991) Peripheral Manipulation, 3rd edn. Oxford: Butterworth Heinemann, pp. 85–97.

Noyes FR (1977) Functional properties of knee ligaments and alterations induced by immobilization: a correlative biomechanical and histological study in primates. Clin Orthop 123: 210–242.

Romness DW, Rand JA (1988) The role of continuous passive motion following total knee arthroplasty. Clin Orthop 226: 34–37.

Steffen TM, Mollinger LA (1995) Low-load prolonged stretch in the treatment of knee flexion contractures in nursing home residents. Phys Ther 75: 895–897.

Strickland JW (1987) Biological basis for hand splinting. In: Fess EE, Phillips CA (eds) Hand Splinting Principles and Methods. St Louis: CV Mosby.

Trudel G, Uhthoff HK (2000) Contractures secondary to immobility: is the restriction articular or muscular? An experimental longitudinal study in the rat knee. Arch Phys Med Rehab 81: 6–12.

Warren GC, Lehmann JF, Koblanski JM (1976) Heat and stretch procedures: An evaluation using rat nail tendon. Arch Phys Med Rehabil 57: 481–487.

Woo SL, Gomez MA, Woo YK, Akeson WH (1982) Mechanical properties of tendons and ligaments, II: the relationships of immobilisation and exercise on tissue remodelling. Biorheology 19: 397–408.

Muscle

Alter MJ (1988) Science of Stretching. Champaign, IL: Human Kinetics Publishers.

Booth FW (1977) Time course of muscular atrophy during immobilisation of hindlimbs in rats. J Appl Physiol 43: 656–661.

De Deyne PG (2001) Application of passive stretch and its implications for muscle fibres. Phys Ther 81: 819–827.

Goldspink G, Williams P (1990) Muscle fibre and connective tissue changes associated with use and disuse. In: Ada L, Canning C (eds) Key Issues in Neurological Physiotherapy. Oxford: Butterworth Heinemann.

Haggmark T, Jansson E, Erikson E (1981) Fiber type, area metabolic potential of the thigh muscle in man after knee surgery and immobilisation. Int J Sports Med 2: 12–17.

Herbert R (1988) The passive mechanical properties of muscle and their adaptations to altered patterns of use. Aust J Physio 34: 141–148.

Herbert R (1990) Human strength adaptations – implications for therapy. In: Ada L, Canning C (eds) Key Issues in Neurological Physiotherapy. Butterworth Heinemann.

Herbert R, Balnave RJ (1993) The effect of position of immobilisation on resting length, resting stiffness and weight of the soleus muscle of the rabbit. J Orthop Res 11: 358–366.

Huxley HE (1969) The mechanism of muscular contraction. Science 164: 1356.

Ilizarov GA (1991) Transosseous Osteosynthesis. Theoretical and Clinical Aspects of the Regeneration and Growth of Tissue. New York: Springer-Verlag

Ilizarov GA (1997) The principles of the Ilizarov method. Bull Hosp Jt Dis 56: 49–53.

Ingemann-Hansen T, Halkjaer-Kristensen J (1980) Computerised tomographic determination of human thigh components. The effects of immobilisation in plaster and subsequent physical training. Scand J Rehabil Med 12: 27–31.

Kyberd PJ, Williams PE, Simpson AHRW, Goldspink G, Kenwright J (1994) The response of mammalian muscle to distraction – a study in the rabbit. Proc Instn Mech Engrs 208: 111–118.

Lowe DA, Always SE (2002) Animal models for inducing muscle hypertrophy: are they relevant for clinical applications in humans? J Orthop Sports Phys Ther 32: 36–43.

McDonagh MJ, Davies CT (1984) Adaptive responses of mammalian skeletal muscle to exercise with high loads. Eur J Appl Physiol Occup Physiol 52: 139–155.

Rose SJ, Rothstein JM (1982) Muscle mutability. Part 1: General concepts and adaptations to altered patterns of use. Phys Ther 62: 1773–1787.

Sargeant AJ, Davies CTM, Edwards RHT, et al. (1977) Functional and structural changes after disuse of human muscle. Clin Sci Mol Med 52: 337–342.

Schumacher B, Keller J, Hvid I (1994) Distraction effects on muscle. Acta Orthop Scand 65: 647–650.

Simpson AHRW, Williams PE, Kyberd P, Goldspink G, Kenwright J (1995) The response of muscle to leg lengthening. J Bone Joint Surg [Br] 77-B: 630–636.

Thompson LV (2002) Skeletal muscle adaptations with age, inactivity and therapeutic exercise. J Orthop Sports Phys Ther 32: 44–57.

Warren GL, Ingalls CP, Lowe DA, Armstrong RB (2002) What mechanisms contribute to the strength loss that occurs during and in the recovery from skeletal muscle injury? J Orthop Sports Phys Ther 32: 58–64.

Williams PE (1988) Effect of intermittent stretch on immobilised muscle. Ann Rheum Dis 47: 1014–1016.

Williams PE (1990) Use of intermittent stretch in the prevention of serial sarcomere loss in immobilised muscles. Ann Rheum Dis 49: 316.

Altered Exercise Tolerance: Cardiovascular Rehabilitation

Angela J. Woodiwiss

INTRODUCTION

Physiotherapists are an integral part of the team of health-care professionals involved in the management of patients with diseases of the cardiovascular system, including coronary heart disease, heart failure and hypertension. The various disorders of the cardiovascular system are defined and their pathophysiology discussed in Chapter 12.1 (Cardiovascular Disorders).

Most patients with cardiovascular disorders benefit from some form of habitual exercise, not only with respect to improved fitness (exercise tolerance) but also from the important lifestyle, dietary and psychological changes which accompany regular physical activity. Throughout this chapter the term physical activity implies *aerobic* (isotonic or endurance) exercise. The benefits of *anaerobic* (isometric or resistance) exercise (performed in moderation) will be discussed separately at the end of this chapter.

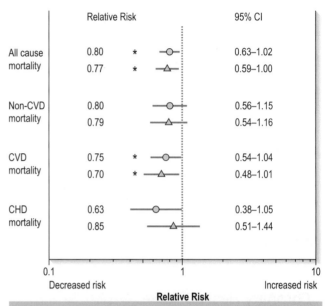

Figure 9.1.1. The effects of physical activity on relative risk of mortality in persons with moderate versus lowest (●) and highest versus lowest (▲) physical activity. Values are adjusted for age, baseline disease and lifestyle factors including cigarette smoking and alcohol consumption. CVD, cardiovascular disease; CHD, coronary heart disease; CI, confidence interval; *$p < 0.05$. (Data from Bijnen et al., 1998.)

General benefits from physical activity in patients with cardiovascular disease

Physiological:	Establish neurohormonal balance to conserve oxygen for myocardium. Alter heart rate and blood pressure to decrease work of myocardium. Enhance contractility of the myocardium. Improve myocardial circulation and metabolism.
Dietary:	Normalize blood lipid profile. Establish more favourable blood clotting characteristics. Establish more favourable body composition.
Psychological:	Provide favourable outlet for stress and tension.

The benefits of physical activity collectively contribute toward primary and secondary prevention of cardiovascular diseases by reducing risk factors. Hence the benefits of physical activity in persons with cardiovascular disease include a reduction in cardiovascular mortality, reduction in symptoms, improvements in exercise tolerance and functional capacity and improvements in psychological well-being and quality of life.

Over the past 10 years there has been a major international focus on both the risks and benefits of exercise, as well as on the relationship between physical activity and cardiovascular health in all age groups. Based on data from more than 40 epidemiological studies, physical inactivity and a sedentary lifestyle are recognized as major risk factors for the development of coronary heart disease, adverse cardiovascular events and mortality from cardiovascular diseases. Physical inactivity is directly associated with increased mortality from cardiovascular disease, in that the increase in mortality is evident even after correction for the association between cardiovascular disease and lifestyle factors including smoking, elevated blood pressure and alcohol consumption (Figs 9.1.1 and 9.1.2). Thus regular aerobic exercise, regardless of whether it is occupational or leisure time activity, confers many health benefits from both a primary and a secondary preventative perspective. Furthermore, as regular physical activity reduces symptoms associated with the various cardiovascular diseases, its benefits can also be perceived as therapeutic. Given that currently 44% of all deaths in the European Union are attributed to cardiovascular diseases and that <20% of the adult population partake in regular sustained physical activity (30 minutes of exercise at any intensity, 5 times per week), it is imperative that patients with cardiovascular disease partake in physical activity programmes.

In order to encourage physical activity in patients with cardiac diseases, specific cardiac rehabilitation programmes have been developed. Cardiac rehabilitation is regarded as a long-term process which includes all the requirements of good patient care. A rehabilitation programme thus includes concern

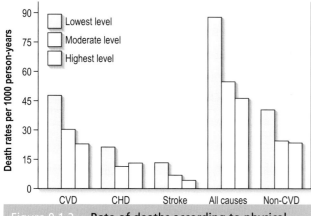

Figure 9.1.2. Rate of deaths according to physical activity level. (Data from Bijnen *et al.*, 1998.)

for both the patient's physiological and psychological status. This is best summarized by the definition of rehabilitation given by the European Office of the World Health Organization (WHO Regional Office for Europe, 1969):

The rehabilitation of cardiac patients can be defined as the sum of activities required to ensure them the best possible physical, mental and social conditions so that they may, by their own efforts, resume as normal a place as possible in the life of the community.

Requirements of good patient care

- Accurate assessment of each patient's physiological and emotional limitations and potentials at periodic intervals using objective tests.
- Continuous education of patients as regards diet and lifestyle modification, as well as the benefit of regular physical exercise.
- Well-supervised programmes of physical activity.
- Awareness of day-to-day interactions of the patient with his disease, physician, spouse and family, and how his occupation may influence the success or failure of rehabilitation.

Importantly the reported reductions in mortality have been highest (approximately 25%) in cardiac rehabilitation programmes that have included the control of cardiovascular risk factors other than physical inactivity. Thus it is imperative that cardiac rehabilitation programmes include patient education. The goal of cardiac rehabilitation is to aid the patient with cardiovascular disease to return rapidly to a normal or pre-illness lifestyle and to a productive, active and satisfying role in society. Hence a successful rehabilitation programme will enable the individual to enjoy life to the fullest physical and mental capacity (with due allowances for

impairments) and most importantly it will include vigorous efforts to reverse or to prevent the progression of the underlying disease process.

The focus of this chapter is to provide the reader with:

1. the justifications for encouraging people with cardiovascular diseases to exercise regularly
2. insights into the mechanisms of the benefits of various types of regular activity
3. guidelines for exercise prescriptions
4. important precautions and restrictions (recommendations) pertaining to specific cardiovascular disease entities.

These four topics will be discussed separately for the three main cardiovascular disease entities for which exercise therapy is currently recommended, namely:

- coronary heart disease
- chronic heart failure
- hypertension.

CORONARY HEART DISEASE

In the term coronary heart disease (CHD) are included:

- coronary artery disease (CAD)
- myocardial ischaemia (MI)
- percutaneous transluminal angioplasty (PTCA)
- coronary artery bypass graft (CABG) surgery.

These entities and their pathophysiology are discussed in Chapter 12.1.

Justifications for encouraging regular exercise

Persons with coronary artery disease experience a gradual decline in their degree of fitness because they are unwilling and possibly afraid to exercise owing to the signs and symptoms (angina, dyspnoea and fatigue) of their disease. However, a reduction in physical activity leads to worsening of fatigue, a decline in effort tolerance and more difficulty experienced whilst performing physical activities, which in turn results in a person further reducing the amount of activity performed. A break in this vicious cycle (Fig. 9.1.3) is thus vitally important.

In the early phase after acute myocardial infarction (MI), percutaneous transluminal angioplasty (PTCA) or coronary artery bypass graft (CABG) surgery, muscular, neuromuscular and cardiovascular functions deteriorate due to inactivity. Consequently, a person's exercise tolerance declines and eventually their ability to perform activities of regular daily living is compromised. In other words, a similar vicious cycle to that described above for patients with coronary artery disease would occur if rehabilitation was not commenced.

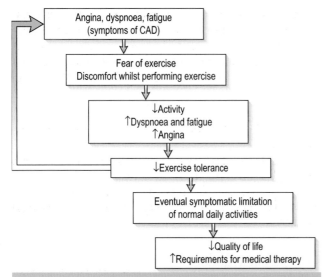

Figure 9.1.3.   Flow diagram depicting the progressive changes that occur in the absence of intervention in persons with coronary artery disease (CAD).

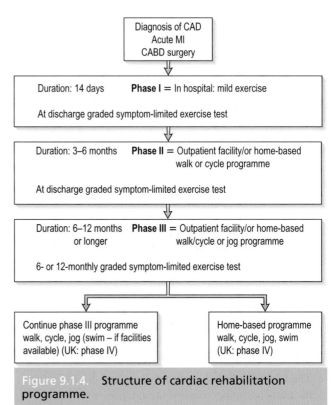

Figure 9.1.4.   Structure of cardiac rehabilitation programme.

Rehabilitation after acute MI, PTCA or CABG surgery consists of three phases (Fig. 9.1.4):

- *phase I*: low-level physical activity = in hospital
- *phase II*: intermediate level of physical activity = after discharge and prior to phase III
- *phase III*: high-level physical activity = 3 to 6 months after hospitalization

In the UK rehabilitation consists of four phases, the above three phases followed by phase IV, which is a long-term maintenance phase. Elsewhere in the world phase IV is considered as part of or an extension of phase III (Fig. 9.1.4).

In addition to the exercise component, rehabilitation programmes also include an important patient-education component. Education programmes are primarily designed to:

1. allay a patient's fears and concerns related to their disease and its associated symptoms
2. assist patients to deal with their disease
3. promote lifestyle changes.

The education programmes run parallel with the exercise programmes within each of the phases. In essence phase I education comprises all three components, whereas phase II and III aim to reinforce and reiterate education, especially in terms of lifestyle changes to promote secondary prevention of disease.

The specific benefits and thus the justification for each of these phases of rehabilitation will be discussed, as well as the possible mechanisms of these benefits. With respect to rehabilitation in patients with coronary artery disease, these three phases are generally followed depending on the patient's initial level of fitness. That is, if a patient is severely debilitated

they would begin exercise according to a phase I programme, whereas fitter patients are more likely to commence exercise according to phase II or III guidelines.

Phase I

Forty years ago convalescence after MI or CABG surgery comprised several weeks of complete bed rest. Currently, after diagnosis of CAD if severe, and following acute MI or CABG surgery, early ambulation or mobilization is advised and is generally begun in the intensive care unit. This involves a low-level physical activity programme consisting mainly of personal care activities, and flexibility and range of motion exercises (for details see 'Guidelines for exercise prescriptions').

Benefits, their mechanisms and hence justification of phase I programme

Moving a patient from the bed to a chair is important as external cardiac work is less in the seated than in the supine position. Thus stress on the heart is transiently reduced whilst sitting. This reduction in workload on the heart is beneficial for cardiac repair in the first few days after MI or CABG surgery. Activity limits the hypovolaemia of protracted bed rest and the resulting orthostasis. Furthermore, even low-level exercise limits the deterioration in oxygen transport capacity and effort tolerance that occurs during sedentary periods of even one week. The incidence of pulmonary atelectasis and thromboembolic complications is reduced in patients who are mobile in comparison to those who remain sedentary. Early activity thus prevents further deconditioning and disability and improves functional status of the patient at the time of discharge. In addition, physical activity results in a reduction in anxiety and depression. Because many psychotropic drugs may have adverse cardiovascular effects (particularly on heart rate (HR), blood pressure (BP) and cardiac rhythm), the reassurance offered by progressive physical activity, which improves the patient's self-confidence and self-image, is an important approach to limiting psychological complications and hence the need for psychotropic medications. Phase I programmes substantially improve recovery after acute MI or CABG surgery and contribute to a more rapid and more complete return of patients to work. In addition, phase I programmes facilitate the current trend to earlier hospital discharge with its associated savings in medical care costs and potentially improved usage of hospital beds.

Summary of benefits of phase I programmes
- ↓ external cardiac work
- ↓ hypovolaemia and orthostasis
- ↓ deterioration of oxygen transport
- ↓ deterioration in effort tolerance
- ↓ risk of pulmonary atelectasis and thromboembolic complications
- ↓ anxiety and depression
- ↑ functional status.

Phase II
The main purpose of phase II programmes is to continue the prevention of deconditioning during the completion of the recovery process. Thus, such programmes bridge the gap between phase I (low-level activity) and phase III (relatively high-level activity) rehabilitation programmes. At the end of the phase II rehabilitation programme a *symptom-limited maximal graded exercise test* is performed to evaluate the current status of the patient in terms of conditioning. This test serves to assess whether a patient is ready to make the transition from a phase II to a phase III rehabilitation programme (for more details see 'Guidelines for exercise prescriptions').

Phase III
It is currently accepted by physicians and cardiologists that patients be referred to long-term (phase III) rehabilitation programmes from 3 to 6 months post MI or post CABG surgery. In addition most patients diagnosed as having CAD are referred to phase III programmes because of the long-term general benefits which slow down the progression of disease (secondary prevention). The phase III rehabilitation programme is usually conducted at a community centre or recreation hall under the supervision of specifically trained medical and allied medical personnel. Patients are generally required to attend supervised exercise sessions at least three times per week.

Exercise consists of walking and/or jogging at a particular level appropriate for each patient. Exercise intensity is prescribed according to HR, which is easy for patients to monitor themselves and thus ensure that they maintain their prescribed exercise intensity (for more details see 'Guidelines for exercise prescriptions').

Benefits, their mechanisms and hence justification of phase III programme
The benefits of phase III programmes are fairly extensive. The responses to training in patients with CAD, MI or CABG surgery include changes in psychological status and metabolic parameters, as well as a large variety of physiological adaptations to training.

Psychological benefits
Both short- and long-term psychological changes have been demonstrated in patients with CHD taking part in a rehabilitation programme. Initially these patients were significantly more tense, aloof, fickle and emotional than healthy individuals; but after a single day of training, they became more ambitious, self-assertive and relaxed than a group of sedentary patients with CHD. Decreases in anxiety and fear have also been reported after exercise training. Self-confidence is increased, a more balanced emotional stability is achieved and socio-economic status is improved as a consequence of the effects of improved psychological status on work performance. In addition, the emotional responses to sudden unexpected psychological stresses are lessened. This effect is important as such emotional triggers have been associated with worsening angina and acute MI.

Summary of psychological benefits
- enhanced feelings of energy, enthusiasm and well-being
- decreased depression
- enhanced self-image
- less 'strain' resulting from psychological 'stress'
- better relaxation and sleep
- more satisfactory sexual responses
- less craving for stimulants and tranquillizers.

Effects of training on metabolic parameters
The effects of physical activity on metabolic parameters in cardiac patients are an important consideration as metabolic parameters such as blood cholesterol levels are cardiovascular risk factors. Other metabolic parameters, such as blood lactate, are important indicators of fitness level.

1. Blood lipids and lipoproteins. Elevated levels of blood cholesterol have been identified as a primary causal agent in the pathogenesis of CAD. However, the different forms in which cholesterol is transported in the blood are more critical in the development of CAD than total cholesterol itself. High levels of *high density lipoprotein cholesterol* (HDL-cholesterol) seem to lower the incidence of CAD; whereas elevated levels of *low density lipoprotein cholesterol* (LDL-cholesterol) are related to a higher incidence of CAD. Results of the Lipid Research Clinics Programme (1984) have shown that the lowering of total cholesterol and LDL-cholesterol levels through medication and diet decreases the incidence of death from CAD by 24% and of non-fatal MI by 19% compared to a placebo group. LDL-cholesterol may contribute to CAD by its ability to infiltrate the arterial intima (inner lining) and thus cholesterol is deposited on the endothelium of the artery. This results in narrowing of the arterial lumen and finally extensive arterial occlusion. Conversely, HDL-cholesterol may exert its protective effect by transporting cholesterol away from the arterial wall to the liver for catabolism and excretion (see Ch. 12.1).

Differences in the reported effects of training studies on blood cholesterol may be the result of variations in the characteristics of subjects, the type of exercise training programmes, measurement procedures or control group selection. However, in a statistical analysis of the summary findings of many studies, it was found that on average total cholesterol decreased by 10 mg/dl, total *triglycerides* (TG) dropped by 15.8 mg/dl, HDL-cholesterol increased by 1.2 mg/dl, LDL-cholesterol decreased by 5.1 mg/dl and the ratio of total cholesterol to HDL-cholesterol declined by 0.48 mg/dl. A positive relationship was noted between the magnitude of the above changes and initial lipid levels, age, frequency of exercise training, duration of the exercise training programme, loss of body weight and loss of body fat during training.

The primary and secondary protective effect of habitual physical activity on the development of CAD is thus in part related to the effect it has on blood lipid levels. Total cholesterol, TG and LDL-cholesterol levels are generally lowered by regular participation in a physical exercise training programme, whereas HDL-cholesterol is increased. Physical activity has been shown to favourably modify abnormalities in lipid concentrations in patients with CHD and thus to decrease the rate of progression of coronary atherosclerosis. The changes in lipid profile are strongly associated with dietary changes and loss of body weight subsequent to exercise training.

2. Blood lactate. The measurement of blood lactate (lactic acid) concentration at increasing levels of exercise gives an indication of an individual's level of fitness. From these measurements the lactate turn point or *onset of blood lactate accumulation* (OBLA) can be determined. The lactate turn point or OBLA is the percentage of *maximum oxygen consumption* (V_{O_2max}, for a description of what a V_{O_2max} test involves see 'Maximum oxygen consumption test' box) or *peak* V_{O_2} (symptom-limited maximal V_{O_2}), at which the lactate concentration begins to rise rapidly. At lower work intensities there is no detectable increase in lactic acid concentration, since lactic acid production is balanced by its

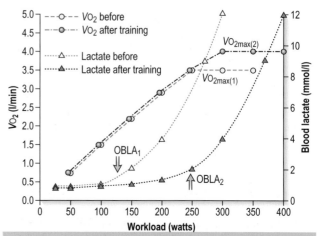

Figure 9.1.5. Graph showing the relationship between V_{O_2} and workload, and blood lactate concentrations and workload. $V_{O_2max(1)}$ is the V_{O_2max} achieved before training and $V_{O_2max(2)}$ is the V_{O_2max} achieved after a period of exercise training. OBLA$_1$ (OBLA before training) occurs at about 50% of $V_{O_2max(1)}$ and OBLA$_2$ (OBLA after exercise training) occurs at about 88% of $V_{O_2max(2)}$.

removal. However, at higher workloads lactic acid is produced at a greater rate than it can be removed, which results in an increase in lactic acid concentration in the blood. In a sedentary person, the lactate turn point occurs at about 40 to 55% of V_{O_2max}, whereas in highly trained individuals lactate only starts to increase at 75 to 90% or more of V_{O_2max} (Fig. 9.1.5). Thus, the fitter an individual becomes, the greater the intensity of exercise he or she can perform without a marked increase in lactic acid concentration. Through physical exercise training it is possible to shift the lactate turn point to the right, thereby extending the scope of aerobic metabolism. As occurs in normal healthy individuals, in patients with CHD the lactate concentration increases significantly less during exercise following even 4 to 6 weeks of exercise training. In other words, the lactate concentration in these patients is significantly less at both a submaximal workload and a symptom-limited maximal workload (peak V_{O_2}) after a period of exercise training.

Maximum oxygen consumption test (V_{O_2max})

The maximum oxygen consumption test (V_{O_2max}) is a test of endurance or fitness. V_{O_2max} is the maximum amount of oxygen in millilitres that a person can use in one minute per kilogram of body weight. Although values of V_{O_2max} are largely genetically determined, they can be modified by exercise training. Fitter individuals have higher V_{O_2max} values and can exercise more intensely than those who are less fit. Many studies show that $V_{O_{2max}}$ can be increased by exercising at an intensity of between 65 and 85% of maximum heart rate for at least 20 minutes, 3 to 5 times per week.

For a $V_{O_{2max}}$ test, exercise is usually performed on a treadmill (or sometimes a stationary cycle). The exercise workloads are selected to gradually progress in increments from moderate to maximal intensity exercise. These increments are achieved by increasing the speed and/or the gradient of the treadmill. A full 12-lead ECG is monitored for the duration of the test. During the course of the test the subject breathes through a mask containing a one-way valve. Oxygen uptake is calculated from measures of oxygen and carbon dioxide in the expired air and minute ventilation. The subject is considered to have reached their $V_{O_{2max}}$ if several of the following occur:

- a plateau in oxygen uptake
- maximum heart rate is achieved (plateau in heart rate)
- attainment of a respiratory exchange ratio or respiratory quotient (the ratio of the volume of carbon dioxide produced to the volume of oxygen consumed perunit of time) of $\geqslant 1.5$
- exhaustion.

In patients with cardiovascular disease, often the test is terminated due to the appearance of symptoms of angina, ECG changes or shortness of breath. In these circumstances the maximum oxygen consumption attained is termed the peak V_{O_2} or symptom-limited V_{O_2}.

Summary of benefits on metabolic parameters

- ↓ LDL cholesterol
- ↓ triglycerides
- ↓ total cholesterol
- ↑ HDL cholesterol
- ↑ HDL:LDL cholesterol
- ↓ lactate at a submaximal workload
- ↓ lactate at peak V_{O_2}.

Physiological benefits

In patients with CHD an improvement in exercise capacity following exercise training has been demonstrated by many research workers. This improvement in exercise capacity may be achieved by peripheral and/or cardiac adaptations to exercise training. In patients with CHD, physical training may improve oxygen-extracting capacity in the peripheral muscles and may influence the peripheral circulation. The cardiac work performed at a given external workload (i.e. submaximal exercise), may decrease and thus symptoms provoked by coronary insufficiency (e.g. angina pectoris, fatigue and dyspnoea), will not appear until heavier workloads are performed. Possible mechanisms for this improvement in cardiac work include an increase in the vascularization of the myocardium,

a higher pain threshold, lower levels of anxiety and a decrease in sympathetic tone.

Myocardial hypertrophy. The results of the earlier studies in patients with CHD indicated that the benefits of endurance training were largely a result of peripheral physiological changes and were not usually associated with any marked direct cardiac effect. However, subsequent studies have reported an increase in *left ventricular end-diastolic volume* (LVEDV) or *left ventricular end-diastolic dimension* (LVEDd, as an indicator of LVEDV) and posterior wall thickness at rest after training. The discrepancies in the data can probably be attributed to differences in training intensity and duration. In the studies reporting no changes, the training was generally of mild to moderate intensity (i.e. at 60% of peak V_{O_2}) and brief in duration; whereas in the studies reporting increases in cardiac dimensions, patients were required to perform high intensity exercise (i.e. at 50 to 70% of peak V_{O_2} for the first 3 months and at 70 to 80% of peak V_{O_2} for the rest of the training period) for a longer duration. Changes in LVEDd (or LVEDV) and wall thickness at rest have been attributed to 'volume overload hypertrophy', as has been shown to occur in normal subjects after exercise training. Volume overload hypertrophy is defined as hypertrophy in which the increment in diastolic filling volume exceeds the increase in ventricular wall thickness (h) and hence the *wall thickness to radius ratio* (h/r) is either decreased or unchanged compared to the non-trained state. This *exercise-induced cardiac hypertrophy* (physiological hypertrophy or athlete's heart) is considered a normal adaptation to the chronic volume overloads imposed by increased blood volume (see below) and venous return during exercise. In addition, increases in LVEDV have been reported during maximal exercise in patients after training. Although, no changes have been reported in LVEDV during submaximal exercise, the increase in LVEDV during maximal exercise probably serves as further evidence of volume overload ventricular hypertrophy as occurs in normal individuals after training.

Vascularization of the myocardium. Exercise training is reported to improve myocardial perfusion in patients with CHD. The mechanisms which mediate the apparent improvement in myocardial perfusion have long been debated. Both a repression of coronary artery stenosis and an improvement of coronary collateralization (development of new branches) have been suggested as potential adaptations. However, the changes observed in coronary artery diameter are small and hence this factor is unlikely to explain the substantial increase in myocardial perfusion and angina threshold which occurs as a consequence of exercise training. Evidence of the formation of coronary collaterals subsequent to exercise training remains controversial. An alternative possible explanation for the improvement in myocardial perfusion is related to changes in luminal diameter of epicardial vessels in response to mechanical (flow-mediated) or agonist-mediated (endogenous or pharmacological) stimuli. The influence of both mechanical and agonist-mediated stimuli on coronary vasomotion is dependent on endothelial *nitric oxide* (NO) synthesis or release as the final common pathway. Patients with CHD are said to have endothelial dysfunction in that atherosclerotic vessels in these patients vasoconstrict (rather than vasodilate) in response to acetylcholine infusion. Endothelial dysfunction occurs as a result of decreased concentrations of bioactive NO at vascular smooth muscle cells. Concentrations of NO can be affected by alterations in the availability of its precursor L-arginine; in *endothelial nitric oxide synthase enzyme* (eNOS); and in NO breakdown velocity related to *reactive oxidative species* (ROS). Reactive oxygen species (or *superoxides*) are chemical species containing nitrogen and oxygen or oxygen only with unpaired electrons. As electrons prefer to pair up to form stable two-electron bonds, these chemical species are very reactive and hence give rise to oxidative reactions. The consequence of such reactions is the oxidation damage of cellular macromolecules. Exercise training in patients with CAD is reported to enhance eNOS and extracellular *superoxide dismutase enzyme* expression, thereby attenuating the premature breakdown of NO by ROS. Superoxide dismutase is the biological enzyme which scavenges superoxides and then converts these superoxides into less reactive species. Consequently both local NO production and half-life are increased, resulting in an improvement in endothelium-dependent vasodilation in response to either blood flow or acetylcholine. It is presumed that these functional changes resulting in improved myocardial perfusion occur rather rapidly after the initiation of exercise training, although no studies have investigated the exact time course so far.

Blood volume. Although no studies of changes in blood volume have been reported in CHD patients, it is generally assumed that exercise training in these subjects results in an increase in total body blood volume, as occurs in normal subjects after training.

Peripheral adaptations and oxygen consumption. Reports are consistent in their findings of enhanced peak V_{O_2} in CHD patients after training. This increase in peak V_{O_2} ranges from 19% to 54% (a mean change of about 35%). These large increases found in CHD patients can probably be attributed to the extremely unfit state of these patients before the commencement of training (i.e. they have a large scope for improvement). Increases in the symptom-limited maximal workload achieved on an exercise ECG test have also been demonstrated after training.

The increase in peak V_{O_2} in CHD patients appears to be primarily due to a widening of the A-V_{O_2}d (*arterio-venous oxygen difference* (enhanced oxygen extraction)). An increase in peak V_{O_2} of 23% and a corresponding increase of 18% in A-V_{O_2}d has been reported. This increase in A-V_{O_2}d appears to be specific to the trained muscles, and thus is most likely the result of local mitochondrial changes that allow the muscle

to function at a lower oxygen saturation. These results suggest that the improvements in peak V_{O_2} are mediated by exercise-induced adaptations in the skeletal muscle and alterations in the responses of the endocrine and autonomic systems to exercise, rather than by adaptations of the heart. Mitochondrial, enzymatic and histological changes, no different from those that occur in normal subjects after exercise training, take place in the trained muscles of patients with CHD. These changes result in an enhanced capacity of the mitochondria to generate ATP aerobically. Consequently, after training, a lower rate of muscle oxygen utilization can be achieved at the same ADP concentration. This may explain the decreases in submaximal V_{O_2} observed in CHD patients after training. It is postulated that such peripheral changes ultimately result in a reduction of myocardial work, thereby enhancing the haemodynamic and metabolic reserve capacities.

Adaptations in skeletal muscle as a consequence of exercise training

↑ size and number of mitochondria
↑ myoglobin content
↑ size of skeletal muscle capillary bed
↑ number of oxidative mitochondrial enzymes
↑ number of type IIA and type I muscle fibres (aerobic) relative to type IIB muscle fibres (anaerobic)

Changes in sympathetic and parasympathetic tone. A decrease in the plasma levels of noradrenaline (norepinephrine) at rest and a reduction in both noradrenaline and adrenaline (epinephrine) levels during submaximal exercise occur after training in CHD patients. This catecholamine response to exercise training is similar to that reported in normal adults. These findings suggest that the training-induced sinus bradycardia that occurs in CHD patients after training is the result of downregulation of cardiac beta-adrenergic receptors and consequently a decrease in sympathetic activity. Training also has effects on intrinsic cardiac components (i.e. on the sinu-atrial node). A greater degree of inhibition of the sinu-atrial node by the vagus nerve (PNS) occurs after exercise training.

Changes noted at rest. In CHD patients both LVEDV and *stroke volume* (SV) are increased at rest. Heart rate, however, is decreased. Thus *cardiac output* (CO) must be maintained by the increase in SV with a reduction of intrinsic cardiac work (i.e. decreased HR). In the studies in which no changes in resting LVEDV or SV were evident after training, the subjects only performed mild to moderate exercise for a short duration.

Changes noted during submaximal exercise. As occurs in normal subjects, CHD patients can perform a given submaximal work load at a lower HR than that observed before training. CO is again maintained by increasing SV. In some studies decreased SV and CO were reported to be maintained after training. Also submaximal V_{O_2} is reported to be decreased after training. If V_{O_2} at a given submaximal workload is decreased then blood flow is autoregulated in proportion to the needs of the tissue. Since submaximal HR decreases at a given submaximal workload, this workload can be performed at a lower myocardial oxygen consumption. After training, BP and HR are lower at any given workload and thus the myocardial oxygen consumption (as reflected by the *rate pressure product*, R-PP) is lowered. This allows a higher intensity of exercise to be achieved before the precipitation of angina.

Changes noted during maximal exercise.   It is important to note that in patients with CHD maximal exercise is not an absolute maximum but a symptom-limited maximum. Symptom-limited maximal HR and SV are increased and thus CO is increased. Also since HR is increased, R-PP is increased (i.e. myocardial oxygen consumption is greater). Peak V_{O_2} is increased due to peripheral adaptations to exercise training. The magnitude of this improvement is dependent on the initial value of peak V_{O_2}, the intensity, duration and frequency of each training session, as well as the total length of the training programme. Patients are also able to reach a higher level of peak V_{O_2} before symptoms of angina or dyspnoea occur. This can most probably be attributed to the training-induced reduction in resting myocardial oxygen consumption (i.e. HR × SBP (systolic blood pressure)), and downward shift in the linear increase in myocardial oxygen consumption with increasing workloads (or increasing V_{O_2}). An alteration in the pain threshold is unlikely, since after training patients do not show a greater degree of ST-segment depression at the onset of angina pectoris than that before training. The enhancement in myocardial oxygen delivery is likely to be achieved by an increase in the flow capacity of existing collateral vessels rather than by the growth of new collateral vessels (see 'Vascularization of the myocardium' above).

Summary of physiological benefits of exercise in patients with CHD

- ↑ minimum work rate required to induce ST-segment depression or angina
- ↓ heart rate at rest and at a submaximal workload
- ↓ in systolic blood pressure at rest and at a submaximal workload
- ↑ peak systolic blood pressure
- ↑ left ventricular wall thickness and left ventricular mass
- ↑ left ventricular end-diastolic volume and diameter
- ↑ myocardial perfusion
- possible ↑ ejection fraction at submaximal workload
- ↓ noradrenaline (norepinephrine) and adrenaline (epinephrine) concentrations at rest and at a submaximal workload

- ↓ myocardial oxygen consumption at a submaximal workload
- ↑ peak oxygen consumption (V_{O_2} peak)

Guidelines for exercise prescriptions

Phase I

Exercise within a phase I programme progresses slowly during the in-hospital period, starting from low-level activities in the intensive care unit and then progressing to more active exercise in the ward. Phase I activities range in level from 1 to 3 METs (one MET is about 3.5 ml O_2/kg body weight/min) provided these activities can be done without angina, significant arrhythmias or related symptoms.

Phase I training programme		
Day 1	'Passive/Assisted active' exercise	Passive range of movements Self-feeding Bedside commode Bed to chair Remain seated in armchair for ± 20 min 3–4 × per day Static muscle exercises Low-level active exercises, e.g. ankle exercises
	'Active' exercise	Active range of movement: progress to mild arm and leg resistance Bed-bath with minimal assistance Bed to chair often during day Walk slowly within ward (2× daily) for distance of about 30 metres Dress, shave, comb hair Bath in tub with assistance
	'Resistive' exercise	Active range of movement: progress to use of trunk as well as 1 or 2 weights for arms and legs Progress walking to about 60 metres Incorporate stairs – down 2 flights; up 1 flight Dress fully Walk to and sit in visitors room at least twice a day

About day 10–14

Discharge graded exercise test[a]

Education | Allay fears associated with intensive care unit
Understanding signs and symptoms of disease (e.g. living with angina, dyspnoea)
Relaxation skills
Dietary advice
Advice on cessation of smoking
Medications
Advice regarding sexual activities
Hospital discharge and transition to home convalescence

[a] *Recommended. Performed on completion of phase I. Enables physician to determine whether patient can tolerate low-level (3–5 METs) exercise without angina, significant arrhythmias or related symptoms.*

Phase II

Phase II is a multifaceted approach which allows diversity to satisfy the unique needs and interests of each patient. The phase II programme consists of either a programme of walking or a stationary bicycle-exercise programme, either of which may be performed at home or at a rehabilitation facility. Importantly both modes of exercise should be preceded by a warm-up period and followed by a cool-down period.

In the home programme the patient should ideally report back to the hospital/physician at periodic intervals for a progress check and possible change of exercise prescription. These periodic checks allow the physician to individualize the patient's rehabilitation programme so that the patient can proceed at a rate that is appropriate for him or her.

High-risk patients (those that experience symptoms at low levels of exercise) are advised to continue their rehabilitation, i.e. from phase I to phase II, in a phase II outpatient clinic where monitoring staff and equipment are available.

The phase II programme is terminated by a graded symptom-limited maximal graded exercise test which serves to assess whether a patient is ready to make the transition from a phase II to a phase III programme. In addition, this test is used for evaluating the status of the patient in terms of recommendations for returning to work or for self-monitored rehabilitative exercises.

Phase III

Phase III programmes encourage regular continued exercise either in an outpatient facility or by means of a home-based

Phase II training programme

Week 1   *Walking*   *Bicycle*

Walking	*Bicycle*
Treadmill graded exercise test at discharge HR = 60% symptom-limited maximal or predicted max	Bicycle graded exercise test at discharge HR = 60% symptom-limited maximal or predicted max
Daily walking schedule progressing from 2 blocks (±0.25 km) daily to 10 blocks (±1 km) daily	Bicycle ×12 min daily at HR ⩽60% of predicted maximum (patient must be asymptomatic)
Walk distance of about 1 km in 20 min, rest and walk back distance of 1 km in 20 min	Increase exercise duration to 14 min daily and intensity to HR <65% of predicted maximum (patient must be asymptomatic)
Walk distance of 2.5 km in 35 min, rest and walk back distance of 2.5 km in 35 min	Increase exercise duration to 16 min daily and maintain intensity at HR <65% predicted maximum (patient must be asymptomatic)
	Increase exercise duration to 20 min daily and intensity to HR <70% predicted maximum (patient must be asymptomatic)

Weeks 12–24   Graded symptom-limited maximal exercise test to assess level of function Phase III rehabilitation/work/retirement/rehabilitation programme at home

programme. Those patients that can attend an outpatient facility are encouraged to do so on a 3–4 times per week basis. Exercise of an endurance type (i.e. walking or jogging) is usually performed for 30–40 minutes preceded by a 10–15 minute warm-up period and followed by 10–15 minutes of cool-down. Exercise intensity is prescribed based on a percentage of symptom-limited maximum HR. Patients are taught to monitor their own HR in order to ensure that they maintain their prescribed intensity of exercise during each training session. Initially exercise begins at a HR of ⩽60% of symptom-limited maximum and progresses to a HR of ⩽75% of symptom-limited maximum. Once the patient has achieved a certain level of fitness and the cardiologist is satisfied that the patient's cardiovascular response to exercise is relatively stable, he or she can be put onto the maintenance phase of rehabilitation. Often at this stage patients leave the outpatient exercise facility and are confident to continue exercise on their own at home. Initially patients are required to attend the rehabilitation centre once a week and then once a month for a routine medical check-up and for their log book in which they record exercise intensity and duration to be assessed. Patients are encouraged to exercise but also cautioned not to increase intensity or duration too rapidly. At various intervals, usually 6- or 12-monthly, graded symptom-limited maximal exercise tests are performed in order to assess the patient's fitness such that their exercise prescription can be altered appropriately to achieve maximum benefit. Education regarding dietary modification, lifestyle changes and smoking cessation is continued during the phase III programme. Often the spouse may be involved in educational programmes at this stage. The spouse may also be instructed in cardiopulmonary resuscitation.

Motivation of patients to continue to adhere to rehabilitation programmes often becomes a challenge at the phase III level. If a patient is attending an outpatient clinic various 'competitions' with rewards can be devised to encourage continued progression with regard to exercise fitness, loss of weight and regular attendance. Spousal support is of prime importance.

Before entry into a phase III training programme a thorough evaluation is performed. This consists of an appropriate history and physical examination, physiological appraisal, blood lipid profile, respiratory function test and an exercise *electrocardiogram* (ECG) test on an ergometer or treadmill to determine symptom-limited maximal physical working capacity. From the results of this initial evaluation each patient's exercise prescription is calculated individually. The major components of this exercise prescription are the intensity, duration, frequency and mode of exercise performed. Other important factors to be considered are the time elapsed since the acute MI, PTCA or CABG surgery, the individual's current physical working capacity and any specific recommendations from the physician, such as physical limitations or symptoms, to be aware of during exercise.

Intensity of training

Training-induced physiological changes depend primarily on the intensity of the exercise performed during the training period. In general, the magnitude of such changes is directly related to the intensity of the work performed. This relationship is a function of age, initial level of physical fitness, and perhaps several other lifestyle factors. In order for training-induced changes to occur exercise training must be performed consistently at a level of physical activity higher than that experienced during normal daily activity. Thus the individual must maintain, throughout each training session, a specific intensity of exercise which lies within the accepted training sensitive zone for that individual's initial level of physical fitness. The training sensitive zone for a sedentary individual or cardiac patient is from 57% to 78% of symptom-limited maximal aerobic capacity. Since it is impractical to consistently record aerobic capacity during exercise training, the monitoring of HR is used as an effective alternative. This is based on the fact that the percentages of maximal oxygen consumption and heart rate are linearly related. This relationship is independent of gender and age. Thus the training sensitive zone corresponds to approximately 70% to 85% of symptom-limited maximal HR. The lower percentage ensures that a training effect will be induced, provided that the individual trains above this level. The higher percentage provides a margin for safety as well as ensuring that the exercise performed is aerobic and not anaerobic. Since the intensity of training is dependent on the individual's initial physical condition, the *training heart rate* (THR) generally used for cardiac patients and sedentary individuals varies from 65% to 85% of symptom-limited maximal HR and from 80% to 90% of maximal HR for more highly trained persons. Each individual's symptom-limited maximal aerobic capacity and HR are generally determined from the initial exercise ECG test performed before entry into the phase III training programme.

The use of HR as a measure of intensity of exercise is appropriate for two reasons. Firstly, cardiac work (or myocardial stress) is reflected with a high degree of accuracy by HR alone. Thus by maintaining a constant THR during exercise, the work of the heart can be maintained at a constant level. Secondly, the THR concept allows for a natural adjustment to the change in training state. As the individual becomes better conditioned he or she will perform the same level of exercise at an increasingly lower HR. The individual must therefore perform at an increasingly higher level of exercise in order to maintain the specific percentage of symptom-limited maximal V_{O_2} (i.e. THR).

Duration of each training session

The training duration threshold level is influenced by the intensity and frequency of training, and the individual's initial level of fitness. Activity of lower intensity generally requires exercise for a relatively longer duration than activity of higher intensity. In poorly conditioned persons, exercise at 60% of symptom-limited maximal HR for only 5 minutes per session is likely to produce some training effect, whereas in athletes, unless exercise training is performed frequently at greater than 85% of maximal HR for at least 45 minutes no training effects will occur.

Frequency of training

Although the frequency of training is an important factor in causing cardiovascular improvements, this factor is considerably less important than either the intensity or the duration of exercise. In studies where total work was kept constant there were no differences between the improvements in *maximum oxygen consumption* (VO_{2max}), when training was performed two versus four times per week, or three versus five times per week. Also, using interval training, reports indicate that training twice weekly resulted in changes in peak VO_2 or VO_{2max} similar to those observed in persons who trained five times per week. Although increasing the frequency of exercise training does not seem to affect changes in physiological function, it is an important consideration if exercise is used as a means of weight control. Exercising five or six times per week represents a considerable caloric expenditure in comparison to training only twice weekly. However, an important consideration is that training less than twice weekly does not produce adequate changes in either aerobic capacity or body composition. Whether training occurs on consecutive or alternate days has no effect on improvements in peak VO_2 or VO_{2max}.

Mode of training

If intensity, frequency and duration are kept constant, the effects of training are similar, provided that the exercise performed involves the use of large muscle groups in a rhythmic aerobic nature. Walking, running, swimming and rope skipping are all excellent examples of such rhythmic aerobic activity. The mode of training is particularly important in cardiac patients. Aerobic activities result in much smaller increments in BP and HR than do strenuous isometric activities. Consequently sudden stop-and-go anaerobic activities, as well as strenuous isometric exercises, are more likely to place large oxygen demands on the myocardium than are aerobic activities. Therefore focusing on anaerobic activities alone is likely to be hazardous for the cardiac patient, whose cardiovascular function is already compromised. Furthermore isometric training alone results in increases in muscle strength, without concomitant increases in cardiovascular function. Other potential detrimental effects of strenuous isometric exercise are the provocation of dangerous Valsalva manoeuvres, and alterations in the responses of cardiac rhythm and BP to exercise. (The benefits of anaerobic activities performed in conjunction with aerobic activities are discussed at the end of this chapter.)

Specificity of training

Although different types of training may produce similar effects, the magnitude of these changes may vary considerably depending on the mode of testing used. This phenomenon is termed the specificity concept. For example, individuals trained on a bicycle show greater improvements when tested on a bicycle than when tested on a treadmill. Similarly, persons trained by running show the greatest improvements when tested by performing exercises involving the leg muscles rather than the muscles of the upper body.

Duration of exercise training

In some normal individuals, training-induced changes (e.g. peripheral changes) may occur in the initial 4 to 6 weeks, although other changes (e.g. cardiac changes) will not manifest themselves for months or even years. However, the rate as well as the magnitude of change can vary considerably among individuals. Some persons will demonstrate large changes quickly, while others may show slow progress initially and then advance more rapidly only much later on. The rate of improvement for uncomplicated cardiac patients is comparable to adaptation in sedentary normal individuals. Training adaptation appears to be affected by both age and initial level of physical condition. In essence the benefits of physical activity do not accrue overnight, but require an extended period of time, probably 6 months or longer, to become apparent.

The physiological effects from regular participation in a programme of gradually increasing levels of physical activity are usually detected within a few weeks. Additional physiological effects may be evidenced as long as the intensity and duration of activity is increased. Since physical activity may offer a preventative as well as a therapeutic advantage to many cardiac patients, cardiac rehabilitation should involve ongoing, longitudinal programmes.

Progression from phase III training programme

Most patients who attain an 8 MET level of performance can safely progress to unsupervised exercise and hence cardiac rehabilitation can continue at home. Most home programmes initially involve walking progressing to jogging or stationary bicycle activities. As the level of fitness improves, recreational activities are included to add variety to the exercise programme. Effective and safe recreational endurance activities include rope-jumping (12 METs), bicycling (3.5–5.7 METs), skating (5.5 METs), rowing (6–7 METs), swimming (4.5–7 METs) and aerobic dancing (6 METs). The specific exercise regimen varies with the goals and needs of each patient, their age, health status, fitness level, personal preferences, acessibility to exercise facilities, prior exercise capacity and skills.

Precautions and contraindications

Phase I
Precautions
- HR should *not* exceed 120 beats/min at any time.
- Physical activity should *not* be associated with chest pain, palpitations, dyspnoea or excessive fatigue.
- Dysrhythmias (abnormalities in cardiac rhythm observed on the ECG) should *not* occur.
- ST-segment displacement on ECG should *not* occur.
- SBP should *not* decrease by more than 10 to 20 mmHg (as this indicates an inadequacy of cardiac output to meet the demand imposed by exercise).

- Should any of the above occur, it signifies that the workload intensity is too great. The patient's physical activity plan needs to be revised to meet a less demanding level.

Contraindications
Patients who have:

- significant dysrhythmias
- shock
- persistent chest pain
- recurrent chest pain
- class IV heart failure
- acute systemic illness or fever
- uncontrolled diabetes mellitus
- recent embolism
- thrombophlebitis (superficial venous thrombosis with inflammation)
- active pericarditis or myocarditis
- moderate to severe aortic stenosis
- regurgitant valve disease requiring surgery.

Exercises to avoid
Isometric exercises and upper arm exercises should be avoided as they elicit a minimal increase in heart rate with a significant increase in systolic blood pressure. This results in a sudden increase in afterload to the heart which is not well tolerated by an ischaemic myocardium, hence resulting in angina pectoris and often in life-threatening cardiac dysrhythmias.

Phases II and III
- Precautions and restrictions as for phase I above apply.
- In addition, exercise should be dynamic, involving rhythmic repetitive movements of large muscle groups, including arms at this stage.
- Isotonic exercises are encouraged because they increase heart rate and stroke volume with little associated change in blood pressure.
- Isometric exercises should be limited because they increase systolic blood pressure and hence may provoke angina, left ventricular dysfunction and arrhythmias.
- Age predicted target heart rate should *not* be used to prescribe exercise intensities for patients with CHD, as age predicted maximums are based on maximum oxygen consumption and not peak oxygen consumption. The optimal intensity of exercise should approximate 57–78% of the individual's peak oxygen consumption, which corresponds to a heart rate between 70 and 85% of symptom-limited maximum.
- Although an increase in either the duration or the frequency of exercise can be substituted to compensate for a modest decrease in exercise intensity, this is not recommended as it is associated with orthopaedic and musculoskeletal injuries as well as poorer adherence to the exercise regimen.
- As various medications may alter the heart rate response to exercise, when exercise testing is being performed to determine an exercise prescription, patients should be receiving those medications that they will be taking during the exercise programme.
- Exercise should *not* be performed at levels higher than those prescribed as higher intensities are likely to elicit inappropriate cardiovascular responses. This is important for patient safety by preventing undue stresses on the heart.

Environmental factors also need to be considered in phase II and III programmes as often the patients will be exercising outside. Exercise in the *cold* presents few problems as individuals can add layers of clothing; however, they should be careful not to overdress as this would lead to overheating and sweating and thereby possible chilling of the patient.

Heat, however, is of concern, particularly with high humidity. Increases in humidity limit the volume of sweat that can be evaporated and hence reduce the degree of cooling. Heat stress results in an increase in sympathetic nervous system activity which in turn causes an increase in HR and vasoconstriction of splanchnic and renal beds. Heat stress combined with exercise imposes demand on both the thermoregulatory and the cardiovascular system to vasodilate skin and muscle circulatory beds respectively. This sets up a competition for the available cardiac output. The consequences of such competition would be hyperthermia, tachycardia, reduced work capacity and ultimately circulatory collapse. The main concern is to maintain stroke volume. Therefore patients are advised to avoid exercising in the heat of the day when humidity is high and to ingest fluids both before and during exercise.

High altitude imposes significant stress on the myocardium due to reduced oxygen availability as a consequence of reductions in the partial pressure of oxygen in proportion to the increment in altitude. Hence patients are advised not to exercise at very high altitudes or alternatively to reduce their exercise intensity when exercising at high altitudes.

CHRONIC HEART FAILURE

At the outset it is important to note that currently exercise therapy is only recommended for patients with *chronic* not acute heart failure. Furthermore, as the evidence available to date emanates from studies in selected patients, it is *not* correct to state that exercise training should be incorporated as a therapeutic measure for all patients with heart failure. Patients who have been included in exercise training studies had chronic heart failure which was congestive, ischaemic or idiopathic in origin; were generally in New York Heart Association (NYHA) functional class II and III; had been clinically stable for the previous 3 months; had left ventricular ejection fraction of <40% and were in normal sinus rhythm. Some studies also incorporated patients with stable heart failure in NYHA functional class I. Therefore the benefits and mechanisms of exercise training in such patients only will be discussed.

The guidelines of the European Working Group are followed in the section on exercise prescription and recommendations for exercise training in patients with heart failure.

Over the past decade, traditional medical teaching and advice regarding physical activity in patients with chronic heart failure have changed. It is now believed that bed rest and exercise restriction may lead to deconditioning and increased morbidity. Recent studies in both asymptomatic patients with left ventricular dysfunction and patients with moderate symptomatic heart failure support this concept.

Justifications for encouraging regular exercise

In the syndrome of heart failure, two of the main symptoms experienced by patients are fatigue and limitations in exercise capacity. These symptoms are caused not only by the impaired mechanical performance of the heart, but also by abnormalities in peripheral blood flow, endothelial function, skeletal muscle and lung function in chronic heart failure.

Accordingly therapeutic strategies aimed at improving muscle function or exercise tolerance are likely to provide symptomatic improvements in patients with heart failure. In other words physical training is likely to be beneficial. Indeed, patients with chronic heart failure show improvements in symptoms, exercise tolerance and functional capacity in response to exercise training, even though left ventricular systolic function appears to be unaffected.

Most of the studies conducted in patients with stable chronic heart failure have reported significant increases in peak oxygen consumption (V_{O_2}), workload or exercise duration. In addition, increases in V_{O_2} around the anaerobic threshold (as determined by both ventilatory and lactate indices) were reported. Overall the benefits of the various exercise training programmes (ranging in duration from 1 to 6 months) were an improvement in physical performance similar in magnitude to that resulting from angiotensin-converting enzyme inhibitor therapy. The magnitude of these increases amounts to on average an increase in peak V_{O_2} of at least 2 ml/kg/min and an increase in exercise time of about 1.5 minutes. Although, these increments are small in terms of magnitude, patients with chronic heart failure are severely limited in their activities by symptoms of fatigue and/or dyspnoea. Hence, these benefits are indeed of both clinical and therapeutic relevance.

In addition to therapeutic benefits, exercise training improves prognosis (secondary prevention) in patients with heart failure. Various indicators of prognosis are reported to be altered in a favourable manner subsequent to exercise training. Examples of such prognostic indicators (V_E/V_{CO_2} slope; peak V_{O_2} and sympathetic overactivity) are defined and discussed below. As the ventilatory response to exercise is exaggerated in patients with heart failure, the slope of the relationship between minute ventilation and carbon dioxide production (V_E/V_{CO_2} slope) is used as an indicator

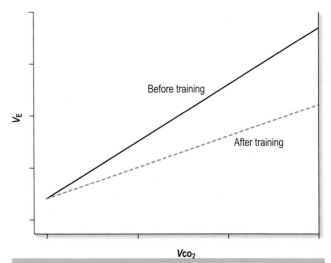

Figure 9.1.6.   The effects of exercise training on the slope of the relationship between V_E and V_{CO_2}.

of prognosis – the greater the slope, the worse the prognosis. Exercise training significantly reduces minute ventilation during submaximal workloads and thereby reduces the V_E/V_{CO_2} slope (Fig. 9.1.6). Furthermore, a reduction in V_E/V_{CO_2} slope at maximal workloads has also been reported after exercise training in patients with heart failure. Another important predictor of prognosis in chronic heart failure is peak V_{O_2}; the lower the peak V_{O_2} the worse the prognosis. Exercise training at low intensity even of fairly short duration in patients with heart failure substantially enhances peak V_{O_2}. After only 6 weeks of exercise training (at low intensity) increases in peak V_{O_2} from as much as 11 to 15 ml/kg/min have been reported.

Other prognostic indicators are abnormalities (decreases) in the variability of heart rate and increased plasma concentrations of noradrenaline (norepinephrine) (sympathetic overactivity). Following exercise training in patients with heart failure, heart rate variability is enhanced and the resting concentrations of both adrenaline (epinephrine) and noradrenaline (norepinephrine) are decreased. These data suggest that exercise training has the capacity to moderate the sympathetic overactivity which occurs in heart failure. Indeed, alterations in the autonomic balance subsequent to exercise training result in an increase in parasympathetic drive and a reduction in sympathetic overactivation. Such alterations are important in that they reduce not only vascular resistance, and hence afterload imposed on the heart, but also the myocardial wall stress. Improvements in HR variability subsequent to exercise training also contribute favourably to reductions in myocardial wall stress. These changes allow the same amount of work to be achieved at a lower metabolic cost (oxygen consumption) to the heart. As exercise training results in improvements in various indicators of prognosis in heart failure, it is fair to say that exercise training has beneficial effects on the progression of chronic heart failure and thereby improves prognosis.

Despite improvements in the efficiency of skeletal muscle metabolic processes and hence a reduction in the symptoms associated with heart failure, concerns have been raised as to the long-term impact of physical exercise programmes on the progression of unfavourable ventricular remodelling in heart failure. It has been argued that training programmes may be harmful in patients with heart failure because the ventricles would be exposed to periodic increases in wall stress during acute bouts of exercise which may represent a stimulus for progressive left ventricular enlargement. However, several studies in patients with heart failure of various aetiologies report an increase in left ventricular ejection fraction associated with no change in end-diastolic volume and a reduction in end-systolic volume after 6 months of exercise training. In comparison in groups of patients with heart failure who did not take part in exercise training programmes, both end-diastolic and end-systolic diameters were increased, revealing a progression of deleterious remodelling, which was associated with no change in left ventricular ejection fraction. It is likely that exercise-training-induced reductions in myocardial wall stress, as discussed above, contribute to the prevention of an unfavourable ventricular remodelling. Hence, asymptomatic patients with left ventricular dysfunction who perform regular exercise while receiving optimal medical treatment may well derive benefit from exercise training with no impairment in ventricular function or geometry.

Mechanisms of benefits

The benefits of exercise training programmes appear to be primarily related to changes in the oxidative capacity of skeletal muscle and peripheral haemodynamics. As the main symptoms of heart failure are fatigue, dyspnoea and limitation in exercise capacity, it stands to reason that exercise programmes would be beneficial. In patients with heart failure the vasodilatory capacity of skeletal muscles is blunted during exercise, which contributes to the increased total peripheral resistance and peripheral hypoperfusion. Hence, patients with heart failure exhibit subnormal peripheral blood flow in response to exercise-induced vasodilation. The primary reasons for this reduction in blood flow are a decreased release of endothelium-derived relaxing factor (nitric oxide vasodilator system) from arterioles in metabolically active skeletal muscle and an exaggerated increase in the systemic release of the vasoconstrictor neurohormones (associated with the sympathetic overactivity which occurs in heart failure), such as endothelin, noradrenaline, renin, angiotensin II and vasopressin.

Exercise training is reported to result in improvements in peripheral haemodynamics in patients with heart failure. Leg blood flow is increased at maximal exercise, whilst vascular resistance is decreased during submaximal exercise. Although not many studies have investigated the mechanisms of these improvements subsequent to exercise training, there is evidence that regular physical exercise can improve endothelial dysfunction, reduce peripheral vascular resistance and thereby enhance skeletal muscle blood flow in patients with heart failure. However, it is not yet known whether these benefits are predominantly due to reductions in vasoconstrictors, tone, improvements in large vessel function or enhanced endothelial vasodilator function. In support of the latter mechanism, it has recently been shown that exercise corrects the impaired endothelium-dependent vasodilation of skeletal muscle vasculature in patients with heart failure. Furthermore, basal production of endothelial nitric oxide is reported to be improved. These changes in the endothelial function of the vasculature in the skeletal muscles of the lower limbs were associated with changes in peripheral resistance. Thus in heart failure exercise therapy is believed to exert its primary effects on the endothelial function of peripheral resistance vessels, thereby contributing to a reduction in peripheral resistance both at rest and at peak exercise.

Furthermore, exercise training may exert its effects by attenuating the sympathetic overactivity which occurs in patients with heart failure. It has been noted that similar to the effects reported in healthy subjects, exercise training in patients with heart failure results in an attenuation of the sympathetic overactivity by an increase in vagal tone. However, these effects cannot be the sole contributor to the reduction in peripheral vascular resistance, as exercise-induced decreases in plasma catecholamine concentrations were not correlated with decreases in vascular resistance.

In addition to the abnormalities in peripheral haemodynamics, a reduction in exercise tolerance and evidence of early muscle lactate release (low VO_2 at which lactate starts to accumulate) despite normal skeletal muscle blood flow occurs in patients with heart failure. This early dependence on anaerobic metabolism is related to alterations in mitochondria, skeletal muscle fibre dimension and number, and deficits in oxidative and glycolytic enzymes. Furthermore, excessive early depletion of high energy phosphate bonds, an excessive early intramuscular acidification, together with defects in beta-oxidation of fatty acids and an increase in amino acid utilization have been reported. It is well known that exercise training programmes in healthy individuals result in an increase in resting levels of *anaerobic substrates* (ATP, CP, free creatine and glycogen), glycolytic and oxidative capacity, number of mitochondria, capacity to mobilize and oxidize for (enhance utilization of fatty acids), and size and number of skeletal muscle fibres. In patients with heart failure, increases in mitochondrial abundance and improvements in oxidative metabolism of skeletal muscle have been demonstrated. Blood lactate concentrations are decreased during submaximal exercise. Moreover, correlations between changes in the volume density of mitochondria and changes in both peak oxygen uptake and lactate threshold have been reported. Interestingly, a close correlation has been noted between changes in venous lactate and both adrenaline (epinephrine) and noradrenaline (norepinephrine) after exercise training in patients with heart failure.

Specific benefits and hence the justification for regular exercise in patients with heart failure

Abnormality	Exercise-induced benefit
↓ peripheral blood flow	↑ peripheral blood flow
↓ endothelial function	↑ endothelial dependent vasodilation
	↑ endothelial NO
↑ SNS (sympathetic nervous system) activity	↓ SNS activity
	↑ vagal tone
↓ skeletal muscle metabolism	
↓ skeletal muscle	↑ anaerobic substrates
↓ high energy phosphates	↑ glycolytic and oxidative capacity
↓ beta-oxidation of fatty acids mitochondrial abnormalities	↑ mitochondria
	↑ muscle fibres
	↑ fatty acid oxidation
↓ glycolytic and oxidative enzymes	
Lung function	
↓ Vo_2/dyspnoea minute ventilation V_E/Vco_2 slope	↑ peak Vo_2
	↓ submaximal Vo_2
	↓ V_E/Vco_2 slope

Guidelines for exercise prescriptions

In general, data indicate that in heart failure, low-intensity exercise programmes at about 50% of peak exercise capacity are effective. The level of exercise intensity is important to note as the maintenance of an exercise training programme can be problematic in patients with heart failure as they are severely limited by symptoms of fatigue and dyspnoea. In the exercise training studies performed to date in patients with NYHA Functional Class (FC) I, II or III heart failure, exercise intensity ranged from 50 to 80% of maximum; exercise type included cycling, rowing, walking, swimming or ball games, exercise sessions lasted 30–60 minutes and were performed 3–5 times per week. Benefits were noted after 1–6 months of participation in an exercise training programme; however, to maintain these benefits continuation with the exercise programme is required. It is important to note that only those patients with NYHA FC I, II and III heart failure who had been stable on standard medical therapy for the previous 3 months, had a left ventricular ejection fraction lower than 40% and were in

sinus rhythm, were included in these studies. Hence exercise prescription at this stage should be limited to such patients only. Studies remain to be performed in other patients with more severe heart failure.

Intensity of training

The intensity of exercise recommended for patients with stable chronic heart failure is at 50% of maximum short-term exercise capacity. The steep ramp test is used to determine a patient's maximum short-term exercise capacity. To perform the steep ramp test the patient starts with unloaded pedalling for 3 minutes. This is then followed by 25 W increments in workload every 10 seconds. The rapid increase in workload allows many patients to achieve workloads of 150 to 200 W during a period of 60 to 90 seconds without complications. The exercise intensity is then calculated as 50% of the maximum workload achieved. In order to assist patients to monitor their own exercise intensity when walking, heart rate should be recorded during the steep ramp test. The heart rate which corresponds to 50% of maximum workload is then given to the patient as the target heart rate.

Duration of each training session

In patients with heart failure, interval rather than steady-state exercise has a more pronounced training effect on their exercise capacity. As most of the benefits of exercise training in patients with heart failure occur in peripheral muscles, it is important that training methods incorporate intense exercise stimuli on peripheral muscles. Such effects can be achieved by interval rather than steady-state exercise without inducing a greater cardiovascular stress. Interval training consists of short bouts of exercise (30 s) followed by short recovery periods (60 s). This is achieved by for example cycling at 50% of maximum short-term exercise capacity for 30 s followed by pedalling at 10 W for 60 s, the latter period of very slow activity representing the recovery period. With respect to walking, the recovery period would entail walking at the slowest speed possible for 60 s. During each exercise session lasting about 15 minutes, the exercise and recovery periods should be repeated about 10–12 times.

Frequency of training

The duration and frequency of the exercise programme prescribed to the patient depends on the individual's baseline clinical and functional status. Patients with chronic heart failure whose functional capacity is <3 METs (about 25–40 W) benefit from multiple (3 to 5/day) short daily exercise sessions of 5–10 minutes each. For those patients with a functional capacity of 3–5 METs (about 40–80 W) 1–2 sessions/day of 15 minutes each are recommended, and for patients with a functional capacity of >5 METs (about >80 W) 3–5 sessions per week of 20–30 minutes each are appropriate.

Mode of training

Due to the pathophysiology of heart failure only a few selected modes of aerobic exercise should be performed. Cycle ergometry is recommended as the most favourable type of initial exercise because it allows exercise to be performed at low workloads which are exactly reproducible. In addition, heart rate and blood pressure can be monitored. Cycling must be performed on an indoor cycle ergometer. Environmental factors such as slopes and head winds produce too great a cardiovascular stress for patients with heart failure. Furthermore, even cycling outdoors at slow speeds (<12 km/hour) on a flat track involves head winds which substantially increase the work intensity. Thus the latter exercise is *only* recommended for patients whose heart failure has been clinically stable for a prolonged period of time and who have a high level of exercise capacity or exercise tolerance.

Walking is also recommended for patients with chronic stable heart failure as it provides a wide range of workloads (from very slow speeds of <50 m/min to faster speeds of about 100 m/min). Patients can monitor their own heart rate and thereby ensure that they do not exceed their prescribed exercise intensity. As the lowest limit of speed that allows for comfortable movement during jogging is 80 m/min, jogging is not advisable for patients with chronic heart failure.

Swimming should be avoided because of the hydrostatically induced volume shifts that occur during this activity even at low intensities. These volume shifts increase the volume loading of the left ventricle with consequent increments in pulmonary capillary wedge pressure and oedema.

Rate of progression of exercise training

This discussion is analogous to the phase I, II and III programmes for patients with CHD. The rate of progression of exercise training in patients with heart failure needs to be tailored individually for each patient according to their baseline clinical status, functional capacity, adaptability to the training programme, age and possible presence of additional diseases. In general progression should be according to three stages, namely the initial stage, the improvement stage and the maintenance stage.

During the *initial stage* (about 4 to 6 weeks in duration) the intensity of exercise should be kept at a low level (2 to 3 METs) until a duration of 10–15 minutes is achieved. Thereafter the duration and frequency should be increased according to the patient's clinical status and symptoms.

In the *improvement stage* the primary aim is to gradually increase the intensity of exercise. The secondary aim is to increase the duration of each exercise session up to a maximum of 30 minutes. Despite the primary aim of this stage being to increase exercise intensity, the general principles of progression of exercise training should be followed in the order of duration, then frequency, then intensity.

The *maintenance stage* usually begins after the first 6 months of training. In this stage the patient continues to exercise

in order to maintain exercise capacity and to prevent or slow down muscle wasting and loss of aerobic capacity with progression of heart failure. Only minor adjustments to their exercise programme will need to be made as further improvements in exercise capacity at this stage are likely to be minimal.

Exercise prescription for patients with heart failure

Initial and improvement stages

Functional capacity of patient	Number of bouts of interval training	Duration	Frequency
<3 METs	3–7	5–10 min	3–5×/day
3–5 METs	10	15 min	1–2×/day
>5 METs	13–20	20–30 min	3–5×/week

Interval training = cycle or walk at 50% of maximum short-term exercise capacity for 30 s followed by cycle at low intensity or walk very slowly for 60 s

Maintenance stage

NYHA FC	Intensity	Number of bouts	Duration	Frequency
Normal and I	>7 METs	20–25	30–35 min	5×/week
II	≥5 METs	13–20	20–30 min	1–2×/day
III	≥2 METs	5–10	10–15 min	3×/day

Isometric exercise training

Although the benefits of isometric exercises are discussed in general at the end of this chapter, as skeletal muscle atrophy characteristically occurs in patients with heart failure the specific effects and hence indications for isometric exercises in these patients will be discussed here. During *sustained* isometric hand grip exercises lasting more than 3 minutes, harmful cardiovascular responses have been found to occur. However, *submaximal* isometric exercises performed in *rhythmic sequences* increase muscle strength without producing harmful increments in cardiovascular stress. The amount of cardiovascular stress incurred during rhythmic isometric exercises depends upon the muscle group involved and the mass of the muscle involved. For example, double arm exercise will result in greater cardiovascular stress than single arm exercise and similarly leg exercise produces greater cardiovascular stress than does arm exercise. The rhythmic isometric sequences prescribed should therefore consist of short bouts of isometric exercises using small muscle groups in one limb, small number of repetitions and an exercise to recovery ratio of 1:2. For example, 2 sets of about 12 one leg presses each, at 60% of one repetition maximum, lasting about 60 s each, interspersed with a rest period of 120 s.

Respiratory muscle training

As respiratory muscles show the same pathophysiological changes as do skeletal muscles, respiratory muscle training is recommended for patients with heart failure. Respiratory muscle strength and endurance is increased by resistive inspiratory muscle exercises. These exercises are best performed using devices that make inhaling more difficult. Examples of such devices are small hand-held incentive spirometers or peak inspiratory flow meters containing a breathing gauge. The patient exhales and then inhales forcefully through the tube using the pressure of inhalation to raise the gauge to the highest possible level. Inspiratory exercises should be performed for a minimum of 20–30 min/day (generally in 2 sessions of 15 min each) for 3 to 5 days/week. The intensity should be at about 25–35% of maximum inspiratory pressure measured at functional residual capacity. The general progression of duration, frequency then intensity should be followed. In addition exercises to strengthen abdominal muscles are recommended. For example, in the supine position with knees bent and abdomen pulled in close to the spinal column (pelvic tilt) raise head and shoulders towards knees while exhaling.

Precautions and contraindications

Precautions

Exercise should not be performed if:

- there is a body mass increase $\geqslant 1.8$ kg over the previous 1 to 3 days (such an increase in body mass is likely to indicate the presence of oedema and hence unstable heart failure)
- supine resting heart rate $\geqslant 100$ beats/min
- there are complex arrhythmias at rest.

Systolic blood pressure should not decrease during exercise. Ventricular arrhythmias should not appear with exercise.

Contraindications

The contraindications listed for patients with CHD are also applicable here. Additional contraindications are:

- progressive worsening of exercise tolerance
- dyspnoea at rest or exertion over the previous 3 to 5 days
- significant ischaemia at low exercise intensities (<2 METs).

Despite the benefits noted in studies in patients with stable chronic heart failure, concern has been expressed by the European Society of Cardiology that this evidence should not be interpreted to mean that exercise training should be incorporated as a therapeutic measure for all patients with heart failure. To reiterate, only those patients who are in stable chronic heart failure and NYHA functional class I, II or III should be considered. It is strongly advised that careful consultation with the patient's physician should precede any recommendation to a patient to start an exercise training programme. Furthermore, it is recommended that exercise training be performed in specialized centres.

With regard to types of exercise, currently the effects of only aerobic exercise training have been examined in patients with chronic heart failure. Isometric exercise (weight lifting) training which specifically improves muscle strength is not as yet advocated for patients with chronic heart failure because of concerns related to the haemodynamic responses to such exercise (see end of this chapter).

The long-term effects of exercise training in heart failure are currently unknown. Studies are required in order to assess the possible effects of exercise training on mortality and morbidity. Although more studies are required to better define the possible long-term risks of exercise training in patients with heart failure, the evidence to date does not indicate harm from exercise training.

ESSENTIAL HYPERTENSION

In the general population, elevated blood pressure is increasingly common and is an important risk factor for coronary heart disease and stroke. Despite the use of antihypertensive medications the rates of hypertension control remain suboptimal, which subsequently impacts negatively on the incidence of coronary heart disease and stroke. The Sixth Report of the Joint National Committee on the Prevention, Detection, Evaluation and Treatment of High Blood Pressure (JNC-VI) and the World Hypertension League now recommend several lifestyle modifications as adjunctive therapy to standard medications. Furthermore, daily physical activity in combination with dietary modifications is recommended as the first-line approach (prior to the commencement of pharmacological therapy) to the management of mild and borderline essential hypertension.

The justifications for the recommendation of exercise as part of the management of high blood pressure, the mechanisms of blood pressure reductions with physical activity, examples of exercise prescriptions and precautions will be discussed.

Justifications for encouraging regular exercise

With respect to essential hypertension, the benefits of exercise training are of both a primary and a secondary preventative nature. Less active and less fit persons have a 30–50% greater risk of developing high blood pressure. Indeed, data from cross-sectional studies revealed that blood pressure and consequently the incidence of essential hypertension was lower in fitter and hence more physically active persons (Fig. 9.1.7). Furthermore, regular physical activity helps to reduce blood pressure in persons who already have elevated blood pressure. Hence, regular exercise is important not only in the

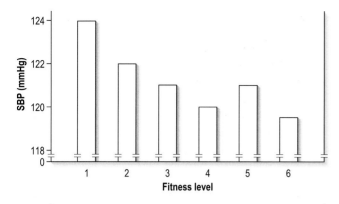

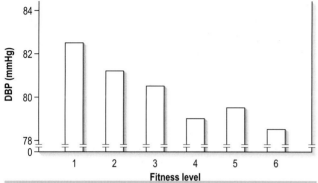

Figure 9.1.7.   The effects of physical fitness (an index of physical activity) on systolic (SBP) and diastolic blood pressure (DBP) in a cross-sectional study of young men. Fitness level 1 indicates the least fit and fitness level 6 the most fit. (Data from Beilin, 1994.)

words the decrease in blood pressure is greater for hypertensives than it is for normotensives. In hypertensives regular physical activity has a greater impact on systolic than on diastolic blood pressure with falls of 11 and 6 mmHg respectively. These apparently small reductions in blood pressure are indeed clinically significant. Such reductions in blood pressure reduce the need for medication in borderline hypertensives and the number of medications required to control blood pressure in moderate to severe hypertensives. Furthermore, these reductions in blood pressure are likely to impact favourably on cardiovascular morbidity and mortality.

Mechanisms of benefits

One of the possible reasons for the reduction in blood pressure from exercise training was postulated to be the concomitant reduction in body weight. However, in a review of the studies performed to date, although in about half of the studies reductions in blood pressure were accompanied by weight loss, the remainder of the studies showed no change in body weight or even increases in body weight. Hence the reductions in blood pressure due to exercise training can be regarded as being largely independent of changes in body weight. Nevertheless, whilst short-term (up to 6 months) reductions in blood pressure are independent of weight loss, long-term falls in blood pressure in physically active persons are more likely to be a combination of both exercise and weight loss. Furthermore, despite independent effects of exercise training and weight loss on blood pressure (at least in the short term), these effects are also additive, thus producing greater reductions in blood pressure when in combination. Hence dietary advice and education is an important component of exercise rehabilitation programmes for hypertensive patients.

The main factors postulated to be part of the mechanism of blood pressure reduction following regular physical activity include changes in the secretion of noradrenaline (norepinephrine) and adrenaline (epinephrine), and changes in cardiac output and peripheral vascular resistance. Regular exercise in hypertensive subjects results in a fall in the concentration of noradrenaline which is not always accompanied by a fall in the concentration of adrenaline. The decreases in the concentration of catecholamines are indicative of a reduction in sympathetic nervous system activity following exercise training in individuals with hypertension. Attenuation of sympathetic nervous system activity contributes toward a lowering of total peripheral resistance and a possible rise in cardiac output. Although evident in some studies, the changes in peripheral resistance and cardiac output are not as consistent as the changes in the concentration of noradrenaline.

Another potential mechanism is changes in the renin–angiotensin–aldosterone system through its effects on blood volume, peripheral resistance and hence blood pressure. In normotensive subjects, exercise training is accompanied by changes in the renin–angiotensin–aldosterone system. Plasma

prevention of the development of hypertension, but also in the therapeutic management of hypertension.

From epidemiological studies it is evident that blood pressure is an important determinant of cardiovascular morbidity and mortality. The positive association between the level of blood pressure and the number of cardiovascular events suggests that decreasing the blood pressure of a subject can favourably affect their prognosis. As yet there are no data showing a direct link between regular physical activity and the incidence of strokes. However, as coronary heart disease contributes to the occurrence of stroke, and regular physical activity reduces the risk of coronary artery disease, it is likely that encouraging people with hypertension to exercise regularly will reduce the incidence of stroke.

In most of the studies performed to assess the effects of exercise training on blood pressure the sample sizes have been relatively small (from 11 to 105 persons) and the majority of those studied were male. Nevertheless the data appear convincing. From an assessment of the well-controlled studies in either normotensives or hypertensives, mean decreases in systolic and diastolic blood pressures of about 6 and 7 mmHg respectively were reported. However, the fall in blood pressure was greater in those with higher baseline values, due to there being a greater opportunity for improvement. In other renin concentrations at rest are reduced and plasma angiotensin II concentrations are lower during exercise, suggesting that exercise training suppresses the renin–angiotensin–aldosterone system. Whether such changes occur in hypertensive subjects following exercise training is not known. Similarly, endothelial responses to nitric oxide (another system implicated in the pathophysiology of hypertension) may be altered by regular exercise. However, whether such effects occur is as yet unknown. Hence further studies are warranted to examine the mechanisms responsible for blood pressure reductions following regular exercise training in hypertensive subjects.

Guidelines for exercise prescriptions

In general falls in systolic and diastolic blood pressure of about 11 and 6 mmHg respectively are reported following aerobic exercise of low (40–60% HR_{max} or 30–50% VO_{2max}) to moderate (60–80% HR_{max} or 50–70% VO_{2max}) intensity. It has been suggested that at higher intensities of exercise training (>80% HR_{max} or >70% VO_{2max}) the effects on blood pressure may be lost. All studies showing reductions in blood pressure utilized activities that used large muscle groups. In general most participants exercised at about 50–70% VO_{2max} and cycling, walking or jogging were the most frequent forms of exercise. Exercise was performed at least three times per week for about 1 hour. However, in obese individuals (because of the concomitant effects of exercise on weight reduction) daily activity appears to give a greater reduction in blood pressure than does activity performed three times per week.

Due to the usual coexistence of obesity and physical inactivity, and the additive effects of weight reduction and exercise on blood pressure, exercise training programmes for patients with hypertension should incorporate an educational component. The focus of such educational programmes should be recommendations to reduce caloric intake and avoidance of foods with high fat and salt content (both are risk factors for hypertension as well as coronary heart disease).

Intensity and mode of training

As discussed, moderate intensity exercise (50–70% VO_{2max}) is more effective than vigorous exercise (>70% VO_{2max}) in lowering blood pressure in hypertensive patients. Hence dynamic exercise such as walking, cycling, non-competitive swimming or slow jogging should be prescribed. In order to ensure that exercise is being performed at moderate intensity heart rate should not exceed 75% of maximum. This intensity of exercise corresponds to an energy equivalent of approximately 4 METs for women and 6 METs for men.

Duration of each training session

The duration of each exercise session significantly influences the blood pressure lowering effects of exercise. Decreases in systolic blood pressure and/or diastolic blood pressure are 94% guaranteed if exercise is performed for 50–60 minutes per session. Reductions in blood pressure are not as consistently observed if exercise is performed for only 30–40 minutes. Therefore, it is recommended that each exercise session last at least 50–60 minutes.

Frequency of training

Significant reductions in blood pressure have consistently been reported provided that a patient exercises at least 3 times per week. The differences observed in blood pressure reductions after exercising 3 times per week versus exercising more than 3 times per week are minimal. Consequently for hypertensive patients the recommendation is that exercise should be performed 3 to 4 times per week. Daily exercise, although necessary for concomitant weight reduction, is not essential to obtain an independent antihypertensive effect.

Duration of exercise training

For patients with essential hypertension progression with exercise follows the three stages namely: initial stage, improvement stage and maintenance stage (see 'Exercise prescription for patients with heart failure' box). Exercise should be prescribed individually for each patient according to their functional capacity, severity of hypertension, presence of concomitant diseases, presence of obesity and whether they are being treated with a beta-adrenergic blocking agent (an attenuation of the blood pressure lowering effect has been observed in patients being treated with beta-adrenergic blockers). The general principles of exercise progression should be followed within each of these stages. In other words the order of duration, then frequency, then intensity should be adhered to. The initial stage is generally 4–6 weeks in duration. Provided that exercise is continued in the maintenance phase, the reductions in blood pressure will be maintained. Importantly if exercise is stopped for a duration of >8–10 weeks the antihypertensive effect will no longer be observed.

> **Exercise prescription for hypertensives**
>
> Cycling, brisk walking, slow jogging or swimming (non-competitive)
> 50–70% VO_{2max} or 60–80% HR_{max} (moderate intensity)
> (4 METs for females and 6 METs for males)
> 50–60 minutes per day
> 3 to 4 times per week

Precautions and contraindications

Data are lacking on specific precautions with regard to exercise in persons with hypertension. Hence the precautions and recommendations for phase II and III rehabilitation for coronary heart disease patients should be followed. In particular, the following should be avoided as they are accompanied by elevations in blood pressure (more in systolic than diastolic):

- forceful isometric exercises, especially upper arm exercises
- exercise in excessive heat
- exercise at higher intensities than those prescribed.

These precautions are especially relevant to those patients with moderate to severe or uncontrolled hypertension.

Exercise testing in order to determine exercise prescriptions should be performed whilst patients are receiving the antihypertensive medication that they will be taking while exercising. Exercise should be dynamic, involving rhythmic repetitive movements of large muscle groups including the arms. In obese subjects, cycling or non-competitive swimming is recommended in preference to walking or jogging in order to avoid orthopaedic injuries.

ISOMETRIC OR RESISTANCE EXERCISE

Resistance or isometric exercise involves sustained muscle contraction against an immovable load with no change in length of the involved muscle and no joint motion. In response to isometric exercise, stroke volume is largely unchanged and only moderate increases in cardiac output occur. Possibly due to reflex vasoconstriction, blood flow to non-contracting muscles does not increase. The vasoconstriction and modest rises in cardiac output in combination result in large increases in blood pressure. Thus a significant pressure load is imposed on the heart. Consequently isometric exercise has traditionally been discouraged in patients with cardiovascular diseases.

However, it has now been found that isometric exercise generally fails to elicit angina pectoris, ischaemic ST-segment depression or ventricular arrhythmias in selected low-risk patients with coronary heart disease. Hence, it is believed that resistance exercise in combination with aerobic exercise is less hazardous in certain patients than was previously presumed. Hence, patients with good aerobic fitness and normal left ventricular function can safely perform resistance exercise within their exercise rehabilitation regimen. However, the safety of resistance training in moderate- to high-risk patients with coronary artery disease requires investigation. Furthermore patients in heart failure (i.e. with left ventricular dysfunction) should be advised NOT to perform isometric exercises. Resistance training in combination with aerobic exercises has been found to be safe in patients with mild controlled hypertension; but is not recommended for those patients with moderate to severe or uncontrolled hypertension.

Justifications for encouraging resistance exercises

The development of endurance, joint flexibility and muscle strength are all important components of a comprehensive exercise training programme, especially as people age. Although isometric exercise alone is not known to lower cardiovascular risk, the use of light weights is beneficial in developing muscle strength and joint flexibility. As many activities of daily living as well as leisure activities require static efforts, improvements in muscle strength are invaluable to the patient. As the pressure response to resistance exercise is largely proportionate to the percentage of maximal voluntary contraction, increases in muscle strength will result in a given degree of static exercise representing a lower percentage of maximal voluntary contraction. Thus the heart rate and blood pressure responses to a given degree of static exercise will be less after resistance training. Consequently myocardial oxygen demands during daily activities such as carrying groceries or lifting moderate to heavy objects will be decreased compared to before resistance training.

Guidelines for exercise prescriptions

In low-risk patients with coronary heart disease and in patients with mild controlled hypertension the guidelines shown in the box are recommended.

Resistance exercise programme

1 set of 10–15 repetitions
8–10 exercises (minimum of one exercise per major muscle group)
2–3 days per week
40–60% of one repetition maximum (one repetition maximum = maximum weight that could be used to complete one repetition)

Importantly, only isometric exercise in combination with dynamic aerobic exercise is recommended. The safety and efficacy of isometric exercise alone in patients with cardiovascular diseases has not yet been established.

COMPLIANCE OR ADHERENCE TO REHABILITATION PROGRAMMES

Adherence to an exercise regimen is of primary importance in order to obtain the maximum benefits thereof. Common reasons for patients to drop out of an exercise programme include difficulties with transportation, poor motivation and lack of cooperation. Since the main reasons for drop-out seem to be psychological, in order to increase compliance patient education is vitally important. Forums for the social interaction of participants and opportunities for interactions with the patient's spouse and family should be provided. Feedback between the patient and the programme personnel should be given on a regular basis in order to instil motivation and encourage cooperation. In essence compliance or adherence to an exercise programme is improved if rehabilitation is an enjoyable experience in which understanding and learning occurs. In order to achieve this active involvement of the patient at all levels is mandatory.

Generally physical activity is more likely to be maintained if an individual:

- perceives a net benefit
- chooses an activity that they enjoy
- feels competent doing the activity
- feels safe doing the activity
- can easily access the activity on a daily basis
- can fit the activity into their daily schedule
- does not perceive that the activity generates financial costs that they are unwilling to bear
- experiences a minimum of negative consequences related to the activity (e.g. injury, loss of time)
- perceives the activity to be accompanied by pleasurable social interaction.

REFERENCES AND FURTHER READING

Arroll B, Beaglehole R (1992) Does physical activity lower blood pressure: a critical review of the clinical trials. J Clin Epidemiol 45: 439–447.

Beilin LJ (1994) Non-pharmacological management of hypertension: optimal strategies for reducing cardiovascular risk. J Hypertens 12 (Suppl 10): S71–81.

Bijnen FCH, Caspersen CJ, Feskens EJM, et al. (1998) Physical activity and 10-year mortality from cardiovascular diseases and all causes. Arch Intern Med 158: 1499–1505.

Cléroux J, Feldman RD, Petrella RJ (1999) Recommendations on physical exercise training. CMAJ 160(Suppl 9): S21–S28.

Ehsani AA, Martin WH III, Heath GW, Coyle EF (1982) Cardiac effects of prolonged and intense exercise training in patients with coronary heart disease. Am J Cardiol 50: 246–254.

Fletcher GF, Balady G, Froelicher VF, et al. (1995) Exercise standards. A statement for healthcare professionals from the American Heart Association. Circulation 91: 580–615.

Gielen S, Schuler G, Hambrecht R (2001) Exercise training in coronary artery disease and vasomotion. Circulation 103: e1–e6.

Goldman MA (1981) Cardiac rehabilitation: state of the art. Geriatrics 36: 103–112.

Hagberg JM, Ehsani AA, Holloszt JO (1983) Effect of 12 months of intense exercise training on stroke volume in patients with coronary artery disease. Circulation 67: 1194–1199.

Haskell WL (1979) Mechanisms by which physical activity may enhance the clinical status of cardiac patients. In: Heart Disease and Rehabilitation. Boston: Houghton Mifflin, pp. 276–296.

Haskell WL (1981) Influence of habitual physical activity on blood lipids and lipoproteins. In: Physical Conditioning and Cardiovascular Rehabilitation. New York: Wiley, pp. 87–102.

McKelvie RS, Teo KK, McCartney N, et al. (1995) Effects of exercise training in patients with congestive heart failure: a critical review. J Am Coll Cardiol 25: 789–796.

Pollock ML, Franklin BA, Balady GJ, et al. (2001) Resistance exercise in individuals with and without cardiovascular disease. Circulation 101: 828–833.

Redwood DR, Rosing DR, Epstein SE (1972) Circulatory and symptomatic effects of physical training in patients with coronary artery disease and angina pectoris. N Engl J Med 286: 959–965.

Tavazzi L, Giannuzzi P (2001) Physical training as a therapeutic measure in chronic heart failure: time for recommendations. Heart 86: 7–11.

Wenger (1979) Rehabilitation of the patient with acute myocardial infarction: Early ambulation and patient education. In: Heart Disease and Rehabilitation. Boston: Houghton Mifflin, pp. 446–462.

Wenger NK (1986) Rehabilitation of the coronary patient: status 1986. Prog Cardiovasc Dis 29: 181–204.

Wilson PK, Edgett JW, Porter GH (1979) Rehabilitation of the cardiac patient: Program organisation. In: Heart Disease and Rehabilitation. Boston: Houghton Mifflin, pp. 379–394.

Working Group on Cardiac Rehabilitation and Exercise Physiology and Working Group on Heart Failure of the European Society of Cardiology (2001) Recommendations for exercise training in chronic heart failure patients. Eur Heart J 22: 125–135.

Altered Exercise Tolerance: Pulmonary Rehabilitation

Carolyn Mason

INTRODUCTION

Chronic obstructive pulmonary disease (COPD) features as one of the leading causes of morbidity, mortality and economic burden throughout the world. Airway obstruction and chronic bronchitis are typical features of the disease, which frequently coexist in the lungs of those who suffer from the condition. COPD is not, however, a disease that is exclusive to the lungs. Decades of research have demonstrated that it is a multisystem disorder that has profound effects throughout the body. Accordingly, the management of patients with chronic lung disease has evolved and become a focus of expertise for healthcare disciplines, much of which has been packaged into comprehensive pulmonary rehabilitation programmes. In consequence, advances have been made in many aspects of care including pharmacological therapy, dietetics and nutrition, ventilatory management, exercise training, psychosocial care and smoking cessation. Exercise therapy as a component of pulmonary rehabilitation has, like its counterparts, matured in its profile and exegesis over the years. It has developed from a treatment option that was practised because it appeared to improve the psychological outlook of the patient, to one that is utilized because it has a sound scientific background with a robust physiological evidence base.

The traditional concepts which explored the pathophysiological mechanisms of exercise intolerance in patients with COPD focused on the lungs. However, mounting evidence of improper function of skeletal muscles in COPD has led researchers to the conclusion that muscular dysfunction could be an additional fundamental and potentially reversible source of exercise intolerance in this group of patients. This chapter considers the current knowledge concerning the mechanisms that predispose to respiratory and skeletal dysfunction and exercise limitation in COPD. It then explores how and why exercise can be utilized as a therapeutic option to challenge the progression of disability which COPD causes.

EXERCISE LIMITATION AND RESPIRATORY/PERIPHERAL MUSCLE DYSFUNCTION IN COPD

Exercise limitation in COPD

Dyspnoea

Dyspnoea has been identified as the overriding complaint and the major disabling symptom of most patients with COPD (American Thoracic Society, 1999a). Dyspnoea is a clinical term for breathlessness, a subjective feeling of discomfort which is associated with the effort in breathing or with the urge to breathe. It is a complex symptom that may occur in healthy and diseased individuals in response to psychological, social and environmental factors such as emotion, exercise or an increase in altitude. In the healthy population the sensation of dyspnoea though variable in intensity is generally reversible and short-lived. In contrast, for those who suffer from cardiopulmonary conditions such as COPD, dyspnoea can become chronic and the symptoms which it gives rise to may feel out of control.

In the disease state of COPD dyspnoea is often linked with the phenomena of hypoxaemia, hypercapnia, metabolic acidosis, failure of the central ventilatory drive and an exceptional mechanical load on the ventilatory muscles induced by airway obstruction and chronic bronchitis. Dyspnoea induced in this way is frequently regarded as a cause for exercise intolerance and reduced quality of life in patients with COPD. The traditional interpretation of the pathological sequelae suggests a downward spiral or vicious circle. This represents a situation whereby patients with COPD have a derangement in their respiratory mechanics leading to a feeling of breathlessness, which may cause them to stop exercising before the skeletal muscles reach their functional limits. Because activity is associated with dyspnoea the patients assume a sedentary lifestyle. This further reduces patients' tolerance to exertion, resulting in the patients becoming housebound, isolated and thoroughly depressed as they try desperately to avoid any activities that may invoke the intolerable dyspnoea caused by these activities (Fig. 9.2.1).

In the past pulmonary rehabilitation including exercise therapy has been prescribed in order to break this vicious circle and it appears to have been successful. However, questions have arisen as to why patients have demonstrated functional improvement in their exercise tolerance, as reduced exercise capacity has only a weak relationship to lung function impairment. Moreover, pulmonary rehabilitation does nothing to improve lung function. Patients who have had their lung function restored to near normal through lung transplantation have not demonstrated that they are able to achieve their predicted exercise capacity following surgery.

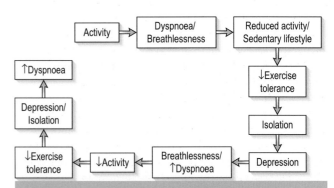

Figure 9.2.1.   Cycle associated with dyspnoea. Because activity is associated with dyspnoea, the patient assumes a sedentary lifestyle. This further reduces the patient's tolerance to exertion, which may result in the patient becoming isolated or housebound.

Muscle dysfunction

Recent studies have demonstrated that peripheral skeletal muscles are compromised in patients with COPD. This may play an important role in the exercise limitation that is experienced by this population. There is evidence to suggest that approximately equal numbers of people terminate their exercise routine as a result of the limitations imposed by their leg effort as those that terminate their exercise due to the experience of dyspnoea.

Whether dyspnoea or leg pain is the cause of the loss of exercise tolerance, functional ability and reduced quality of life, it is essential that there is an understanding of the causative factors of the disability.

Mechanisms which predispose to respiratory/peripheral muscle dysfunction and exercise limitation in COPD

Respiratory muscle dysfunction

The cause of exercise limitation in patients with COPD is the subject of much debate. Excessive inspiratory muscle loading and reduced pulmonary capacity are frequently cited in explanation of this. Pathophysiological changes in patients with COPD lead to an imbalance in *respiratory muscle load* (Pbreath) and *capacity* (Pmax) (Fig. 9.2.2). This manifests itself in low respiratory muscle strength and endurance.

Respiratory muscle load

Lung *hyperinflation* has profound effects on the respiratory muscle load. It compromises the function of the muscles of inspiration in particular, the function of the expiratory muscles being relatively well preserved.

As pathological processes are not constant throughout the lungs, differential elastic recoil properties exist which results in an uneven distribution of ventilation. Emphysematous lung is more compliant than normal lung at low lung volume, therefore it responds to small changes in pressure by expanding to a larger volume (Fig. 9.2.3). When a greater pressure is exerted the emphysematous portion becomes hyperinflated and accepts less volume change per unit of pressure change. In this state the emphysematous lung operates with reduced dynamic compliance. It behaves as a 'stiff' lung, which is under-ventilated in comparison to the normal lung. In cases of severe airflow limitation the time required to empty the lungs is greater than the time available for expiration. The patient initiates his next breath before reaching the normal end-expiratory lung volume or functional residual capacity (FRC). *Dynamic hyperinflation* is the term used to describe the breath stacking increase in FRC that occurs as a result of incomplete expiration.

Ventilation/perfusion

As lung emptying is not terminated at end expiration, a residual positive pressure remains in the airways. This has

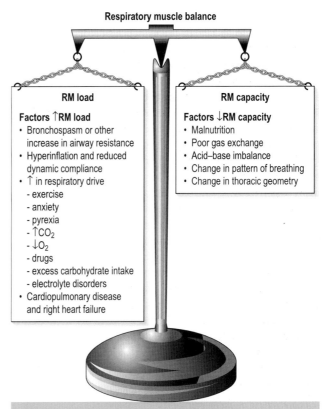

Respiratory muscle balance

RM load	RM capacity
Factors ↑RM load	**Factors ↓RM capacity**
• Bronchospasm or other increase in airway resistance	• Malnutrition
• Hyperinflation and reduced dynamic compliance	• Poor gas exchange
• ↑ in respiratory drive	• Acid–base imbalance
- exercise	• Change in pattern of breathing
- anxiety	• Change in thoracic geometry
- pyrexia	
- ↑CO_2	
- ↓O_2	
- drugs	
- excess carbohydrate intake	
- electrolyte disorders	
• Cardiopulmonary disease and right heart failure	

Figure 9.2.2. Pathophysiological changes in patients with COPD which lead to an imbalance in respiratory muscle (RM) load and RM capacity.

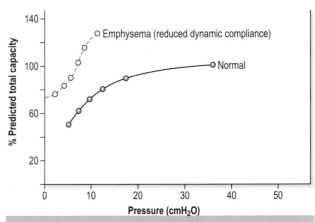

Figure 9.2.3. Pressure–volume curves of the lung. Emphysematous lung is more compliant than normal lung at low lung volume. It responds to small changes in pressure by expanding to a larger volume. When a greater pressure is exerted, the emphysematous portion becomes hyperinflated and accepts less volume change per unit of pressure change. The resultant pressure–volume curve is displaced to the left and has a steeper slope than that of the normal lung.

been termed 'intrinsic positive end-expiratory pressure' (intrinsic PEEP or auto PEEP). In the presence of PEEP, *transmural* pressure is profoundly increased in the emphysematous region, which predisposes to the perfusion being even more compromised than ventilation. This results in a high ventilation:perfusion ratio and a consequence of increased physiological dead space. In parallel, constricted airways in other regions of the lung may prevent adequate ventilation of relatively well-perfused alveoli. This will produce a concomitant ventilation:perfusion mismatch which may further result in hypoxaemia (Fig. 9.2.4). Alveolar ventilation must be sufficient to deliver adequate oxygen to the pulmonary capillaries and to eliminate the carbon dioxide that is produced. Insufficient oxygen levels will result in constriction of the pulmonary capillary bed, increased pulmonary artery pressure, right-sided heart failure, cardiac arrhythmia and eventually death. Hypoxaemia also results in impaired cognitive function as a result of a lack of oxygen to the brain. As ventilatory demand increases, as in the case of advancing disease or with exercise, so does the work of breathing and for patients with COPD the control of ventilation and perfusion becomes even more of a challenge. This is exacerbated by the change in lung mechanics and altered respiratory muscle capacity.

Respiratory muscle capacity

The most important muscle of inspiration is the diaphragm, a mobile structure that is composed of long downward fibres, which extend from a non-contractile central tendon to attach to the lower ribs and the upper lumbar spine. Like all skeletal muscles, the diaphragm is governed by the length–tension relationship. At an optimal length the actin and myosin muscle filaments of the diaphragm are capable of shortening up to 40% between full expiration and end inspiration. If the muscle is working at a shorter length the tension produced is much less for the same level of neural activation. When the thorax is in a state of hyperinflation, the reduced length of the diaphragm mainly affects its vertical displacement, the so-called 'zone of apposition'. As the diaphragm works like a piston, the more profound the hyperinflation, the tighter the diaphragm, causing the zone of apposition to disappear. This generates a reduced respiratory muscle capacity. An ineffective breathing pattern is produced as muscle fibres pull the ribs in an expiratory rather than an inspiratory direction. Respiratory muscle dysfunction may degenerate into respiratory fatigue and failure if the hyperinflation becomes severe. In advanced COPD the respiratory muscles are chronically overworked in this fashion. They have little to offer the body in response to the demands imposed by exercise.

Contradictory evidence claims that failure of the generation of transdiaphragmatic pressure (P_{di}) is not clinically important in patients with COPD. Alternatively it is proposed that compensatory adaptation occurs in the diaphragm of these patients. The assumption is that the diaphragm is trained by chronic overload rather than fatigued. Cellular adaptations of the diaphragm including a shift to the more fatigue-resistant slow twitch fibre profile have been postulated in explanation of this observation.

Muscular fibre typing and the diaphragm

Fibre typing is mainly performed histochemically and is based on the differences between fibres in myosin ATPase activities or immunocytochemistry. The adult mammalian skeleton is supported by muscle that is composed of three myosin heavy chain isoforms, namely *I, IIa* and *IIb/x*.

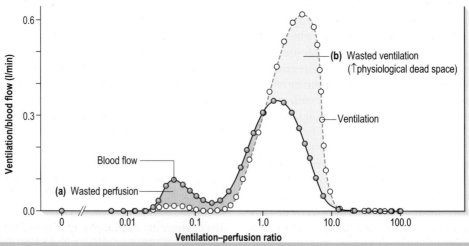

Figure 9.2.4.   Distribution of ventilation–perfusion ratios in emphysema. Some ventilation and blood flow go to compartments of the lung where the ventilation–perfusion ratio is near normal. (a) Considerable blood flow is being delivered to areas where constricted airways prevent adequate ventilation of relatively well-perfused alveoli. (b) Overheated and underperfused units where alveolar walls may have been destroyed and capillaries obliterated.

- *Fibre type I* has a slow twitch and develops at a relatively small tension. It depends on aerobic metabolism and is fatigue resistant.
- *Fibre type IIb/x* has a fast twitch and develops large tensions. Its energy conversion is based on anaerobic, glycolytic metabolism and so is susceptible to fatigue.
- *Type IIa* has a fibre type which lies somewhere between types I and IIb/x. It has fast twitch properties, develops under a moderate tension, is relatively resistant to fatigue and is capable of working under both aerobic and anaerobic conditions.

(Muscle fibre types are discussed in detail in Chapter 5.)

In healthy subjects the diaphragm has approximately 50% type I (slow twitch) fibres, 25% type IIb/x (fast twitch), and 25% type IIa (intermediate twitch) fibres. Some authors believe that in patients with COPD there is a reduction in the proportion of fast twitch fibres resulting from a shift from type IIb/x to type I (slow twitch, small tension) fibres. This accounts for the impaired force-generating capacity of the diaphragm; it also implies that the diaphragm becomes more fatigue resistant in patients with COPD.

Additional muscles of respiration

Other muscles assist the diaphragm with the effort of inspiration and as such are agonists in quiet breathing. The scalene and parasternal muscles are thus described as primary muscles of respiration. In addition, the sternomastoid, latissimus dorsi, trapezius external intercostal and pectoralis minor muscles, not active in quiet breathing in normal subjects, augment respiratory muscle force with increased ventilatory loads and thus are described as accessory muscles of respiration.

In COPD, patients increase their thoracic volume using their accessory muscles. The accessory muscles, including the sternocleidomastoid, assist in raising the ribs, which contributes to a stretch of the lungs and an increased intrapulmonary volume. In the absence of a normally functioning diaphragm this allows the intrapulmonary pressure to drop relative to atmospheric pressure, encouraging some air to enter the lungs along a pressure gradient. At the same time the intrapleural pressure declines relative to atmospheric pressure. Exhalation is primarily a passive process, which relies on the elastic recoil of the lungs. In COPD, however, the abdominal muscles frequently act as accessory muscles to expiration as their contraction can facilitate expiration by contributing to the generation of gastric pressure required for diaphragmatic contraction to be effective. Contraction of the internal intercostals, rectus abdominis and internal and external oblique muscles lowers and deflates the rib cage during exhalation, which decreases both the thoracic and intrapulmonary volume. This compresses the alveoli and raises the intrapulmonary pressure. At the same time the intrapleural pressure rises. Air leaves the lungs along a pressure gradient.

The proportion of type I (slow twitch, small tension) fibres in both the internal and external intercostal muscles has been demonstrated to be the same in both patients with COPD and normal subjects, suggesting that accessory muscles of respiration do not show the type IIb/x to type I fibre shift that occurs in the diaphragm. Rather they conform to the behaviour of peripheral skeletal muscles. However, in the clinical examination of patients with COPD, there is a tendency for the sternocleidomastoid muscle to be described as being hypertrophied. This is possibly as a result of the perception that this muscle works hard in the hyperinflated state. As this is not physiologically proven, the prominence of the sternocleidomastoid may be attributed to the presence of exaggerated pleural pressure swings discussed above, which are easily discerned in the cachexic COPD patient.

Competing dual roles of the muscles of respiration

The respiratory muscles are unique, as their roles are not confined to ventilation. The diaphragm for example contributes to:

- postural stabilization of the torso
- parturition, defecation and micturition through its ability to raise intra-abdominal pressure.

The rib cage muscles also:

- maintain upper body posture
- assist in movement of the thorax
- support the upper limbs in unsupported arm movement.

The muscles of the face and upper airway required for the performance of speech, mastication and facial expression also assist in the maintenance of respiration when there is an increased ventilatory load.

In normal subjects the respiratory muscles are able to maintain ventilation over other non-ventilatory activities. However, when the respiratory muscles are required for the performance of respiratory *and* tonic functions, their ability to assist ventilation may be compromised. Here the muscles that are participating in respiration have to have a high degree of coordination in order to perform their additional non-ventilatory work. If muscle function becomes dyscoordinated, then dysfunction results. This has been demonstrated in patients with COPD who perform unsupported arm exercise. Exercises such as grooming lead to early fatigue of the muscles involved in the task but also to dyssynchrony between the rib cage and the diaphragm–abdomen. Dyssynchrony occurs when movement between the thoracic cage and the abdomen is poorly coordinated. *Abdominal paradoxical breathing* occurs when the diaphragm is fixed and has little vertical displacement. The resultant decrease in pleural pressure is transmitted across the diaphragm to the abdomen, leading to a reduction in abdominal pressure and inward displacement of the abdominal wall during inspiration (Figs 9.2.5 and 9.2.6).

The dyssynchrony which may be perceived as dyspnoea, early fatigue and limited exercise endurance has also been observed in normal individuals breathing against increased

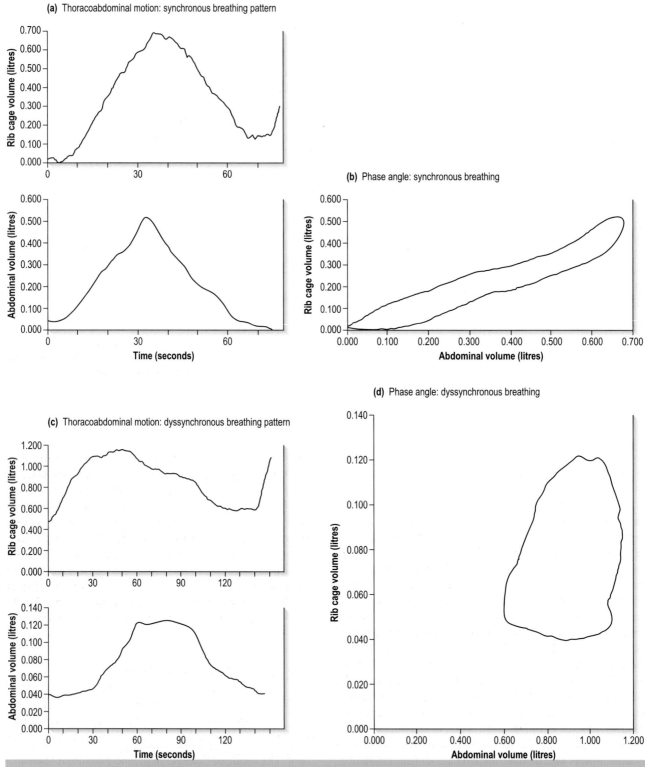

Figure 9.2.5.   Analogue waveforms and phase angles of rib cage and abdomen excursion with synchronous breathing (a, b), and dyssynchronous breathing (c, d). (Adapted from Breslin, 1996.)

loads, and in patients with COPD breathing during voluntary hyperventilation.

Additional mechanisms have been postulated for the reduced capacity and the dyscoordinated and dysfunctional action of respiratory muscles in COPD. These include the competing outputs of the driving centres of respiration in the brain in addition to diverse effects such as malnutrition, corticosteroids, poor cardiovascular status and electrolyte

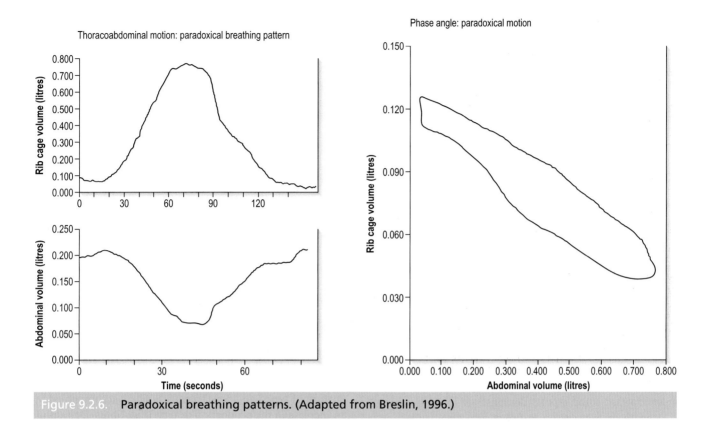

Figure 9.2.6.   Paradoxical breathing patterns. (Adapted from Breslin, 1996.)

disturbances. As these also affect the peripheral muscles of the body they will be discussed later in this chapter.

Control of ventilation

For ventilation to take place it is necessary to move air into and out of the lung. This is achieved by the action of the muscles of respiration on the rib cage and abdomen under the control of the respiratory centres. The respiratory cycle is regulated by a complex array of centrally organized neurons which coordinate and maintain rhythmic breathing; this generally goes unnoticed but can be overridden by cortical control. The central controller of the respiratory centre is located in the medulla and integrates input from the periphery and other parts of the nervous system. This generator then distributes its output, by the conducting nerves to the respiratory muscles, which shorten and deform the rib cage and the abdomen altering intrathoracic pressures and allowing air to move into or out of the lungs.

Patients with COPD have an increased neural drive to their respiratory muscles which seems to be emphasized in hypercapnic patients, possibly as a result of afferent activity from mechanical receptors in the lungs and chest wall and from chemoreceptors detecting hypoxia. The increased respiratory drive maybe required to overcome increased airway resistance in an attempt to compensate for the mechanically disadvantaged diaphragm and chest wall. Alternatively it has been suggested that the automatic and voluntary ventilatory

pathways are different and that the ventilatory and tonic functions of the respiratory muscles are driven from different central nervous areas, integrated at the spinal level. Some authors suggest that muscle dyssynchrony in COPD can be caused by competing outputs of the separate driving centres that control rhythmic breathing and tonic activities of the accessory muscles and the diaphragm. When the load is increased, for example during exercise, there is even greater competition placed upon the driving centres of the bi-functional respiratory muscles, which could be a further predisposing factor for the dyspnoea experienced when patients with COPD exercise.

Peripheral muscle dysfunction

Distribution of muscle weakness

Many patients with COPD will stop exercising because of peripheral muscle fatigue rather than dyspnoea. This observation has stimulated renewed interest in the physiological function of limb muscles and a growing realization that COPD is a multi-organ system disease.

The presence and distribution of peripheral muscle weakness in patients with COPD remains a source of debate:

- Some have found a significant degree of weakness of the quadriceps femoris muscle.
- Others have observed no significant difference in quadriceps strength in patients with COPD compared with matched control subjects.

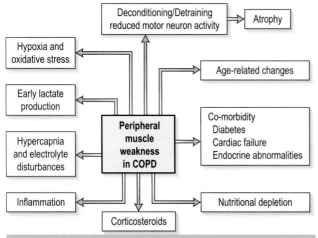

Figure 9.2.7. Some of the documented causes of peripheral muscle dysfunction in patients with COPD. These may vary from muscle to muscle and from patient to patient. Many of the factors are interrelated.

- With regard to upper and lower limb distribution of weakness, there are studies that have showed no statistically significant difference between arm and quadriceps muscles.
- In contrast, some reports demonstrate lower quadriceps strength in comparison to upper arm and trunk muscle strength in COPD patients.
- Proximal muscle strength may be affected more than distal muscles as the latter can retain their function with little impact on ventilatory requirement.
- Reduced handgrip has been demonstrated in patients who suffer with COPD.

Causes of peripheral muscle weakness

The causes of peripheral muscle dysfunction are various (Fig. 9.2.7) and will probably differ from muscle to muscle and patient to patient. Different mechanisms may be involved in weakness of each of the muscle groups. Susceptibility to steroids, cardiac failure, endocrine abnormalities, hypoxaemia, hypercapnia, age and a poor nutritional state will all be considered. In most, however, deconditioning is a crucial component.

Deconditioning and muscle atrophy

Some theorists propose that the preferential distribution of muscle weakness to the lower limbs in comparison to the upper limbs and to the respiratory muscles could be related to differences in accustomed level of activity between the muscle groups. This suggests that muscle bulk will be better preserved in the upper limbs, as they are more functionally involved in the activities of daily living. In contrast, other theories suggest that there is only a modest reduction in peripheral muscle strength in patients with COPD and that this is comparable

between the upper and lower limbs. Further there is a belief that patients with COPD avoid the use of their proximal upper limb muscles as this tends to induce breathlessness, whereas there is more preservation of distal limb function as the muscles of the distal upper extremity are utilized with less symptomatic effect.

With regard to the muscles of inspiration, respiratory muscle weakness can contribute to exercise limitation, but it is unlikely to be as a result of deconditioning. As discussed earlier in this chapter, the diaphragm is probably not disused in COPD and a kind of endurance training effect may even occur. Equally the pectoralis major and the latissimus dorsi as accessory muscles of respiration assist breathing manoeuvres and positions to reduce breathlessness. They are therefore generally over-stimulated rather than under-utilized in COPD.

Detraining

Detraining causes muscle weaknesses because of reduced motor neuron activity and muscle wasting or atrophy. In general atrophy is reversible and affects both type I and type IIa fibres with a distinct preference for type I fibres. In patients with COPD it has been reported that there is a reduced proportion of type I and type IIa muscle fibres accompanied by an increase in the proportion of type IIb/x fibres. Detraining causes a decline in the activity of enzymes involved in the oxidative energy conversion in both type I and type II fibres and consequent early lactic acidosis irrespective of whether there is any change in fibre composition. (This is discussed in more detail later in this chapter under 'Muscle bioenergetics and early lactate production').

Age-related changes

Muscle force is known to decrease by 30–40% between 30 and 80 years of age. Strength is said to be greatest between the ages of 20 and 30 when the cross-sectional area of muscle is at its greatest. Thereafter strength in muscle gradually declines until middle age, when the decline becomes more rapid. The associated reduction in muscle mass of up to 50% has been attributed to a reduction in cross-sectional area of all muscle fibres but particularly of the fast twitch type IIb/x fibres, which results in a proportionate increase in the area occupied by slow twitch type I fibres. Age-related atrophy is related to motor unit remodelling. Under normal circumstances this is a cyclical process involving end-plate repair and reconstruction. This occurs at the neuromuscular junction and involves the processes of selective denervation of muscle fibres, which is followed by terminal sprouting of axons from adjacent motor units. Generally type I motor units increase in size as there is selective denervation of the type II fibres and faster reinnervation by collateral sprouting from type I motor units. As a result, some muscles have been shown to reduce their motor units by 75% with increasing age.

In the seventh decade of life the mean area of type II fibres decreases by approximately 15% and the percentage of type II fibres decreases by 40%. Strength loss among the older population can be directly associated with their limited mobility and physical performance. Elderly bedridden patients can lose virtually all of their type IIa fibres.

Although the effects of ageing on skeletal muscle in patients with COPD is unknown, it is likely that strength loss through age-related atrophy compounds the susceptibility of these patients to early fatigue. Moreover it has been suggested that there may be a specific myopathy associated with COPD. It is also recognized that peripheral muscle function may be adversely affected by factors such as malnutrition, hypoxia, hypercapnia and drug therapy, yet to be discussed in this chapter. The effects of smoking, though not considered here, must also not be ignored.

Nutritional depletion

The relationship between weight loss and COPD has been recognized since the late nineteenth century. Originally perceived to be a terminal progression of the disease process, little interest was given to nutrition and COPD, but in recent years indications that mortality could be reduced by weight gain after nutritional support has renewed interest and changed concepts in the management of the disease. As previously mentioned, the most prominent symptoms of COPD are dyspnoea and impaired exercise capacity. Over the last decade research has consistently demonstrated that skeletal muscle weakness contributes to these symptoms and in particular that there is a relationship between COPD, skeletal muscle mass and peripheral skeletal muscle dysfunction.

Nutritional depletion commonly occurs in patients with COPD, usually as a consequence of the conflict which occurs between the individual's desire to breathe, the desire to eat and the physical inability to achieve both of these objectives at the same time. Systemic inflammation, common in COPD, may also affect the patient's appetite and dietary intake mediated by the appetite-regulating hormone *leptin*. In the presence of a normal or above normal dietary intake, patients with COPD may also lose weight as a result of a raised total and resting energy expenditure. The total daily energy expenditure is due to the increased oxygen cost of breathing associated with hyperinflation during exercise. The suggested contributors to raised resting energy expenditure are the thermogenic effects of systemic inflammation and of the bronchodilating agents which are commonly utilized to treat the airway narrowing characteristic of the disease.

Body composition

The effects of nutritional depletion on peripheral skeletal muscle must be considered in addition to disuse. Body weight is often used as a determinant of nutritional status but it fails to take into account the differences in body composition between individuals. Determination of body composition with respect to nutritional depletion is important, however, as it allows one to distinguish between the different patterns of weight loss:

- predominant loss of fat mass
- predominant loss of fat-free mass
- or a combination of both.

Depleted fat-free mass (FFM) is associated with reductions in muscle mass, exercise capacity and exercise response; however, the mechanical effectiveness of the remaining muscle is not affected. Patients with a reduced FFM have a low peak oxygen consumption and peak work rate and early onset of lactic acid compared with patients with adequate nutrition.

Muscle morphology and nutritional depletion

With regard to muscle morphology the effects of nutritional depletion are more significant on type II fibres, causing reduction of their cross-sectional area. This results in the relative preservation of slow oxidative fibres, which have a greater resistance to fatigue than the fast twitch fibres. Although the tension of the muscles generated during basal activities is well preserved, the power potential may be impaired as progressively more fast twitch fibres are recruited. This has been demonstrated in clinical studies that have investigated the effects of nutritional depletion on peripheral skeletal muscle function using neurophysiological tests. Here nutritional depletion was associated with a reduction in force at higher stimulation frequencies, slowing of the relaxation rate after supramaximal stimulation and a reduction in muscle endurance. Studies have demonstrated that nutritional depletion not only decreases peripheral muscle function but also affects respiratory muscle mass and strength. In particular, body weight reduction has been related to decreases in diaphragm muscle mass, intercostal muscle fibre size, and sternomastoid thickness.

Muscle wasting can occur as part of overall body weight loss, but it can also occur in patients with COPD of normal weight, suggesting that muscle wasting can occur independently of fat loss. In an attempt to explain this phenomenon researchers have deduced that disturbances can occur in the metabolism of protein in patients with COPD. In particular, there are disturbances in plasma and muscle amino acid levels in these patients. This could be related to the process of inflammation rather than to a loss in body weight.

Inflammation

Local and systemic inflammation is characteristic of patients with COPD and can be a cause of oxidative stress. Chemicals released by immune cells throughout a period of inflammation can modulate various cellular processes including carbohydrate metabolism, calcium homeostasis, mitochondrial oxygen consumption and membrane transport. Monocytes and macrophages, for example, produce *cytokine tumour necrosis factor α* (TNF-α) which may in turn induce oxidative stress in myocytes (described in Ch. 2). This is a phenomenon that has been detected in the blood of patients with COPD, especially in those who have had considerable weight loss or muscle wasting.

Hormonal influences

Normal muscle growth is dependent upon adequate levels of anabolic hormones whilst an absence of anabolic hormones results in muscle wasting. Skeletal muscle dysfunction in patients with COPD may be caused by reduced levels of circulating anabolic hormones within the blood.

Growth hormone or *somatotropin* is secreted by the anterior pituitary gland. This is controlled by neural input to the hypothalamus from stimuli such as anxiety, stress and physical activity. In the adult, growth hormone facilitates protein synthesis and subsequent muscle hypertrophy and its release can cause a decrease in carbohydrate breakdown and subsequent mobilization and use of lipids as an energy source.

Although there are some direct effects on the muscle, the major effect of growth hormone is on the liver. Growth hormone causes the liver to produce a group of small peptides called *somatomedins*, which have a potent effect on cellular proliferation. Resembling proinsulin in structure these peptides, originally discovered in plasma, were termed *insulin-like growth factors (IGFs)* because of the similar effect to insulin on growth. There are at least four somatomedins, but by far the most important is *somatomedin C* also known as *insulin-like growth factor 1 (IGF-1)*.

Testosterone, secreted by the testes in men, also has a substantial anabolic effect on muscle. In addition to its role in development of the secondary sex characteristics, it contributes to the sex differences in muscle mass and strength through its tissue-building role. Testosterone causes increased deposition of protein in the tissues throughout the body, including an increase of up to 50% in the contractile proteins of the muscles. Women also have circulating levels of testosterone, but in far less magnitude than that present in men, roughly only 10%. There is evidence to suggest that patients with COPD demonstrate substantially reduced levels of both IGF-1 and testosterone, which may contribute to their muscle dysfunction.

Hypercapnia and electrolyte disturbances

Patients with COPD may have tissue hypoxia, hypercapnia and premature lactic acid production in addition to electrolyte and acid–base imbalances. Electrolyte and acid–base imbalance may alter the resting membrane potential and inhibit normal production of any muscle action potential. In addition, the accumulation of lactic acid and other metabolic end-products can contribute to muscle dysfunction.

Hypercapnia

Hypercapnia, either chronic or acute, is frequently present in patients with COPD. If acute, hypercapnia can contribute to intracellular acidosis. In the skeletal muscles of individuals with respiratory failure this has been associated with reduced

potassium and magnesium content and with a reduced efflux of lactate and pyruvate. Such conditions within the muscle reduce the intracellular pH, which can have a detrimental effect on the contractility of the muscle through the following mechanisms:

- decreasing the affinity of the troponin for calcium
- increasing the binding of calcium by the sarcoplasmic reticulum
- reducing the rate of glycolysis and thus ATP resynthesis.

Within the respiratory system hypercapnic disturbances can affect the functioning of the muscles that contribute to ventilation. With particular regard to the work of breathing, hypercapnia has been associated with a decrease in contractility and endurance time of the diaphragm in normal subjects. Investigators have shown that hypercapnia reduces the capacity of the diaphragm to generate force during voluntary contraction. In addition, when breathing was performed against resistance, hypercapnia produced electromyographic changes consistent with diaphragmatic muscle fatigue. In contrast others have found that exercise capacity is similarly reduced in eucapnic and hypercapnic patients with severe stable COPD, but that hypercapnic patients achieve lower ventilation with exercise. They found that respiratory muscle function as respiratory muscle strength, and ventilatory recruitment at rest and during exercise are equally affected in eucapnic and hypercapnic patients. Consequently, an elevated carbon-dioxide level is not an important cause of respiratory muscle weakness in patients with stable COPD. The suggestion is that hypercapnia in patients with COPD is more likely as a result of the inability of the patient to increase ventilation. They attribute this to the mechanical changes incurred by progressive airflow obstruction and the failure of the lungs to wash out the carbon dioxide produced at an increased level of physiological ventilatory drive.

Several theories exist which suggest that in COPD, chronic alveolar hypoventilation occurs in association with hypercapnia, as the result of a breathing strategy developed by patients to avoid fatigue of weakened muscles working against high inspiratory loads, fatigue and ultimate respiratory failure.

Muscle bioenergetics and early lactate production

Early lactate acidosis has been suggested as a factor that negatively influences the exercise capacity of patients with COPD. Since premature lactic acidosis represents an imbalance between lactic acid production and the body's ability to clear lactic acid it is important to discern the factors that define both the rate of lactic acid production and clearance in COPD.

Under normal conditions stored glycogen in muscle can be split into glucose, which then can be used for energy. There are two stages to this process:

- Glycolysis is the initial stage, completed in the absence of oxygen, in which each glucose molecule is split into two pyruvic acid molecules and energy is released to form four adenosine triphosphate (ATP) molecules for each original glucose molecule.

- The second part of the reaction occurs when the pyruvic acid enters the mitochondria of the muscle cell and forms more ATP molecules by reacting with oxygen in the tricarboxylic acid cycle (TCA) or citric acid/ Krebs cycle.

In circumstances where there is insufficient oxygen for the second stage to occur, most of the pyruvic acid is converted to lactic acid, which diffuses out of the muscle cells into the interstitial fluid and blood.

Generally muscle lactic acid production will increase when the rate of pyruvate production by glycolysis exceeds the rate of pyruvate oxidation by the Krebs cycle. This can occur as a result of many factors in patients with COPD. These include:

- the effects of hypoxia
- impaired oxidative muscle metabolism
- hypercapnia of the exercising peripheral skeletal muscles.

Significantly the fibre type and distribution in peripheral skeletal muscle is important as the ratio of oxidative to glycolytic fibres is fundamental to the range over which lactic acidosis can move during exercise.

- *Type IIb* fibres with their high concentration of glycolytic enzymes and *La-dehydrogenase–M isozyme* and low mitochondrial content favour glycolytic or anaerobic energy production. They therefore produce lactate when stimulated.
- In contrast *type I* fibres are predominantly aerobic in their metabolic capacity having high mitochondrial density and enzyme activity.

Type I fibres have greater lactate and pyruvate oxidative capacity than do type IIb fibres during exercise. Oxidative type I fibres therefore play an important role in clearance of lactate produced by the glycolytic type IIb/x fibres during exercise.

Since COPD patients, in particular those with emphysema, have physical inactivity related reduction in the percentage of type I fibres in their skeletal muscles there is a general shift to a more glycolytic and less oxidative capacity in these areas. Also, as there is a reduced percentage of type I fibres there is less capacity for these patients to reduce the enhanced levels of lactate produced by the type IIb fibres during low level exercise. The loss of fatigue resistance associated with the diminished concentration of type I fibres might contribute to the observed loss of exercise tolerance and the enhanced levels of lactic acid in the legs of these patients (Fig. 9.2.8). This reduction in oxidative capacity does not occur in the diaphragm. As previously stated, it is believed that here hypoxia may cause an endurance training effect due to an increase in ventilation which results in a shift towards more aerobic metabolism.

Early lactic acidosis during exercise in patients with COPD (in particular those with emphysema, and physical inactivity)

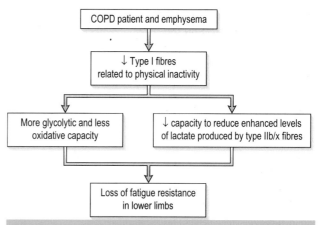

Figure 9.2.8.   Contribution of a reduction of type I fibres to the loss of fatigue resistance in the lower limbs.

has been related to the reduction in the patients' muscle glutamate (GLU). Glutamate is an amino acid that is required within skeletal muscle to contribute to energy production through transamination. Decreased availability of oxygen reduces glutamate metabolism, which reduces the muscle's capacity to resist the production of lactate. The reduced intracellular glutamate levels in COPD have been attributed to a decreased capacity for membrane transport of GLU into the muscle and/or to increased intramuscular GLU degradation.

Lactic acid as a ventilatory stimulant

In addition to the local effects that lactic acid has on the exercising muscle, it must be considered that lactic acid is also, indirectly, a ventilatory stimulant which may further impair the exercise tolerance of COPD patients. Almost all of the lactic acid generated in anaerobic metabolism is buffered to lactate in the blood by sodium bicarbonate. However, the excess non-metabolic carbon dioxide released in this reaction stimulates pulmonary ventilation, allowing carbon dioxide to be released into the atmosphere.

Hypoxia and oxidative stress

Under normal circumstances the majority of oxygen consumed during energy metabolism combines with hydrogen in the mitochondria to form water. However, 2–5% of the oxygen will form *oxygen free radicals* such as *superoxide*, *hydrogen peroxide* and *hydroxyl* due to electron 'leakage' at various steps in the electron transport chain. It is the accumulation of these free radicals that increases the potential for cell damage or oxidative stress within the body. Substances that are particularly affected by oxidative stress are DNA, protein and lipid containing structures such as the bi-layer membrane, which helps to protect the cell from noxious agents. Although there is no way to abate the production of free radicals from oxygen reduction, the body has a natural defence system against their damaging effects within the cells. Such defence comes in the form of *antioxidant scavenger enzymes* and *antioxidant vitamins* that protect the plasma membrane by reacting with and removing the free radicals.

Despite the wide understanding that physical activity is beneficial, negative effects are being investigated based on the observation that oxygen flux to muscles can increase tremendously during exercise, resulting in greater propensity towards oxidative stress. Elevated aerobic metabolism in exercise increases the production of free radicals, which could overwhelm the body's natural defence mechanisms and predispose to pathology.

During exercise oxygen free radicals can be produced in various ways:

- An electron leak in the mitochondria where the superoxide radicals are produced.
- During intense exercise alterations in blood flow and oxygen supply result in periods of underperfusion and reperfusion, which promotes free radical production.

The suggestion is that the risk is proportional to the intensity of exercise and the individual's state of training. As exhaustive exercise in untrained individuals is more likely to produce oxidative damage to active muscles, the question arises as to whether deconditioned patients with COPD are at risk in undertaking exercise training within a pulmonary rehabilitation programme.

Dealing with free radicals

Some authors suggest that for disease-free individuals, the body's normal antioxidant defences are adequate to cope with the excess of free radicals that are produced during exercise. Alternatively where there is repeated exposure to oxidative stress, during for example long-term physical training, the defence system is 'upregulated' against oxygen free radicals in that concentrations of scavengers and activities of antioxidant enzyme increase. In contrast, where there has been disuse of muscles, as in patients with COPD, the antioxidant-stimulating trigger will be removed, resulting in low antioxidant status and the potential for tissue damage, in particular to the malfunction of ATP generation.

This is compounded by chronic hypoxia which itself has also been demonstrated to predispose to myopathy of skeletal muscles. Hypoxia reduces the antioxidant stimulating trigger as less oxygen is available to form reactive oxygen species. Studies of myocardium have revealed that when the muscle reperfuses following a period of ischaemia, free radicals are formed which may damage proteins and membranes. This has the effect of overloading the mitochondria with calcium, which inhibits the production of ATP. Although the latter studies were conducted on cardiac tissue, there is an assumption that adaptation to hypoxia in patients with COPD makes muscles more vulnerable to oxidative stress. A similar study reported an increased antioxidant activity of muscle in

patients exposed to acute hypoxia. The suggestion here is that there is a shift to glycolytic metabolism, which reduces the oxidative capacity of the skeletal muscle. In animal studies, rats were exposed to intermittent hypoxia and it was found that the citric acid cycle activity was reduced whereas glycolytic metabolism was enhanced, resulting in an increased ratio of lactate to pyruvate. It is the subsequent increase in lactate production and the consequent fall in muscle pH that may cause exercise intolerance in this group of patients.

Peripheral oxygen supply

Debate remains with regard to whether the oxygen supply to the periphery is compromised in patients with COPD and whether this has any impact on the formation of oxidative stress and the accumulation of lactic acid within the tissues.

Cardiovascular effects.   There is a great deal of evidence to support the presence of abnormal cardiovascular function in patients with COPD, which may limit the capacity to exercise in these patients. Several studies have associated a decreased cardiac output during exercise in patients with COPD and expiratory flow limitation. Pathology within the lungs predisposes to raised pulmonary vascular resistance and an increase in pulmonary artery pressures. The right ventricular end-diastolic volume is increased but the right ventricular ejection fraction fails to increase, so there is a decrease in the left ventricular end-diastolic, end-systolic and stroke volumes.

Authors have linked cardiovascular and lung mechanical abnormalities and have suggested that exercise limitation in COPD occurs as result of the dynamic interaction between disordered right heart function and ventilation. In addition other research has implied that impairment of oxygen delivery may impact upon the exercise performance. These authors have demonstrated that the best predictor of maximal uptake of oxygen in COPD is the amount of oxygen delivered to the tissues per heart beat (oxygen pulse), which in turn is dictated by the degree of pleural pressure swing during exercise. In COPD, as a result of the increased work of breathing, it has been postulated that there is a redistribution of blood flow towards the respiratory apparatus, creating the possibility that oxygen supply to the peripheries is reduced during exercise. If the ventilatory muscles are unloaded, their perfusion is reduced, allowing more blood to flow to the skeletal muscles and yielding greater exercise power and less lactateamia for the same cardiac output. Should this be the case, the exercise capacity in patients with COPD is limited by the same process as in health and indeed chronic heart failure, that is, by a cardiac output which is insufficient to match the demands of the entire body.

In contrast, some studies report that bulk oxygen transfer to the lower extremities appears to be adequate, suggesting that a biochemical abnormality in exercising muscles is a possible cause of muscle dysfunction in COPD.

Muscle capillary density.   It has been reported that the muscle capillary density per unit surface area in the vastus lateralis falls in patients with COPD. As the number of mitochondria per unit surface area was unchanged, the capillary/mitochondria ratio was also decreased in comparison to age-matched normal subjects. A lower number of capillary contacts in combination with a reduced level of myoglobin has also been found in the vastus lateralis muscle of patients with COPD. This may contribute to the reduced oxygen delivery within muscles in these patients as there is an increased distance for oxygen diffusion between the blood and the tissues.

Corticosteroids

Inflammatory changes within the airways of patients with COPD are associated with airway narrowing and often results in bronchospasm. Although this provides justification for the role of corticosteroids in COPD, the deleterious effects that their use may induce has meant that their role is still controversial. Muscle weakness has been discovered as one of the various side effects as a result of the use of corticosteroids. Animal and clinical models have shown that both peripheral and respiratory muscles are affected by prolonged use of corticosteroids. Acute and chronic myopathies have been described.

Acute myopathy.   Acute steroid myopathy, the more rare of the two, presents as a profound general muscle weakness associated with the administration of high doses of intravenous corticosteroids. Affected muscles show local and diffuse necrosis and atrophy of all fibres associated with *rhabdomyolysis* and high levels of serum *creatinine kinase* and *myoglobinuria*. Acute steroid myopathy of this type has not been described in patients with COPD.

Chronic myopathy.   In contrast, chronic steroid myopathy is much more common and occurs after prolonged administration of lower doses of oral fluorinated corticosteroids. This presentation is often one of proximal weakness and is frequently found in patients with COPD independent of their degree of airflow obstruction (estimated by percentage prediction of FEV_1). In these patients, functional and histological characteristics are demonstrated. As well as peripheral muscle weakness, the levels of La-dehydrogenase–M isozyme are increased, as is the amount of creatinine that is excreted in the urine. Myopathy ensues, biopsies of which exhibit an increase of connective tissue between fibres and an increase in subsarcolemmal and central nuclei. In addition there is diffuse atrophy of muscle fibres, with relative preservation of type IIa and type I fibres compared with type IIb/x fibres. This could be associated with, or compounded by, the effects of poor nutrition, which is also a cause of type IIb/x fibre atrophy.

Animal models provide the majority of the data that explain the specific mechanism of steroid-induced damage to skeletal muscles. Corticosteroids appear to affect the production of contractile proteins and the turnover of biochemical substrates in skeletal muscle. Studies on rat diaphragms have demonstrated that corticosteroids can affect the function of IGF-1, particularly in type II muscle fibres. This inhibits protein synthesis by downregulating peptide initiation on the *ribosomes*. In addition, corticosteroids can accelerate myofibrillar and soluble protein degradation in skeletal muscle by the increased action of *cytoplasmic protease*. Studies on rabbit diaphragm have also demonstrated that steroid myopathy can affect carbohydrate metabolism and predispose to reduced glycolytic and increased concentrations of intramuscular glycogen. This is as a result of the failure of the phosphorylation process which inevitably predisposes to the inability to reform glucose. This may explain why corticosteroids have been associated with the diminished production of energy in skeletal muscle.

Summary and therapeutic implications

- Dyspnoea, reduced quality of life and impaired exercise tolerance are common symptoms of patients with COPD. Although classically described as a pathological process that takes place within the pulmonary system, the evidence suggests overwhelmingly that COPD is not a disease that is exclusive to the lung. Indeed the complaints that patients suffer are the consequence of multifactorial physiological and psychological mechanisms, which are manifested throughout the body.

- Treatment for dyspnoea in patients with COPD should focus on the specific mechanism that contributes to the individual patient's symptoms. For some symptoms, such as bronchospasm, this may be obvious but for others it may be difficult to be sure of the exact factors that are fundamentally accountable for the clinical features manifested. The selection of the appropriate therapeutic intervention therefore becomes problematic.

- Various approaches to the treatment of COPD have been described which are targeted at the pathophysiological mechanisms that exacerbate the symptoms. They focus on reduced ventilatory demand, reduced ventilatory impedance, improvement of muscle function and alteration of the central perception of dyspnoea (American Thoracic Society, 1999a).

- Pulmonary rehabilitation has been developed in an attempt to gear interventions towards the accumulating evidence that COPD is a multisystem disease. The unique problems and needs of each patient are as such implemented by a multidisciplinary team of healthcare professionals. On the basis of this statement the American Thoracic Society developed the following definition of pulmonary rehabilitation in 1999:

Pulmonary rehabilitation is a multidisciplinary programme of care for patients with chronic respiratory impairment that is individually tailored and designed to optimize physical and social performance and autonomy. (American Thoracic Society, 1999b)

THE PRACTICE OF PULMONARY REHABILITATION

Pulmonary rehabilitation aims to reduce the symptoms, increase the functional ability and generally improve the quality of life of patients who suffer from chronic obstructive pulmonary diseases. Unfortunately, much of the damage that occurs to the lung itself is irreversible. However, benefits are still possible as much of the disability and handicap associated with COPD is related to the secondary effects of the disease. These, discussed in the first half of this chapter, include:

- excessive exertional dyspnoea
- loss of skeletal and respiratory muscle function
- a reduction in fat-free mass
- loss of confidence
- social isolation.

Pulmonary rehabilitation programmes vary in structure and organization throughout Britain, and also throughout the world. Whilst differences amongst countries reflect contrasts in the organization of the healthcare systems, politics and tradition, differences within Britain reflect variation in staff availability, type of patient and funding.

Comprehensive pulmonary rehabilitation programmes generally include a host of therapeutic interventions each of which is targeted on the pathophysiological mechanisms that can predispose to dyspnoea. The multidisciplinary team often includes physicians, physiotherapists, occupational therapists, psychologists and social workers. The therapeutic interventions are delivered within four major components of pulmonary rehabilitation. These are:

- exercise training
- education
- psychological/behavioural intervention
- outcome assessment.

Of the therapeutic options available, exercise training is considered to be the foundation of pulmonary rehabilitation. There is no evidence to suggest that it has any effect on the underlying respiratory impairment, but there is considerable evidence that demonstrates its positive effects on dyspnoea, functional ability and psychological state. Outcome measurements for pulmonary rehabilitation are usually primarily those related to an improvement in exercise capacity and health-related quality of life. Secondary outcomes are related to education and psychosocial support including compliance with medical therapy and knowledge about the disease.

Exercise

The effects of systemic exercise have been the subject of much debate. In the normal population there are physiological and psychological benefits. These include:

- an increase in $V_{O_{2max}}$
  - increase in blood volume
  - increase in haemoglobin
  - increase in stroke volume
  - decrease in heart rate
  - increase in extraction and utilization of oxygen by peripheral muscles
- decrease in blood pressure
- increase in muscular strength and endurance
- improved balance and coordination
- improved stride length and gait coordination
- loss of adipose tissue and change of body composition
- improved psychological state.

Who benefits?

There is some debate with regard to the type of patients who would benefit most from pulmonary rehabilitation. The contention surrounds those patients who are deemed too well or ironically too unwell to gain returns. Traditionally and largely as a result of the expense incurred, pulmonary rehabilitation is not prescribed until there are significant symptoms with an advanced stage of the disorder, that is, moderate or severe disease. This, despite the fact that patients with so-called mild disease have a reduced quality of life and physical capacity to work. Conversely, there is a perception that patients with the most severe disease may be too ill to exercise. Patients with severe cardiac failure or major locomotor disorders and severe co-morbidity are often excluded because it is believed that they cannot exercise with sufficient intensity. Contemporary thought, in contrast, suggests that similar gains in physical performance and health-related quality of life can be achieved in patients with mild, moderate and severe disease after exercise training.

In patients with COPD the benefits that can be achieved through exercise will depend to a certain extent on the severity of the pathological process that has taken place throughout the lungs. Patients with mild COPD are likely to experience similar advantages from exercising as their 'normal' counterparts. However, those with more advanced disease are said to be able to increase their exercise tolerance and feeling of well-being with little or any increase in their maximal oxygen uptake. All patients with COPD regardless of their level of disability should therefore be referred for exercise rehabilitation or be encouraged to begin exercise training on their own.

Physiological benefits of exercise

Proposed mechanisms of exercise that improve the quality of life of all patients with COPD are said to include:

- better motivation
- desensitization to dyspnoea
- reduction of the sense of leg effort.

To this end there is a wealth of evidence to support the concept that exercise programmes are capable of inducing physiological changes in the peripheral and respiratory muscles that improve the exercise tolerance of patients with COPD.

With the understanding that muscle atrophy due to impaired physical activity is one of the principal causes of muscle dysfunction in COPD, it is reasonable to assume that exercise training could contribute to an improvement in performance of patients who suffer with this condition. Furthermore, muscle biopsies taken before and after rigorous endurance training programmes have proved that there is an increase in the concentration of enzymes facilitating oxidative metabolism.

Training-induced increases in the cross-sectional areas of oxidative fibres and elevated oxidative enzyme activities have been found in the quadriceps muscle of trained patients with COPD. Equally, after an endurance training programme it has been demonstrated that there is a smaller increase in arterial lactate acid accumulation during exercise which is also associated with a lower level of carbon dioxide output and ventilatory requirement. The resulting decrease in ventilatory requirement allows patients with COPD to sustain a given level of exercise for a longer period of time. There is also evidence to suggest that there is better aerobic function of muscles after the onset of constant work rate exercise as the kinetics of oxygen uptake are faster. This may be attributed to the fact that muscle capillaries and myoglobin levels are higher after training, thereby improving the transport of oxygen to exercising muscles.

In peripheral muscles, training induces a partial improvement of the oxidative capacity in combination with increased exercise performance. Prolonged endurance training gives rise to an increased percentage of type I and type IIa fibres which is accompanied by greater oxidative capacity resulting in higher fatigue resistance. As fatigue is the main limiting factor in peripheral muscle performance, an endurance protocol may be the most suitable for improving the exercise capacity of limb muscles in patients with COPD.

In contrast to the effect on peripheral muscles, there is little convincing data with regard to the effect of exercise on the oxidative capacity of respiratory muscles. Some evidence does exist which suggests that training the respiratory muscles may improve its performance even though a real clinical benefit may be in doubt. Until recently it was believed that general exercise training programmes can lead to small improvements in respiratory strength and endurance in normal subjects, and in patients with cystic fibrosis, but improvements

in patients with COPD have been negligible. In a more recent study the researchers discovered that general exercise training, targeted at the highest possible intensity, improves inspiratory muscle strength and endurance and increased expiratory muscle strength in patients with chronic airflow limitation. In this study patients were subjected to a graduated training programme that incorporated elements of both endurance training and strength training. Static expiratory muscle strength increased in parallel with increased inspiratory muscle strength, supporting evidence that expiratory muscle recruitment in conjunction with accessory muscle recruitment during inspiration often occurs in patients with COPD who exercise. This was manifested in reduced ventilation after training as a result of improved efficiency and reduced breathing frequency. It is suggested that this process contributes to the unloading of the overworked, overburdened mechanically compromised diaphragm in these hyperinflated patients and hence contributes to the strength and endurance of the respiratory mechanism.

Unfortunately, despite these claims, the researchers were unable to demonstrate any relationship between improved muscle function, improved symptoms and improved exercise performance. This was possibly because the sample size was too small or because the patients who were entered onto the trial were not sufficiently compromised with regard to their pre-existing inspiratory muscle strength. Whilst reduced ventilatory demand can contribute to improved exercise endurance times, other 'non physiological' factors may also contribute to symptom alleviation. The development of increased tolerance to stimuli that promote dyspnoea and altered perceptual response to evoked sensations are offered as additional explanations.

The magnitude of the ventilatory muscle functional improvement was comparable to that achieved by specific inspiratory muscle training. Inspiratory muscle training is a type of resistance training in which the inspiratory muscles are subjected to an increased pressure load, and has previously probably demonstrated the best effects. As this is a kind of power training effect, the suggestion is that training of the diaphragm should focus more on strength than endurance. Ventilatory muscle training will be discussed in more detail later in this chapter.

Principles of training

The major objective of the exercise component of pulmonary rehabilitation is to facilitate biological adaptations that will improve the performance of specific tasks in just the same way as it would in an elite athlete. The physiological improvements in muscle function can therefore only be brought about by a rigorous programme of endurance training that is underpinned by the physiological principles of exercise prescription. Consequently to train patients with COPD several principles of physiological conditioning should be incorporated into the carefully planned workout programmes.

Overload principle

Patients with COPD are often severely deconditioned. It was initially believed therefore that they could not exercise to sufficient intensity to induce a physiological training effect. Ironically the converse of this is true. Even some of the sickest patients with COPD are able to train closer to their maximal capacity than healthy subjects. Studies that fail to show such adaptations probably involved an insufficient training stimulus.

In order to enhance any physiological improvement and to precipitate a training response an exercise overload, specific to the activity, must be applied. Exercising beyond the level of intensity that is normally performed can induce training effects that enable the body to function more efficiently. Achieving the appropriate overload for any individual requires the manipulation of training frequency, intensity and duration in addition to some consideration of the mode or the specificity of the exercise. In healthy subjects, a submaximal heart rate of 60–90% or 50–80% of the maximal oxygen uptake is generally targeted in order to achieve aerobic training. This level is sustained for 20–45 minutes and repeated a minimum of three times per week.

In patients with COPD, the prevailing thought has been that ventilatory limitations preclude the level of aerobic training required to achieve beneficial physiological adaptations. However, over the years it has become apparent that this concept is incorrect and strong support has been gained for the view that patients with COPD can benefit from an exercise-training programme. It has been proven that the larger the number of sessions and the greater the intensity of the sessions as a function of maximal performance, the better the results will be in terms of physiological adaptations in this group of people.

In their work, Belman and Kendregan (1982) exercised patients at 30% of their maximal intensity four times a week for 6 weeks, with a load that was increased as tolerated by the patient. In this study, a significant improvement on the endurance time was observed in only 8 out of the 15 participants. In contrast, other studies have demonstrated that patients with COPD are able to train closer to their maximum capacity than healthy subjects and that studies that had previously failed to show such metabolic adaptations probably involved an insufficient training stimulus. Casaburi and co-workers (1991) studied 19 patients with moderate COPD before and after they were assigned to either a low intensity (50% of maximal) or high intensity exercise programme (80% of maximal). These workers demonstrated that the high intensity programme was more effective than the low intensity programme. They observed a drop in ventilatory requirement for exercise after training that was proportional to the drop in lactate at a given work rate. It should be noted that the patients who underwent this study showed 'moderate' airflow obstruction and were relatively young, the mean age being 49 years. Significantly, perhaps consideration should also be made as to whether training a patient with COPD to 80% of the maximum work load is realistic given the gruelling nature of exercising to this intensity. Such expectations might negatively impact on the patients' long-term adherence with exercise. Given that Cassaburi and colleagues also deduced that programmes that had supervised training sessions were more effective than those that were self-monitored, perhaps a lower intensity might be more effective and achievable for self-motivated groups. In contrast and with regard to older populations, Roomi and co-workers (1996) provided evidence that significant improvements could be made in exercise tolerance when patients over 70 years of age used self-prescribed dyspnoea levels to limit their exercise. It should be noted that throughout the prescription of intensity of exercise consideration must be given for the nature of the pathological processes of COPD and the amount of airflow limitation which is present. Kearan and co-workers (1991) have established that prolonged respiratory activity can increase ventilation and dyspnoea and also that dyspnoea can be more affected by increases in exercise intensity than by increments in the duration of exercise.

Specificity of training

Adaptations in the metabolic and physiological systems depend not only on the intensity of overload imposed but also on the type of exercise. Training specificity refers to the observation that a specific exercise stress will induce a specific adaptation. Strength training will produce a strength power adaptation associated with an increase in size of muscle cells and number of myofibrils. Specific aerobic or cardiovascular exercise will elicit endurance-training adaptations. Such modifications would include an increase in the size and number of type I fibres and the transformation of type IIb/x fibres to type IIa fibres, increasing their oxidative capacity. Some crossover effect has been demonstrated as a result of exercise of similar muscle groups. An increase in walking distance can be achieved after cycle ergometer training, but this effect would not be achieved following upper extremity training.

Length and reversibility

Most pulmonary rehabilitation programmes utilize endurance training. The frequency varies between two and five times a week, the duration lasting in the region of 30–60 minutes. The programme is generally sustained for approximately 8–12 weeks or until a targeted load is reached. The reversibility principle of the training effect states that the results of conditioning decline after training ceases. In fit individuals the training effects are maintained only as long as exercise is continued. The same principle applies to patients with COPD. In most cases therefore the pulmonary rehabilitation programme is followed by a home maintenance course. Failure to comply with a maintenance prescription following the completion of a rehabilitation programme has explained in part the reductions in timed walk and exercise endurance in some groups of patients, although deterioration in the chronic lung condition could contribute to these results.

Throughout, training levels in excess of 60% of the maximal load are recommended, although consideration and flexibility is required for the number of patients who are unable to train at this intensity. Interval training is used as an alternative for these patients. Here patients perform 2–3 minutes of high intensity of exercise (up to 80% of their maximal exercise capacity) alternating with equal periods of rest for a total of approximately 30 minutes. Studies have been conducted which compare interval training with continuous training in patients with COPD. It was observed that there was no significant difference between the groups although there was a trend towards greater oxidative adaptive changes in the groups that undertook continuous exercise compared with the interval-training group.

Monitoring

The target level of exercise training should be a percentage of the maximum work capacity ($V_{O_{2max}}$), for example 60% of the maximal oxygen consumption. In many centres exact metabolic measurements are not possible for the duration of the rehabilitation programme, so a compromise is made by the implementation of an associated measure such as the shuttle walk test. More frequently the submaximal heart rate is used to estimate the training intensity. The reliability of either of these methods is considered to be limited as there is an understanding that it is breathlessness and its sensory consequences that curtails patients' ability to exercise rather than their heart rate. In addition, there can be discrepancies between heart rate and work rate among and within subjects, caused by the affects of cardiac and lung disease or their therapy.

The Borg scale has been adapted for use as an alternative. The Borg scale of breathlessness is used to provide symptom-limited exercise prescription (Fig. 9.2.9). It is based on the perception of dyspnoea represented on a visual analogue scale. The exerciser rates his exertion on a numerical scale. The exercise levels that correspond to higher levels of energy expenditure and physiological strain result in a higher rating of perceived exertion (RPE, 13 or 14 on the Borg scale). This would correspond to an exercise heart rate of about 70% of maximum. More moderate exercise levels would correspond to lower scores on the Borg scale. An RPE of around 11 corresponds to the lactate threshold in both the fit and the unfit.

The Borg scale has proved to be an inexpensive and reliable way to contribute to the monitoring and prescription of exercise in most settings. However, it is also subject to flaws in reliability. The utilization of this method fails to recognize that approximately equal numbers of people terminate their exercise routine as a result of the limitations imposed by their leg effort as those that terminate their exercise due to the experience of dyspnoea. In addition, as dyspnoea is a subjective perception, fear and anxiety, particularly at the beginning of a programme, may cause exercise to be terminated before a sufficient intensity of training has been reached.

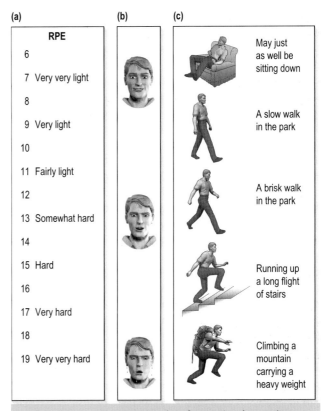

Figure 9.2.9. The Borg scale of perceived exertion. (a) The Borg scale is used to obtain the rate of perceived exertion (RPE) during exercise. (b, c) Illustrative and descriptive adaptations can provide useful alternatives to the original scale.

Type of training

Lower extremity training

Lower extremity endurance exercise. Many pulmonary rehabilitation programmes include lower limb endurance exercise. They have been proven to be beneficial for patients with COPD in terms of increased exercise endurance, and less dyspnoea both during exercise and when completing activities of daily living. Cycle ergometry, stair climbing, treadmill walking or ground-based walking are the exercise methods classically used, either individually and continuous, or incorporated into a circuit. The physiological mechanism by which such exercise brings about improvements is the subject of some debate. A drop in heart rate with exercise has led some researchers to surmise that the training effect may be related to a decrease in exercising lactate levels. Evidence supporting this theory and the development of a skeletal muscle adaptation to lower limb endurance training in COPD patients arises from studies which demonstrate that patients show a reduction in exercise lactic acidosis and ventilation that is proportional to the intensity of the training.

Strength training. Skeletal muscle weakness has been reported to be a serious problem in patients with COPD and the many factors such as loss of fat free mass, ageing, inflammation, the effect of steroids and immobility which contribute to this have been discussed. As the contractile properties of muscle are said to be preserved in weakened muscle, the concept of strength training appears to be a rational one. However, the effect of this method of training in the limbs of patients with COPD has not been widely researched. One study refers specifically to the effects of weight lifting on patients with COPD whilst a second evaluates whether strength training is a useful addition to aerobic training in patients with COPD.

In the former randomized controlled trial an 8-week training strategy was employed, which included one exercise for the arm and two for the legs along with a control group. On completion of the training period muscle strength had increased from 14 to 40% depending on the muscle group evaluated. There was also an associated increase in the submaximal endurance time for whole body exercise and a measured improvement in quality of life. In the latter study 45 patients with COPD were randomized to a 12-week period of aerobic training alone or combined with strength training. Muscle resistive exercises induced less dyspnoea than cycle ergometry, helped motivate and maintain patient interest and could help to increase bone density. The addition of strength training to aerobic training in patients with COPD was associated with a significant increase in muscle strength and mass, but it did not provide additional improvement in exercise capacity or quality of life.

Other reports mention the incidental effects that the more typically utilized endurance exercises have on strength of muscle. The whole body exercise training targeted at the highest tolerable intensity leads to consistent improvements in peripheral muscle strength and endurance in COPD, though no explanation is offered as to why this might be so. Some would suggest that if weakness is a cause of exercise limitation then the patient may benefit from strength training, whilst patients who suffer from dyspnoea may benefit from a more endurance-based training programme. Perhaps a combination of the two philosophies would be the most appropriate, encouraging a total body/fitness approach. More research would be useful in this area.

Upper extremity training

The upper and lower fibres of trapezius, latissimus dorsi, serratus anterior, subclavius, pectoralis minor and major are all muscles that have insertions both around and beyond the thorax. Such multisite attachments allow these muscles to have dual roles, contributing both to the functions of respiration and to the maintenance of posture. Depending on their point of anchorage the muscles may contribute to movements and functions of the upper limbs or they may exert a pulling force on the rib cage which in the event of increased ventilatory requirement assists in the generation of inspiratory pressures.

Some patients with COPD are reliant upon the use of their accessory muscles to augment ventilation; therefore when they perform tasks with their upper limbs, their ability to breathe becomes compromised and they report a greater degree of dyspnoea. Tasks that require unsupported arm exercise pose particular problems for this group of patients. Unsupported arm exercise is problematic as the respiratory muscles are called upon to perform their dual roles at the same time. The increased demand incurred during unsupported arm exercise causes the patient to adopt a rapid shallow breathing pattern, which may result in severe dyspnoea and dyssynchronous breathing.

The dyssynchrony of breathing allied with upper limb activity has been associated with the transfer of work back to the diaphragm, which is already working at a mechanical disadvantage in the COPD disease state. In addition significant increases in VO_2, VCO_2, heart rate and V_E have been demonstrated. There is a suggestion that if ventilatory requirement could be reduced or if the upper limbs could be trained to do more work, then the exercise tolerance in this group of patients could be improved.

Unsupported arm exercise.   Studies of arm training using arm ergometry or unsupported arm exercises such as lifting a piece of dowel and proprioceptive neuromuscular facilitation have demonstrated improved performance on arm-specific endurance exercises and decreased metabolic and ventilatory requirements for arm activities. Changes in the patient's ability to perform three tasks of daily living (dish washing, cleaning windows and shelving groceries) were, however, less apparent. It was felt that the failure to demonstrate an improvement of triceps oxidative capacity in patients with COPD was as a result of the low training intensity that was employed. When compared, although unsupported arm training and ergometry both improved the total exercise endurance time, it was concluded that arm exercise against gravity may be more effective in training patients as these resemble more closely the activities of daily living. It should be noted that no correlation between the improvement of upper limb function and health-related quality of life (HRQL) has been described.

Adjuncts to exercise

Ventilatory muscle training

Patients with COPD experience increased resistance to airflow, air trapping and hyperinflation of the lung. Hyperinflation places the inspiratory muscles in a position of mechanical disadvantage, which results in an inability of the muscles to perform what has become an increased task of breathing. As the inspiratory muscles become weakened and compromised there is an increased sensation of dyspnoea, a limitation in exercise tolerance and a possible rise in arterial carbon dioxide levels. The magnitude of breathing (*P*breath) becomes greater than the strength to perform the task of breathing (Pimax). Ventilatory muscle training in patients with respiratory disease is said to cause an increase in strength or endurance of the respiratory muscles, which will lower the Pbreath/Pimax, reduce the severity of dyspnoea and improve exercise capacity. Specific exercise training for respiratory muscles is now a common feature of many pulmonary rehabilitation programmes. The suggestion is that increased respiratory muscle strength will translate into increased exercise tolerance by a reduction in dyspnoea. Further increased strength and endurance of the diaphragm may enable greater tolerance of higher inspiratory loads.

Respiratory muscle strength is commonly estimated by measuring maximal negative inspiratory pressure (Pimax) from residual volume or functional residual capacity. Inspiratory muscle training (IMT) is generally initiated at low intensities, then gradually increased to achieve 60–70% of Pimax. The minimum load to achieve a training effect is 30% of the Pimax.

As with all muscles, the muscles of respiration can be trained for both strength and endurance, with similar physiological adaptations taking place. The most common methods of inspiratory muscle training are the threshold loading and the resistive loading techniques. Analogous with strength training of peripheral muscles that require high workloads and few repetitions, strength training of respiratory muscles requires a maximal inspiratory effort against an occluded airway (threshold training). Similarly, where endurance training of peripheral muscles requires low to moderate workloads with high repetitions, endurance training of respiratory muscles requires the performance of a maximal sustainable ventilation of approximately 15 minutes (resistive training).

With regard to effect, several authors have demonstrated that targeted inspiratory muscle training may enhance respiratory function when used either alone or in conjunction with a general exercise programme. In each instance variable results have been achieved. The Pimax was the most frequently used outcome measure. Alternatively or in addition, the level of dyspnoea, exercise capacity and HRQL were used as outcome measures in some cases. In the studies where Pimax was measured as an outcome variable, significant increases occurred in the experimental group. The findings in the groups, which did not demonstrate an increase in Pimax, suggest that the training stimulus in these groups was inadequate to induce the expected physiological training response, that is, over 30% of the baseline Pimax. This is confirmed in a review in which the authors document that training intensity is often below that required to achieve physiological effects and that changes in breathing pattern during training alter the resistance provided. Levels of dyspnoea, exercise capacity and HRQL have been investigated to a lesser extent. Consequently there is little evidence on the benefit for functional outcomes and health status. The available evidence appears to suggest that the overall improvements in respiratory muscle

function, dyspnoea and exercise tolerance support the addition of targeted IMT to a pulmonary rehabilitation programme. The evidence that IMT confers any additional benefit over exercise alone is, however, unequivocal. Improvements in exercise capacity in terms of $V_{O_{2max}}$ have not been demonstrated persuasively.

Oxygen therapy

The value of long-term oxygen therapy for the increased survival and improvement in quality of life for patients with COPD and hypoxaemia has long been well documented. These have included an improvement in pulmonary hypertension, appetite, meal-related symptoms, neuropsychiatric and cognitive function. More recently it has been advocated that the acute supplementation of oxygen can also optimize the effects of pulmonary rehabilitation in those patients who are symptomatic at rest. Exercise performance might be enhanced with the benefit of supplemental oxygen during training sessions, whilst supplementary oxygen may improve the patient's tolerance to dyspnoea. Although the benefits for patients who are normoxic at rest but desaturate during exercise is less clear, it is reasonable to assume that performance is also likely to be improved in this group. The mechanisms by which supplemental oxygen will improve exercise tolerance is said to include the reduction of minute ventilation during exercise, the relief of pulmonary vasoconstriction and the improvement of systemic oxygen delivery through an increased arterial oxygen content and cardiac output. It appears that supplemental oxygen has a greater effect on exercise endurance than on muscle strength. Exercise endurance improves when there is greater limb muscle oxygen utilization through the enhancement of limb muscle oxidative capacity.

Early falls in muscle intracellular pH, a reduced Pi/PCr (inorganic phosphate/phosphocreatine) ratio and a reduction in the resynthesis of PCr was demonstrated after exercise in COPD patients as compared to age-matched control subjects, yet these were partially resolved when oxygen was administered to the patient during exercise. Similarly, it has been ascertained that the supplementation of oxygen during exercise can improve ATP production from oxidative phosphorylation. Improved peripheral muscle loading has been suggested as a mechanism by which this can be achieved. However, there is also contradictory evidence which suggests that cellular respiration and mitochondrial function is independent of oxygen delivery. Lactate output from the muscles has shown no relationship to oxygen delivery, implying that the failure of oxidative metabolism in peripheral muscles lies with its inability to extract oxygen rather than the inability of the lungs to provide oxygen to it. Similarly, although more contentious, the partial pressure of oxygen in the gracilis muscle of animal models has been found to be higher than the value when respiration in isolated mitochondria becomes impaired. Further, a dimension which has not yet been explored in full is the notion that limb muscle aerobic function may actually be increased in the presence of carefully controlled hypoxic situations, suggesting that supplementing oxygen to patients undergoing rehabilitation could be counterproductive.

Although there is no evidence yet to suggest that this is the case in COPD, results indicative of this phenomenon have been demonstrated from studies investigating alternative hypoxic conditions such as in the presence of peripheral vascular disease and high altitude. In consideration of these results it is suggested that this may limit the performance benefit of supplementary oxygen to COPD patients, and that pulmonary rehabilitation programmes should rather address the problem of muscle dysfunction in COPD.

Non-invasive positive pressure ventilation

For patients with stable COPD and chronic hypercapnia, non-invasive pressure support ventilation (NPSV) has become a useful adjunct to therapy. Its clinical effects include an improvement in arterial blood gases and unloading of the muscles of inspiration, with a consequent reduction in dyspnoea. As excessive inspiratory muscle loading has been postulated as a cause of exercise limitation in patients with COPD, attempts have been made to counter this effect by unloading the ventilatory muscles during exercise using inspiratory pressure support. In investigating this theory, positive results have been reported indicating that inspiratory pressure support during cycle training and treadmill walking respectively was associated with increased exercise tolerance and a lessening of the perception of breathlessness. The evidence suggests that in patients with COPD who perform steady state treadmill exercise, the absolute pressures generated by the inspiratory muscles stop increasing well in advance of the termination of exercise, the effect being most marked in the diaphragm. In contrast, abdominal expiratory muscle pressure generation and minute ventilation continue to increase until the point of exercise limitation. The provision of inspiratory pressure support reduces both inspiratory and expiratory muscle use. This could contribute to a reduction in lactate accumulation and carbon dioxide generation and ultimately lessen the perception of dyspnoea, which would thus improve the training benefit of pulmonary rehabilitation. Unfortunately although this information is of huge scientific interest, it is believed that this treatment is unlikely to provide pragmatic benefits to patients due to the practical obstacles which would arise in providing ventilation during a pulmonary rehabilitation class and at home.

Hormone supplementation

Patients with COPD are known to develop atrophy of their muscles and it is with regard to this that investigations have taken place to identify the effect of the administration of growth hormone, both in conjunction with an exercise programme and alone. Although conclusive in their own right, none of these studies reach consensus. This has promoted debate on

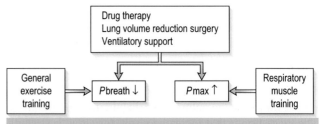

Figure 9.2.10.   Therapeutic options which aim to correct the balance between respiratory muscle load (Pbreath) and capacity (Pmax) in COPD.

the cost-effectiveness of growth hormone supplementation, which has thus far rendered the treatment non-justifiable in terms of cost.

Other adjuncts

In addition to oxygen therapy, ventilatory muscle training and non-invasive positive pressure ventilation, several other adjuncts have been investigated with regard to the enhancement of physical and physiological performance of patients with COPD. These include the addition of psychological support, acupressure, nutritional supplementation, neuromuscular electrical stimulation, volume reduction surgery and the advent of modernized and novel drug and therapeutic options, including the use of performance enhancing drugs. Clearly a thorough understanding of the limitations which each individual with COPD has to exercise and muscle performance will be required in order to match the most appropriate and useful therapeutic adjuncts to the exercise component of the pulmonary rehabilitation programme (Fig. 9.2.10).

Conclusion

Exercise as a component of pulmonary rehabilitation is sufficiently grounded in sound physiological evidence to command respect for its use in the treatment of patients with COPD. There is little doubt that muscles are responsive to training but it must be recognized that there are a multitude of other factors that will mediate muscle weakness. Such factors include extent of the disease, nutritional status, hypoxia, hypercapnia, inflammatory mediators and circulating hormones, the effects of which should all be addressed as much as possible alongside the prescription of the exercise programme. When designing rehabilitation programmes for patients with COPD, it is essential to reflect upon what could be considered as the broader consequences of the disease and to construct a treatment regime that will be of greatest benefit to each patient. A wholly individualist and pragmatic approach therefore needs to be adopted.

REFERENCES AND FURTHER READING

Aliverti A, Macklem PT (2001) How and why exercise is limited in COPD. Respiration 68: 229–239.

American Thoracic Society (1999a) Dyspnea: mechanisms, assessment, and management: A consensus statement. Am J Respir Crit Care Med 159(1): 321–340.

American Thoracic Society (1999b) Official statement on pulmonary rehabilitation. Am J Respir Crit Care Med 159: 1666–1682.

American Thoracic Society and European Respiratory Society (1999) Skeletal muscle dysfunction in chronic obstructive pulmonary disease. Am J Respir Crit Care Med 159(4): S2–S40.

Arora N, Rochester D (1982) Effect of body weight and muscularity on human diaphragm muscle mass, thickness and area. J Physiol 52: 64–70.

Arora N, Rochester D (1984) Effect of chronic airflow limitation on sternocleidomastoid muscle thickness. Chest 85(suppl): 58S–59S.

Barnes PJ (2001) Future advances in COPD therapy. Thematic Review Series. Respiration 68: 441–448.

Bauldoff GS, Hoffman L, Sciurba F, Thomas Z (1996) Home based, upper-arm training for patients with chronic obstructive pulmonary disease. Heart Lung, J Acute Crit Care 25(4): 288–294.

Begin P, Grassino A (1991) Inspiratory muscle dysfunction and chronic hypercapnia in chronic obstructive pulmonary disease. Am Rev Respir Dis 143: 905–912.

Belman MJ, Kendregan BA (1982) Physical training fails to improve ventilatory muscle endurance in patients with chronic obstructive pulmonary disease. Chest 93: 688–692.

Belman MJ, Botnick WC, Nathan SD, et al. (1994) Ventilatory load characteristics during ventilatory muscle training. Am J Respir Crit Care Med 149(4): 925–929.

Bernard S, Leblanc P, Whittom F, et al. (1998) Peripheral muscle weakness in patients with chronic obstructive pulmonary disease. Am J Crit Care Med 158(2): 629–634.

Bernard S, Whittom F, LeBlanc P, et al. (1999) Aerobic and strength training in patients with chronic obstructive pulmonary disease. Am J Respir Crit Care Med 159(3): 896–901.

Berne RM, Levy MN (1990) Principles of Physiology. International Student Edition. London: Wolfe.

Berry MJ, Rejeski WJ, Adair NE, Zaccaro D (1999) Exercise rehabilitation and chronic obstructive pulmonary disease stage. Am J Respir Crit Care Med 160(4): 1248–1253.

Bianchi L, Foglio K, Pagani M, et al. (1998) Effects of proportional assist ventilation on exercise tolerance in COPD patients with chronic hypercapnia. Eur Respir J 11: 422–427.

Boggard HJ, Dekker BM, Arntzen BW, et al. (1998) The haemodynamic response to exercise in chronic obstructive pulmonary disease: assessment by impedance cardiography. Eur Respir J 12: 374–379.

Bradley BL, Garner AE, Billiu D, et al. (1978), Oxygen assisted exercise in chronic obstructive lung disease. Am Rev Respir Dis 118: 239–243.

Braun NM, Arora NS, Rochester DF (1982) The force–length relationship of the normal human diaphragm. J Appl Physiol 53: 405–412.

Breslin EH (1996) Respiratory muscle function in patients with chronic obstructive pulmonary disease. Heart Lung 25(4): 271–287.

Burdet L, deMuralt B, Schutz Y, Pichard C, Fitting JW (1997) Administration of growth hormone to underweight patients with COPD. Am J Crit Care Med 156: 1800–1806.

Cambach W, Chadwick-Straver RVM, Wagenaar RC, Van Keimpema ARJ, Kemper HCG (1997) The effects of a community based pulmonary rehabilitation programme on exercise tolerance and quality of life: a randomised controlled trial. Eur Respir J 10: 104–113.

Campbell JA, Hughes RL, Sahgal V, Frederikson J, Shields TW (1980) Alterations in intercostal muscle morphology and biochemistry in patients with obstructive lung disease. Am Rev Respir Dis 122: 679–686.

Carrieri-Kohlman V, Stulbarg MS (2000) Dyspnoea: assessment and management. In: Hodgkin JE, Celli BR, Connors G (eds) Pulmonary Rehabilitation: Guidelines to Success, 3rd edn. London: Lippincott Williams & Wilkins.

Carurana-Montaldo B, Gleeson K, Zwillich C (2000) The control of breathing in clinical practice. Chest 117: 205–225.

Casaburi R (1993) Exercise training in chronic obstructive lung disease. In: Casaburi R, Petty TL (eds) Principles and Practice of Pulmonary Rehabilitation. Philadelphia: WB Saunders, pp. 317–321.

Casaburi R (2000) Skeletal muscle function in COPD. Chest Suppl 117: 267S–271S.

Casaburi R, Patessio A, Ioloi F, et al. (1991) Reductions in exercise lactic acidosis and ventilation as a result of exercise training in patients with obstructive lung disease. Am Rev Respir Dis 143: 9–18.

Casaburi R, Goren S, Bhasin S (1996) Substantial prevalence of low anabolic hormone levels in COPD patients undergoing rehabilitation (abstract). Am J Crit Care Med 153: A128.

Casaburi R, Porszasz J, Burns MR, et al. (1996) Physiologic benefits of exercise training in rehabilitation of severe COPD patients. Am J Respir Crit Care Med 155: 1541–1551.

Casaburi R, Carithers E, Tosolini J, Phillips J, Bhasin S (1997) Randomised placebo controlled trial of growth hormone in severe COPD patients undergoing endurance training. Am J Crit Care Med 155: A498.

Cassart M, Pettiaux N, Gevenois PA, Paiva M, Estenne M (1997) Effect of chronic hyperinflation on diaphragm length and surface area. Am J Respir Crit Care Med 156: 504–508.

Celli B (2000) Pathophysiology of chronic obstructive lung disease. In: Hodgkin JE, Celli BR, Connors GL (eds) Pulmonary Rehabilitation: Guidelines to Success, 3rd edn. London: Lippincott Williams & Wilkins.

Connett RJ, Gayeski TEJ, Honig CR, et al. (1984) Lactate accumulation in fully aerobic working dog gracilis muscle. Am J Appl Physiol 246: H120–H128.

Coppoolse R, Schols A, Baarends E, et al. (1999) Interval versus continuous training in patients with severe COPD: a randomised controlled trial. Eur Respir J 14: 258–263.

Corbucci GG, Menichetti A, Cogliati A, Ruvolo C (1995) Metabolic aspects of cardiac and skeletal muscle tissues in the condition of hypoxia, ischaemia and reperfusion, induced by extracorporeal circulation. Int J Tissue React 17: 219–225.

Couser Jr JI (2000) Pharmacological therapy. In: Hodgkin JE, Celli BR, Connors GL (eds) Pulmonary Rehabilitation: Guidelines to Success, 3rd edn. London: Lippincott Williams & Wilkins.

Couser J, Martinez F, Celli B (1992) Respiratory response to arm elevation in normal subjects. Chest 101: 336–340.

Criner GJ, Celli BR (1988) Effect of unsupported arm exercise on ventilatory muscle recruitment in patients with severe chronic airflow obstruction. Am Rev Respir Dis 138: 856–867.

De Godoy I, Donahoe M, Calhoun WJ, Mancino J, Rogers RM (1996) Elevated TNF-α production by peripheral blood monocytes of weight losing COPD patients. Am J Respir Crit Care Med 153: 633–637.

De Troyer A, Kelly S, Zin W (1983) Mechanical action of intercostal muscles on the ribs. Science 220: 87–88.

Decramer M, Lacquet LM, Fagard R, Rogiers P (1994) Corticosteroids contribute to muscle weakness in chronic airflow obstruction. Am Rev Respir Dis 150: 11–16.

Decramer M, de Bock V, Dom R (1996) Functional and histologic picture of steroid induced myopathy in chronic obstructive pulmonary disease. Am J Respir Crit Care Med 153: 1958–1964.

Dyer CAE, White R (2001) Pulmonary rehabilitation: the evidence base. Gerontology 47(5): 231–236.

Engelen MP, Schols AM, Lamars RJ, Wouters EF (1999) Different patterns of chronic tissue wasting among patients with chronic bronchitis. Clin Nutr 18(5): 275–280.

Engelen J, Schols A, Does JD, Wouters E (2000) Skeletal muscle weakness is associated with extremity fat free mass but not with airflow obstruction in patients with chronic obstructive pulmonary disease. Am J Clin Nutr 71(3): 733–738.

Engelen MPKJ, Schols AMWJ, Does JD, et al. (2000) Exercise-induced lactate increase in relation to muscle substrates in patients with chronic obstructive pulmonary disease. Am J Crit Care Med 162(5): 1697–1704.

Ferguson GT, Irvin CG, Cherniack RM (1990) Effects of corticosteroids on diaphragm function and biochemistry in the rabbit. Am Rev Respir Dis 141: 156–163.

Ferreira IM, Brooks B, Lacasse Y, et al. (2000) Nutritional support for individuals with COPD: a meta-analysis. Chest 117: 672–678.

Fitting JW (2001) Respiratory muscles in chronic obstructive pulmonary disease. Swiss Med Wkly 131: 483–486.

Fulco CS, Rock PB, Cymerman A (2000) Improving athletic performance: is altitude resistance or altitude training helpful? Aviat Space Environ Med 71: 162–171.

Garrod R, Wedzicha W (2002) Pulmonary rehabilitation: a multidisciplinary intervention. In: Pryor JA, Prasad SA (eds) Physiotherapy for Respiratory and Cardiac Problems: Adults and Paediatrics, 3rd edn. London: Churchill Livingstone.

Garrod R, Paul EA, Wedzicha JA (2000) Supplemental oxygen during pulmonary rehabilitation in patients with chronic obstructive pulmonary disease and exercise hypoxaemia. Thorax 55: 539–543.

Gosker HR, Wouters EFM, van der Vusse G, Schols AMWJ (2000) Skeletal muscle dysfunction in chronic obstructive pulmonary disease and chronic heart failure: underlying mechanisms and therapy perspectives. Am J Clin Nutr 71: 1033–1047.

Gosselink R, Troosters T, Decramer M (2000) Distribution of muscle weakness in patients with stable chronic obstructive pulmonary disease. J Cardiopulm Rehabil 20: 353–360.

Grimby G, Danneskiold-Samsoe B, Hvid K, Saltin B (1982) Morphology and enzymatic capacity in arm and leg muscles in 78–82 year old men and women. Acta Physiol Scand 115: 124–134.

Guyton AC, Hall JE (1996) Textbook of Medical Physiology, 9th edn. Philadelphia: WB Saunders.

Hamilton AL, Killian E, Summers E, Jones NL (1995) Muscle strength, symptom intensity and exercise capacity in patients with cardiorespiratory disorders. Am J Respir Crit Care Med 152: 2021–2031.

Hamilton AL, Killian KJ, Summers L, Jones NL (1996) Symptom intensity and subjective limitation to exercise in patients with cardiorespiratory disorders. Chest 110: 1255–1263.

Hards JM, Reid WD, Pardy RL, Pare PD (1990) Respiratory muscle fibre morphometry. Correlation with pulmonary function and nutrition. Chest 97: 1037–1044.

Heunks LMA, Viña J, van Herwaarden CLA, et al. (1999) Xanthine oxidase is involved in exercise induced oxidative stress in chronic obstructive pulmonary disease. Am J Physiol – Regulatory, Integrative and Comparative Physiology 277(6): R1697–R1704.

Horowitz MB, Littenberg B, Mahler DA (1996) Dyspnea ratings for prescribing exercise intensity in patients with COPD. Chest 109(5): 1169–1175.

Hughes RL, Katz H, Sahgal V, et al. (1983) Fibre size and energy metabolites in five separate muscles from patients with chronic obstructive lung disease. Respiration 44: 321–328.

Jansson E, Johansson J, Sylven C, Kaijser ML (1988) Calf muscle adaptation in intermittent claudication: side differences in muscle metabolic characteristics in patients with unilateral arterial disease. Clin Physiol 8: 17–29.

Ji LL (1995) Exercise and oxidative stress: role of the cellular antioxidant systems. Exerc Sport Sci Rev 23: 135.

Juan G, Calverley C, Talamo C, Schnader J, Rousson C (1984) Effect of carbon dioxide in diaphragmatic function in human beings. N Engl J Med 310: 874–879.

Kearon MC, Summers E, Jones N, et al. (1991) Effort and dyspnea during work of varying intensity and duration. Eur Respir J 4: 917–925.

Keilty S, Ponte J, Fleming T, et al. (1994) Effect of inspiratory pressure support on exercise tolerance and breathlessness in patients with severe stable COPD. Thorax 49: 990–994.

Killian KJ, Martin DH, Summers E, Jones NL, Campbell EJM (1992) Exercise capacity and ventilatory, circulatory and symptom limitation in patients with chronic airflow limitation. Am Rev Respir Dis 146: 935–940.

Kim MJ, Larson JL, Covey MK, et al. (1993) Inspiratory muscle training in patients with chronic obstructive pulmonary disease. Nurs Res 42: 356–362.

Kutsuzawa T, Shioya S, Kurita D, et al. (1992) P-NMR Study of skeletal muscle metabolism in patients with chronic respiratory impairment. Am Rev Respir Dis 146: 1019–1024.

Kyroussis D, Polkey MI, Hamnegård C-H, et al. (2000) Respiratory muscle activity in patients with COPD walking to exhaustion with and without pressure support. Eur Respir J 15: 649–655.

Lacasse Y, Guyatt G, Goldstein RS (1997) The components of a respiratory rehabilitation programme: a systematic review. Chest 111(4): 1077–1088.

Larsson L, Grimby G, Karlsson J (1990) Muscle strength and speed of movement in relation to age and muscle morphometry. J Appl Physiol 46: 451–456.

Levine S, Kaiser L, Leverovich J, Tikunov B (1997) Cellular adaptations in the diaphragm in chronic obstructive pulmonary disease. N Engl J Med 337: 1799–1806.

Levy RD, Ernst S, Levine SM, et al. (1993) Exercise performance after lung transplantation. J Heart Lung Transplant 12: 23–33.

Lopes J, Rissell DM, Whitwell J, Jeejeebhoy KN (1982) Skeletal muscle function in malnutrition. Am J Clin Nutr 36: 602–610.

Maa SH, Gauthier D, Turner M (1997) Acupressure as an adjunct to the pulmonary rehabilitation programme. J Cardiopulmon Rehabil 17(4): 268–276.

Mador MJ, Kufel TS, Pineda LA, et al. (2001) Effect of pulmonary rehabilitation on quadriceps fatiguability during exercise. Am J Respir Crit Care Med 163(4): 930–935.

Mahler DA (2000) Ventilatory muscle training. In: Hodgkin JE, Celli BR, Connors GL (eds) Pulmonary Rehabilitation: Guidelines to Success, 3rd edn. London: Lippincott Williams & Wilkins.

Maltais F, Leblanc P, Simard C, et al. (1996) Skeletal muscle adaptation to endurance training in patients with chronic obstructive pulmonary disease. Am J Respir Crit Care Med 154: 442–447.

Maltais F, Jobin J, Sullivan MJ, et al. (1998) Metabolic and haemodynamic responses of lower limb exercise in patients with COPD. J Appl Physiol 84: 1573–1580.

Mannix E, Boska M, Galassetti P, et al. (1995) Modulation of ATP production by oxygen in obstructive lung disease as assessed by P-MRS. J Appl Physiol 78: 2218–2227.

Martinez FJ, Vogel PD, Dupont DN, et al. (1993) Supported arm exercise vs unsupported arm exercise in the rehabilitation of patients with severe chronic airflow obstruction. Chest 103: 1397–1402.

Mayer M, Rosen F (1977) Interaction of glucocorticoids and androgens with skeletal muscle. Metabolism 26: 937–962.

McComas AJ (1996) Skeletal Muscle Form and Function. Champaign, IL: Human Kinetics.

Montes de Oca M, Celli BR (2000) Respiratory muscle recruitment and exercise performance in eucapnic and hypercapnic severe chronic obstructive pulmonary disease. Am J Crit Care Med 161: 880–885.

Montes de Oca M, Rassulo J, Celli BR (1996) Respiratory muscle and cardiopulmonary function during exercise in severe COPD. Am J Respir Crit Care Med 154: 1284–1289.

Morrison DA, Adcock K, Collins CM, et al. (1987) Right ventricular dysfunction and exercise limitation in chronic obstructive pulmonary disease. J Am Coll Cardiol 9: 1219–1229.

Nedder JA, Jones PW, Nery LE, Whipp BJ (2000) Determinants of the exercise endurance capacity in patients with chronic obstructive pulmonary disease: the power duration relationship. Am J Respir Crit Care Med 162(2): 497–504.

Nedder JA, Sword D, Ward SA, Mackay E (2002) Home based neuromuscular electrical stimulation as a new rehabilitative strategy for severely disabled patients with chronic obstructive pulmonary disease (COPD). Thorax 57(4): 333–341.

Neff TA, Petty TL (1970) Long term continuous oxygen therapy in chronic airways obstruction: mortality in relationship to corpulmonale, hypoxia and hypercapnia. Ann Intern Med 72: 621.

O'Donnell DE, McGuire M, Samis L, Webb KA (1998) General exercise training improves ventilatory and peripheral muscle strength and endurance in chronic airflow limitation. Am J Respir Crit Care Med 157(5): 1489–1497.

Orenstein DM, Franklin BA, Doershuk CF, et al. (1981) Exercise conditioning and cardiopulmonary fitness in cystic fibrosis: the effect of a three month supervised running programme. Chest 80: 392–398.

Pape GS, Friedman M, Underwood LE, Clemmons DR (1991) The effect of growth hormone on weight gain and pulmonary function in patients with chronic obstructive lung disease. Chest 99: 1495–1500.

Pastoris O, Dossena M, Foppa P, et al. (1995) Modifications by chronic intermittent hypoxia and drug treatment on skeletal muscle metabolism. Neurochem Res 20: 143–150.

Payen JF, Wuyam B, Levy P, et al. (1993) Muscular metabolism during oxygen supplementation in patients with chronic hypoemia. Am Rev Respir Dis 147: 592–598.

Peche R, Estenne M, Gevenois PA, et al. (1996) Sternomastoid muscle size and strength in patients with severe chronic obstructive pulmonary disease. Am J Crit Care Med 153: 622–628.

Polkey MI, Hawkins P, Kyroussis D, et al. (2000) Inspiratory pressure support prolongs exercise induced lactataemia in severe COPD. Thorax 55(7): 547–549.

Pouw EM, Schols AMWJ, van der Vusse GJ, Wouters EFM (1996) Muscle adenine nucleotide status in COPD (abstract). Am J Respir Crit Care Med 153: A453.

Pouw EM, Schols AMWJ, Deutz EP, Wouters EFM (1998) Plasma and muscle amino acid levels in relation to resting energy expenditure and inflammation in stable, chronic, obstructive pulmonary disease. Am J Crit Care Med 158(3): 797–801.

Rannels SR, Rannels DE, Pegg AE, Jefferson LS (1978) Glucocorticoid effects on peptide chain initiation in skeletal muscle and heart. Am J Physiol 235: E134–E139.

Reid MB (1996) Reactive oxygen and nitric oxide in skeletal muscle. New Physiol Sci 11: 114–119.

Reid W, Samrai B (1995) Respiratory muscle training for patients with COPD. Phys Ther 75(11): 70–79.

Richardson RS, Sheldon J, Poole DC, et al. (1999) Evidence of skeletal muscle metabolic reserve during whole body exercise in patients with chronic obstructive pulmonary disease. Am J Crit Care Med 159: 881–885.

Riera H, S, Rubio TM, Ruiz FO, et al. (2001) Inspiratory muscle training in patients with COPD: effect of dyspnea, exercise performance and quality of life. Chest 120(3): 748–756.

Ries AL, Ellis B, Hawkins RW (1988) Upper extremity exercise training in chronic obstructive pulmonary disease. Chest 93: 688–692.

Ries AZ, Kaplan R, Linberg T, et al. (1995) Effects of pulmonary rehabilitation on physiologic and psychosocial outcomes in patients with chronic obstructive pulmonary disease. Ann Intern Med 122: 823–827.

Robinson EP, Kjeldgaard JM (1982) Improvement in ventilatory muscle function with running. J Appl Physiol 52: 1400–1406.

Rochester DF, Braun NM (1985) Determinants of maximal inspiratory pressure in chronic obstructive pulmonary disease. Am Rev Respir Dis 132: 42–47.

Roomi J, Johnson MM, Waters K, et al. (1996) Respiratory rehabilitation, exercise capacity and quality of life in chronic airways disease in old age. Age Ageing 25: 12–16.

Rooyackers JM, Dekhuijzen PN, Van Herwaarden CL, et al. (1997) Training with supplemental oxygen in patients with COPD and hypoxaemia at peak exercise. Thorax 55: 539–543.

Schols AMWJ, Soeters PB, Dingemans ANC, et al. (1993) Prevalence and characteristics of nutritional depletion in patients with COPD eligible for pulmonary rehabilitation. Am Rev Respir Dis 147: 1151–1156.

Schols AMWJ, Creutzberg EC, Buurman WA, et al. (1999) Plasma leptin is related to pro-inflammatory status and dietary intake in patients with chronic obstructive pulmonary disease. Am J Respir Crit Care Med 160: 1220–1226.

Serres I, Gautier V, Varray A, Prefaut C (1998) Impaired skeletal muscle endurance related to physical inactivity and altered lung function in COPD patients. Chest 113: 900–905.

Simard C, Maltais F, Leblanc P, Simard M, Jobin J (1996) Mitochondrial and capillarity changes in vastus lateralis muscle of COPD patients: electron microscopy study. Med Sci Sports Exerc 23: S95.

Similowski T, Yan S, Gauthier AP, Macklem PT, Bellemare F (1991) Contractile properties of the human diaphragm during chronic hyperinflation. N Engl J Med 325: 917–923.

Simpson K, Killian KJ, McCartney N, Stubbing DG, Jones NL (1992) Randomised controlled trial of weight lifting exercise in patients with chronic airflow limitation. Thorax 47: 70–75.

Singh SJ, Morgan MDL, Hardman AE, et al. (1994) Comparison of oxygen uptake during a conventional treadmill test and the shuttle walk test in chronic airflow limitation. Eur Respir J 7: 2016–2020.

Smith K, Cook D, Guyatt GH, et al. (1992) Respiratory muscle training in chronic airflow limitation: a meta-analysis. Am Rev Respir Dis 145: 533–539.

Stewart RL, Lewis CM (1986) Cardiac output during exercise in patients with COPD. Chest 89: 199–205.

Sullivan SD, Ramsey SD, Lee TD (2000) The economic burden of COPD. Chest Supplement 117: 5S–9S.

Vale F, Reardon JZ, ZuWallack RL (1993) The long term benefits of outpatient pulmonary rehabilitation on exercise endurance and quality of life. Chest 103: 42–45.

Wasserman K, Sue DY, Casaburi R, Moricca RB (1989) Selection criteria for exercise training in pulmonary rehabilitation. Eur Respir J Suppl 7: 604S–610S.

Whittom F, Jobin J, Simard PM, et al. (1998) Histochemical and morphological characteristics of the vastus lateralis muscle in patients with chronic obstructive pulmonary disease. Med Sci Sports Exerc 30: 1467–1474.

Zack MB, Pelange AV (1985) Oxygen supplemented exercise of ventilatory and non ventilatory muscles in pulmonary rehabilitation. Chest 88(5): 669–675.

PREGNANCY

Physiology of Pregnancy

Richard Craven

10

INTRODUCTION

The successful establishment of pregnancy creates a parabiotic relationship between the mother and the fetus that will be maintained for 9 months. Conventionally the 9 months of pregnancy are divided into three trimesters of 3 months. During the pregnancy the fetus develops and then grows, and is dependent on maternal support for its metabolic needs. To this end the fetus, or more accurately the feto-placental unit or conceptus, will influence maternal metabolism to meet these needs. Maternal physiology is therefore significantly altered during pregnancy with profound changes in the physiology of the endocrine, renal, respiratory, cardiovascular and musculoskeletal systems.

Establishment of pregnancy

In animals pregnancy might be timed from mating, since mating almost invariably leads to pregnancy. In the human this tight correlation is lost. Perhaps the fertilization of the oocyte marks the effective beginning of pregnancy. However, in humans, of every 100 fertilized oocytes, 31 fail to implant, so fertilization is not the effective beginning of pregnancy. The implantation of the embryo into the wall of the uterus is the point at which the embryo is able to direct the maternal physiology, and, although there are still embryos that will be lost post implantation, it is this event more than any other that marks the beginning of pregnancy. Although fertilization may not mark the beginning of pregnancy it is nevertheless a convenient point to start considering the processes that culminate in implantation and the shift for the embryo from a free existence in the uterus to the parabiotic existence that characterizes pregnancy.

Fertilization

The fusion of the sperm and the oocyte occurs in the fallopian tube. The oocyte has not yet completed meiosis. It completed the first meiotic division just prior to ovulation and has stopped again at the second metaphase stage. The oocyte is surrounded by the zona pellucida, which is an acellular barrier made up of a mucopolysaccharide ground substance containing proteins. Thus the first encounter the sperm has with the oocyte is with the zona pellucida. Proteins in the zona react with proteins in the sperm membrane and as a result of this interaction the sperm is able to penetrate the zona and then bind to the plasma membrane of the oocyte. This binding triggers the completion of meiosis in the oocyte, and at the same time the head of the sperm enters the oocyte, and the two pronuclei are formed. This process is illustrated in Figure 10.1. The two pronuclei, that of the sperm and that of the oocyte, fuse forming the zygote, which then begins to divide. These divisions are called cleavage divisions. These continue as the embryo moves down the fallopian tube (Fig. 10.2). By the time the embryo reaches the uterus, about 4 days following ovulation, it has gone through several cleavage divisions, passed through the morula stage and is now more than a simple ball of cells. It has differentiated into the blastocyst. This is a hollow ball of cells with at least two distinct cell types: an outer layer of cells, the trophoblast or trophectoderm, and the inner cell mass. The cells of the trophectoderm are polar – they have orientation; and they have an outer surface that is specialized for contact. The inner cell mass will give rise to the fetus, and, in combination with the trophectoderm, to the placenta, and the fetal membranes. The blastocyst itself has orientation. It can now be oriented by the inner cell mass end and the non-inner cell mass end. Implantation is orientated such that the inner cell mass end is closest to the uterine wall.

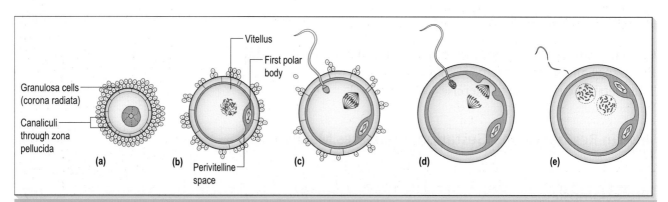

Figure 10.1.   Fertilization: (a) primary oocyte; (b) secondary oocyte formed by the completion of the first meiotic division, first polar body pinched off; both oocyte and polar body now have a haploid number of chromosomes; (c) second meiotic division stimulated by the sperm binding to the oocyte membrane, and penetrating the oocyte; (d) second polar body forming; (e) male and female pronuclei formed. (Reproduced with permission from Llewellyn-Jones, 1999.)

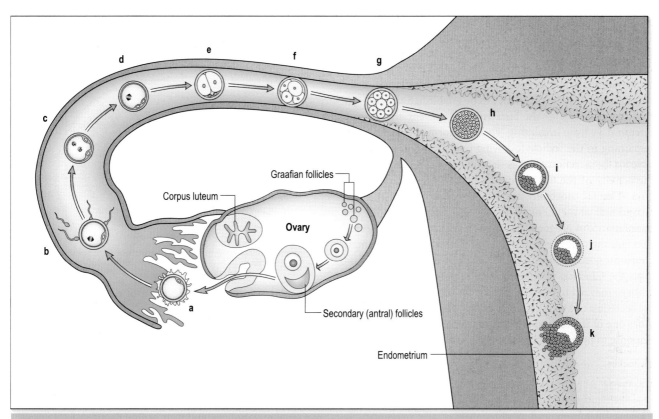

Figure 10.2.   Development of the ovum and its passage through the fallopian tube into the cavity of the uterus: (a) unsegmented oocyte; (b) fertilization; (c) pronuclei formed; (d) first spindle division; (e) two cell stage; (f) four cell stage; (g) eight cell stage; (h) morula; (i) and (j) blastocyst formation; (k) zona pellucida lost and implantation occurs. (Reproduced with permission from Llewellyn-Jones, 1999.)

Implantation

The blastocyst is a free-living organism and has derived its nutrients from its environment. To continue to develop and grow it needs the support of the maternal organism. To achieve this it must make contact with the mother, and create the appropriate alterations in her physiology. Implantation is the process by which this is accomplished. The initial alterations in maternal physiology are local. The pre-implantation embryo alters the activity of the endometrial epithelial cells (EEC), by altering the activity of the molecules which regulate cell adhesion and apoptosis (programmed cell death) in the EEC, creating the conditions for the initial phase of implantation which is attachment. Following attachment the trophoblast cells kill the modified EEC and invade the endometrium. The trophoblast flows into the tissue of the endometrium followed by the inner cell mass. The trophoblast is differentiating. The leading edge, as it invades the maternal tissue, becomes transformed into a syncytium (a multinucleate mass of cytoplasm formed by the fusion of cells), the syncytiotrophoblast. This, with extra-embryonic mesoderm, and endoderm from an outgrowth from the posterior end of the primitive gut, will develop into the placenta (Fig. 10.3).

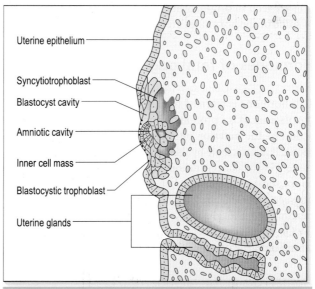

Figure 10.3.   Section of a 7½ day human ovum partially implanted in the endometrium. The embryo is represented by the inner cell mass; the blastocyst has collapsed. (Reproduced with permission from Llewellyn-Jones, 1999.)

It is the syncytiotrophoblast (trophectoderm) that is the source of the placental hormones that will regulate maternal physiology. Implantation will occur 5–7 days following the mid-cycle surge in luteinizing hormone (LH). It is following implantation that the first overt change in the maternal physiology occurs. For the pregnancy to be established the embryo must achieve two goals. First it must prevent the corpus luteum (CL) from involuting. The CL is formed from the cells remaining in the follicle following ovulation and is responsible for the secretion of progesterone. Second, it must prolong the activity of the CL beyond its normal lifespan of 12–14 days. The CL normally secretes progesterone during the second half of the menstrual cycle, and it is essential for the maintenance of pregnancy. If at any stage progesterone secretion fails then the pregnancy will fail. The secretion of human chorionic gonadotrophin (hCG), by the trophectoderm, sustains the CL. It is possible that interferons secreted by the embryo may act to prevent the involution of the CL, but it is the secretion of hCG that prolongs the life of the CL and provides one of the earliest alterations in maternal physiology in response to pregnancy, the suspension of the menstrual cycle.

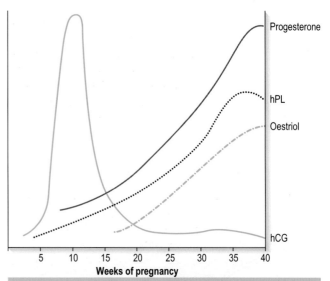

Figure 10.4.   Oestriol, progesterone, hCG (human chorionic gonadotrophin) and hPL (human placental lactogen) plasma levels in pregnancy. (Reproduced with permission from Llewellyn-Jones, 1999.)

ENDOCRINE CHANGES

The establishment and maintenance of the pregnancy is dependent on the feto-placental unit signalling its presence to the mother, and then influencing maternal metabolism to meet its metabolic requirements. There are thus major changes in maternal endocrinology associated with pregnancy. Some of the hormones found in the maternal circulation are fetal in origin, others maternal. The changing levels of some of the hormones are summarized in Figure 10.4.

Hormones of fetal origin

Human chorionic gonadotrophin (hCG)

This hormone is secreted by the syncytiotrophoblast cells of the placenta. It is a protein hormone, similar in structure and action to the anterior pituitary hormone, luteinizing hormone. It is detectable by the tenth day following the midcycle surge. Plasma concentrations rise rapidly to week 8 of pregnancy, remaining constant between weeks 8 and 12, declining between weeks 12 and 18. From week 18 to term its levels remain constant. The role of HCG is to maintain the life of the CL, and ensure that the CL continues to produce progesterone until the placenta can take over production.

Human placental lactogen (hPL)

This is a peptide hormone that is also synthesized and secreted by the syncytiotrophoblast. It may be detected by the third week post conception, but by the third trimester placental production may reach between 1 and 3 g per day. It is the most abundant peptide hormone in primates. While human

placental lactogen is found primarily in the maternal circulation, it is also found in the fetal circulation. It will affect maternal metabolism, and thus indirectly affect fetal growth, but it also has direct effects on fetal growth and development. In the fetus it stimulates amino acid transport, cell proliferation, thymidine incorporation (which is a measure of protein synthesis), and the stimulation of somatomedin-C, and insulin-like growth factor-1 (IGF-1) in fetal fibroblasts. There are hPL receptors on fetal muscle cells, and it stimulates the growth of fetal hepatocytes, and DNA synthesis in fetal connective tissue.

In addition to these direct effects on the fetus, hPL will affect maternal metabolism. In the fasting state it stimulates lipolysis, leading to an increase in plasma levels of free fatty acids in the maternal circulation. These may be used as an alternative energy source sparing glucose for the fetus. In the fed state hPL stimulates glucose uptake, and increases fat deposition, ensuring adequate triglyceride for the mother in the fasted state. Human placental lactogen is an insulin antagonist, and will reduce glucose tolerance. Thus it acts to help maintain glucose availability for the fetus.

Placental growth hormone (pGH)

Placental growth hormone has been characterized during the last 10 years. It is a peptide hormone essentially similar to pituitary growth hormone. It is the product of the GH-V gene expressed in the syncytiotrophoblast. It is secreted in a non-pulsatile manner from the placenta, in contrast to the pulsatile pattern of secretion of pituitary growth hormone. By 15–20 weeks of gestation and continuing to term pGH will have replaced pituitary growth hormone in the maternal circulation. Its secretion into the maternal circulation seems to be a reflection of placental growth. In contrast to hPL the actions of pGH are on maternal metabolism where it stimulates maternal plasma IGF-1 levels. It seems to do this independently of the endogenous maternal IGF-1 levels. Maternal levels of pGH and IGF-1 rose steadily during pregnancy in a pregnant woman with acromegaly in spite of initially high levels of maternal IGF-1.

Hormones of maternal origin

The steroids progesterone and oestrogen both rise during pregnancy. Progesterone levels increase from approximately 11 ng/ml measured in the mid-luteal phase of the menstrual cycle to levels between 125 and 299 ng/ml. Oestrogens also rise from levels of approximately 0.2 ng/ml in the luteal phase of the cycle to 15 ng/ml during late pregnancy. Progesterone is essential for the maintenance of the pregnancy and if its secretion fails then pregnancy will also fail. Maternal cortisol levels rise during pregnancy, partly caused by the decrease in metabolism of cortisol, and partly caused by the threefold increase in the plasma cortisol-binding protein transcortin stimulated by oestrogen.

Prolactin

Prolactin levels rise during pregnancy from 10 to 200 ng/ml. In combination with hPL it prepares the mammary glands for lactation.

Thyroid hormone

The thyroid gland may be enlarged in 50% of pregnant women, as a result of diffuse hyperplasia. The circulating levels of thyroid hormone rise during pregnancy. This may be caused in part by the rising levels of oestrogen increasing the sensitivity of the pituitary to hypothalamic *thyroid releasing hormone*. The increase in oestrogen also results in an increase in the plasma levels of thyroid binding globulin. The ultimate effect of the increase in the levels of thyroid hormone is an increase in basal metabolic rate (BMR) evident by the sixteenth week of pregnancy, which may rise by 10–30% by the end of the third trimester.

Parathyroid hormone

There is an increase in the size of the parathyroid glands, and an increase in circulating parathyroid hormone, resulting in an increase in Ca^{2+} levels. In spite of this there can be an increase in muscle cramps in late pregnancy (see 'Musculoskeletal changes').

Relaxin

Relaxin is a polypeptide hormone secreted by both the CL and the placenta. Relaxin levels rise during the first trimester, then fall during the second trimester to levels which remain constant until term.

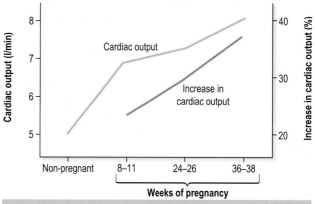

Figure 10.5.   Cardiac output in pregnancy. (Reproduced with permission from Llewellyn-Jones, 1999.)

As the feto-placental unit grows and develops the maternal physiology becomes increasingly altered to accommodate and support this growth.

One of the main consequences of supporting the growing fetus is a major readjustment in fluid volume dynamics.

FLUID VOLUME DYNAMICS

Simple statistics reflect the changes in cardiovascular physiology which occur during pregnancy:

- Cardiac output will rise by 25–50% and may reach 7 l/min (Fig. 10.5).
- Blood volume rises by some 42%.
- Red blood cell volume rises by an average of 25%, which, in combination with the rise in blood volume, results in a decreased haematocrit and decreased blood viscosity (Fig. 10.6).
- There is a decrease in systemic vascular resistance.

The reduction in vascular resistance will contribute to the reduction in mean arterial pressure reported in early pregnancy. Many of the changes in cardiovascular physiology are seen within the first 8 to 15 weeks of pregnancy, at a time when the conceptus is still small. They may therefore reflect preparatory alterations in cardiovascular physiology and not reactive changes.

The alterations in the cardiovascular functional parameters are part of a more general alteration in extracellular fluid volume during pregnancy. Pregnancy is not a steady state, and while cardiovascular changes may be detected early in pregnancy, within the first trimester, there is an increase in weight that continues throughout pregnancy. This weight increase will be approximately 11 kg. Between 6 and 8 kg of the overall increase in weight is accounted for by an expansion of the extracellular fluid (ECF) volume of 6–8 litres. This

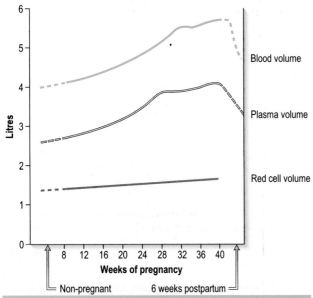

Figure 10.6.   Blood changes in pregnancy; the relatively smaller increase in red cell volume compared with overall blood volume will result in a decrease in haematocrit and blood viscosity. (Reproduced with permission from Llewellyn-Jones, 1999.)

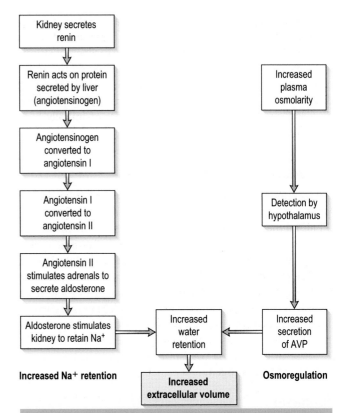

Figure 10.7.   Mechanisms of extracellular fluid volume regulation by the kidneys; renin–angiotensin–aldosterone regulation of Na$^+$ retention; regulation of water retention by arginine vasopressin (AVP).

increase in ECF volume is usually achieved without an increase in blood pressure. This is achieved by a parallel decrease in vascular resistance. The increase of volume without a concomitant increase in blood pressure represents a substantial readjustment of volume homeostasis. There is a significant relationship between the expansion of the ECF volume and the growth of the fetus. In pregnancies in which there is intrauterine growth retardation (IUGR) plasma volume is reduced.

What are the changes that produce this expansion of ECF volume? In the non-pregnant individual the ECF volume is maintained within very narrow limits by the interplay between pressure-sensitive receptors in the atria and great vessels, and the response to plasma osmolarity by the hypothalamus. The hypothalamus is also sensitive to information from the pressure sensors. The executive system that translates the output from the sensing systems is the kidney, and it is the regulation of sodium excretion by the kidney that is the major mechanism for the regulation of ECF fluid volume (see Ch. 8), supported by the regulation of water loss by arginine vasopressin (AVP). The mechanisms are summarized in Figure 10.7. Renin is an enzyme secreted by the kidney. It acts on a protein (angiotensinogen) secreted by the liver, converting it to angiotensin I. This, in turn, is converted to angiotensin II by angiotensin-converting enzyme in the lungs. Angiotensin II stimulates the adrenal cortex to produce the steroid hormone aldosterone. Aldosterone stimulates sodium retention by the kidney, which results in the isotonic retention of water, and a consequent increase in extracellular fluid volume. Alterations

in plasma osmolarity are sensed by the hypothalamus, which responds by altering the secretion of AVP. An increase in plasma osmolarity will cause the release of AVP, which stimulates the kidney to retain more water. Reduction in plasma osmolarity reduces the secretion of AVP and stimulates water loss by the kidney.

To achieve a volume expansion of 7–8 litres the pregnant woman must be in positive Na$^+$ balance. In fact she must retain some 900 mmol of sodium over the pregnancy, equivalent to a positive sodium balance of 2–4 mmol per day. In addition, there is an increase in renal blood flow with a concomitant increase in glomerular filtration rate (GFR). The increase in GFR means that there is a substantial increase in the amount of sodium filtered (the filtered load). The filtered load for sodium rises from 20 000 mmol per day to 30 000 mmol per day. To maintain a positive sodium balance and thus gain volume in the face of such a dramatic tendency to lose sodium represents a massive realignment of renal function. In addition to the development of this potentially sodium-wasting situation, which itself would prevent volume expansion, there is a decrease in plasma osmolarity. Plasma osmolarity decreases by 8–10 mOsm/kg below the non-pregnant values. This decrease is apparent by the fifth

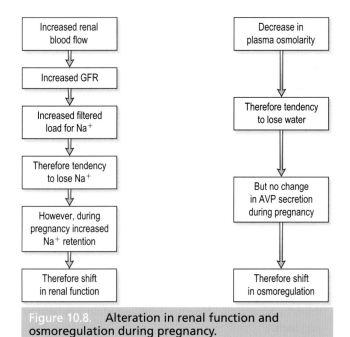

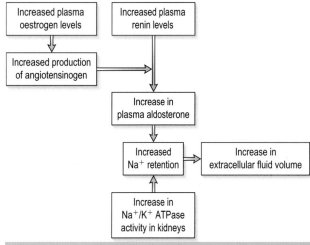

Figure 10.8.   Alteration in renal function and osmoregulation during pregnancy.

Figure 10.9.   Mechanisms contributing to the positive sodium balance of pregnancy.

week of pregnancy, reaching a minimum by week 10 and remaining at this level for the remainder of the pregnancy. In the non-pregnant condition this decrease in osmolarity would inhibit the secretion of AVP, which, in turn, would stimulate the loss of water and prevent fluid volume expansion. Similarly the fluid volume expansion itself should inhibit AVP secretion. However, there appears to be no reduction in AVP secretion during pregnancy as pregnant women are not polyuric. This suggests that in addition to alteration in renal function there is a shift in osmoregulation (Fig. 10.8). However, although volume homeostasis appears to be shifting during the pregnancy, the homeostatic mechanisms remain functional. Pregnant women respond to sodium loading and the alterations in hydration status in the normal way. It would seem therefore that there is a resetting of the reference point at which the systems involved in the control of both sodium and AVP are set, which allows the fluid volume expansion.

How do these control systems adapt to allow the fluid volume expansion?

Sodium retention

Sodium retention is increased in the face of several sodium-wasting changes.

- Increased GFR increases the filtered load.
- The increased plasma blood flow results in a decrease in filtered fraction which itself exacerbates the sodium wasting of the increased GFR. This tendency is reversed in late pregnancy.
- The high levels of progesterone secreted during pregnancy stimulate sodium loss, by antagonizing the actions of the mineralocorticoids (aldosterone) and by reducing the ability of the nephron to reabsorb sodium.

The activity of renin–angiotensin–aldosterone system seems to be altered at two levels during pregnancy. While there is always an appropriate response of plasma renin to sodium loading, the plasma renin is always higher during pregnancy than in the non-pregnant woman. This resetting of the system is essential as it allows the normal homeostatic controls to remain functional. There also seems to be a dissociation between aldosterone and renin. Aldosterone levels rise during the first trimester preceding that of renin. The proportional increase in aldosterone is much greater than that of renin.

In addition to the alterations in the renin–aldosterone axis, there is also an increase in the number of Na^+/K^+ ATPase sites in the kidney during pregnancy. This will increase the capacity of the kidney to remove sodium from the tubular fluid. Oestrogen, which is also secreted during pregnancy, will stimulate the liver to increase the production of angiotensinogen. Thus there are changes that increase the stimulus to retain sodium and a concomitant increase in the ability to pump sodium. These changes are summarized in Figure 10.9.

Osmoregulation

Even with the increase in sodium retention there is still a decrease in osmolarity. Thus the fluid volume expansion cannot be generated solely by the increased sodium retention. There must be a contribution from simple water retention. The osmolarity of the body fluid is very closely regulated, and the normal responses of pregnant women to water deprivation and loading suggest that this tight control is maintained during pregnancy, albeit at a new level. How then might osmoregulation be reset in the pregnant woman?

There are two major mechanisms for the regulation of osmolarity: the response to changes in osmotic pressure controlled by the hypothalamus, and the response to volume changes sensed by the pressure sensing systems. The alteration in osmolarity occurs during the first trimester. This might suggest that it is a response to the hormones of early pregnancy. One of the major pregnancy-specific hormones is human chorionic gonadotrophin (hCG). hCG can decrease the level at which a reduction in plasma osmolarity will stimulate the release of AVP. The specific action of hCG is supported by the fact that there is no similar reduction in the osmotic threshold in pseudopregnancy, when chorionic gonadotrophin is not produced.

The fluid volume expansion seen during pregnancy is not normally associated with an increase in blood pressure. While this may be in part attributed to the decrease in arterial resistance, there is also a resetting of the baroreflex during pregnancy. This will effectively reset the sensitivity of the AVP response to changes in volume. Such a resetting of the system still allows for a normal response to volume changes. Studies have shown that AVP was secreted in response to a 7% reduction in plasma volume, which was a similar response to that seen in the non-pregnant state, but the plasma volume at which the AVP secretion occurred was greater than in the non-pregnant state.

The alteration in fluid volume dynamics required by pregnancy is brought about by alterations in renal function, and by resetting the sensitivity of the osmoregulatory systems.

MUSCULOSKELETAL CHANGES

One of the inevitable changes that occur during pregnancy is weight gain. This in itself will have effects on the musculoskeletal system, but the change in centre of gravity caused by the growing gravid uterus, and the compensatory lumbar lordosis, will exacerbate these effects dramatically. Almost all pregnant women will have some musculoskeletal problem associated with their pregnancy. Some of the more common complaints are back pain, posterior pelvic pain and leg cramps. In addition to the musculoskeletal complaints associated with pregnancy per se, pregnancy will also affect existing complaints.

One of the major changes contributing to alterations in the musculoskeletal system during pregnancy is the secretion of the hormones of pregnancy. There is increasing joint laxity as the pregnancy progresses. Oestrogen will reduce fibroblast proliferation and reduce collagen synthesis in the anterior cruciate ligament, and reduce its tensile strength.

- Relaxin is a major contributor to the increased joint laxity recorded during pregnancy. Some 70% of pregnant women complain of low back pain and this appears to be associated with increased joint laxity. Plasma relaxin is significantly elevated in patients with low back pain compared to those who do not report low back pain.
- Leg cramps occur in 15–30% of pregnant women. They are forceful tetanic contractions. Their cause is not clear, but may involve a calcium deficiency later in pregnancy.
- Carpal tunnel syndrome may occur in 1–25% of pregnant women.

The effects of pregnancy on existing musculoskeletal conditions are varied.

- Scoliosis seems not to be affected by pregnancy. The increasing levels of relaxin during pregnancy might be expected to contribute to the condition, but there seems to be no acceleration of the scoliotic curves during pregnancy.
- Spondylolisthesis and spondylolysis are not affected by pregnancy.
- Ankylosing spondylitis is largely unaffected by pregnancy.
- Rheumatoid arthritis will show remission in some two-thirds of women who have the condition when they become pregnant.

While there are demonstrable effects of pregnancy on the tensile strength of the ligaments with consequent effects on joint laxity, the effects of pregnancy on the skeletal system itself are less clear. The combination of the increase in parathyroid hormone secretion, the demands of the developing fetus for calcium, and the increase in GFR would suggest that the pregnant woman would be in a potentially negative calcium balance. The incidence of muscle cramps and their link with low calcium would tend to support this hypothesis. Such a condition, if it exists, might therefore be expected to lead to a loss of bone as increasing levels of calcium were mobilized, which in turn would be reflected in a decrease in bone mineral density associated with pregnancy. It is difficult to study bone mineral density in the pregnant woman because of the ethical problems of gratuitous exposure to radiation that is involved in such studies. Clinical observations give conflicting data:

- Adolescent mothers, matched for body mass index (BMI), total body bone mineral content and sporting activity at 12 years of age, showed a significant decrease in hip bone density compared with non-pregnant controls. However, it is possible that in these individuals who became pregnant between 16.5 and 19.5 years of age, the effects of pregnancy per se on bone density may well have been complicated by the underlying developmental dynamic of calcium metabolism.
- Measurement in the bone density of the calcaneus using ultrasound showed a decrease in bone mineral density during the third trimester. Bone metabolism was also increased.
- In contrast, a longitudinal study using dual density X-rays to measure the bone density of the distal radius, in which the bone mineral density of 22 women was measured several

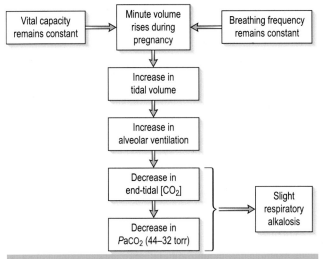

Figure 10.10. Summary of the respiratory changes during pregnancy.

times between the first trimester and 24 months postpartum, showed no decrease in bone mineral density during pregnancy.

Study differences may be explained by the use of different technologies, different sites of measurement and different times during the pregnancy.

RESPIRATORY CHANGES IN PREGNANCY

As pregnancy advances, the gravid uterus pushes up into the abdomen and in pushing up against the diaphragm reduces the vertical height of the chest by some 4 cm. In compensation there is an increase in the anteroposterior and transverse diameters of some 10 cm. The vital capacity remains constant. The minute volume rises during pregnancy, but breathing frequency remains the same. This inevitably means an increase in tidal volume, which may rise by about 30%. The increase in tidal volume results in an increase in alveolar ventilation. This in turn will result in a reduction in end-tidal $[CO_2]$ and the $PaCO_2$ may decrease from 44 to 32 torr, resulting in a slight respiratory alkalosis (Fig. 10.10).

As previously discussed, in addition to the changes in respiratory function there is also a change in BMR. Oxygen consumption (VO_2) at rest increases between 16 and 20% over the non-pregnant state, with increases from 182 ml/kg in the non-pregnant state to 380 ml/kg at 32 weeks of pregnancy. The increase in resting oxygen consumption during pregnancy is not surprising. As the fetus grows, its demand for oxygen will rise and will be reflected by the increase in maternal resting oxygen consumption. Whether the increase in thyroid hormone discussed earlier is proactive or reactive is not clear.

With the change in cardiovascular and respiratory functions, and the increase in BMR, it is interesting to explore the effects of pregnancy on the economy of exercise, the metabolic response to exercise and the capacity for exercise.

PREGNANCY AND EXERCISE

Exercise in the non-pregnant state will induce marked changes in the subjects' physiological parameters. Cardiac output, oxygen consumption, minute volume, breathing frequency all rise. The same responses are recorded during pregnancy. The responses of heart rate, stroke volume and cardiac output to mild exercise (30 watts on a bicycle ergometer) seem to be the same in late gestation as they are postpartum. However, pregnancy per se may affect the metabolic responses to exercise.

Changes in oxygen consumption during submaximal work

The alterations in oxygen consumption during submaximal work, not surprisingly, will be affected by the type of work done. Oxygen consumption can be increased by approximately 10% compared with the non-pregnant state for equivalent work rate undertaken on a treadmill. The pregnancy-induced changes in oxygen consumption for non-load-bearing work are very much reduced when they are present at all. Studies in which women are asked to work at light to moderate intensities on a bicycle ergometer during pregnancy report either an increase in oxygen consumption, no change or a decrease in oxygen consumption compared with the non-pregnant state and for equivalent workloads. Although the effects of pregnancy on the economy of exercise are equivocal there does seem to be an improvement in aerobic capacity as a result of pregnancy. Anaerobic threshold, the respiratory compensatory threshold (the respiratory compensatory threshold is the level of exercise when the excess CO_2 produced by buffering the exercise-induced increase in blood lactate begins to induce hyperventilation) and post-exercise blood lactate concentrations are all improved during pregnancy.

Pregnancy and work capacity

Work capacity is measured by the maximal amount of oxygen an individual can consume (VO_{2max}). Maximal oxygen consumption may be estimated from submaximal exercise tests. Estimation of VO_{2max} from submaximal exercise depends on the fact that there is a linear relationship between workload and oxygen consumption in the non-pregnant woman. If this relationship were to change during pregnancy then these estimations would become invalid. Pregnancy does not appear to alter this relationship. Thus estimates of VO_{2max} from submaximal exercise in pregnancy are valid.

Such estimations suggest that there is no pregnancy-dependent decrease in $V_{O_{2max}}$. Direct measurements of $V_{O_{2max}}$ are ethically questionable, and thus less common, but do provide a direct measure of the work capacity of the pregnant woman. Incremental maximal oxygen uptake tests carried out on either a bicycle ergometer or a treadmill suggest that there is no difference in $V_{O_{2max}}$ during the first, second and third trimesters or postpartum.

The metabolic response to exercise

The metabolic response to exercise during pregnancy does appear to change. During pregnancy the resting levels of plasma triglycerides, free fatty acids and ketones rise, while the fasting plasma glucose levels fall. Exercise will result in an exaggerated fall in blood glucose compared with the non-pregnant state. In response to 30 minutes of moderate exercise (heart rate of between 130 and 140 beats per minute), plasma glucose levels decrease by 25% in the second trimester and by 32% in the third trimester, compared with a decrease of 16% in the non-pregnant state. Exercise will produce a more marked reduction in plasma glucose in the pregnant than in the non-pregnant state. This decrease seems to be insulin independent and to be a post-receptor phenomenon. With the marked changes in physiology produced by exercise, regular exercise by the mother may have the potential to harm the developing fetus. By diverting blood to the exercising muscle, the fetus may be deprived of oxygen. The exaggerated decrease in plasma glucose produced by exercise during pregnancy may also adversely affect the fetus. Is exercise during pregnancy harmful to the fetus?

Regular exercise during pregnancy, especially in those women who exercised regularly before becoming pregnant, seems to have no adverse effects either during early pregnancy or on the outcome of the pregnancy.

INSULIN RESISTANCE AND GESTATIONAL DIABETES MELLITUS

Pregnancy is characterized by a state of insulin resistance. As pregnancy progresses, women show a reduced glucose tolerance to a glucose load compared to non-pregnant women. Although the increased insulin resistance seen in pregnancy may be considered diabetogenic, only 2–5% of pregnant women develop gestational diabetes mellitus (GDM); the majority retain a normal glucose tolerance, which though reduced is still within normal limits.

Insulin regulates the uptake of glucose by binding to a receptor (see Ch. 4). The insulin receptor is located in the cell membrane and belongs to a class of receptors known as receptor tyrosine kinases (Fig. 10.11). Once insulin binds to the receptor the tyrosine kinase is activated and will phosphorylate, and thus activate in turn, a series of signalling proteins

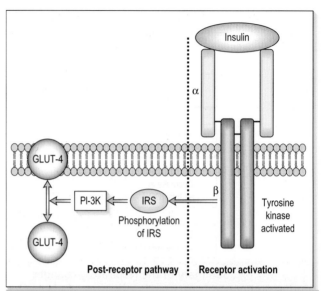

Figure 10.11.   Interaction of insulin with its receptor; the insulin receptor is a tyrosine kinase consisting of two α and two β units; the activated tyrosine kinase phosphorylates the insulin receptor substrate protein (IRS); IRS activates the enzyme phosphatidylinositol-3-kinase (PI-3K); PI-3K is responsible for inserting the glucose transporter GLUT-4 into the membrane; this facilitates the uptake of glucose by the cell.

within the cell. These proteins are known as insulin receptor substrate (IRS) proteins. The IRS proteins will activate an enzyme, phosphatidylinositol-3-kinase (PI-3K). This enzyme is responsible for stimulating the insertion of the glucose transporter protein GLUT-4 into the cell membrane and so facilitating glucose uptake by the cell.

Insulin resistance is increased in pregnancy, but to a much greater extent in women who develop GDM compared to those who show normal glucose tolerance. Insulin binding to its receptor is unchanged by pregnancy when compared to the non-pregnant state. It also is unchanged in women who develop GDM. This observation suggests that pregnancy-dependent insulin resistance represents an alteration in the events that occur after insulin has bound to the receptor.

Post-receptor changes during pregnancy include:

- A decrease in receptor tyrosine kinase activity. This decrease is greater in women who develop GDM.
- A 22% reduction in IRS proteins during a normal pregnancy, and a 44% reduction in GDM.
- A reduction in the expression of the GLUT-4 gene in fat cells during pregnancy. This reduction is more pronounced in women with GDM.
- There is no change in the activity of PI-3K during pregnancy.

There is therefore a reduction in the capacity of the post-receptor pathway, which would lead to an increase in insulin resistance, and this is more pronounced in women with GDM.

Several hormones rise dramatically during pregnancy (see above). Some of these will alter insulin sensitivity and might contribute to the increase in insulin resistance.

- Cortisol increases glucose production by the liver. It will decrease the activity of the insulin receptor by reducing its level of phosphorylation, and it reduces the amount of IRS protein in muscle cells.
- Human placental lactogen reduces glucose transport in fat cells without altering insulin binding to its receptor.

The increase in insulin resistance during pregnancy is associated with beta cell hypertrophy in the pancreas and increase in their sensitivity to glucose. This increase in secretory capacity allows the maintenance of normal glucose tolerance in spite of the increased resistance. In women who develop GDM, there seems to be a reduction in the capacity to secrete insulin.

Insulin resistance seems to arise from an alteration in post-receptor events, which may be affected by the hormones of pregnancy. In women who develop GDM this alteration is exaggerated and not accompanied by a parallel increase in insulin-secreting capacity.

PRE-ECLAMPSIA

Pre-eclampsia is a multisystem disorder peculiar to pregnancy. It has been described in pregnancies in which there has been trophoblastic tissue, i.e. placental tissue, but not fetal tissue, which indicates that pre-eclampsia is a disease of the placenta. It is a complication in 6–8% of all pregnancies, and is a major cause of maternal mortality, and fetal morbidity and mortality. Pre-eclampsia can result in intrauterine growth retardation with a consequent reduction in birth weight of between 5 and 23%. There is no current effective treatment for pre-eclampsia, and because it is a disease of the placenta, delivery is the only effective cure.

There are three major diagnostic symptoms, all of which spontaneously resolve at delivery:

- new onset hypertension: blood pressure ≥140/90 in previously normotensive women
- new onset proteinuria, >300 mg/24 hours.
- new onset oedema.

Pre-eclampsia is considered to be a disease of first pregnancy. A woman who has had a normal first pregnancy has a substantially reduced risk of developing the disease in a second or subsequent pregnancies. However, if the second or subsequent pregnancy is by a new partner then the risk of developing pre-eclampsia rises dramatically. The risk of developing pre-eclampsia is also increased by the use of barrier methods of contraception. In contrast, the risk of developing pre-eclampsia is inversely proportional to length of cohabitation

prior to the pregnancy. These observations suggest an immunological component in the onset of the disease, and that exposure to novel paternal antigens is a contributory factor. Perhaps pre-eclampsia is better considered as a disease of primipaternity (the first pregnancy by that father) rather than primiparity (the first pregnancy). Paradoxically the increased risk of developing pre-eclampsia associated with pregnancy by a new partner may not be because of maternal exposure to paternal antigens which are incompatible, but because the paternal antigens are too compatible with the maternal antigens. Human leucocytic antigens (HLA) are the major tissue compatibility antigens (see Ch. 2). Sharing of maternal and paternal HLA can lead to adverse pregnancy outcomes including pre-eclampsia. To establish and sustain a pregnancy a mother needs to establish and maintain an immune tolerance. This appears to be established by the placental expression of paternal HLA, which stimulates the maternal immune system. If there is HLA sharing then this stimulus may be lacking and lead to the initiation of, or a predisposition to, pre-eclampsia. This explanation is supported by the observation that women with pre-eclampsia, who would therefore be expected to share HLA with their partner, have a 30% reduction in risk of pre-eclampsia in a subsequent pregnancy if that pregnancy is with a new partner. In contrast, women whose first pregnancy is normal, who therefore do not share HLA with their partner, have an increase in risk of pre-eclampsia if a subsequent pregnancy is with a new partner. The apparent protection from pre-eclampsia afforded by increased exposure to semen would also support this explanation. If sharing HLA reduces the stimulus required to induce immune tolerance, then repeated exposure to paternal antigens would increase the stimulus, and reduce the risk of pre-eclampsia.

PREGNANCY AND BREAST CANCER

Pregnancy per se appears to have no direct link with the risk of developing breast cancer. There is no correlation between the risk of developing the disease and the time interval since the last full term pregnancy. However, it is well established that there is a strong relationship between the age at which the first pregnancy occurs and the risk of subsequently developing breast cancer. The earlier the first pregnancy occurs the less the risk of developing breast cancer, compared with the nulliparous state. As the age at which the first pregnancy occurs increases so does the risk of developing breast cancer, until in women whose first pregnancy occurs at or after 35 years of age the risk is as great or greater than that of the nulliparous woman.

The mechanism of the protective effect of pregnancy is not clear. It is believed that the hormones of pregnancy induce maturation and development of the mammary tissue that reduces its susceptibility to tumorigenesis.

FURTHER READING

Introduction

Hill JA (2001) Maternal-embryonic cross talk. Ann N Y Acad Sci 943: 17.

Johnson MH, Everitt BJ (2000) Essential Reproduction, 5th edn. Oxford: Blackwell Science.

Llewellyn-Jones D (1999) Fundamentals of Obstetrics and Gynaecology, 7th edn. Edinburgh: Mosby.

Pinon R Jr (2002) Biology of Human Reproduction. Sausalito, CA: University Science Books.

Roberts RM, Farin CE, Cross JC (1990) Trophoblast proteins and maternal recognition of pregnancy. Oxf Rev Reprod Biol 12: 147.

Roberts RM, Xie S, Mathialagan N (1996) Maternal recognition of pregnancy. Biol Reprod 54: 294.

Simon C, Dominguez F, Remohi J, Pellicer A (2001) Embryonic regulation of endometrial molecules in human implantation. Ann N Y Acad Sci 943: 1.

Endocrine changes

Alsat E, Guibourdenche J, Coutourier A, Evain-Brion D (1998) Physiological role of human placental growth hormone. Mol Cell Endocrinol 140: 121.

Lacroix MC, Guibourdenche J, Frendo JL, Evain-Brion D (2002) Human placental growth hormone – a review. Placenta 23 Suppl A: S87.

Laros RK (1987) Physiology of normal pregnancy. In: Wilson JR, Carrington ER (eds) Obstetrics and Gynecology, 8th edn. St Louis: CV Mosby, p. 251.

Szlachter BN, Quagliarllo J, Jewdewicz R, et al. (1982) Relaxin in normal and pathogenic pregnancies. Obstet Gynecol 59: 167.

Walker WH, Fitzpatrick SL, Barrera-Saldans HH, Resondez-Perez D, Sanndes GF (1991) The human placental lactogen genes: structure, function, evolution and transcription regulation. Endocr Rev. 12: 316.

Fluid volume dynamics

Brown MA, Gallery EDM (1994) Volume homeostasis in normal pregnancy and pre-eclampsia: physiology and clinical implications. Baillière's Clin Obstet Gynecol 8: 287.

Capeless EL, Clapp JF (1989) Cardiovascular changes in early phase pregnancy. Am J Obstet Gynecol 161: 1449.

Chesley LC (1972) Plasma and red cell volumes during pregnancy. Am J Obstet Gynecol 112: 440–450.

Chesley LC (1975) Cardiovascular changes in pregnancy. Obstetrics and Gynecology Annual (ed. RM Wynn).

Clapp JF, Seaward BL, Sleamaker RH, Hiser J (1988) Maternal physiologic adaptations to early human pregnancy. Am J Obstet Gynecol 159: 1456.

Dunlop W (1980) Serial changes in renal haemodynamics during normal human pregnancy. Br J Obstet Gynaecol 88: 1.

Dunlop W, Davison JM (1987) Renal haemodynamics and tubular function during pregnancy. Baillière's Clin Obstet Gynecol 1: 769.

Lindheimer HD, Barron WM (1993) Water metabolism and vasopressin secretion during pregnancy. Baillière's Clin Obstet Gynecol 8: 311.

Sturgiss SN, Dunlop W, Davison JM (1994) Renal haemodynamics and tubular function in human pregnancy. Baillière's Clin Obstet Gynecol 8: 209.

Sodium retention

Oparil S, Erlich EN, Lindheimer MD (1974) Effect of progesterone on renal sodium handling in man: relation to aldosterone secretion and plasma renin activity. Clin Sci Mol Med 49: 139.

Osmoregulation

Davison JM, Shiells EA, Philips PR, Lindheimer MD (1990) Influence of humoral and volume factors on altered osmoregulation of normal human pregnancy. Am J Physiol 258: F900.

Duvekot JJ, Peeters LLH (1994) Renal haemodynamics and volume homeostasis in pregnancy. Obstet Gynecol Surv 49: 830.

Leduc L, Wasserman N, Spillman T, Cotton DB (1991) Baroreflex function in normal pregnancy. Am J Obstet Gynecol 165: 886.

Theunissen IM, Parer JT (1994) Fluid and electrolytes in pregnancy. Clin Obstet Gynecol 37: 3.

Musculoskeletal changes

Heckman JD, Sassard R (1994) Musculoskeletal considerations in pregnancy. J Bone Joint Surg Am 76: 1720.

Huston LJ, Greenfield ML, Wojtys EM (2000) Anterior cruciate ligament injuries in the female athlete. Clin Orthop. Mar (372): 50–63.

Ireland ML, Ott SM (2000) The effects of pregnancy on the musculoskeletal system. Clin Orthop Mar (372): 169–179.

Lloyd T, Lin HM, Eggli DF, et al. (2002) Adolescent Caucasian mothers have reduced adult hipbone density. Fertil Steril 77: 136–140.

MacLennan AN, Nicholson R, Green RC, Bath M (1986) Serum relaxin levels and pelvic pain of pregnancy. Lancet 8501: 243.

Matsumoto I, Kosha S, Noguchi S, et al. (1995) Changes in bone mineral density in pregnant and post partum women. J Obstet Gynecol 21: 419.

Yamaga A, Michigoshi I, Minaguchi H, Sato K (1996) Changes in bone mass as determined by ultrasound and biochemical markers on bone turnover during pregnancy and puerperium. J Clin Endocr Metabol 81: 752.

Respiratory changes

Lotgering FK, Gilbert RD, Longo LD (1985) Maternal and fetal responses to exercise during pregnancy. Physiol Rev 65: 1.

Pernoll ML, Metcalfe J, Kovach PA, Wachtel R, Dunham MJ (1975) Ventilation during rest and exercise in pregnancy and post partum. Respir Physiol 25: 295.

Revelli A, Durando A, Massobrio M (1992) Exercise and pregnancy: a review of maternal and fetal effects. Obstet Gynecol Surv 47: 355.

Spatling L, Fallenstein F, Huch A, Huch R, Rooth G (1992) The variability of cardiopulmonary adaptation to pregnancy at rest and during exercise. Br J Obstet Gynaecol 99 (suppl 8): 1.

Pregnancy and exercise

Bessinger RC, McMurray RG, Hackney AC (2002) Substrate utilization and hormonal responses to moderate intermittent exercise during pregnancy and after delivery. Am J Obstet Gynecol 186: 757.

Clapp JF (1989) Oxygen consumption during treadmill exercise before, during and after pregnancy. Am J Obstet Gynecol 161: 1458.

Lotgering FK, Gilbert RD, Longo LD (1984) The interactions of exercise and pregnancy: a review. Am J Obstet Gynecol 149: 560.

Lotgering FK, van Doorn MB, Struijik PC, Pool J, Wallenburg H (1991) Maximal aerobic exercise in pregnant women: heart rate, O_2 consumption, CO_2 production and ventilation. J Appl Physiol 70: 1016.

Lotgering FK, Struijik PC, van Doorn MB, Spinnewijn WE, Wallenburg HC (1995) Anaerobic threshold and respiratory compensation in pregnant women. J Appl Physiol 78: 1772.

McMurray RG, Hackney AC, Katz VL, Gall M, Watson WJ (1991) Pregnancy-induced changes in the maximal physiological response during swimming. J Appl Physiol 71: 1454.

Wolfe LA, Walker RM, Bonen A, McGrath MJ (1994) Effects of pregnancy and chronic exercise on respiratory responses to graded exercise. J Appl Physiol 76: 1928.

The metabolic response to exercise

Clapp JF (1989) The effects of maternal exercise on early pregnancy outcome. Am J Obstet Gynecol 161: 1453.

Clapp JF (1990) The course of labor after endurance exercise during pregnancy. Am J Obstet Gynecol 163: 1799.

Lotgering FK, Gilbert RD, Longo LD (1984) The interactions of exercise and pregnancy: a review. Am J Obstet Gynecol 149: 560.

Revelli A, Durando A, Massobrio M (1992) Exercise and pregnancy: a review of maternal and fetal effects. Obstet Gynecol Surv 47: 355.

Insulin resistance and gestational diabetes

Kuhl C (1991) insulin secretion and insulin resistance in pregnancy and gestational diabetes mellitus. Diabetes 40 (suppl 2): 18.

Yamashita H, Shao J, Friedman JE (2000) Physiologic and molecular changes in carbohydrate metabolism during pregnancy and gestational diabetes mellitus. Clin Obstet Gynecol 43: 87.

Pre-eclampsia

Dekker GA (1999) Risk factors for pre-eclampsia. Clin Obstet Gynecol 42: 422.

Li D-K, Wi S (2000) Changing partners and the risk of preeclampsia/eclampsia in the subsequent pregnancy. Am J Epidemiol 151: 57.

Norwitz ER, Robinson JN, Repke JT (1999) Prevention of pre-eclampsia: Is it possible? Clin Obstet Gynecol 42: 436.

Odegaard RE, Vatten LJ, Nilsen ST, Salvessen KA, Austgulen R (2000) Preeclampsia and fetal growth. Obstet Gynecol 96: 950.

Pregnancy and breast cancer

Chie WC, Hsieh CC, Newcomb PA, et al. (2000) Age at any full-term pregnancy and cancer risk. Am J Epidemiol 151: 715.

Cohn BA, Cirillo PM, Christianson RE, van den Berg BJ, Siiteri PK (2001) Placental characteristics and reduced risk of maternal breast cancer. J Natl Cancer Inst 93: 1133.

Cumming P, Stanford JL, Daling JR, Weiss NS, McKnight B (1994) Risk of breast cancer in relation to the interval since the last full term pregnancy. BMJ 308: 1672.

Ewertz M, Duffy SW, Adami H-O, et al. (1990) Age at first birth, parity and risk of breast cancer: A meta-analysis of 8 studies from the Nordic countries. Int J Cancer 46: 597.

McPherson K, Steel CM, Dixon JM (1994) Breast cancer – Epidemiology, risk factors and genetics. BMJ 309: 1003.

DISORDERS OF THE SYSTEMS

The Nervous System: The Pathophysiology of Pain

Sue Syndica-Drummond

INTRODUCTION

It could be said that pain is all in the mind. Would you agree or would you yell in indignation from the reality of experience?

This section looks at how the physiology of the powerful sensation of pain can be both friend and foe, guiding us through survival or destroying our lives. Indeed the integration of sensation in the brain and our response to that sensation provides clues to how we perceive self and how complex psychological and physical processes occur.

In common with nerve transmission throughout the body, integration of pain sensation requires the circuit of sensor, transmission and synapse with cells in the spinal cord, thus evoking a reflex response as well as passing information to the brain. The brain assimilates that information and evokes a response to that pain.

Features of the pain mechanism

The model neuron (Fig. 11.1.1) represents the complex communication system that enables the body automatically to control its many homeostatic systems *and* to sense, process and respond to many stimuli including self-generated impulses.

The afferent system consists of the sensor (receptor sites), the transmitter (neuron cell body and processes) and the processor (spinal cord synaptic junctions and brain).

The spinal cord will integrate a reflex reaction (Fig. 11.1.2) and/or regulated response. The brain coordinates the reflex response to bring about the desired action (Fig. 11.1.3).

The key to understanding this system is to understand the significance of the structure of the neuron in relation to its axon size, and the effect of the chemicals or neurotransmitters, both at the origin of a signal and at the point of synapse or junction with other neurons.

NEUROANATOMY AND PAIN TRANSMISSION

What is pain?

Pain is an unpleasant sensory and emotional experience with actual or potential tissue damage, or described in terms of such damage. Pain is always subjective. … Many people report pain in the absence of tissue damage or any likely patho-physiological cause … there is no way to distinguish their experience from that due to tissue damage. (International Association for the Study of Pain)

This means: *pain is what the patient says it is.*

Basic pain mechanisms

In normal circumstances pain sensation stimulates a reaction to move away from the source of tissue damage, and if tissue damage has occurred encourages rest to allow healing of the damaged area. Pain is thus designed to be protective.

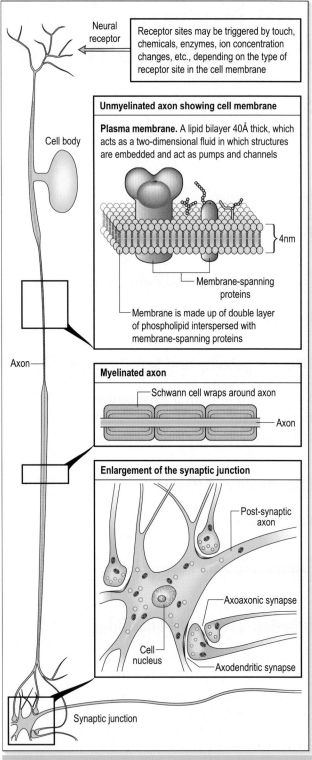

Figure 11.1.1.   Diagram of a model neuron.

Consider a person who stands on a sharp metal object that cuts the foot. The response can be broken down into the component physiological responses.

Firstly recall the normal nerve transmission mechanisms. When sufficient stimulus initiates an action potential, an

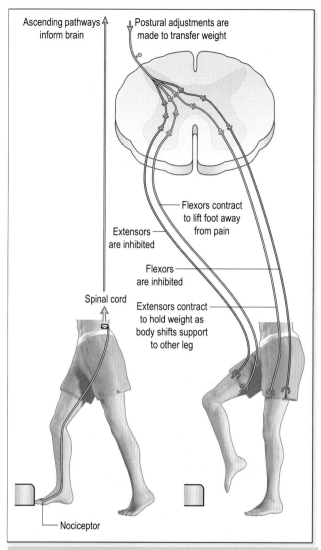

Figure 11.1.2.   Diagram of the withdrawal reflex.

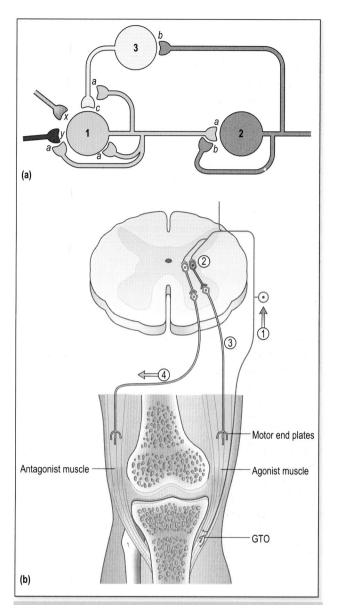

Figure 11.1.3.   (a) Simplified scheme of neuronal interconnections in the CNS. Neurons 1, 2 and 3 are shown releasing transmitters a, b and c, respectively, which may be excitatory or inhibitory. Boutons of neuron 1 terminate on neuron 2, but also on neuron 1 itself, and on presynaptic terminals of other neurons that make synaptic connections with neuron 1. Neuron 2 also feeds back on neuron 1 via interneuron 3. Transmitters (x and y), released by other neurons are also shown impinging on neuron 1. Even with a such a simple network, the effects of drug-induced interference with specific transmitter systems can be difficult to predict. (Reproduced with permission from Rang et al., 2003.) (b) Reflex effects of Golgi tendon organ (GTO) stimulation. (1) Agonist contraction excites GTO afferent which (2) excites inhibitory internuncial synapsing on (4) homonymous motor neuron and (3) excites excitatory internuncial synapsing on (4) motor neuron supplying antagonist. (Reproduced with permission from FitzGerald and Folan-Curran, 2001.)

impulse is transmitted along the axon to produce neurotransmitters at the next synaptic junction (Fig. 11.1.4).

'Nociceptor' is the name given to a neuron whose function is to receive and transmit pain sensations.

Afferent sensory fibres consist of three types:

- Aβ are low threshold, myelinated type II fibres, fast conducting (>40 m per second). L-glutamate is the transmitter. The axon is 3 μm in diameter and provides touch sensation.
- Aδ are high and low threshold type III fibres, fast conducting (10–40 m per second). The axon is 3 μm in diameter and senses first sharp pain.
- C fibres are high threshold, unmyelinated, slow conducting (<2 m per second) type IV fibres. Substance P and calcitonin gene-related peptide (CGRP) are the neurotransmitters (i.e. peptides), the axon is 0.5 μm in diameter and sensing second dull spreading pain.

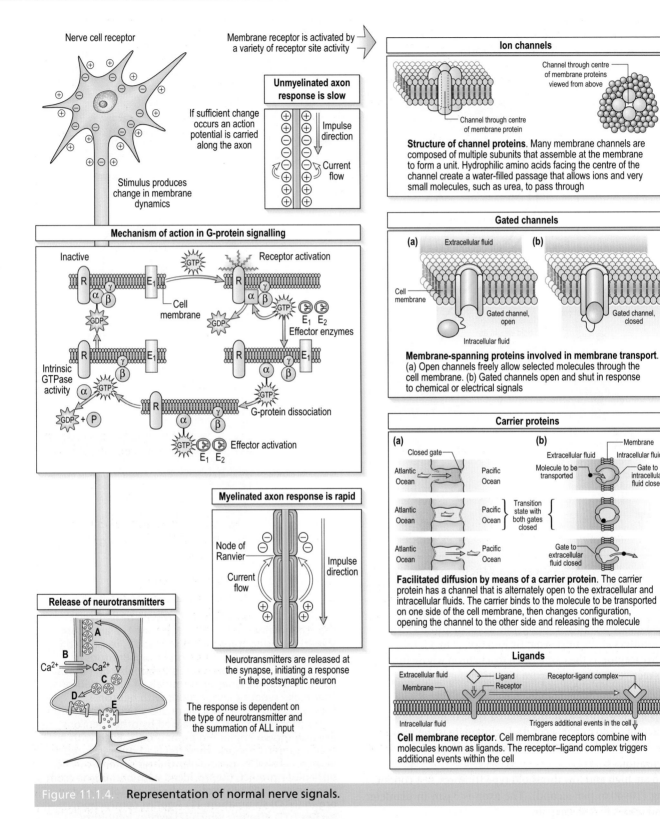

Figure 11.1.4.   Representation of normal nerve signals.

Sensations in the peripheral areas are conveyed through the afferent nervous system. The Aβ fibres are not part of nociceptor perception but influence nociceptor transmission to the higher centres. These fibres respond to light touch. The Aδ fibres (also known as A-mechanoheat or type III fibres) can be broken down into fibres that respond to sustained stimulation and fibres that convey immediate sharp pain initiating a withdrawal reflex. These fibres are unimodal.

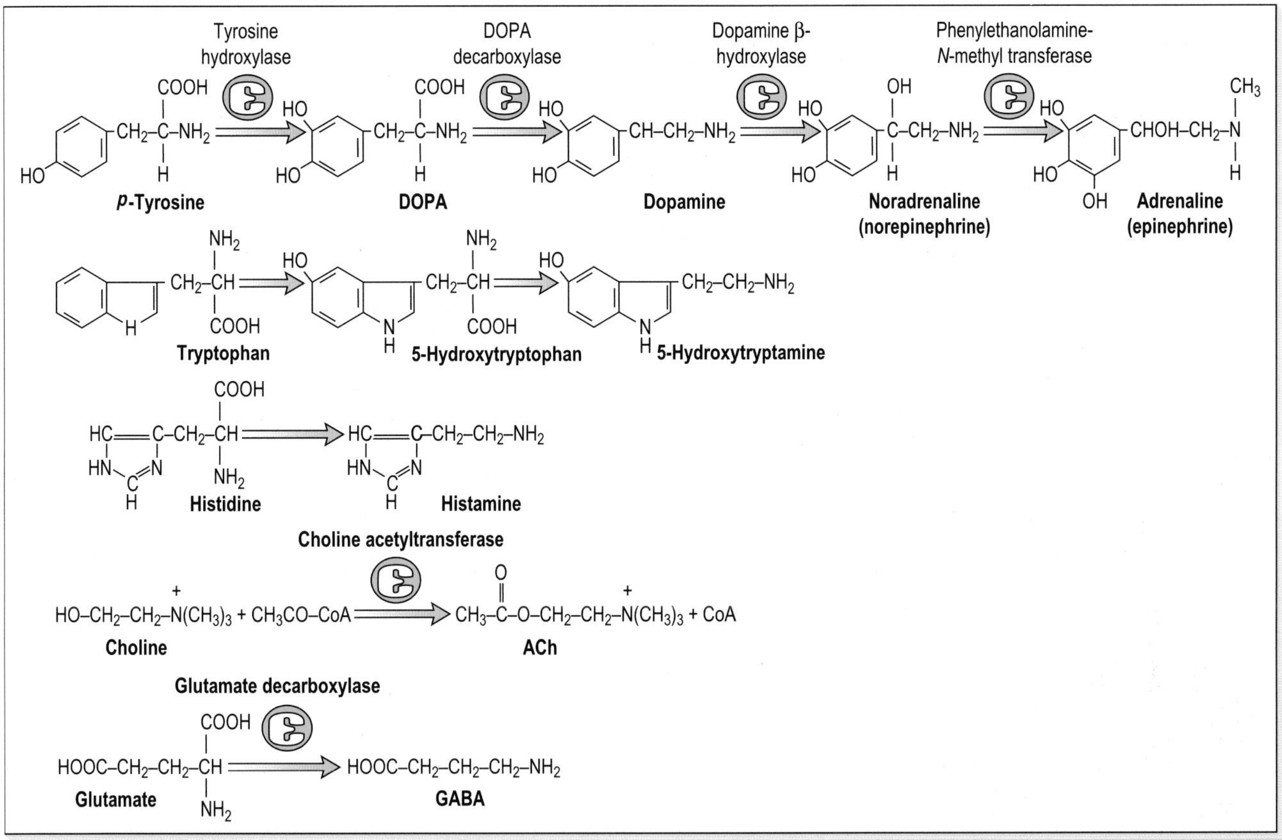

Figure 11.1.5.   Synthesis of neurotransmitters. Pathways of synthesis of neurotransmitters are simple. (Reproduced with permission from Baynes and Dominiczak, 1999.)

C fibres respond to noxious thermal, noxious mechanical and noxious chemical stimuli and may also be called polymodal and C-mechanoheat.

In addition, there are neurons called wide-dynamic-range neurons that respond to a wide range of stimulus intensities, giving a very accurate and differential response. If sufficient stimulus of the nociceptors occurs, two basic types of fibres will transmit signals to the spinal cord: fast small myelinated Aδ fibres and slow smaller unmyelinated C fibres. The initial response to the pain is via the pain receptors which generate an action potential in the Aδ fibres. These nociceptors are perceived first because the axons transmit the signal more rapidly than the C fibres.

The response in the spinal cord will depend on the quantity and type of neurotransmitter produced in the cord by the afferent fibres (Fig. 11.1.5 and Table 11.1.1).

Excitatory post-synaptic action potentials are generated by glutamate for fast and brief patterns and by peptides for slow extended patterns.

Different chemicals instigate a response in the C fibres. Some of these substances are produced by tissue damage. Pain input after tissue-damaging stimuli have ceased does have a purpose. The purpose of sharp localized pain identification

Table 11.1.1.   Classification of neurotransmitters (Baynes and Dominiczak, 1999)

Group	Examples
Amines	Acetylcholine (ACh) Noradrenaline (norepinephrine), adrenaline (epinephrine), dopamine, 5HT
Amino acids	Glutamate, GABA
Purines	ATP, adenosine
Gases	Nitric oxide
Peptides	Endorphins, tachykinins, many others

is to stimulate the withdrawal response, e.g. to stop full weight being placed on an injured foot and increasing the damage to the area. In addition, if pain sensations are maintained for a longer period the drive will be to protect the area. This will allow healing of delicate new tissue. This 'after pain' is the major function of the C fibre nociceptors system. It is essential to understand the role of neurotransmitters if the full implication of pain sensation is to be understood (Fig. 11.1.6). The type of neurotransmitter release causes what is known as sensitization.

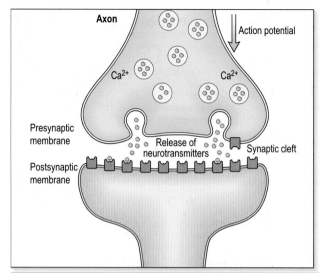

Figure 11.1.6.   Effect of the action potential at the synapse. An action potential passing down an axon to the axon terminal or region with similar function (e.g. axonal varicosities) changes membrane polarization, resulting in Ca²⁺ entry into the cell. This triggers the fusion of neurochemical-containing vesicles and cell membrane and the release of neurochemical (neurotransmitter) into the synaptic cleft. The neurotransmitter diffuses across the cleft and binds to specific receptors on the postsynaptic membrane to initiate a response in the postsynaptic neuron. (Reproduced with permission from Page et al., 2002.)

NEUROANATOMY AND SENSITIZATION

When the nociceptor is stimulated sufficiently to initiate an action potential in the afferent system the stimulus is sent via the dorsal horn ganglion to the substantia gelatinosa area of the spine, where the signal is processed prior to the perception of pain in the higher centres of the brain (Fig. 11.1.7).

The spinal cord pathway of physiological pain transmission

The Aδ fibres synapse in the II and V lamina of the substantia gelatinosa. They cross to the contralateral spinothalamic tract and if sufficient stimulus is applied will register in the ventrobasal nuclei of the thalamus and then project forward to the sensory cortex. The area of the sensory cortex responsible for perception of the relevant areas of the body is in the homunculus as shown in Figure 11.1.8.

If, for example, a man cut his foot not in the 21st century, but in the Stone Age while hunting a sabre-toothed tiger. He has cut his foot and his reflex withdrawal has thrown his spear aim off so that he misses the tiger. The hunter is now the hunted. Thanks to the inhibition of the pain fibres, our ancestor can run away with no awareness of the pain and escape.

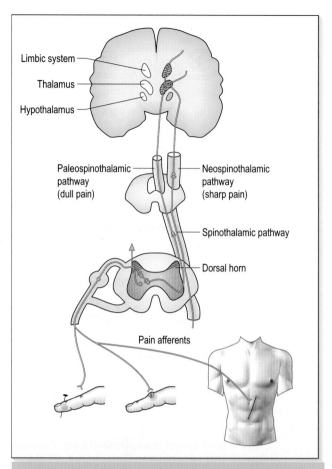

Figure 11.1.7.   Diagram of a spinal cord segment. Shaded areas are rich in opioid receptors. Opioid receptors are also found in medullary areas and the spinal cord. This shows in simplified form the pathways activated following stimulation of peripheral nociceptive nerve terminals. Many mediators are involved during afferent stimulation of the nociceptive pathway. Mediator release (bradykinin, 5-hydroxytryptamine, prostaglandins) stimulates the nerve terminals of pain fibres. Onward afferent transmission of ascending nerve impulses at the synapses in the dorsal horn involves neuropeptides such as substance P. Hyperexcitability of pain fibres can also be promoted by other mediators. The ascending pathways innervate areas of the midbrain and thalamus. (Reproduced with permission from Waller et al., 2001.)

An explanation for this mechanism is proposed in the pain gate theory of Melzack and Wall (1965) (Fig. 11.1.9).

The pain gate mechanism

To summarize, the perception of pain firstly consists of a sharp stabbing pain designed to allow us to withdraw from the source of damage. (Aδ fibre transmission mediated by L-glutamate.) A dull spreading pain designed to encourage rest follows this. Tissue damage releases neurotransmitters

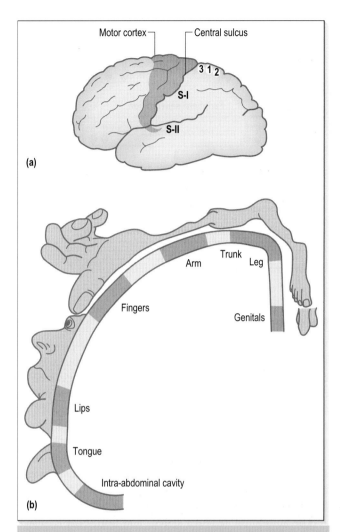

(a)

Motor cortex — Central sulcus

3 1 2
S-I
S-II

(b)

Arm   Trunk   Leg
Fingers
Genitals
Lips
Tongue
Intra-abdominal cavity

Figure 11.1.8. The sensory homunculus. (a) The somatosensory cortex is divided into primary (S-I) and secondary (S-II) areas which are closely associated with the posterior parietal cortex and the motor cortex. S-I is histologically divided into four (Brodmann areas 3a, 3b, 1 and 2). (b) In coronal section the S-I cortex is topographically (*topos* – a place) organized as a distorted map of the body with areas proportionate to the sensory importance of the body parts. The largest areas in the cortex are reserved for the fingers, lips, tongue and genitalia. This differential sensitivity has been represented as a homunculus. (Reproduced with permission from Davies et al., 2001.)

(peptides), which stimulate C fibres and produce pain. Rest allows for healing.

The full response depends on the *overall* effect of the summation of input of both excitatory and inhibitory neurotransmitters. Other sensations can influence the perception by closing the pain gate.

Now let us consider what will happen to our ancestor when he has escaped the tiger, and fear is no longer overriding the

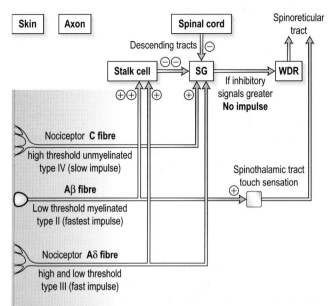

Skin   Axon   Spinal cord   Spinoreticular tract

Descending tracts

Stalk cell   SG   WDR
If inhibitory signals greater
No impulse

Nociceptor **C fibre**
high threshold unmyelinated type IV (slow impulse)

Aβ fibre
Low threshold myelinated type II (fastest impulse)

Nociceptor **Aδ fibre**
high and low threshold type III (fast impulse)

Spinothalamic tract touch sensation

Figure 11.1.9. The pain gate mechanism. The fast fibre input, via the stalk cells, generates inhibitory neurotransmitters in the substantia gelatinosa (SG). This, combined with the descending pathways from other nerve roots via interneurons and the direct inhibition from the higher centres, effectively 'closes the pain gate'. WDR, wide dynamic range.

pain perception of the tissue damage inflicted on his foot. He will now suffer what is known as *pathological* pain. When tissue is damaged the cells in the area go through the normal changes that initiate inflammation in preparation for healing (see Ch. 1 for details). These changes stimulate firing of the C fibres.

Pathological pain

Mediated by chemical changes in the tissue or central nervous system via a variety of neurological responses, e.g. inflammatory response. There is tissue damage.

Physiological pain

Mediated by high threshold nociceptors (Aβ and Aδ) where the size of the response depends on the size of the stimulus. There is no tissue damage.

This process of chemical changes initiated by the inflammatory response causes what is known as *sensitization*. The basic mechanism of sensitization in its simplest form is the *triple response.* This is a simple tissue reaction to stimulation of the skin:

- a nociceptor is activated
- a chemical neurotransmitter called substance P is released
- substance P causes local vasodilatation redness, oedema and flare from the area of stimulation.

When the stimulation is stronger this process spreads to the C fibre mechanism.

Peripheral sensitization

- Mechanical damage causes cell injury.
- Plasma leakage releases cytokinins, prostanoids, K^+ and H^+ ions, macrophages, mast cells, platelets and monocytes.
- These substances stimulate the C fibres.

Local stimulation initiates a response in the C fibres, which pass to the substantia gelatinosa. If sufficient signal is transmitted pain is registered via the opposite spinoreticular tract within the reticular formation of the brain. The mechanism of peripheral sensitization can also occur within the spinal cord leading to central sensitization. As a result pain may be reported in the absence of tissue damage. This is known as allodynia and hyperaesthesia.

Definition of pathological pain terms

- *Allodynia.* Reduced threshold to elicit pain. Touch is felt as pain.
- *Hyperalgesia.* Increased response to painful stimuli. Pain response is far greater than normal for a given stimulus.
- *Persistent pain.* Sustained response to transient stimuli, e.g. a pin prick continues to be painful.
- *Referred pain.* Spatial spread of pain sensation to uninjured tissue, e.g. pain from the heart is felt in the left arm in angina.
- *Neuropathic pain.* Pain perceptions induced by changes in the central nervous system or neurons.

Mechanism of central sensitization

When sensitization extends to the spinal cord so that the perception of pain is far greater than the original input, a mechanism called 'wind up' is said to occur (Fig. 11.1.10).

Wind up may be perpetuated by changes in the brain and spinal cord (which are explained later), where the neuron mechanism changes so that normal non-pain sensations provoke pain, and pain may even be perceived without any direct stimulation of the nociceptive pathways.

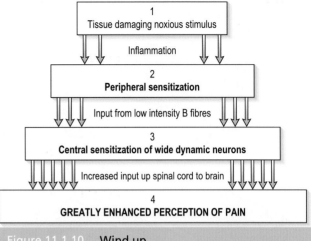

Figure 11.1.10.   Wind up.

Referred pain

Referred pain is defined as the spatial spread of pain sensation to uninjured tissue. For example, a nerve root trapped by a facet joint locking, or a protruding disc is registered by the brain as a barrage of pain signals and inflammatory neurotransmitters coming from the sensory distribution of that nerve root. If the fifth lumbar nerve root is trapped, pain is registered in the foot and front of the shin.

In other words, the pain is referred from the source of stimulation at the nerve root to the area of sensory distribution of that nerve in the foot. The brain will only recognize the area on the skin supplied by that nerve afferent.

The autonomic nervous system and hormonal feedback loops control visceral functional activity. Visceral pain tends to be diffuse and difficult to localize. It can be referred to other deep viscera, deep non-visceral structures and the skin, and tends not to be somatotopically organized.

Neuropathic pain

Neuropathic pain occurs where changes in the neuron or central nervous system generate pain perceptions in the absence of nociceptor input or tissue damage. The nervous system is particularly vulnerable to these changes when the mediators stimulating pain perceptions are peptides.

Peptides such as endorphins and tachykinins (substance P, neurokinin A and neurokinin B) cause C fibre transmission, which, if not controlled by the pain gate, will initiate stimulation of wide dynamic neurons. These neurons will alter their stimulation mechanism to respond to multiple sources of stimulation. This is the physiological mechanism of allodynia, hyperaesthesia and neuropathic pain.

The understanding of the mediators responsible for signalling in the nervous system becomes poorer when we examine the slow long-term synaptic transmission

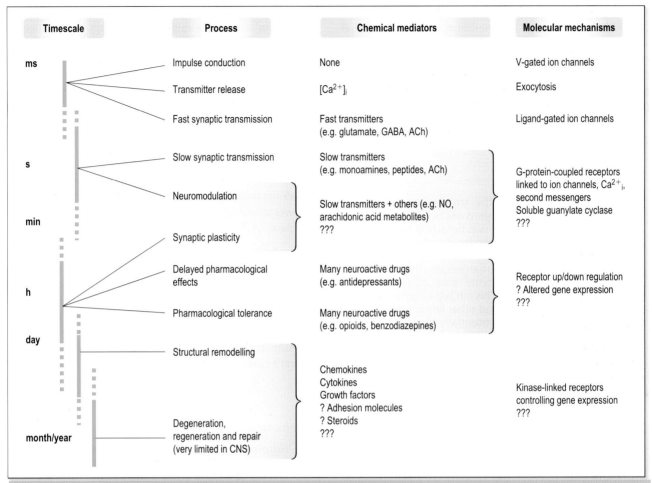

Timescale	Process	Chemical mediators	Molecular mechanisms
ms	Impulse conduction	None	V-gated ion channels
	Transmitter release	$[Ca^{2+}]_i$	Exocytosis
	Fast synaptic transmission	Fast transmitters (e.g. glutamate, GABA, ACh)	Ligand-gated ion channels
s	Slow synaptic transmission	Slow transmitters (e.g. monoamines, peptides, ACh)	G-protein-coupled receptors linked to ion channels, Ca^{2+}_i, second messengers Soluble guanylate cyclase ???
min	Neuromodulation	Slow transmitters + others (e.g. NO, arachidonic acid metabolites) ???	
	Synaptic plasticity		
h	Delayed pharmacological effects	Many neuroactive drugs (e.g. antidepressants)	Receptor up/down regulation ? Altered gene expression ???
	Pharmacological tolerance	Many neuroactive drugs (e.g. opioids, benzodiazepines)	
day	Structural remodelling	Chemokines Cytokines Growth factors ? Adhesion molecules ? Steroids ???	Kinase-linked receptors controlling gene expression ???
month/year	Degeneration, regeneration and repair (very limited in CNS)		

Figure 11.1.11.   Chemical signalling in the nervous system. Knowledge of the mediators and mechanisms becomes sparser as we move from the rapid events of synaptic transmission to the slower ones involving remodelling and alterations of gene expression. ACh, acetylcholine; GABA, gamma-aminobutyric acid; NO, nitric oxide; ???, areas of uncertainty. (Reproduced with permission from Rang et al., 2003.)

Causes of neuropathic pain

Complex regional pain syndrome
Malignant infiltration
Painful diabetic neuropathy
Phantom pain
Postherpetic neuralgia
Radicular pain
Trigeminal neuralgia
Post-stroke pain
Multiple sclerosis

---

requiring remodelling and alterations of gene expression. These mechanisms are certainly responsible for chronic pain and an understanding of the mechanisms is essential if suitable treatments are to be given to help control pain (Fig. 11.1.11).

The autonomic nervous system is not usually considered as a mechanism involved in pain generation and perception, as it is considered to be an 'effector' system that responds to the demands of the sensory and central nervous system producing an effect on the tissues it supplies, such as smooth muscle and glands. However, the autonomic nervous system causes nervous and secretory changes that influence the nociceptors.

THE REALITY OF PAIN

When we perceive any sensation we know that several areas of the brain respond to that sensation. When a monkey observes another monkey feeding not only does his visual cortex respond but also the area of the motor cortex that would be responsible for initiating the same movement, except that the movement is not carried out. This means that the monkey sees the feeding actions and also feels the movements that bring about the action.

Pain perception not only requires input from the nociceptors but also requires the emotional significance of that sensation for perception to have any reality. This significance requires experience to give depth of meaning, and that meaning is dependent on external factors such as the response from others, the implications of the sensation and the social expectations of the experience.

We know that the sensation of pain is designed to be protective and that inhibition of pain is necessary in some circumstances.

Ramachandran describes the story of Livingstone who 'saw his arm being ripped off but felt no pain or even fear. He felt like he was detached from it all, watching it all happen'. A similar situation occurs in soldiers in battle or sometimes to women being raped. During such dire emergencies, the anterior cingulate gyrus in the frontal part of the brain becomes extremely active. This inhibits or temporarily shuts down the amygdala and other limbic emotional centres, which suppresses potentially disabling emotions like anxiety and fear – temporarily. But at the same time, the anterior cingulate gyrus allows one to be extremely alert and vigilant so that the appropriate action can be taken.

The summation of this perception is real, with tangible changes in the periphery, spine and the brain that can be measured by the action of the neurons and the neurotransmitter/receptor mechanisms. The perception of pain, however, is not a simple trigger of stimulus and awareness, but comprises a multitude of neuronal activities where the action of the brain is as significant as the stimulus or indeed lack of stimulus in the peripheral neurons.

Pain physiology and psychology

Pain patients often come from families that include a member suffering from pain or illness. Studies done do not indicate that family size or order of birth is of significance. However, it is conceivable that spouses reinforce pain behaviour in partners, and illness behaviour may be rewarded within the family system in general. Although the evidence concerning family systems theory is contentious, it is feasible that this theory may partly explain why an individual develops chronic pain and why the family helps that person to perpetuate pain behaviour. It can be tentatively concluded that a chronic pain sufferer may significantly subscribe to poor marital relationships, poor sexual adjustment and high levels of emotional distress.

We know that pain is perceived in the brain and is influenced by emotion and the summation of the input of the neurotransmitters produced by nociceptors. The perception of pain is clearly influenced by the understanding of what that pain means, and is often influenced by unspoken beliefs and reinforcements not necessarily easily accessible to modification by conscious thought or action.

Pain is a subjective experience that can be perceived directly only by the sufferer. It is a multidimensional phenomenon that can be described by pain location, intensity, temporal aspects, quality, impact and meaning. Pain does not occur in isolation but in a specific person in psychosocial, economic and verbal and non-verbal expression of pain. (NIH Consensus Development Conference, 1987)

The primary concept to understand when trying to make sense of pain and the psychology of pain is that pain pathways are bi-directional. With this in mind assessment of pain must encompass more than a measurement of pain intensity and frequency, and must include awareness of culture, personality, gender, mood, social implications of disability and the influence of 'significant others' in the sufferer's environment.

Pain measurement questionnaires

- *Hospital Anxiety and Depression Scale (HADS).* Assesses an individual's level of depressions and anxiety (Zigmund and Snaith, 1983).
- *McGill Pain Questionnaire (MPQ).* Self-reporting questionnaire assesses different components of reported pain. Sufficiently sensitive to detect differences between various pain relief methods and able to provide information regarding effects of specific treatment on sensory, affective and evaluative dimensions of pain. Also assesses how the pain changes over time and what things increase it (Melzack, 1975).
- *Pain Cognition List.* Measures cognitions about chronic pain (Vlaeyen J et al., 1990).
- *Pain Coping Strategies Questionnaire (CSQ).* Assesses an individual's use of coping strategies when pain is experienced, and the extent to which these are effective in controlling and or reducing pain. (Rosenteil and Keefe, 1983).
- *Pain Self Efficacy Questionnaire (PSEQ).* Assesses an individual's confidence in their ability to cope with activities despite their pain.
- *Pain Stages of Change.* Assesses an individual's readiness to adopt a self-management approach to the chronic pain situation (Kerns et al., 1997).

The only conclusion we can draw is that pain is what the individual says it is. The difference between imaginary pain and real pain cannot be determined.

ABNORMAL PAIN PERCEPTIONS

Sensitization is the foundation of chronic pain, and abnormal pain perceptions such as phantom limb pain, neuropathic pain and centrally mediated pain. These arise because of modulation of pain signals.

Drugs, acupuncture, cognitive influences and other psychological and physical influences can modulate pain.

Phantom limb pain occurs when a limb has been severed and the nerve supplying that area is stimulated. Although the limb is absent the brain perceives the signal from the nerve as pain originating from the area that nerve would normally supply, say the thumb or hand of the non-existent limb. This occurs because although the limb is severed the sensory cortex still has neurons responsible for organizing perceptions from the relevant area of the body.

When normal input does not occur the brain and central nervous system will seek a stimulus to replace that input. This may be in the form of:

- hyperaesthesia from adjacent nerves
- spinal cord sensitization triggering pain response in the absence of tissue damage
- nociceptor stimulus, or growth of damaged or severed nerves producing 'buds' or neuromas in response to nerve damage.

This requirement for normal perception includes not just sensation but also the emotional feel of the sensation.

In a condition called prosopognosia the sufferer is unable to recognize people's faces; not because he cannot see them but because damage to the fusiform gyrus in the temporal lobe makes it impossible to connect the visual imprint with the memory of that face. The fusiform gyrus, once a visual image is recognized, sends a signal to the amygdala, the area of the brain that is the gateway to the limbic system. The limbic system is the emotional core of the brain. A patient may therefore look at his mother but not 'feel' that she is his mother. However when he speaks to his mother on the telephone his perception will be completely normal, as the connection from sound to the emotions is not affected.

Melzack identifies a concept of a 'neuromatrix' in which he describes the impact of the development of the gate theory by research specifically examining phantom limb and body pain: 'the anatomical substrate of the body-self is a large widespread network of neurons that consist of loops between the thalamus and cortex as well as between the cortex and limbic system. I have labelled the entire network, whose special distribution and synaptic links are initially determined genetically and are later sculpted by sensory inputs, as a *Neuromatrix*.' Melzack describes work done by himself and Loeser indicating that pain could be generated by the brain itself, in the absence of a spinal gate as occurs in paraplegics. Citing many other researchers, he goes on to propose that phantom pain becomes comprehensible once we recognize that the brain generates the experience of the body. It is this response of the brain (and spinal cord) that appears to stimulate the suffering of chronic pain compared to acute pain arising from trauma to the body.

For treatment purposes, pain is often classified as acute pain or chronic pain:

- *Acute pain* has a protective function and resolves after removal of the stimulus and after tissue healing has occurred. Signs include: increased respiration, pulse, blood pressure; dilated pupils; diaphoresis; restlessness, distraction, worry, distress.
- *Chronic pain* persists after the removal of or in the absence of a noxious stimulus. It may occur because of intermittent or constant stimulus. Signs include: normal respiration, pulse, blood pressure, pupil size; no diaphoresis; reduced or absent physical activity, despair, depression, hopelessness.

PHYSIOLOGY AND PHARMACOLOGY

Transduction is the term used to describe the conversion of stimulus (mechanical, thermal or chemical) into neural activity. This activity requires sufficient stimulus to generate an action potential, i.e. the threshold of stimulation must be reached. All mechanisms require a specialized transducer molecule that undergoes a transformation that directly or indirectly opens the sodium channels in the receptor membrane. Transducer molecules vary according to the type of stimulus they transduce, different receptors having varying degrees of specificity for different types of stimuli. Receptors that respond to only one type of stimuli are termed unimodal. Polymodal receptors respond to two or more types of stimuli.

Nociceptors have a highly complex structure and function reflecting their specialized transduction properties. Some nociceptors are polymodal (C fibres), while non-nociceptor sensory receptors are unimodal, with high sensitivity and a low activation threshold. Nociceptors require high stimulus energy for activation.

Recall Figure 11.1.4 showing membrane activity stimulated by a variety of receptor sites, such as ion channels, gated channels, carrier proteins and ligands. The structure of the membrane proteins will determine the receptor site activity and what can influence its open or closed state.

When signals are passed to the central nervous system via *transduction* of the receptor mechanisms, processing or *abstraction* extracts the relevant information. Control or *modulation* of the signal allows the signals to be enhanced or reduced, affecting the perception of pain.

Modulation can be exogenous or endogenous. Drugs can be used to reduce the signal, as can cognitive influences, such as distraction. Endogenous opioid peptide-related neurotransmitters are produced in the midbrain to facilitate descending pain modulation. Anxiety and fear can enhance pain, and descending facilitation of pain signals may play a large part in chronic pain states, so that neural activity in the spine is facilitated continuously rather than being inhibited.

Nociceptive pathways consist of three ascending tracts: neospinothalamic tract, the paleospinothalamic tract and the spinobulbar pathway (Table 11.1.2). These all travel in the anterolateral quadrant of the spinal cord.

Pain therefore comprises the sensory discriminatory aspect and the motivational–affective aspect. This allows exact location and characterization of pain especially in the skin but less exactly in the deeper tissues such as viscera, as well as incorporating an emotional response to nociceptive input. Overlying both of these perceptions is the cognitive–evaluative processing, such as cultural and anxiety-related influences, as previously discussed.

The higher centres affect pain perception by modulation of nociceptive input, usually in the spinal cord via the descending tracts (Table 11.1.3) but also within the brain, with linkages between the emotional limbic system and other centres.

How can the receptor sites be influenced? Receptors can be activated by an agonist, blocked by an antagonist, or influenced by a partial antagonist or agonist, e.g. opiate μ receptors stimulated by morphine or blocked by naloxone.

An *agonist* is a neurotransmitter, a drug or other molecule that stimulates receptors to produce a desired reaction. An *antagonist* is a drug or other molecule that blocks receptors.

For example, morphine is an agonist, and naloxone is an antagonist. Opioid receptors are found in many locations, as shown in Figure 11.1.12.

Enzymes can be inhibited by blocking of normal reaction, production of an abnormal metabolite by use of a false substrate or an active drug being produced by the use of a pro-drug (Fig. 11.1.13), e.g. cyclo-oxygenase inhibited by aspirin.

There are four basic families of receptor–effector linkage, the type of receptor influencing the time it takes for the cellular effect to be seen from activation of the receptor sites. Channel-linked receptors involved in nerve action potential generation may only take milliseconds, while the pain-relieving effects of anti-inflammatory drugs may take hours, or longer in the case of receptors linked to gene transcription as used by steroid drugs. Figure 11.1.14 presents a summary of the

Table 11.1.2.   The three ascending tracts

Neospinothalamic tract	Paleospinothalamic tract	Spinobulbar pathway
Sensory discriminatory aspect of pain	Motivational affective aspect of pain – subjective elements of sensory input	Activate descending modulation of nociception
Goes to the ventrolateral and ventromedial portion of thalamus, then projects to the parietal lobe of the cerebral cortex	Goes to the intralaminar portion of the thalamus, then projects to the limbic system and cortex	Spinoreticular tract ascends to the medulla. Spinomesencephalic tract goes to the midbrain. Projects to the thalamus – may influence the motivational–affective component of pain

Table 11.1.3.   Descending pathways modulating pain

Corticospinal tract	Lateral vestibulospinal tract	Lateral reticulospinal tract	Catecholaminergic pathways
Pathway for facilitation of flexor response, and inhibition of extensor response	Pathway for facilitation of extensor response and inhibition of the flexor response	Synapses in lamina IV to VI involved in pain perception	Pass from pons and medulla to lamina I to VI. Act to modulate sensory perception

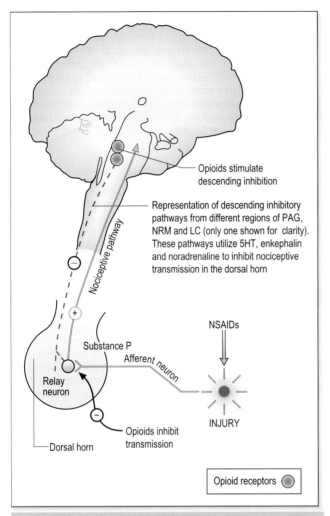

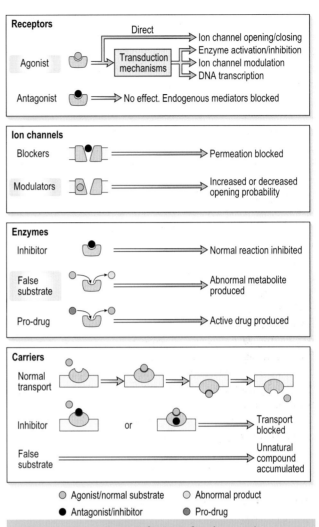

Figure 11.1.12. Transmitters and receptors for pain perception. The nociceptive pathways use a variety of transmitter substances, and promoters of transmission in neurons, substance P, other neuropeptides and nitric oxide all appear to be involved. The afferent pathways are subject to inhibitory control. Opioids act at opioid receptor-rich sites in the periaqueductal grey matter (PAG), the raphe magnus nucleus (NMR) and other spinal sites to stimulate descending inhibitory fibres that inhibit nociceptive transmission in the dorsal horn. Descending pathways from the locus coeruleus (LC) that are noradrenergic are also involved. Opioids also act directly in the dorsal horn to inhibit transmission. The inhibitory pathways associated with 5-hydroxytryptamine (5HT) and noradrenergic neurons may also explain the analgesic properties of antidepressants and anticonvulsants in certain types of pain. NSAIDs, non-steroidal anti-inflammatory drugs. (Reproduced with permission from Waller et al., 2001.)

Figure 11.1.13. Types of target for drug action. (Reproduced with permission from Rang et al., 2001.)

mediators likely to generate the action potential in a nociceptive fibre and the point of action locally of steroids and NSAIDs. Understanding these actions will help allied health professionals in advising clients who may become impatient with slow results from prescribed drugs.

Chemical signalling in the central nervous system is complex and although we understand much about synaptic transmission and neuromodulation, much less is known about long-term adaptive processes. As discussed by Rang et al. (2003) chemical mediators in the brain produce slow and long-lasting effects, often at considerable distance from their site of release. The term neuromodulator is used to describe a neuronally released mediator the actions of which do not conform to the original neurotransmitter effect. This term covers neuropeptide mediators and mediators such as nitric oxide and arachidonic acid metabolites. In general neuromodulation relates to synaptic plasticity. When patients complain of pain many factors influence this perception. The mechanisms influencing synaptic plasticity bring home the reality that pain is indeed all in the mind, but the perception of pain can never be described as imaginary.

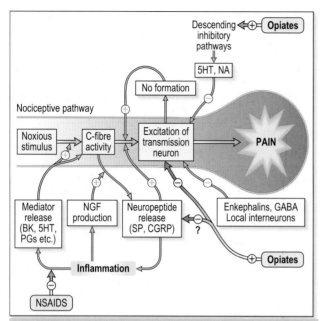

Figure 11.1.14. Summary of modulatory mechanisms in the nociceptive pathway. 5HT, 5-hydroxytryptamine; NA, noradrenaline; BK, bradykinin; PGs, prostaglandins; NGF, nerve growth factor; SP, substance P; CGRP, calcitonin gene-related peptide; GABA, gamma-aminobutyric acid; NSAIDs, non-steroidal anti-inflammatory drugs; NO, nitric oxide. (Reproduced with permission from Rang et al., 2003.)

The physiology of physical treatments for pain

Heat

This therapy works through modulation of the pain signals at the spinal cord via the Aδ fibres, where the heat sensation blocks the C fibre input via the pain gate mechanism. Heat also stimulates local vasodilatation, improving the removal of exudates and providing nutrients for tissue regeneration. It aids muscle relaxation, by reducing the firing of secondary spindle afferent endings, and it allows the tendon extensibility to increase.

Cold

Cryotherapy inhibits nerve conduction, particularly in the small Aδ fibres, controlling pain and reducing muscle spasticity. It increases viscosity in tissues, reduces metabolism and although useful in haemostasis, helping to control tissue exudates, it does not benefit healing in the long term. Following initial vasoconstriction, increased blood flow to a small localized area can be increased by local application of cold as the body will respond to increase the temperature of a small isolated area of temperature reduction by vasodilatation.

Massage

Massage will control pain through the pain gate mechanisms, improvement of local tissue fluid exchange, and removal of tissue exudates and oedema. Specific techniques of massage, manipulation and passive stretching will also reduce muscle spasm, fibrous adhesions and lengthen shortened muscles, fascia and tendons. Reduction of exudates and restoring normal muscle tone has a direct effect of reducing pressure on nerves.

Transcutaneous nerve stimulation

TNS works through the pain gate mechanisms described and may also influence the endogenous endorphin response (see below).

Acupuncture

The pain gate mechanism is thought to explain some of the effects of acupuncture. This may be via the stalked cells in the substantia gelatinosa, which inhibit C fibre pain transmission. The stalked cells fire most effectively at 3 Hz. It is known that the endogenous endorphins are influenced by the application of acupuncture. The neurotransmitters 5-hydroxytryptamine (5HT), β endorphin, enkephalin and dynorphins are known to be involved during acupuncture. High frequency electrostimulation (around 200 Hz) of acupuncture points is known to release dynorphins and 5HT, while low frequency stimulation (around 4 Hz) releases β endorphin, enkephalin and dynorphins.

Exercise

Suitable strengthening and mobilizing exercises will reduce pain by the release of endorphins, encouraging feelings of well-being, improved nutrition and circulation to the tissues, improved stability of joints, and stretching of shortened muscles, fascia and tendons. Psychologically, empowerment through achieving exercise targets and the establishment of coping mechanisms, and strategies to achieve goals despite pain perception, assist the modulation of nociceptor input as discussed in this chapter.

REFERENCES AND FURTHER READING

Baynes J, Dominiczak M (1999) Medical Biochemistry. St Louis: Mosby.

Benjamin S, Mawert J, Lennon S (1992) The knowledge and beliefs of family care givers and chronic pain patients. J Psychosom Res 36(3): 211–217.

Bliss T, Collingridge GL (1993) Synaptic model of memory: long term potentiation in the hippocampus. Nature 361: 31–38.

Coderret J, Vaccarino AL, Melzack R (1990) Central nervous system plasticity in tonic pain response to subcutaneous formalin injection. Brain Res 535: 155–158.

Cooper JR, Bloom FE, Roth RH (1996) The Biochemical Basis of Neurophysiology. New York: Oxford University Press.

Davies A, Blakeley AGH, Kidd C (2001) Human Physiology. Edinburgh: Churchill Livingstone.

Ell K (1996) Social Networks, Social Support and Coping with Serious Illness: The Family Connection. Oxford: Pergamon Press.

FitzGerald MJT, Folan-Curran J (2001) Clinical Neuroanatomy and Related Neuroscience. Philadelphia: Saunders.

Fozard JR (ed.) The Peripheral Actions of 5-Hydroxytryptamine. Oxford: Oxford University Press.

Gifford L, Thacker M (2002) A clinical overview of the autonomic nervous system, the supply to the gut and mind-body pathways. Topical Issues in Pain. Physiotherapy Pain Association, 3: 23–51.

Gifford L (ed.) (2002) Topical Issues in Pain 3 and 4. Physiotherapy Pain Association.

Hewitt DJ The use of NMDA-receptor antagonists in the treatment of chronic pain. Clin J Pain 2000 16: supplement 73–79.

Kelly WJ (ed.) (2001) Professionals Handbook of Drug Therapy for Pain. Springhouse, PA: Springhouse Corp., pp. 9–10.

Kerns RD, Rosenberg R, Jamison RN, et al. (1997) Readiness to adopt a self management approach to chronic pain: The pain stages of change questionnaire. Pain 72: 227–234.

Malenka RC, Nicoll RA (1993) NMDA-receptor-dependent synaptic plasticity: multi forms and mechanisms. Trends Pharmacol Sci 11: 22–24.

Melzack R (1975) The McGill Pain Questionnaire: major properties and scoring methods. Pain 1(3): 277–299.

Melzack R (1996) Gate control theory: on the evolution of pain concepts. Pain forum. Official Journal of the American Pain Society 5: 128–138.

Melzack R, Loeser JD (1978) Phantom body pain in paraplegics: evidence for a central generating mechanism for pain. Pain 4: 195–210.

Melzack R, Wall PD (1965) Pain mechanisms: A new theory. Science 50: 971–979.

Njobvu P, Hunt I, Pope D, Macfarlane G (1999) Pain among ethnic minority groups of South Asian Origin in the United Kingdom; A review. Rheumatology 38: 1184–1187.

Oxford Pain Internet Site. www.jr2.ox.uk/bandolier/booth/painpag/index.html.

Page C, Curtis M, Sutter MC, et al. (2002) Integrated Pharmacology. Edinburgh: Mosby.

Ramachandran VS (2003) Reith lectures 2003. http://www.bbc.co.uk/radio4/reith2003/.

Rang HP, Dale MM, Ritter JM (2001) Pharmacology, 4th edn. Edinburgh: Churchill Livingstone.

Rang HP, Dale MM, Ritter JM, Moore P (2003) Pharmacology, 5th edn. Edinburgh: Churchill Livingstone.

Reiss D (1981) The Family's Construction of Reality. Cambridge, MA: Harvard University Press.

Report of the Working Party on Pain after Surgery (1990).

Rosensteil AK, Keefe FJ (1983) The use of coping strategies in chronic low back pain patients: Relationships to patient characteristics and current adjustment. Pain 17: 33–44.

Sear JW (1998) Recent advances in and developments in the clinical use of i.v. opioids during the preoperative period. Br J Anaesth 81(1): 38–50.

Snelling J (1990) The role of the family in relation to chronic pain; review of the literature. J Adv Nurs 15: 771–776.

Thompson H (March 2002) Notes, Leicester University MSc Pain Management.

Tremont-Lukats IW, Megeff C, Backonja MM (2000) Anticonvulsants for neuropathic pain syndromes. Clin J Pain 16: supplement 67–72.

Vlaeyen J, Geurts SM, Kole-Snigders AM, et al. (1990) What do chronic pain patients think of their pain? Towards a pain cognition questionnaire. British Journal of Clinical Psychology 29: 383–394.

Wall PD (1999) Introduction. Textbook of Pain, 4th edn. Edinburgh: Churchill Livingstone.

Waller DG, Renwick AG, Hillier K (2001) Medical Pharmacology. Edinburgh: Saunders.

Watson C The treatment of neuropathic pain: antidepressants and opioids. Clin J Pain 2000 16: supplement 49–55.

Zigmond A, Snaith R (1983) The Hospital Anxiety and Depression Scale. Acta Psychiatr Scand 67: 361–370.

The Nervous System: The Central Nervous System

Udo Kischka

INTRODUCTION

Disorders of the central nervous system (CNS) can be caused by a variety of different processes: vascular disorders, traumatic injury, inflammatory diseases, demyelination, neurodegenerative diseases, tumours, epilepsy. These conditions produce clinical symptoms of different onset: some suddenly, others slowly. However, the kind of neurological symptom which occurs depends not only on the nature of the underlying pathology, but also on the localization of the affected site within the CNS. This is because certain areas of the central nervous system are specialized in processing distinct functions (motor control, sensation, language, etc.). For example, the symptoms caused by an infarction of the left cerebellar hemisphere will be very similar to those of an inflammatory process of the same region, except for the speed of onset. Similarly, any kind of lesion of the spinal cord can disrupt the passing of motor impulses from the brain to the lower motor neurons, and of information from the sensory receptors to the brain.

On the other hand, different parts of the CNS usually work together in neuronal networks to perform a certain function. This can explain the finding that lesions in separate parts of the CNS can sometimes cause similar clinical neurological deficits.

Following injury of the CNS and loss of neurons, the chances of recovery are unfortunately quite limited. CNS neurons are less able to regrow, or to be replaced by new cells, than are cells in other parts of the body.

However, functional recovery (at least partial) can sometimes occur even if the neurons which have died are not replaced. One possible cause for such a functional improvement is the recovery of neurons which were damaged but not destroyed. Another cause is *plasticity*, a property of the CNS which probably involves several mechanisms, such as the formation of new dendrites, and changes in the characteristics of existing synapses. These mechanisms may enable the formation of new pathways of information flow, which can take over some of the lost functions.

VASCULAR DISEASES

This chapter focuses on the most frequent vascular disorders of the CNS: stroke (ischaemic and haemorrhagic), and subarachnoid haemorrhage.

Stroke

Stroke represents the most common cause of death from neurological disease. It is a condition whereby the normal blood flow of the brain is suddenly disrupted. The neurological symptoms that follow are usually also of sudden onset. Two different mechanisms can be distinguished. The most common is a serious drop in blood flow through a brain artery, causing *ischaemia* of the brain tissue which it supplies. The other mechanism is *haemorrhage* when a cerebral artery ruptures, allowing blood to stream out into the surrounding brain tissue.

In the normal state, blood reaches the brain via the two internal carotid arteries (ICA), and two vertebral arteries which join up to form the basilar artery. The ICAs and the basilar artery connect via a ring of arteries called the circle of Willis. From there, several arteries branch out, the biggest of which are the middle cerebral artery (MCA), anterior cerebral artery (ACA) and posterior cerebral artery (PCA). Together with their branches, these arteries supply circumscribed parts of the brain with blood.

Ischaemic stroke

A reduction in blood flow through a cerebral artery which is serious enough to cause ischaemic stroke is in most cases due to either atherosclerosis or an embolus, or a combination of both. There are two possible mechanisms: a complete occlusion of the artery, or a combined effect of serious narrowing of the artery and a drop in blood pressure.

Atherosclerosis is a condition whereby the space within an artery (the lumen) is progressively narrowed over many years by deposits on the inner wall (Fig. 11.2.1). This occurs mainly in places where turbulences in the blood flow damage the inner wall (the intima). Typical areas are branching sites of arteries, for example the splitting of the common carotid artery into the internal and the external carotid arteries. The process starts with fat sticking to the damaged inner walls, and macrophages attaching themselves to the fatty deposits. Over the following years, a chronic inflammatory response develops locally, leading to fibrosis, calcification and the accumulation of even more fat. This whole conglomerate is called *atherosclerotic plaque*. The irregular surface of the plaque attracts blood platelets (thrombocytes) which become activated and trigger the coagulation of erythrocytes, forming a *thrombus*. With time, the atherosclerotic plaque and the thrombus will lead to a narrowing or *stenosis* of the lumen. The stenosis reduces the blood flow through the artery.

In the healthy person, a constant *cerebral blood flow* (CBF) is ensured by a finely tuned mechanism called autoregulation. In the event of a drop in arterial blood pressure with a concomitant fall in *cerebral perfusion pressure* (CPP), the small vessels in the brain react by dilating, thereby reducing the resistance to the blood flow. This mechanism is fast, although sometimes not fast enough, which can be confirmed by anyone who has nearly passed out when getting up too quickly from a reclining position. The mechanism also fails, and more seriously, when the CPP drops to such an extent that the resistance vessels are maximally dilated and cannot dilate further. In this situation, the brain tissue reacts by increasing the extraction of oxygen from the blood. If, however, the fall of

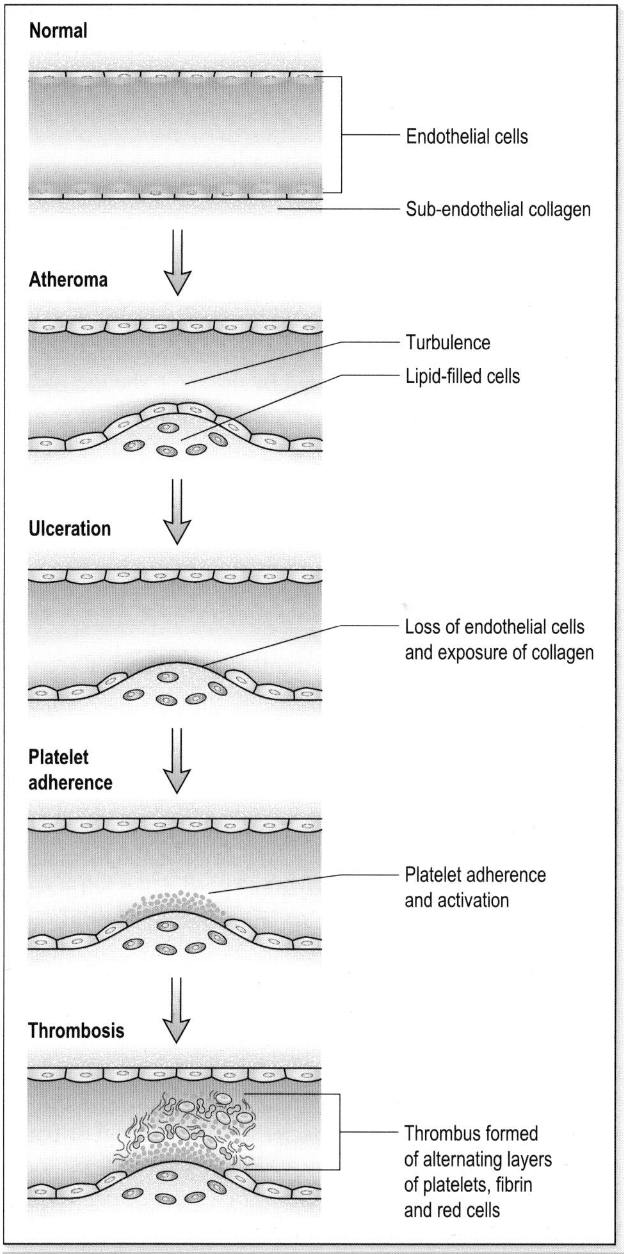
Normal
Endothelial cells
Sub-endothelial collagen
Atheroma
Turbulence
Lipid-filled cells
Ulceration
Loss of endothelial cells and exposure of collagen
Platelet adherence
Platelet adherence and activation
Thrombosis
Thrombus formed of alternating layers of platelets, fibrin and red cells

Figure 11.2.1. Thrombus forming inside an artery. (Reproduced with permission from Underwood, 2000.)

CPP is too steep, this mechanism will also fail. The resulting lack of oxygen supply triggers a chain of events which, within minutes or hours, leads to neuronal death:

- The brain cells lose their ability to uphold protein synthesis.
- Intracellular glucose metabolism has to switch from aerobic to anaerobic, producing increasing amounts of lactate and rendering the intracellular milieu acidic.
- The energy-sources ATP and phosphocreatine cannot be produced any more.
- Consequently, the energy-requiring ion pumps of the cell membranes cease to work, allowing sodium and chloride (and with it, water) to enter, and potassium to leave the cells.
- Calcium enters the cells, exerting a cytotoxic effect.
- The neurotoxic transmitters glutamate and aspartate leak out into the extracellular space.
- Free oxygen radicals and nitric oxide contribute to the cell damage.
- An inflammatory response is started, whereby cytokines activate granulocytes and macrophages to invade the ischaemic area, which probably adds to the death of brain cells.
- *Oedema* develops in and around the infarcted area. *Cytotoxic* oedema refers to swelling of cells by the mechanism described above, and *vasogenic* oedema is caused by impaired function of the *blood–brain barrier*, letting proteins and other substances (together with water) pass into the extracellular space.

This process of neuronal death can affect the whole brain and is then called *hypoxic brain damage*. If, on the other hand, the neuronal death is local, caused by stenosis or occlusion of a single cerebral artery, one speaks of *ischaemic infarction*.

Another potential cause of ischaemic infarction is an *embolus*. This is a particle transported within the bloodstream which is big enough to occlude an artery. Most emboli originate from a thrombus, either on an arterial wall, or in the heart. Common sites of thrombi in the heart are the atria, as well as valves that have previously been damaged, for instance by inflammation (endocarditis). Normally, the atria contract in synchronicity with the ventricles, ensuring a constant smooth blood flow through the heart. In people with atrial fibrillation, whereby the atrial walls are not moving, blood can stagnate inside. Stagnation of blood increases the risk of thrombus formation. If an embolus is transported to the brain, the damage will usually be directly related to its size. However, even a small embolus can cause a large infarction by occluding a large artery which has been stenosed by an atherosclerotic plaque.

Less frequent causes of ischaemic infarction include *vasculitis* (inflammation of the arterial walls), *dissection* (in which the inner layer of the arterial wall rips off), and *vasospasm* (spasm of a cerebral artery, caused for example by an operation on the brain).

When ischaemic infarction has occurred, some limited perfusion of the affected arterial branches can be established by *collaterals*, connections from other arteries. Such collaterals are provided, for example, by the circle of Willis, by connections between the external and the internal carotid arteries through the eye socket, and by small blood vessels on the surface of the brain connecting branches from the MCA, ACA and PCA.

Around the infarcted zone of dead neurons lies an area of neurons on the brink of death, the *penumbra*. Whether or not the neurons of the penumbra will recover depends on the restoration of blood flow. Reperfusion can occur, whereby the thrombus or embolus spontaneously dissolves, but this process may take days by which time it is too late.

Haemorrhagic stroke

When an artery within the brain bursts, blood streams out into the surrounding brain tissue, destroying neurons and other cells in this area. This is called haemorrhagic stroke or intracerebral haemorrhage. The weakness in the arterial wall allowing for such a rupture can be caused by a variety of conditions. The main cause is hypertension which over several years leads to deposits of fat and hyaline in the arterial wall called *lipohyalinosis*. Other possible causes of rupture are congenital deformity of the arterial wall (either arteriovenous malformation or aneurysm), vasculitis or tumour.

In addition to the local destruction of brain tissue, the haemorrhage may, if sufficiently large, create diffuse cerebral damage by increasing the intracranial pressure.

Subarachnoid haemorrhage

The subarachnoid space in between the thin layers of the arachnoid and the pia mater surrounding the brain is filled with cerebrospinal fluid (CSF). Arteries, veins and nerves run through it. Arteries can sometimes develop local dilatations (outpouchings) called *aneurysms*. They typically occur where the walls are less sturdy, close to branching of arteries, and with the aneurysm's growth, the walls become even thinner. Eventually, the aneurysm's wall can rupture, and blood pours into the subarachnoid space. This is in itself a life-threatening situation, but further complications, such as ischaemic infarction (see above), cerebral oedema and *hydrocephalus*, may follow. Normally, CSF is produced inside the ventricles of the brain at the same rate as it is transported into the subarachnoid space, and eventually reabsorbed into the bloodstream. Hydrocephalus occurs when the reabsorption becomes slower than the production, leading to increased CSF pressure.

TRAUMA

Traumatic brain injury

Head injury can be *penetrating* the skull, whereby an object injures the brain directly, or it can be *closed*. In closed head injury, the damage inflicted on the brain is usually due to a combination of mechanisms:

- Focal *contusion* of cells of the brain by it being thrown against the inside of the skull. The brain areas most frequently affected by contusion are the lower parts of the frontal lobes, and the tips of the temporal lobes. In addition to the contusion at the site of impact, the brain is often also injured at the opposite side, called *contre-coup*.
- *Diffuse axonal injury* caused by tearing and shearing forces exerting their effect throughout the whole brain.

- *Haematoma* caused by rupture of blood vessels. This can occur within the brain matter (intracerebral haemorrhage), or between brain surface and skull (subdural haematoma or extradural haematoma).

The injury sets about pathophysiological processes which are probably at least in part similar to those occuring in stroke and lead to neuronal death. They include loss of neuronal functions, disintegration of cellular metabolism, inflammatory response and oedema.

Traumatic brain injury often affects a large cerebral area, and therefore the oedema can be severe and widespread. Because the space for expansion is limited by the skull, the increasing intracranial pressure damages brain cells further. It may also constrict cerebral arteries, causing secondary ischaemic infarctions. In severe cases, the lower parts of the brain can be pushed downward through the foramen magnum, thereby compressing the brainstem, which will lead to the person's death.

Spinal cord injury

Spinal cord injury affects most frequently the cervical region, usually by forced flexion or hyperextension of the neck. The contusion is often accompanied by small haemorrhages, oedema and disintegration of the myelin sheaths surrounding the nerves. The axons die above and below the lesion (Wallerian degeneration). The area of necrosis is called *myelomalacia*. A potential late complication is the formation of a *syrinx*, a space within the spinal cord filled with cerebrospinal fluid. The syrinx can compress cell bodies and axons surrounding it.

INFLAMMATORY DISEASES

Inflammation of the CNS can occur by infection with one of several groups of pathogens: bacteria, viruses, fungi or parasites. The infectious agent can reach it by blood, by local spread from an adjacent structure, or by a penetrating wound. *Meningitis* refers to a condition whereby the meninges covering the central nervous system are inflamed. Inflammation localized in parts of the brain itself is called *encephalitis*, and if the spinal cord is affected, *myelitis*. Bacterial inflammation sometimes forms a local accumulation of pus, called an *abscess* or *empyema*.

The CNS is protected by the blood–brain barrier from pathogens in the blood. However, they can breach it under conditions that are not well understood, but are probably due to certain properties of their surface, or simply due to sheer number of pathogens. Once pathogens have succeeded in invading the CNS, there is little resistance to them entering neurons, astrocytes and oligodendroglia cells, destroying them and using them to replicate and advance. This is because there is only a very rudimentary immune system present in the CNS. The immunological defence against the intruding pathogens is therefore initially weak and takes some time to build up. Complement and immunoglobulin levels are low, but granulocytes and macrophages are present and start with phagocytosis of the pathogens. Breakdown products from brain cells and pathogens provide a chemotactic stimulus for more cells of the immune system (granulocytes, macrophages, T-lymphocytes and B-lymphocytes) to approach and create an inflammatory reaction. The inflammation makes the blood–brain barrier more permeable for the pathogens, but also for the immunological cells, and for complement, which makes the immune response more effective. The B-lymphocytes produce immunoglobulins, and the T-lymphocytes have several functions, including release of enzymes (e.g. perforins) which attack the walls of the pathogens, and of interleukins and interferons which activate macrophages and microglia. They in turn secrete cytokines (interleukins, tumour necrosis factor) which act as pro-inflammatory mediators. Oedema develops in the inflamed area. Unfortunately, the whole of the inflammatory process not only combats the pathogens, but also contributes to the destruction of brain cells.

Meningitis

Meningitis is most frequently caused by viruses or bacteria which colonize the nasal and pharyngeal spaces. When present in sufficient numbers, they can enter the bloodstream and overwhelm the blood–brain barrier.

Viral meningitis is mainly caused by enteroviruses, in particular coxsackie and echovirus. The disease is usually self-limiting.

Bacterial meningitis in the child and adult is most frequently caused by *Streptococcus pneumoniae*, *Neisseria meningitidis* or *Haemophilus influenzae*. The latter used to be responsible for the majority of cases, but has lost some of its influence as a result of vaccination programmes. In neonates and the elderly, *Streptococcus* group B, *Listeria* and Gram-negative bacilli are the main causes.

The most feared complications of meningitis are:

- spreading of the inflammation into the brain, causing encephalitis
- cerebral oedema
- hydrocephalus
- dysfunction of the cerebrovascular system with ischaemic infarction or sinus venous thrombosis.

Encephalitis

Encephalitis is mostly caused by viruses, most frequently herpes simplex. Other common pathogens are varicella zoster, cytomegalovirus and arbovirus. A special feature of the herpes simplex virus is its ability, after an earlier mild infection, to lie dormant within parts of the nervous system, most often in the trigeminal ganglia or the olfactory bulb. In a situation of stress or infection, it can become reactivated and invade the brain, causing encephalitis. The temporal lobes are the parts of the brain most likely to be affected by herpes simplex.

DEMYELINATION

Multiple sclerosis

Multiple sclerosis is an autoimmune disease in which the myelin sheath around neuronal axons is destroyed by the person's own immune system.

The myelin sheath is formed by oligodendrocytes which surround the neuronal axons. Myelin contains a high proportion of lipids in addition to proteins and forms a layer of electrical insulation around the axon, but this layer is interrupted at regular intervals at the nodes of Ranvier where Na^+ and K^+ channels are found. The electrical current in myelinated axons can travel in a saltatory fashion from one node of Ranvier to the next, which makes it much faster than the continuous electrical conduction in unmyelinated fibres.

For reasons that are not yet understood, in multiple sclerosis the person's own immune system directs its defence mechanisms against the myelin sheath around neuronal axons, treating it like foreign antigen and destroying it. The process starts with inflammation: macrophages, microglia, T-lymphocytes and B-lymphocytes cross the blood–brain barrier and accumulate around the small blood vessels. They secrete cytokines (such as interferon) which activate microglia, and they secrete tumour necrosis factor which directly attacks and destroys the myelin. Oligodendrocytes and, in advanced disease, axons also die. The impulse conduction through the affected neurons is slowed down, or even ceases, through short-circuiting or axonal loss. It is likely that, at least in early stages of the disease, the inflammation can self-terminate, and partial remyelination can occur.

A characteristic of multiple sclerosis is the scattered distribution of multiple separate demyelinated areas in the white matter of the brain and/or the spinal cord. This explains the wide variety of neurological deficits observed in this disease. Another characteristic of multiple sclerosis is the course, which in the early stages often runs in *relapses* (deteriorations) followed by *remissions* (improvements) and so on. With advancing disease, it often turns into a chronic progressive course, with slowly worsening symptoms.

As mentioned above, it is not clear what makes the immune system turn against parts of its own host body. Genetic factors and viral infections are being discussed as potentially playing a causative role.

NEURODEGENERATIVE DISEASES

Parkinson's disease

The progressive loss of dopaminergic nigrostriatal neurons is central to Parkinson's disease.

The striatum comprises two parts, the caudate nucleus and the putamen. Together with the globus pallidus, the striatum forms the basal ganglia, a group of large nuclei deep in the cerebral hemispheres. The basal ganglia are strongly

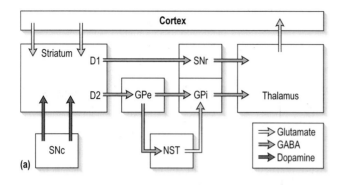

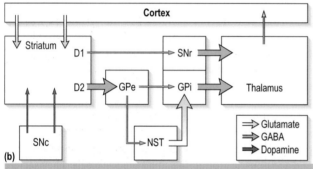

Figure 11.2.2. Neurotransmitter interactions in the healthy person (a) and in Parkinson's disease (b). D1, D1 receptors; D2, D2 receptors; GPe, globus pallidus external segment; GPi, globus pallidus internal segment; NST, nucleus subthalamicus; SNc, substantia nigra pars compacta; SNr, substantia nigra pars reticulata.

connected with the cortex and the thalamus in a system which has been described as cortico-subcortical circuits or loops (Fig. 11.2.2). Some brainstem nuclei, in particular the subthalamic nucleus and the substantia nigra, also have connections with the basal ganglia. This whole system is very likely involved in the initiation and modulation of movement.

Neurons in the substantia nigra, a nucleus in the brainstem, send their axons to the striatum, where they release the neurotransmitter dopamine. In Parkinson's disease, these neurons die, and the dopamine input into the striatum diminishes. Some of the surviving neurons contain inclusions called *Lewy bodies* which are typical but not specific for the disease. The cause of Parkinson's disease is not known, but hereditary as well as environmental factors have been implicated.

Alzheimer's disease

Alzheimer's disease is characterized by progressive death of cortical neurons, accompanied by *senile plaques* and *neurofibrillary tangles* in the cortex.

It is generally a disease of old age, but can also occur in persons under 50. There are two different types: the (significantly

more common) sporadic and the familial one. Although the causes of the sporadic form are not yet understood, this should be helped by studies of the familial forms which have shed light on the pathogenesis of the disease.

In familial Alzheimer's disease, the process probably starts with a genetic disturbance of the metabolism of amyloid which is being formed in excessive quantities from the precursor *amyloid precursor protein* (APP). It is assumed that the amyloid is deposited in different parts of the cortex, leading to the plaques and tangles, and also accumulates in the walls of cerebral blood vessels. The pathological changes and the ensuing cortical atrophy are most pronounced in the temporal and parietal association areas, and in the hippocampus. However, some subcortical nuclei also show the typical pathology, in particular the nucleus basalis of Meynert in the basal forebrain. This sends cholinergic efferent projections diffusely into the neocortex and the hippocampus, where, as a consequence, acetylcholine levels are reduced in Alzheimer's disease. To a lesser extent, two brainstem nuclei, the locus coeruleus and the nucleus raphe, are also affected. They send diffuse projections to the neocortex containing noradrenaline and serotonin, respectively, and consequently, the cortical levels of these neurotransmitters are also reduced. The predominance of pathology in the hippocampus and temporoparietal cortex, which play a major role in memory processes, explains the amnestic symptoms which are the cardinal clinical feature in Alzheimer's disease.

TUMOUR

Tumour growth starts with genetic alterations or mutations within cells, whereby parts of the DNA are rearranged or deleted. These changes can be hereditary or occur at random, and they can also be caused by external influences such as radiation or chemicals. Tumour growth is characterized by uncontrolled replication of cells (*proliferation*), unhindered by the normal inhibitory influences of the surrounding tissue. So far, three classes of genes have been identified as playing a role in the development of tumours:

- *Oncogenes*: when transformed from a deactivated to an activated state, they stimulate cell division.
- *Tumour suppressor genes*: their normal role is to suppress cell division. When such a gene is rendered inactive by mutation, uncontrolled proliferation of cells will occur.
- *Mismatch repair genes*: they usually control the maintenance of the genome and the repair of mutations that have occurred. If these genes are themselves damaged, mutations will not be corrected.

Tumours of the central nervous system can be classified according to different criteria. Table 11.2.1 shows the classification according to the WHO. Primary tumours develop from cells inside the CNS itself, whereas secondary tumours

Table 11.2.1.   World Health Organization (WHO) classification of CNS tumours

1. **Tumours of neuroepithelial tissue**
   Astrocytic tumours
   Oligodendroglial tumours
   Ependymal tumours
   Mixed gliomas
   Choroid plexus tumours
   Neuroepithelial tumours
   Neuronal and mixed neuronal-glial tumours
   Pineal parenchymal tumours
   Embryonal tumours

2. **Tumours of cranial and spinal nerves**
   Schwannoma (neurinoma)
   Neurofibroma
   Malignant peripheral nerve sheath tumour

3. **Tumours of the meninges**
   Tumours of meningothelial cells
   Mesenchymal, non-meningothelial
      Benign neoplasms
      Malignant neoplasms
   Primary melanocytic lesions
   Tumours of uncertain histogenesis

4. **Lymphoma and haemopoietic tumours**
   Malignant lymphoma
   Plasmocytoma
   Granulocytic sarcoma
   Other

5. **Germ cell tumours**
   Germinoma
   Embryonal carcinoma
   Yolk sac tumour
   Choriocarcinoma
   Teratoma
   Mixed germ cell tumour

6. **Cysts and tumour-like lesions**

7. **Tumours of the sellar region**
   Pituitary adenoma
   Pituitary carcinoma
   Craniopharyngioma

8. **Local extensions of regional tumours**
   Paraganglioma
   Chordoma
   Chondroma/chondrosarcoma
   Carcinoma

9. **Metastatic tumours**

10. **Unclassified tumour**

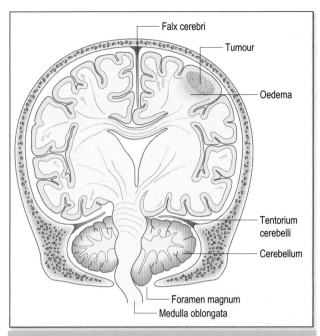

Figure 11.2.3.   Intracerebral tumour. (Reproduced with permission from FitzGerald and Folan-Curran, 2001.)

are metastases from tumours somewhere else in the body. Tumours can be further divided according to the cells from which they arise, such as neurons, astrocytes, meninges or choroid plexus. Tumour *grading* refers to histological examination of the differentiation of the tumour cells. Tumours containing less differentiated (*anaplastic*) cells are more malignant than those with highly differentiated cells. Grade 1 indicates the lowest malignancy, whereas the most malignant tumours are classified as grade 4. Over time, some types of tumours usually undergo malignant transformation (e.g. astrocytomas), whereas others do so only rarely (e.g. meningiomas). Tumour *staging* is not the same as grading. It is based not on characteristics of cells, but on the whole tumour, its size, extent of invasion of other tissues and metastatic spreading.

It is important to realize that the terms 'benign' and 'malignant' refer to a tumour's histological and growth characteristics. This does not mean that a benign intracranial tumour could not be life-threatening. Just like a highly malignant tumour, it can increase the pressure inside the skull (Fig. 11.2.3), causing death by compression of the brain stem.

The largest group of intracranial tumours are metastases, most frequently from carcinoma of the lung or the breast. The most common primary intracranial CNS tumours are gliomas, meningiomas, acoustic neuromas and pituitary tumours.

EPILEPSY

In the living brain, there is a constant flow of information which is maintained by neuronal axons and dendrites transporting electrical impulses, and by neurotransmitters carrying the information across synapses to neighbouring neurons. Normally, these processes occur in an orderly manner, which is astonishing, considering the immense number of neurons (100 billion) in the CNS. During an epileptic seizure, this order is disrupted. A number of neurons start firing spontaneously in a synchronous fashion, and these discharges spread throughout neighbouring parts of the brain, sometimes even the whole brain.

Based on the empirical evidence available today, initiation of seizures probably occurs in groups of neurons (pacemakers) with certain properties, in particular CA3 pyramidal neurons in the hippocampus, and neurons in cortical layers IV and V. These neurons can undergo *paroxysmal depolarization shift* (PDS), a spontaneous change in the electrical potential of their cell membranes, enabling the occurrence of high-frequency burst firing of these neurons. These bursts are followed by hyperpolarization of the membrane. If a sufficient number of neurons fire synchronously in this pattern, the electroencephalogram (EEG) recordings from the surface of the scalp show typical *spike–wave complexes*. Once a critical mass of neurons is exceeded and a large number of bursts follow one another, an epileptic seizure will result. For propagation of burst discharges onto such large numbers of neurons to occur, a lack of the inhibitory neurotransmitter γ-aminobutyric acid (GABA) must be assumed.

Which mechanism actually triggers the start of the initial PDS and the burst firing is still unclear. Findings from cell cultures and animal experiments suggest that a process called *kindling* may play a role, whereby repeated subthreshold stimulation adds up to elicit the processes described above.

SPASTICITY

Spasticity can occur after damage to upper motor neurons. It is therefore considered to be part of a more complex motor disorder, the *upper motor neuron syndrome*, which comprises minus symptoms and plus symptoms (the spasticity):

Upper motor neuron syndrome

Minus symptoms:
- Muscle weakness (paresis or plegia)
- Loss of dexterity
- Mass synergy patterns of movement

Plus symptoms (spasticity):
- Increased muscle tone
- Enhanced tendon reflexes
- Clonus
- Spasms

Minus symptoms

Muscle weakness is called paresis when it is partial, and plegia when a muscle or muscle group cannot be activated at all. The ability to selectively activate certain muscles or muscle groups is reduced, and co-contraction of synergistic and antagonistic muscles occurs. This contributes to mass synergy patterns of movement, and to loss of dexterity, making movements appear clumsy.

Plus symptoms

Characteristic for the increased muscle tone is that it is velocity-dependent. If the spastic muscle is being stretched quickly, it reacts by contracting. However, when stretching the muscle slowly, the spasticity is more easily overcome. This aspect of spasticity is considered to be due to an exaggeration of *tonic stretch reflexes*. Similarly, hyperexcitability of the *phasic stretch reflex* causes increased tendon reflexes, and clonus (rhythmic muscle contractions following stretching of the muscle). Spasms are involuntary muscle contractions which typically start rapidly and subside only slowly. They sometimes occur as a reaction to a subtle stimulus such as light touch, but sometimes without any recognizable cause.

The pathophysiological mechanisms underlying spasticity are poorly understood, but they probably fall into two different categories:

- Changes in interactions between neurons: In the normal state, spinal stretch reflexes (which can be monosynaptic or polysynaptic) are controlled by sensory feedback from the muscle spindles which sense the extent of muscle stretch, and by descending tracts from the brain (Fig. 11.2.4). There are several separate descending tracts, but in the context of spasticity the most important ones are the

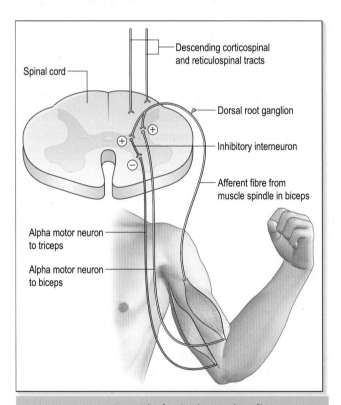

Figure 11.2.4.   Control of spinal stretch reflexes.

corticospinal tract (pyramidal tract), and dorsal and medial reticulospinal tracts which originate in the reticular formation in the brainstem. The dorsal reticulospinal tract has mainly an inhibitory, the medial reticulospinal tract mainly a facilitating effect on spinal reflexes. The corticospinal tract has both facilitating and inhibitory effects. Following a lesion of these tracts, spasticity is caused by loss of inhibition of monosynaptic reflexes, and loss of facilitation of polysynaptic reflexes.

- Changes within the muscle: if a muscle remains in a contracted state (such as in spasticity), its elasticity can slowly diminish both by the formation of links between the actin and myosin, and by fibrosis and atrophy. Over time, irreversible contractures develop.

Case

A 67-year-old man had a left-sided weakness of sudden onset. On arrival at A&E, he was noted to have a dense left hemiparesis with flaccid muscle tone, and reduced sensation of the whole left half of his body. Brain CT scan showed a right-sided ischaemic infarction in the territory of the middle cerebral artery, mainly affecting the right internal capsule. Over the following weeks, his left arm remained plegic, but he slowly regained active movement in his left leg, eventually enabling him to stand, then walk a few steps with the help of physiotherapists. He finally learned to walk independently with a stick. However, the muscle tone in his left arm and leg had steadily increased, so that the spasticity in the arm was in a flexor pattern, and in the leg in an extensor pattern. The severity of the spasticity in his leg could be controlled with physiotherapy, but his left hand was clenched into a tight fist, making hygiene of the palm difficult. He received botulinum toxin injections into the left wrist and finger flexors, followed by intensive stretching exercises and splinting, which resulted in a lasting improvement of the hand posture.

REFERENCES AND FURTHER READING

Barnett H (ed.) (1998) Stroke: Pathophysiology, Diagnosis and Management. Edinburgh: Churchill Livingstone.

Barnes MP, Johnson GR (eds) (2001) Upper Motor Neurone Syndrome and Spasticity: Clinical Management and Neurophysiology. Cambridge: Cambridge University Press.

Donaghy M (ed.) (2001) Brain's Diseases of the Nervous System. Oxford: Oxford University Press.

Fawcett JW, Rosser AE, Dunnett SB (2002) Brain Damage, Brain Repair. Oxford: Oxford University Press.

FitzGerald MJT, Folan-Curran J (2001) Clinical Neuroanatomy and Related Neuroscience. Philadelphia: Saunders.

Underwood JCE (2000) General and Systematic Pathology. Edinburgh: Churchill Livingstone.

The Nervous System: The Peripheral Nervous System

Delva Shamley

DEMYELINATING POLYNEUROPATHIES

Polyneuropathies are disorders of a non-inflammatory nature affecting peripheral nerves. These may be acute or chronic in nature.

Acute inflammatory demyelinating polyneuropathy (AIDP)

Guillain–Barré syndrome

Guillain–Barré syndrome (GBS) is an autoimmune mediated disease of roots and peripheral nerves affecting 1:100 000 people. Most frequently GBS occurs within hours or weeks following a respiratory or gastrointestinal infection. The first symptoms are weakness and tingling in the legs which escalates in the next 2–3 weeks to the point of absent reflexes and ultimately respiratory muscle paralyses (Table 11.3.1). During the course of the disease the myelin sheath, and in some cases the axons, are damaged and destroyed. The subtypes of GBS are shown in Figure 11.3.1.

In the *acute inflammatory demyelinating pattern (AIDP)*, the disease process is characterized by the presence of inflammatory and demyelinating infiltrates into the roots and spinal nerves. The target of these cells appears to be the myelin sheath not the Schwann cell itself (see section on 'Secondary axonal atrophy or axonal loss' for details) but still resulting in the destruction of myelin and altered nerve conduction.

The *acute motor axonal pattern (AMAN)* is characterized by axonal degeneration with pathological changes including: Wallerian degeneration of peripheral nerves, no inflammation, minimal lymphatic response, absent demyelination and macrophages in the periaxonal space (between the axolemma and Schwann cell). Studies have shown complement activation on the nodal axolemma of large motor fibres and IgG and complement binding (see Ch. 2 for details of this process) on internodal axolemma, suggesting an antibody-mediated attack on an axonal epitope (site on the axon that allows binding with a specific antibody). The nodes of Ranvier tend to be the commonest target for this antibody-mediated immune attack. The immune response includes macrophage processes entering the paranodal space (adjacent to nodes of Ranvier) and facilitating the entry of additional macrophages. As macrophages can express major histocompatibility complex (MHC) antigens and costimulatory B7 molecules it is possible that local endoneurial macrophages act as antigen-presenting cells, thereby playing a key role in triggering the autoimmune process (see Ch. 2 for further details). Autoantibodies may guide the macrophages to their myelin or primarily axonal targets, which then attack in a complement-dependent and receptor-mediated manner. The axon is detached from the Schwann cell plasmalemma, eventually causing demyelination and Wallerian degeneration of the

Table 11.3.1.   Clinical features of GBS

- Progressive symmetrical weakness of the limbs
- Paraesthesia in hands and feet
- Back pain in 30% of cases
- Depressed or absent reflexes
- Cranial nerves affected in 50% of cases
- Progression to peak disability in 4 weeks

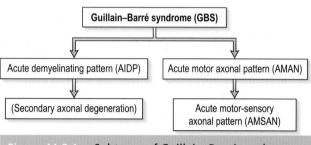

Figure 11.3.1.   Subtypes of Guillain–Barré syndrome.

axon. The similarity between the pathological processes in AMAN and acute motor-sensory axonal pattern (AMSAN) has led to the belief that AMSAN is a more severe manifestation of AMAN.

> *Treatment of AIDP*
>
> - Plasma exchange and intravenous immunoglobulin (IVIG) are used to treat severe AIDP. IVIG exerts a therapeutic effect by complement activation, neutralization of self-antibodies, cytokine inhibition and saturation of Fc receptors on endoneurial macrophages.
> - The use of corticosteroids for GBS is still not proven.

Chronic inflammatory demyelinating polyneuropathy (CIDP)

Chronic inflammatory demyelinating polyneuropathy (CIDP) involves inflammation of the nerve roots, peripheral nerves and spinal ganglia. It is characterized by slowly progressive weakness and sensory dysfunction of the legs and arms and is caused by damage to the myelin sheath. CIDP shares many features with Guillain–Barré syndrome (GBS) and is often considered the chronic version of GBS.

In CIDP several subtypes are emerging in terms of the clinical features (Table 11.3.2), disease course and response to treatment. Patients with CIDP generally demonstrate both proximal and distal weakness. However, some may have mainly

Table 11.3.2.   Clinical features of chronic inflammatory demyelinating polyneuropathy

- Tingling or numbness (beginning in toes and fingers)
- Weakness of arms and legs
- Aching pain in muscles
- Loss of deep tendon reflexes (areflexia)
- Fatigue

distal and others mainly proximal weakness. Classification of these subtypes has not yet emerged and will be dependent on the full knowledge of the pathophysiological mechanisms in each type.

The following evidence seems to support an autoimmune disease mechanism:

- Antimyelin protein antibodies have been implicated in the disease production in some CIDP cases. For example, antibodies to the myelin protein P0 have been shown to cause conduction block and demyelination.
- Schwann cells are able to act as antigen-presenting cells and T-cell responses can be initiated within a nerve. This means that peripheral nerves may similarly be exposed to self-antigen, setting off the T-cell co-stimulatory reaction and a full-blown immune reaction against components of the nerve cell and sheath.
- Transcription factor *nuclear factor κB*, involved in gene regulation of the immune response, is upregulated in CIDP patients.

Diagnostic studies

- *Activity-dependent hyperpolarization* has been shown in patients with CIDP. This hyperpolarization of motor axons is associated with voluntary activity and has been shown to be paralleled by activity-dependent conduction block. This response is similar to the central demyelinating disorder multiple sclerosis.
- *MRI scans* show hypertrophy of nerves.

Secondary axonal atrophy or axonal loss

Secondary axonal atrophy is described in a number of forms of hereditary and acquired demyelinating neuropathies including Guillain–Barré syndrome, hereditary demyelinating neuropathy and chronic inflammatory demyelinating polyneuropathy (CIDP). Patients with demyelinating neuropathies have distally enhanced sensory and motor deficits with the lower limbs being affected earlier and more severely. Electrophysiological nerve examinations show abnormal spontaneous activity and polyphasic motor unit action

potentials occurring after nerve conduction block, indicating that axonal disease is secondary. The deleterious effects of abnormal Schwann cells have been shown in both animal and human studies. These effects include:

- decreased axonal diameter
- increased density of neurofilaments
- decreased neurofilament phosphorylation.

One possible mechanism for the observed Schwann cell–axon interactions may be through the *myelin-associated glycoprotein (MAG)*. MAG is found at the Schwann cell–axon interface of myelinated nerve fibres. A growing body of evidence suggests that MAG is involved in the control of neurofilament spacing through sidearm phosphorylation. Anti-MAG antibodies or the absence of MAG may lead to the observed clinical and experimental findings in demyelinating neuropathies. Axonal atrophy or loss may therefore be secondary to diseased Schwann cells or myelin sheaths.

AXONAL DEGENERATION

Understanding the nature of neuronal cell death has been the focus of enquiries into neurodegenerative disorders. However, the pathology of many neurological disorders includes the degeneration of the nerve process or axon. Several types of axonal degeneration have been identified.

Wallerian degeneration

Wallerian degeneration is the degeneration of a nerve fibre (axon) that has been severed from its nerve cell body (Fig. 11.3.2). Morphological features of Wallerian degeneration include:

- disintegrating endoplasmic reticulum
- degrading neurofilaments
- swollen mitochondria
- granular disintegration and beading of an axon distal to a site of injury with fragments being phagocytosed.

These effects are seen in many neurodegenerative disorders and can be triggered by neurotoxins and by defects in myelin, axonal transport or oxygen delivery. Wallerian degeneration can be seen in the peripheral and the central nervous systems.

'Dying back'

In this case the axon of an unhealthy neuron degenerates over weeks or months, starting distally and spreading towards the cell body (Fig. 11.3.2b). This occurs more commonly in peripheral nerve disorders (caused by toxic, metabolic and infectious conditions, e.g. polyneuropathies of diabetes, alcoholism and AIDS) but also in some CNS neurodegenerative diseases (motor neuron disease, Parkinson's and Alzheimer's disease). There is some evidence to suggest that the absence of nerve growth factor may play a role in this localized degeneration of an axon (Fig. 11.3.2c).

Neither Wallerian degeneration nor 'dying back' occurs as a result of the mechanism of apoptosis (programmed death). Both processes are, however, active and current evidence suggests that the *ubiquitin–proteasome pathway* may play a role in the active process of Wallerian axonal degeneration. Less is known about the mechanism behind axonal loss due to 'dying back'.

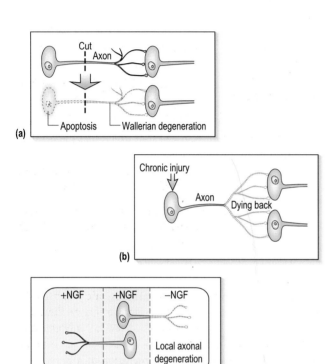

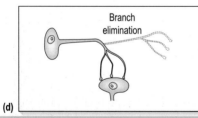

Figure 11.3.2.   The various types of axonal degeneration. (a) When an axon is cut, the isolated distal segment rapidly undergoes Wallerian degeneration. When the axon of a developing neuron is cut, the cell body frequently undergoes apoptosis. (b) In dying-back axonal degeneration, the axonal tree of an unhealthy neuron degenerates, beginning distally and progressing proximally. (c) When the distal part of an axon of a sympathetic neuron is locally deprived of nerve growth factor (NGF) in a three-chamber culture dish, the deprived axon segment degenerates, whereas the rest of the axon and the cell survive. (d) During normal development, inappropriate axonal branches are frequently eliminated: in some cases, at least, this seems to occur by branch degeneration.

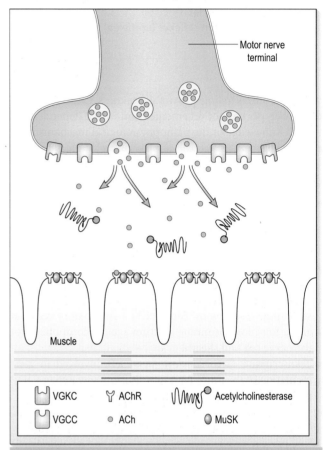

Figure 11.3.3.   Neuromuscular transmission. Neuromuscular transmission depends on the entry of calcium, through voltage-gated calcium channels (VGCCs), into the motor nerve terminal, which leads to the rapid release of 'packets' (or quanta) of acetylcholine (ACh). Acetylcholine binds to postsynaptic ACh receptors (AChRs) and opens the associated ion channels (Fig. 11.3.4). This results in a depolarization that, if sufficient, activates voltage-gated sodium channels (not shown), leading to an action potential in the muscle and muscle contraction. Acetylcholine is destroyed immediately by acetylcholinesterase, and repolarization of the motor nerve terminal results from opening of the voltage-gated potassium channels (VGKCs). It is now clear that AChRs, VGCCs and VGKCs are targets in antibody-mediated neurological diseases. In addition, the muscle-specific receptor tyrosine kinase MuSK has been shown recently to be a target for antibodies in some patients who have myasthenia gravis (MG) without AChR-specific antibodies. In MG (and Lambert–Eaton myasthenic syndrome), some symptomatic improvement can be obtained by inhibition of acetylcholinesterase, thereby prolonging the action of ACh. (Reproduced with permission from Vincent, 2002.)

MONONEUROPATHIES

Compression injuries

Compression of a nerve can occur through trauma or entrapment of a nerve (e.g. carpal tunnel syndrome, compartment syndrome). This may cause anaesthesia or pain if a sensory nerve and loss of function if a motor nerve. The main effect of compression is the loss of blood supply to the nerve and the subsequent loss of oxygen which affects neural transmission. Chronic nerve compression has been shown to be accompanied by progressive demyelination with associated slowing of nerve conduction.

DISORDERS OF THE NEUROMUSCULAR JUNCTION

Myasthenia gravis

Myasthenia gravis (MG) is an autoimmune disorder of the neuromuscular junction. It is associated with the loss of acetylcholine (ACh) receptors which initiate muscle contraction leading to loss of striated muscle function. The disease usually appears between the ages of 15 and 50 years with females being more commonly affected than males. The primary symptom is abnormal fatigue of muscles. Initial movement may be strong but rapidly weakens with symptoms intensifying at the end of a day or following vigorous exercise.

During neuromuscular transmission small 'packets' of ACh are released from the nerve terminal and interact with the postsynaptic membrane (Fig. 11.3.3). This causes miniature endplate potentials and muscle contraction is initiated. In MG patients the size of these endplate potentials is markedly reduced. Either there is a loss of ACh in MG or something is preventing the binding of ACh to the muscle membrane.

Five human ACh receptors (AChR) have been identified and cloned, including the different isoforms for adult and fetal receptors.

MG can be divided into three different forms based on the age of onset, thymic pathology, MHC associations and whether or not there are antibodies specific for non-AChR antigens (Table 11.3.3).

Humoral immunity

The autoantibody associated with MG is produced by B-lymphocytes, defectively controlled by T-lymphocytes because of a thymic disorder (see below). These AChR-specific antibodies produced by B-cells are polyclonal IgG, which react with different binding sites on the surface of AChRs (Fig. 11.3.4). Once bound to the receptor these IgG antibodies can:

- activate the complement system (detailed in Ch. 2) causing lysis of the muscle membrane or
- antibodies specific for the main immunogenic region of the receptor increase the degradation rate of the receptor.

The effect of both these autoimmune reactions is to reduce the number of receptors available to respond to released ACh at the neuromuscular junction.

The role of the thymus

Most affected patients have at least one thymic abnormality, most commonly germinal centres indicating an immune reaction and B-cell cloning. Current evidence indicates that the thymus of MG patients is able to launch an immune response against AChR for the following reasons:

- cultures of thymic cells can produce AChR specific antibodies
- T-cell lines specific for AChRs can be cloned from the thymus

Table 11.3.3. Subgroups of MG patients with AChR-specific antibodies[a]

Subtype of MG	Age at onset	Sex M:F	Typical thymic pathology	MHC association	Associated autoantibodies
Early onset	<41 years	1:3	Hyperplastic	B8, DR3	Might have other tissue-specific antibodies (such as thyroid specific)
Thymoma-associated	Mainly 40–60 years	1:1	Epithelial tumour containing many lymphocytes	No clear association	Antibodies specific for titin and ryanodine receptor are very common. Also, anti-cytokine antibodies
Late onset	>40 years	1.5:1	Normal or atrophied	B7, DR2 in males	Antibodies specific for titin and ryanodine receptor, particularly after 60 years

[a] These subdivisions relate particularly to Caucasians who have generalized myasthenia gravis (MG) and are positive for acetylcholine receptor (AChR)-specific antibodies. These subgroups are not appropriate in patients who have purely ocular MG or who lack AChR-specific antibodies, or possibly in other ethnic populations. F, female; M, male.
Reproduced with permission from Vincent (2002).

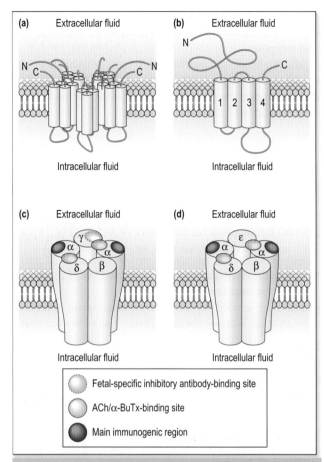

Figure 11.3.4. Fetal and adult forms of the acetylcholine receptor. (a) The acetylcholine receptor (AChR) is a pentameric membrane protein. (b) Each of the subunits consists of an extracellular domain, four transmembrane regions and a cytoplasmic domain. The receptor consists of $(\alpha)_2$, β, γ and δ subunits in the fetal form (c), and $(\alpha)_2$, β, δ and ε subunits in the adult form (d). A large proportion of the antibodies in the sera of myasthenia gravis patients bind to the main immunogenic regions that are on both of the α subunits, to which the sequence $\alpha 64$–76 makes an important contribution. In addition, many patients' antibodies bind to the fetal-specific γ subunit. In some cases, these antibodies inhibit the function of the AChR in vitro, and in pregnant mothers, they can cross the placenta, causing fetal muscle paralysis and severe, and often fatal, deformities. α-BuTx, α-bungarotoxin. (Reproduced with permission from Vincent, 2002.)

Figure legend key:
- Fetal-specific inhibitory antibody-binding site
- ACh/α-BuTx-binding site
- Main immunogenic region

- the level of AChR antibodies drops on removal of the thymus
- thymic myoid cells express AChR on their membranes
- thymic epithelial cells can express AChRs.

In many patients this may be the source of the circulating AChR antibodies which affect the neuromuscular junction (NMJ) throughout the body.

Approximately 10% of patients with MG present with a thymoma, which may precede the onset of MG. The pathology of MG associated with thymoma differs in that the patients also have other autoantibodies which affect intracellular activities in muscle as opposed to NMJ activities. Thymoma MG patients do not necessarily respond to thymectomy and often need additional immunosuppressive therapy.

Maternal transfer of antibodies

Maternal AChR antibodies can cross the placental barrier and affect neuromuscular transmission in the baby. The maternal serum antibodies are biased towards recognizing the fetal form of the AChR, thereby blocking neuromuscular transmission in utero and effectively paralysing the developing fetus.

REFERENCES AND FURTHER READING

Demyelinating polyneuropathy
Chowdhury D, Arora A (2001) Axonal Guillain–Barré syndrome: a critical review. Acta Neurol Scand 103: 267–277.
Griffin JW, Li CY, Macko C, et al. (1996) Early nodal changes in the acute motor axonal neuropathy pattern of the Guillain–Barré syndrome. J Neurocytol 25: 33–51.
Griffin JW, Li CY, Ho TW (1996) Pathology of the motor sensory axonal Guillain–Barré syndrome. Ann Neurol 39: 17–28.
Gorson KC, Allam G, Ropper AH (1997) Chronic inflammatory demyelinating polyneuropathy: clinical features and response to treatment in 67 consecutive patients with and without a monoclonal gammopathy. Neurology 48: 321–328.
Hanemann CO, Gabreel-Festen AAWM (2002) Secondary axon atrophy and neurological dysfunction in demyelinating neuropathies. Curr Opin Neurol 15: 611–615.
Misawa S, Kuwabara S, Mori M, et al. (2001) Serum levels of tumour necrosis factor alpha in chronic inflammatory demyelinating polyneuropathy. Neurology 56: 666–669.
Pollard JD (2002) Chronic inflammatory demyelinating polyradiculoneuropathy. Curr Opin Neurol 15: 279–283.

Wallerian degeneration
Coleman MP, Perry VH (2002) Axon pathology in neurological disease: a neglected therapeutic target. Trends Neurosci 25(10): 532–537.
Hirata K, Kawabuchi M (2002) Myelin phagocytosis by macrophages and nonmacrophages during Wallerian degeneration. Microsc Res Tech 57(6): 541–547.
Jander S, Lausberg F, Stoll G (2001) Differential recruitment of CD8+ macrophages during Wallerian degeneration in the peripheral and central nervous system. Brain Pathol 11(1): 27–38.
Raff MC, Whitmore AV, Finn JT (2002) Axonal self destruction and neurodegeneration. Science 296: 868–871.

Myasthenia gravis
Kornstein MJ, Asher O, Fuchs S (1995) Acetylcholine receptor α-subunit and myogenin mRNAs in thymus and thymomas. Am J Pathol 146: 1320–1324.
Vincent A, Palace J, Hilton-Jones D (2001) Myasthenia gravis. Lancet 357: 2122–2128.
Vincent A (2002) Unravelling the pathogenesis of myasthenia gravis. Nature Rev 2: 797–804.

The Nervous System: Nervous System Reorganization Following Injury

R. Chen, L.G. Cohen and M. Hallett

It is a common clinical observation that functional recovery frequently occurs following a nervous system injury such as stroke, although the extent of recovery is highly variable. Some patients with initial severe hemiparesis may eventually achieve full recovery, while others have little or no improvement and remain severely disabled. There are many reasons for the different degrees of recovery, including age of the patient, location and extent of the lesion as well as individual variations in anatomical and functional connections. An understanding of the mechanisms underlying functional recovery is crucial to develop treatment programmes to improve functional outcome.

There is now considerable evidence that cortical representation of body parts is continuously modulated in response to activity, behaviour and skill acquisition. Reorganization of cortical representation also occurs following a peripheral injury such as amputation or a brain injury such as stroke. These changes in plasticity may account for recovery of function after injury. While it is likely that some of the reorganization following injury takes place in the cortex, plastic changes may also occur in subcortical structures such as the thalamus, brainstem or spinal cord.

REORGANIZATION FOLLOWING PERIPHERAL INJURY

Transient deafferentation

Transient deafferentation can induce rapid reorganization of the adult central nervous system (CNS) and is a useful model to study short-term plasticity changes.

Deafferentation of human limbs is induced by regional anaesthesia or ischaemic nerve block with inflation of a blood pressure cuff above systolic blood pressure. Within minutes after the onset of deafferentation, the motor-evoked potential (MEP) amplitude elicited by transcranial magnetic stimulation (TMS) in the muscle immediately proximal to deafferentation increases several fold, then returns to control values within 20 minutes after termination of ischaemia. This suggests that motor cortex excitability was increased during deafferentation (Fig. 11.4.1). The number of scalp positions that focal TMS could elicit responses to in the muscle immediately proximal to ischaemic block is also increased, which may be due to expansion of muscle representation or increased excitability of the motor system. Studies in humans with magnetoencephalography (MEG) also showed that rapid changes in somatosensory representation occur with deafferentation. Somatosensory-evoked fields produced by finger stimulation can be altered by transient ischaemic deafferentation of the adjacent fingers. The representation of the stimulated finger shifts toward the representation of the deafferented fingers.

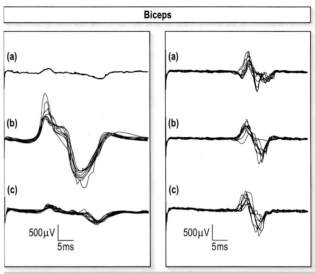

Biceps

Figure 11.4.1.   Effects of transient deafferentation of the forearm in one subject. Deafferentation was induced by a tourniquet placed below the left elbow in combination with regional nerve block of the forearm and hand with administration of lidocaine (lignocaine). Ten superimposed MEPs from TMS before anaesthesia (a), during anaesthetic block (b) and after anaesthesia (c) recorded from the left biceps and right (contralateral) abductor pollicis brevis (APB) muscles are shown on the left. MEP amplitudes from the left biceps and right APB muscles as a function of time course of the experiment are shown on the right. The biceps MEP amplitudes increased during anaesthesia and returned to baseline level within 20 minutes after termination of anaesthetic block. The contralateral APB MEP amplitudes were unchanged throughout the experiment. (Modified from Brasil-Neto et al., 1992.)

Amputation and peripheral nerve lesions

Animal studies

Plasticity of the somatosensory system has been studied extensively, and dramatic changes in the organization map of the SI occur after removal of afferent input. These changes can be reversed after nerve regeneration. Although initial studies suggested that the upper limit of cortical expansion is 1–2 mm, corresponding to the projection zone of single thalamocortical axons, it is now known that long-standing amputation may result in cortical reorganization over a distance of up to 14 mm. In the motor system, changes in cortical representation also occur after peripheral injury. Following amputation or peripheral nerve lesions, the area from which stimulation evokes movements of the adjacent body parts is enlarged and the threshold for eliciting these movements is reduced. These changes begin within hours after the motor nerve lesion.

Human studies

In humans, reorganization of the somatosensory and motor systems also occurs following amputation (Fig. 11.4.2).

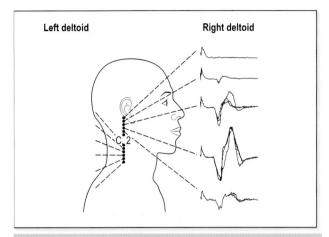

Figure 11.4.2.   Schematic diagram of the head of a right above-elbow amputee. Electromyogram responses from the deltoid muscles evoked by TMS with a focal figure-of-eight coil at equal stimulus intensities from different scalp positions 1 cm apart along the coronal axis are shown. Stimulation at four positions evoked responses from the deltoid muscle on the amputated side, whereas stimulation at only one position evoked responses from the deltoid muscle on the intact side. (Modified from Cohen et al., 1991a.)

Sensations in the phantom limb can be elicited by somatosensory stimulation of the face and upper body in upper-limb amputees, suggesting that the somatosensory representations of the face and upper body may have expanded to occupy the arm and hand area. The extent of shift in cortical representation correlates with the amount of phantom. Results suggest that the excitability of the motor system projecting to the muscle immediately above the amputation is increased.

Cortical reorganization also occurs in humans after peripheral nerve lesions. In patients with facial palsy, TMS and positron emission tomography (PET) studies reveal an enlargement of the hand representation with medial extension into the site of the presumed face area.

Site of reorganization following peripheral lesions

Changes in cortical maps following a peripheral lesion may be the result of reorganization at cortical or subcortical levels. There is evidence that reorganization can occur at multiple levels including the cortex, thalamus, brainstem, spinal cord and peripheral nerves. After chronic partial digit amputation in animals there is both increased branching of the severed digital nerve and increased innervation density in the stump. It has been suggested that the stump may be innervated by neurons that previously had innervated the amputated digit, which may explain the expansion of the cortical map of the stump. Plasticity changes have also been demonstrated in the thalamus, where neuronal recordings show that local

anesthesia induced immediate and reversible reorganization of the ventral posterior medial nucleus. In other situations, reorganization may occur mainly within the cortex. It appears that plasticity changes in the somatosensory system can occur at multiple cortical and subcortical sites, whereas in the visual system reorganization mainly is in the cortex.

REORGANIZATION ASSOCIATED WITH RECOVERY FROM STROKE

Spontaneous recovery usually occurs, although the extent is highly variable. Multivariate analysis suggested that the best predictor of outcome after hemispheric stroke is the severity of initial neurological deficit. Motor recovery occurs predominantly in the initial weeks to first 3 months, but can continue at a slower pace throughout the first year.

Recovery in the first few days may be due to resolution of oedema or reperfusion of the ischaemic penumbra. Much of the recovery after the initial 2 weeks is likely due to brain plasticity, with some areas of the brain taking over the functions previously performed by the damaged regions. Proposed mechanisms of recovery include redundancy of brain circuitry with parallel pathways performing similar functions such that an alternative pathway may take over when another has been damaged, unmasking of previously existing but functionally inactive pathways, and sprouting of fibres from the surviving neurons with formation of new synapses. The mechanisms involved probably depend on the extent of injury. When damage to a functional system is partial, within-system recovery is possible, whereas after complete destruction, substitution by a functionally related system becomes the only alternative.

Factors that determine the severity of deficits and degree of functional recovery

Several studies examined the factors that determine the severity of deficits and the extent of recovery. The influence of lesion size is controversial but the location of the infarct may be more important. Poor motor recovery was associated with more severe damage to the pyramidal tract as measured with magnetic resonance imaging (MRI) or lesion of the parietal lobe. The importance of the pyramidal tract is also demonstrated by several TMS studies. TMS activates pyramidal-tract neurons and the MEP amplitude of hand muscles in response to stimulation of the lesioned cortex correlates with the extent of recovery of hand function.

The role of the affected hemisphere in mediating stroke recovery

Motor recovery following damage to the motor cortex or the pyramidal tract may be mediated by the use of alternative cortical areas in the damaged hemisphere that can access spinal motor neurons. Two general mechanisms are possible here: the use of parallel, redundant pathways or new regions taking over the function of the damaged area. There are several parallel motor pathways in the motor system. In addition to the M1, motor areas have been identified in the premotor cortex, SMA and cingulate cortex. All these motor areas contain somatotopic representations and all contribute to the pyramidal tract. These parallel pathways may substitute for each other in recovery from hemiparesis. Patients with an infarct limited to the anterior or posterior limb of the internal capsule initially had severe motor deficits, but subsequently had excellent recovery. Patients with more extensive lesions of the internal capsule had poor recovery. Further support for the role of alternative motor pathways in functional recovery came from PET studies in patients with good recovery from striatocapsular infarcts. Compared to normal subjects, finger movements of the recovered hand showed greater activation of the anterior aspect of the insular and the inferior parietal cortex, and both areas have direct connections to the premotor cortex (area 6). In some patients, movement of the recovered hand led to increased SMA activation, which may represent a correlate of the reorganization in SMA observed in monkeys with Ml lesions.

There is also evidence for the adjacent cortex taking over the function of the damaged pathways. In patients with lesions limited to the posterior limb of the internal capsule, recovered hand movement led to motor cortex activation that extended laterally to the face area, suggesting that the hand representation shifts toward the face area. This change was not observed in patients with lesions in the anterior limb of the internal capsule. This may be explained by sparing of the pyramidal tract from the face representation in patients with lesions confined to the posterior limb of the internal capsule, since the fibres destined for the face travel to more anterior locations in the internal capsule than fibres for the arm and leg. Thus, the shift of cortical representation following amputation or peripheral nerve lesions may also be present with recovery from stroke.

REORGANIZATION FOLLOWING CENTRAL LESIONS

Spinal cord injury

Several studies showed that spinal cord injury induced reorganization of the sensory and motor systems. In humans, motor reorganization has been demonstrated by TMS in patients with spinal cord injury. In the muscle immediately rostral to the level of injury, MEPs can be elicited from more scalp positions and TMS activated a higher percentage of the motor neuron pool than in normal controls. This again points to increased excitability of the motor system projecting to the

muscle immediately above the level of injury, similar to the findings in amputees. The site of reorganization after spinal cord injury has not been studied in detail. It is possible that cortical mechanisms are important, similar to the reorganization following amputation.

Cerebral palsy

Cerebral palsy refers to non-progressive neurological deficits in children and is usually due to focal brain injury that had occurred in utero or shortly after birth. In patients with congenital hemiplegia, intense mirror movements and relatively good functions of the affected hand, TMS of the unaffected M1 elicited short-latency MEPs from the ipsilateral first dorsal interosseous (FDI) muscle. These patients were considered to have suffered their brain insult before 29 weeks of gestation. In patients with good recovery of the affected hand without mirror movements, stimulation of the affected M1 elicited short-latency MEPs from the affected (contralateral) FDI muscle. Patients with no MEP, from the affected FDI with stimulation of the affected or the unaffected M1 all had poor hand functions. Ipsilateral MEPs with prolonged latencies were found in some patients without mirror movements; these patients had variable degrees of recovery. Thus, it appeared that direct corticospinal projections, as shown by short-latency MEPs, are necessary for good recovery of hand functions and may arise from either the affected or the unaffected hemisphere. Ipsilateral motor pathways from the unaffected hemisphere may play a role in recovery from brain injury occurring early in life. Possible mechanisms include development of new ipsilateral corticospinal projections, double-crossing of contralateral corticospinal fibres and reinforcement of existing ipsilateral corticospinal pathways. Ipsilateral MEPs of prolonged latency may be due to enhanced corticoreticulospinal pathway. The importance of ipsilateral pathways in mediating recovery of function from brain injury early in life was also demonstrated in a functional MRI study in patients with unilateral brain damage in the perinatal period. Finger movements of the affected hand produced widespread activation of the intact, ipsilateral hemisphere.

MECHANISMS OF CORTICAL REORGANIZATION

Mechanisms for short-term changes

The two main mechanisms proposed to explain reorganization after peripheral lesions are unmasking of previous present but functionally inactive connections and growth of new connections (collateral sprouting). Since the growth of new connections takes time, rapid expansion of muscle representation that occurs within minutes to hours following transient deafferentation in humans or nerve lesions in animals probably involves unmasking of latent excitatory synapses.

Unmasking of latent synapses can be due to several mechanisms and include increased excitatory neurotransmitter release, increased density of postsynaptic receptors, changes in membrane conductance that enhance the effects of weak or distant inputs, displacement of presynaptic elements to a more favourable site, decreased inhibitory inputs or removing inhibition from excitatory inputs (unmasking excitation). Among these possibilities, the evidence is strongest for removal of inhibition to excitatory synapses, which is likely due to reduced GABAergic inhibition, in mediating short-term plastic changes.

Role of GABAergic inhibition

Several lines of evidence indicate that modulation of GABAergic inhibition plays a significant role in cortical plasticity. GABA is the most important inhibitory neurotransmitter in the brain. GABAergic neurons constitute 25–30% of the neuronal population in the motor cortex and their horizontal connections can extend up to 6 mm or more. Following application of the GABA antagonist *bicuculline* to the forelimb area of the motor cortex, stimulation of the adjacent vibrissa area led to forelimb movements, suggesting that GABAergic neurons are crucial to the maintenance of cortical motor representations. These changes are similar to the expansion of TMS maps of the involved muscles following transient deafferentation or peripheral nerve lesions. Deafferentation of the somatosensory or visual cortex also led to a reduction in the number of neurons containing GABA or its synthesizing enzyme, glutamic acid decarboxylase.

Mechanisms for long-term changes

Plasticity changes that occur over a longer time probably involve mechanisms in addition to the unmasking of latent synapses. These may include long-term potentiation (LTP), which requires NMDA receptor activation and increased intracellular calcium concentration, and has been demonstrated in the motor cortex. Axonal regeneration and sprouting with alterations in synapse shape, number, size and type may also be involved.

Mechanisms for reorganization in amputees

Both TMS threshold and intracortical inhibition are reduced for the muscle just proximal to the amputation. Therefore, it appears that diminished intracortical inhibition, which may be related to reduced GABAergic inhibition and occurs shortly after deafferentation, persists for prolonged periods after deafferentation. Changes in motor threshold apparently required a longer time to develop, because the motor threshold was unchanged with transient deafferentation. The mechanisms underlying reduction in motor threshold are likely to be separate from those for intracortical inhibition, since the motor threshold is altered by drugs that change membrane excitability, whereas intracortical inhibition is altered by drugs that influence GABAergic mechanisms. Because the excitability of subcortical structures is unchanged, the reduction of motor threshold probably involves enhancement of cortico-cortical connections. Since drugs that block voltage-gated sodium channels raise the motor threshold, one possible mechanism involves changes in sodium channels. Other mechanisms are also possible, including LTP, axonal regeneration and formation of new synapses.

Functional significance of plasticity following injury

The functional role of reorganization following peripheral injury is unclear. It is conceivable that increased cortical representation of the muscle immediately above the amputation may improve motor control of the muscle in an attempt to compensate for partial loss of a limb. Similarly, increased somatosensory representation of the stump may improve sensory perception and discrimination. However, these ideas remain speculative and in most situations, the functional significance of reorganization following peripheral lesions remains to be demonstrated. It appears that plasticity changes can, in some situations, lead to functional improvement, but in other circumstances may have harmful consequences.

There is little doubt that recovery from stroke involves plasticity reorganization of the brain which leads to functional improvement. The challenge is to identify which of the many changes demonstrated are important in mediating recovery. One example is whether activation of the ipsilateral motor cortex with movement of the recovered hand represents involvement of ipsilateral motor pathways in stroke recovery or merely reflects associated movement of the unaffected hand.

ACKNOWLEDGEMENT

This chapter reprinted (in modified form) from Chen et al. (2002), with permission from Elsevier.

REFERENCES AND FURTHER READING

Aizawa H, Inase M, Mushiake H, Shima K, Tanji J (1991) Reorganization of activity in the supplementary motor area associated with motor learning and functional recovery. Exp Brain Res 84: 668–671.

Binkofski F, Seitz RJ, Arnold S, et al. (1996) Thalamic metabolism and corticospinal tract integrity determine motor recovery in stroke. Ann Neurol 39: 460–470.

Brasil-Neto JP, Cohen LG, Pascual-Leone A, et al. (1992) Rapid reversible modulation of human motor outputs after transient deafferentation of the forearm: A study with transcranial magnetic stimulation. Neurology 42: 1302–1306.

Caramia MD, Lani C, Bernardi G (1996) Cerebral plasticity after stroke as revealed by ipsilateral responses to magnetic stimulation. NeuroReport 7: 1756–1760.

Chen R, Corwell B, Hallett M, Cohen LG (1997a) Mechanisms involved in motor reorganization following lower limb amputation. Neurology 48: A345.

Chen R, Samii A, Canos M, Wassermann E, Hallett M (1997b) Effects of phenytoin on cortical excitability in humans. Neurology 49: 881–883.

Chen R, Cohen LG, Hallett M (2002) Nervous system reorganization following injury. Neuroscience 111(4): 761–773.

Cohen LG, Bandinelli S, Findley TW, Hallett M (1991a) Motor reorganization after upper limb amputation in man. Brain 114: 615–627.

Cohen LG, Zeffiro T, Bookheimer S, et al. (1991b) Reorganization in motor pathways following a large congenital hemispheric lesion in man: different motor representation areas for ipsi and contralateral muscles. J Physiol (Lond) 438: 33P.

Cohen LG, Celnik P, Pascual-Leone A, et al. (1997) Functional relevance of cross-modal plasticity in the blind. Nature 389: 180–183.

Corwell BN, Chen R, Hallett M, Cohen LG (1997) Mechanisms underlying plasticity of human motor cortex during transient deafferentation of the forearm. Neurology 48: A345–A346.

Flor H, Elbert T, Knecht S, et al. (1995) Phantom-limb pain as a perceptual correlate of cortical reorganization following arm amputation. Nature 375: 482–484.

Hess G, Donoghue JP (1994) Long-term potentiation of horizontal connections provides a mechanism to reorganize cortical maps. J Neurophysiol 71: 2543–2547.

Kass JH, Florence SL (1997) Mechanisms of reorganization in sensory systems of primates after peripheral nerve injury. In: Freund H-J, Sabel BA, White OW (eds) Brain Plasticity, Advances in Neurology, vol. 73. Philadelphia, PA: Lippincott-Raven, pp. 147–158.

Kalaska J, Pomeranz B (1979) Chronic paw denervation causes an age-dependent appearance of novel responses from forearm in 'paw cortex' of kittens and adult cats. J Neurophysiol 42: 618–633.

Knecht S, Henningsen H, Elbert T, et al. (1996) Reorganization and perceptual changes after amputation. Brain 119: 1213–1219.

Lee RG, van Donkelaar P (1995) Mechanisms underlying functional recovery following stroke. Can J Neurol Sci 22: 257–263.

Manger PR, Woods TM, Jones EG (1996) Plasticity of the somatosensory cortical map in macaque monkeys after chronic partial amputation of a digit. Proc R Soc Lond B263: 933–939.

Nudo RJ, Milliken GW (1996) Reorganization of movement representations in primary motor cortex following focal ischemic infarcts in adult squirrel monkeys. J Neurophysiol 75: 2144–2149.

Pantano P, Formisano R, Ricci M, et al. (1996) Motor recovery after stroke. Morphological and functional brain alterations. Brain 119: 1849–1857.

The Circulatory System: Cardiovascular Disorders

Angela J. Woodiwiss

The term cardiovascular disorders encompasses a myriad of abnormalities ranging from intrinsic cardiac pathologies to those of vascular origin. This chapter discusses disorders with particular reference to those entities that would most commonly be encountered by the rehabilitation practitioner. These cardiovascular disease entities are listed in Table 12.1.1. The pathophysiology of each of these disorders will be described in order to provide the reader with knowledge of the abnormalities associated with each of these disease entities. This knowledge will in turn serve as a basis on which to effectively develop an understanding of the various rehabilitative therapeutic approaches. In addition, a brief overview of the therapeutic approaches in each of these entities is given.

As it is not one of the cardiovascular diseases for which cardiac rehabilitation is currently recommended per se, hypertrophic cardiomyopathy is not included in Table 12.1.1 and is not discussed in Chapter 9.1. However, a mention of hypertrophic cardiomyopathy is pertinent in that this cardiovascular disease is a genetic disorder which has a relatively high frequency among the general population, and is responsible for the majority of sudden deaths in young people. Hence, hypertrophic cardiomyopathy will be briefly discussed at the end of this chapter.

CORONARY HEART DISEASE

Coronary heart (artery) disease is synonymous with ischaemic heart disease as the pathophysiological basis of coronary heart disease is myocardial ischaemia. The term ischaemia refers to oxygen deprivation resulting from reduced perfusion of tissues with blood. Myocardial ischaemia arises when cardiac metabolic demands exceed coronary artery blood supply. This imbalance between oxygen supply and demand is usually related to either an absolute reduction in coronary blood flow or an inability to increase coronary blood flow relative to the needs of the heart. Both of these are most often due to atherosclerotic obstruction of large coronary arteries. More rarely the myocardium can be rendered ischaemic by non-atheromatous coronary artery obstructions such as embolism and coronary

Table 12.1.1.   Cardiovascular disease entities

Coronary heart (artery) disease
    Atherosclerosis
    Angina pectoris
    Myocardial infarction
Heart failure
    Congestive heart failure
    Ischaemic heart failure
    Idiopathic dilated cardiomyopathy
Essential hypertension

artery spasm. The location of atherosclerotic lesions in the coronary circulation and the degree of luminal narrowing that they cause determines whether clinically significant ischaemia occurs. Furthermore, as the adequacy of blood flow is relative to the metabolic demands of the tissue for oxygen, blood flow to the heart may be sufficient at rest, but not during exercise.

Atherosclerosis

Atherosclerosis is the most common form of arteriosclerosis (hardening of the arteries). It contributes toward not only coronary artery disease but also stroke and thereby is responsible for about 80% of all deaths in the United States, Europe and Japan. In atherosclerosis localized plaques or atheromas protrude into the lumen of the artery and thus reduce blood flow. In addition, atheromas serve as sites for thrombus (blood clot) formation which can further occlude the blood supply to an organ.

It is currently believed that atherosclerosis is triggered by damage or an 'insult' to the endothelium. Such insults are produced by hypertension, smoking, high blood cholesterol and diabetes mellitus. Endothelial damage results in the loss of the ability of the endothelial cells to attach to one another and to the underlying connective tissue. Continual exposure of damaged endothelial cells to the shearing stress of blood flow results in cell desquamation (loss of cells). As shearing stresses are highest at branching points of arteries, these are the most common sites of atherosclerosis. As a consequence of cell loss the subendothelial tissue becomes exposed to increased concentrations of plasma constituents (e.g. cholesterol), and a sequence of events including platelet adherence, platelet aggregation, the formation of thrombi (blood clots) and the release of platelet granular components including a potent mitogenic factor occurs. This platelet factor in conjunction with lipoproteins stimulates the migration of smooth muscles from the tunica media to the tunica intima and the subsequent proliferation of smooth muscle cells. These smooth muscle cells then change from a contractile to a synthetic state in which they synthesize and secrete connective tissue proteins. Endothelial cells normally prevent the penetration of circulating blood monocytes and lymphocytes into the media by secreting autocrine regulators. High plasma cholesterol concentrations are known to interfere with this protective function of endothelial cells. In the absence of endothelial protection, lipid-filled macrophages (derived from circulating monocytes in the presence of high circulating cholesterol and triglycerides) and lymphocytes collect within the tunica intima of arteries. This area therefore becomes infiltrated with macrophages and with smooth muscle cells. Thereafter connective tissue from altered smooth muscle cells forms a cap around this area, which is now called a fibrous plaque. As plaques grow they protrude into the lumen of the blood vessel. Once the process of plaque formation is

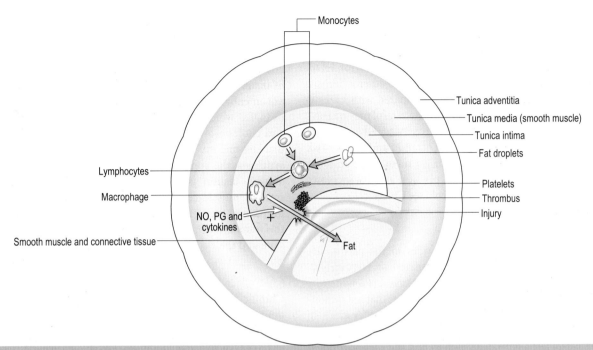

Figure 12.1.1. Diagrammatic representation of the process of atherosclerosis.

triggered (by damage to the endothelium) its progression is maintained by a variety of autocrine regulators including cytokines, nitric oxide (NO) and prostaglandins (PG). Some of these regulators continue to attract monocytes (which become macrophages when they engulf elevated plasma lipids) and lymphocytes to the damaged endothelium. This process of atherosclerosis is summarized diagrammatically in Figure 12.1.1.

Although it is clear that atherosclerosis is accelerated in the presence of high plasma cholesterol concentrations, this process can occur in the presence of normal lipoprotein concentrations. Other factors known to be associated with increased risk of development of atherosclerosis include hypertension, diabetes mellitus, obesity, smoking, age and male gender.

Risk factors for atherosclerosis

Hypercholesterolaemia
Hypertriglyceridaemia
Hypertension
Obesity
Diabetes mellitus
Cigarette smoking
Ageing
Male gender
Genetic (family history of premature atherosclerosis: in females <65 years; in males <55 years)
Physical inactivity
Excessive alcohol consumption
Emotional stress/personality type (type A)

Cholesterol

High plasma cholesterol concentrations are associated with an increased risk of atherosclerosis. Elevations in plasma cholesterol can be produced by a diet rich in cholesterol and saturated fat (such foods as fatty meat, egg yolks, liver and fast-food meals) or as the result of an inherited condition known as familial hypercholesterolaemia (a genetic disorder resulting in the total lack of the receptor for low density lipoproteins). Cholesterol, like other lipids, is transported in the blood attached to carrier proteins. The plasma proteins which transport the majority (two-thirds) of cholesterol are called *low-density lipoproteins* (LDL). Cells in various organs contain receptors for LDL. On binding to its receptor, LDL is engulfed by the cell, where it releases the cholesterol for use by the cell. LDLs are produced in, as well as removed by, the liver.

Regulation of LDL receptor number is an important mechanism for controlling plasma LDL concentrations. The low number of LDL receptors in individuals with familial hyper-cholesterolaemia and in those who eat a diet high in cholesterol and saturated fat results in these people having high plasma cholesterol concentrations. Without LDL receptors, the liver is less able to remove LDL from the blood. Consequently more LDL is available to enter the endothelial cells of arteries.

When endothelial cells engulf LDL, they oxidize it to a product called oxidized LDL. Recent evidence suggests that it is this oxidized LDL which contributes to endothelial cell injury, migration of monocytes and lymphocytes, and thereby progression of atherosclerosis.

In addition to LDL, if cholesterol concentrations are very high, *high-density lipoproteins* (HDL) may also transport cholesterol. The cholesterol in HDL is not taken up into the arterial wall because arterial cells lack the receptor for HDL. Hence this cholesterol does not contribute to atherosclerosis. Indeed a high proportion of HDLs compared with LDLs is advantageous in that it indicates that cholesterol may be travelling away from blood vessels to the liver (via HDLs). Women in general have a higher HDL concentration and a lower risk of developing atherosclerosis than do men. More importantly in both males and females, physical activity increases the ratio of HDL to LDL cholesterol (see Ch. 9).

Hypertriglyceridaemia

Elevated concentrations of triglycerides in the plasma are also an important risk factor for atherosclerosis. Hypertriglyceridaemia is associated with a rise in plasma *very low-density lipoproteins* (VLDLs) as it is these lipoproteins that are responsible for transporting triglycerides to the liver. Elevations in plasma triglycerides are a consequence of overproduction of VLDL (associated with diets high in fats and carbohydrates) or an inability to catabolize VLDL. It is usually when VLDL production rates are elevated that defects in VLDL catabolism manifest (the rate of catabolism cannot be increased in proportion to the increased production). Hypertriglyceridaemia may be the consequence of a genetic defect in VLDL metabolism (familial hypertriglyceridaemia) or may be associated with obesity and diabetes mellitus. In the presence of a damaged endothelium VLDL and triglycerides infiltrate into the tunica media, thereby contributing to atherosclerosis.

Hypertension

High blood pressure is an important risk factor for atherosclerosis with the risk increasing progressively with increasing blood pressure levels. Data from the Framingham Heart Study showed that the incidence of atherosclerosis in middle-aged men with a systolic/diastolic blood pressure (SBP/DBP) >160/95 mmHg was more than five times that in normotensive men (SBP/DBP <140/90 mmHg). Although these data were obtained in men, hypertensive women are also at a higher risk of developing atherosclerosis than are normotensive women. It is thought that diastolic blood pressure is a more important risk factor than systolic blood pressure. However, the reasons for this are as yet unknown.

High blood pressures increase the mechanical stresses imposed on the vasculature. Hence hypertension is likely to enhance atherogenesis by directly damaging the endothelial cells specifically at sites of high pressure. This damage to the endothelium induces platelet aggregation with consequent release of growth-stimulating factors and local thrombus formation. The growth-stimulating factors are thought to contribute to smooth muscle migration into the tunica intima and their synthesis of connective tissue.

Obesity and diabetes mellitus

Obesity commonly produces insulin resistance in peripheral tissues (mainly muscle and adipose tissues) which leads to compensatory hyperinsulinaemia (increased concentration of insulin in the plasma). The consequent effects on the liver are an enhanced production of triglyceride rich lipoproteins (VLDLs) which in turn leads to elevated plasma triglyceride and cholesterol concentrations. In other words obesity and diabetes mellitus are associated with an increased cholesterol synthesis, the consequence of which is atherosclerosis (see above). Insulin is known to stimulate the migration of smooth muscle cells from the tunica media to the tunica intima and their proliferation. Furthermore, insulin enhances the transformation of smooth muscle cells into a synthetic state and their consequent production of connective tissue.

Smoking

Chronic inhalation of smoke is likely to result in repetitive injury to endothelial cells with consequent acceleration of atherogenesis. In addition, smoking is associated with high levels of carboxyhaemoglobin and low oxygen delivery to tissues. The tissue hypoxia which ensues stimulates the proliferation of arterial smooth muscle cells which in turn can migrate into the tunica intima and synthesize connective tissue. Furthermore, hypoxia may diminish the degradative ability of lysosomal enzymes, resulting in impaired degradation of LDLs by smooth muscle cells. Consequently LDLs will accumulate within cells, thereby enhancing the progression of atherosclerosis.

Angina

Angina pectoris is the name given to the substernal pain associated with myocardial ischaemia. This pain may also be referred to the left shoulder and radiate down the left arm. The production of lactic acid as a consequence of anaerobic respiration in ischaemic tissue is one of the factors thought to be responsible for this pain. However, myocardial ischaemia may also be silent in that it is not always associated with pain.

As stated above, inadequate supply of oxygen because of inadequate blood flow to a tissue renders the tissue ischaemic. However, the adequacy of blood flow is relative as it depends on the metabolic requirements of the tissue for oxygen. For example, an obstruction of a coronary artery by atheroma may allow sufficient coronary blood flow at rest but not when the heart is stressed by exercise or emotional conditions. This is due to the increased activity of the *sympathetic nervous system* (SNS) and *renin–angiotensin–aldosterone system* (RAAS) in such conditions. Increased activity in these systems results in arterial vasoconstriction and an augmented heart rate which in turn elevate blood pressure. Consequently the work of the heart is enhanced, thereby raising its oxygen requirements (Fig. 12.1.2).

Furthermore, mental stress can cause constriction of atherosclerotic coronary arteries, leading to ischaemia of heart muscle. The mechanism of this stress-induced vasoconstriction is related to abnormal functioning of the damaged endothelium. In atherosclerotic arteries, the normal vasodilator response to acetycholine is blunted. This abnormal response is probably due to reduced concentrations of the endothelial derived relaxant factor, *nitric oxide* (NO). Reductions in NO concentration have been attributed to:

- decreases in the precursor L-arginine
- decreases in the activity of endothelial NO synthase
- increases in the rate of NO breakdown.

In this regard it is interesting to note that vasodilator drugs often used to treat angina pectoris (including nitroglycerine and sodium nitroprusside) promote vasodilation indirectly through their conversion into nitric oxide, hence relieving the ischaemia and associated pain. As myocardial ischaemia and/or angina often only manifest under stress conditions it is imperative that stress tests are performed in an individual who is suspected to have myocardial ischaemia. Such tests involve an exercise treadmill test at incremental workloads during which a full 12-lead *electrocardiogram* (ECG) is recorded. Myocardial ischaemia can be detected by changes in the ST segments (most commonly ST segment depression) of the ECG (Fig. 12.1.3) and is often accompanied by angina during the stress test.

Myocardial infarction

Myocardial cells are adapted to respire aerobically. Hence, they cannot respire anaerobically for more than a few minutes. Therefore if myocardial ischaemia and anaerobic metabolism continue for more than a few minutes necrosis (cell death) is likely to occur in those areas most deprived of oxygen. A sudden irreversible injury of this kind is called a myocardial infarction, which in lay terms is called a 'heart attack'. Whereas atherosclerosis contributes to chronic myocardial ischaemia, a sudden obstruction of blood flow through coronary vasculature is more likely the consequence of a thrombosis (a clot which has moved from one area of atherosclerosis and lodged in another area of the vasculature – usually at the bifurcation of arteries). Myocardial infarction may also result in ST segment changes (most commonly ST segment elevation) in the ECG (Fig. 12.1.3). Furthermore, the diagnosis of myocardial infarction is aided by the measurement of the concentration of various enzymes in the plasma that were released by the infarcted tissue. In addition, these enzymes give a rough indication as to when the infarction occurred. For example, plasma concentrations of the enzyme *creatine phosphokinase* (CPK, the enzyme that transfers phosphate between creatine and ATP) are increased within 3 to 6 hours after the infarction and *lactate dehydrogenase* (LDH, the enzyme that catalyses the conversion of pyruvic acid to lactic acid) concentrations within 10 to 12 hours. CPK reaches its maximum after 24 to 36 hours and LDH after 48 to 72 hours. CPK returns to normal after 3 days and LDH only after 11 days (Fig. 12.1.4).

Management of patients with coronary heart disease

The management of patients with coronary artery disease includes pharmacological therapy, non-operative dilation of coronary artery stenosis and surgical procedures such as coronary artery bypass graft surgery.

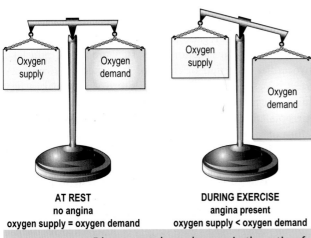

AT REST
no angina
oxygen supply = oxygen demand

DURING EXERCISE
angina present
oxygen supply < oxygen demand

Figure 12.1.2. Diagram to show changes in the ratio of oxygen supply to demand during exercise compared with at rest.

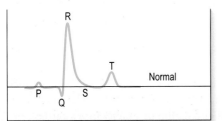
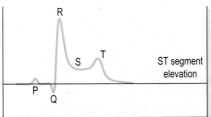
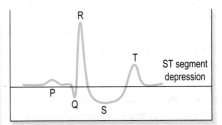

Normal

ST segment elevation

ST segment depression

Figure 12.1.3. Diagrammatic representation of a normal electrocardiogram (ECG) compared with changes observed with myocardial ischaemia (ST segment depression) or myocardial infarction (ST segment elevation).

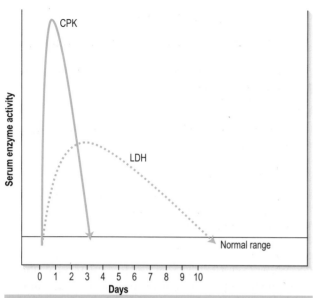

Figure 12.1.4.   Diagrammatic representation of the changes in creatine phosphokinase (CPK) and lactate dehydrogenase (LDH) concentrations during the first 10 days after a myocardial infarction.

Pharmacological therapy

Pharmacological therapy includes the use of nitrates, beta-adrenergic blocking agents, cardiac glycosides, diuretics and calcium channel blockers. Nitrates (nitroglycerine) promote vasodilation via conversion into nitric oxide. Beta-adrenergic blocking agents oppose the effects mediated by cardiac beta-adrenergic receptors namely increases in heart rate, myocardial contractility, cardiac output and myocardial oxygen consumption, and decreases in total peripheral resistance. Cardiac glycosides and diuretics are useful to reduce wall tension if wall tension is elevated by an increased left ventricular end-diastolic filling volume (as a consequence of reduced left ventricular systolic function in the presence of myocardial ischaemia). Calcium channel blockers are potent coronary artery vasodilators thereby improving blood flow in coronary arteries. In addition, calcium channel blockers reduce arterial pressure (via decreasing peripheral resistance) and myocardial contractility thereby reducing myocardial oxygen demand. Hence the myocardial oxygen demand to supply ratio is improved.

Non-operative dilation of coronary artery stenoses

The non-operative procedure to dilate coronary arteries is called *percutaneous transluminal angioplasty* (PTCA). This procedure, performed under local anaesthesia, involves the placement of a radial artery cannula for constant arterial pressure monitoring, and a Swan–Ganz catheter for monitoring of pulmonary artery and capillary wedge pressures

and thereby the monitoring of left ventricular filling pressure. A standard angiographic catheter is inserted percutaneously from the groin or by means of a cutdown from the brachial artery. Following a routine angiogram to visualize the site of the lesion a specialized balloon-tipped catheter is passed from the groin or brachial artery through the coronary artery stenosis over a guide wire. Once the balloon of the catheter is positioned over the stenotic lesion, it is inflated in order to occlude the vessel. With further expansion of the balloon the atherosclerotic plaque responsible for the stenosis splits at its weakest point. This split then allows the tunica media and adventitia to stretch over the expanded dilating balloon. The split occurs in the atherosclerotic plaque and not in the vessel as the former is not elastic. The balloon is then deflated and withdrawn leaving the split atherosclerotic plaque and dilated tunica media and adventitia, thus resulting in an enlarged vessel lumen. Successful PTCA rarely obliterates the coronary artery stenosis completely. However, final pressure gradients across the stenosis are generally less than 10 mmHg in comparison to gradients of 50 mmHg or more prior to PTCA.

Importantly in order to aid the 'splitting' of the atherosclerotic plaque, heparin (an anticoagulant) is given to patients during PTCA. For a few days prior to and up to 6 months after PTCA, antiplatelet agents (aspirin) are given as the presence of the catheter in the vessel lumen is an irritant which can initiate platelet aggregation and the formation of blood clots.

The major complications of PTCA are death, non-fatal myocardial infarction or the need for emergency coronary artery bypass graft surgery due to closure of a coronary artery during the procedure. These complications occur in 9% of all attempts at PTCA. The restenosis rate, as measured by the return of symptoms at one year of follow-up, is between 20 and 30%. The best candidates for PTCA are those patients with isolated one-vessel coronary artery disease as these patients have the lowest complication and restenosis rates.

Coronary artery bypass graft surgery

Coronary artery bypass graft surgery (CABG) involves the use of a section of vein (usually the saphenous) to form a connection between the aorta and the coronary artery distal to the obstructing lesion. Alternatively the end of the mammary artery may be anastomosed to the coronary artery distal to the obstructing lesion. Coronary artery bypass graft surgery is performed under general anaesthesia and involves cardiopulmonary bypass following a midline thoracotomy. Cardiopulmonary bypass is the procedure used to divert blood away from the heart and then return it to the systemic circulation. Cardiopulmonary bypass therefore replaces the function of both the lungs and the heart. Blood is drained from the systemic venous circulation by gravity into a cardiotomy reservoir, from where it is directed through an oxygenator and then returned to the systemic circulation using a centrifugal pump. The operative procedure is preceded by the placement of a radial artery catheter for continuous monitoring of arterial pressure, a Swan–Ganz catheter for the measurement of pulmonary artery and pulmonary capillary wedge pressures before and after bypass as well as for the determination of cardiac output via the thermodilution method. After cardiopulmonary bypass a left atrial catheter is inserted through the right superior pulmonary vein for continuous monitoring of left atrial pressure and temporary pacing wires are attached to the epicardial surface of the right atrium and ventricle for pacing when indicated. Following the operative procedure the patient is carefully monitored in a coronary care intensive care unit (ICU) for approximately 3–5 days provided there are no complications (if complications occur the period in ICU will be longer).

These operations are relatively safe with reported mortality rates of 1% in elective (as opposed to emergency) operations carried out by experienced surgical teams and in patients with near normal left ventricular function. As patency rates of 70–85% are reported at 2–3 years after surgery and angina is abolished or reduced in 85% of patients, coronary artery bypass graft surgery despite its high degree of invasiveness is a viable option especially for those patients in whom PTCA is not indicated. As knowledge about the effect of coronary artery bypass graft surgery on the natural history of coronary artery disease is minimal, such surgery is generally only performed in persons with two- or three-vessel disease and some degree (although small) of left ventricular dysfunction. In some centres patients with lesions in only a single vessel are also considered for surgery, particularly if they are severely symptomatic and/or they have severe lesions in the left anterior descending coronary artery (supplies the anterior surface of the left ventricle and the anterior two-thirds of the interventricular septum) or the left main coronary artery (supplies the lateral and posterior walls of the left ventricle via the left circumflex, and the anterior surface of the left ventricle and the anterior two-thirds of the interventricular septum via the left anterior descending coronary artery). Although it has been suggested that coronary artery bypass graft surgery may favourably affect the natural history of coronary artery disease, this possible beneficial effect remains to be confirmed before coronary artery bypass graft surgery is indicated for asymptomatic or mildly symptomatic patients with coronary artery disease.

HEART FAILURE

There are various forms of heart failure (Table 12.1.2). However, their differences are mainly in terms of aetiology rather than pathophysiology. With respect to pathophysiology there are two main types of heart failure – low output and high output. Low output heart failure encompasses all primary disorders of the heart itself that result in a reduced cardiac output if the disorder is severe enough (Table 12.1.2).

Table 12.1.2.   Causes of heart failure

Low output: decreased ventricular contraction (congestive heart failure)
- Ischaemic heart disease – loss of normally contracting cells
- Secondary to increased workload
  - hypertension
  - valvular disease
- Cardiomyopathy (primary non-ischaemic abnormality in heart muscle)
  - familial
  - idiopathic dilated

High output: excess venous return due to increased vasodilation, increased blood volume, shunts
- Increased vasodilation
  - Hyperthyroidism
  - Beri-beri
  - Severe anaemias
  - Cor pulmonale
- Increased blood volume
  - Renal disease
  - Hepatic cirrhosis
- Shunts
  - Arteriovenous fistulas
  - Paget's disease of bone

High output heart failure occurs in response to non-cardiac disorders and is characterized by an elevated cardiac output. As cardiac rehabilitation has at present only been advised for heart failure of cardiac origin (in particular congestive, ischaemic and idiopathic dilated heart failure), the pathophysiology of only these types of heart failure will be discussed.

Pathophysiology of congestive heart failure

There are numerous classifications of heart failure, but clinically the term heart failure is reserved for circulatory congestion of cardiac origin. The term congestion is used to describe the forms of heart failure which result in increased filling pressures. Failure of the left ventricle raises the pressure in the left atrium, which produces pulmonary congestion and oedema. Similarly failure of the right ventricle raises right atrial pressure, which results in congestion and oedema in the systemic circulation (liver congestion, ascites and pedal oedema). The major cause of congestive heart failure is coronary heart disease (ischaemic heart failure) with less common causes being hypertension, idiopathic dilated cardiomyopathy, valvular abnormalities (aortic valve stenosis, aortic valve incompetence and mitral valve incompetence) and familial cardiomyopathies.

The incidence of congestive heart failure is strongly influenced by age and gender. With respect to age congestive heart failure occurs in 1% of persons under the age of 50 years and approximately doubles for each decade of life. In women the incidence of congestive heart failure is 65% that of men after adjustment for age. Risk factors that predispose patients to the development of congestive heart failure include increased cholesterol concentrations, smoking, essential hypertension, diabetes mellitus and evidence of left ventricular hypertrophy.

In congestive heart failure the physiological alterations that are observed are either primary to the disease process itself or representative of secondary compensatory changes which occur in response to disturbances of the normal circulatory control mechanisms. Consequently the pathophysiological findings in congestive heart failure are a complex inter-relationship between haemodynamic and neurohumoral changes (Fig. 12.1.5). The two major neurohumoral systems involved are the sympathetic nervous system (SNS) and the renin–angiotensin–aldosterone system (RAAS). Other vaso-active substances which are involved include antidiuretic hormone, nitric oxide, endothelin (vasoconstrictor) and prostaglandins.

Contractility of the heart is the central haemodynamic abnormality, which may be the result of myocyte loss (due to ischaemia and necrosis), ischaemic dysfunction due to reduced blood flow, or pump dysfunction due to cardiac remodelling (left ventricular hypertrophy or dilation). Intrinsic myocardial contractility is the strength of contrac-tion of the cardiac myocytes independent of influences such as *heart rate* (HR), afterload (external pressure loading or vasoconstriction) and preload (filling pressure or volume loading). Intrinsic myocyte contractility is distinguished from left ventricular chamber or pump performance which describes the overall function of the heart due to the effects of remodelling as well as myocardial contractility. The Frank–Starling relationship represents normal left ventricu-lar pump function (Fig. 12.1.6a). This relationship is altered by changes in myocardial contractility. A decreased slope indicates a decreased contractility (Fig. 12.1.6a). Changes in the dimension of the heart (cardiac remodelling) also influ-ence this relationship. A right shift with an increased volume intercept occurs in the presence to ventricular dilation (Fig. 12.1.6a). One can use this curve to demonstrate point by point the compensatory changes which occur in a person with congestive heart failure (Fig. 12.1.6b).

With reference to Figure 12.1.6b, point A represents the normal relationship between *stroke volume* (SV) and *left ven-tricular filling pressure* (LVEDP). Immediately after an acute ischaemic episode, for example, myocardial contractility will be decreased and hence there will be a decreased SV for a given LVEDP (point B). As a consequence of the decreased SV, the volume of blood remaining in the LV will be greater than normal (increased *left ventricular end-systolic volume*, LVESV) and hence *filling volume* (LVEDV) will be enhanced. An increase in LVEDV will result in an increase in LVEDP. As the response of the heart to an increased LVEDP is to increase SV, the point on the curve shifts from B to C. Superimposed on these haemodynamic changes are the influences of the neuro-endocrine systems. An increased SNS activity enhances con-tractility and hence results in a shift to point D. Whether point D represents an SV the same as normal or less than normal is dependent upon the extent of the original myocardial insult. Nevertheless point D represents a compensatory change whereby SV is maintained at the expense of an elevated *end-diastolic filling pressure* (LVEDP), which ultimately gives rise to the signs and symptoms associated with heart failure.

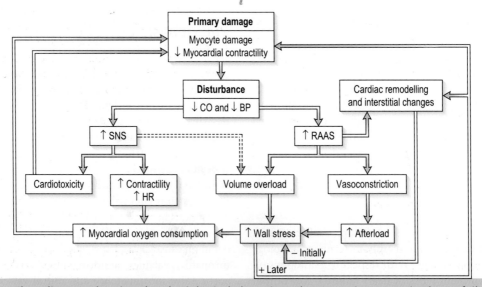

Figure 12.1.5.   Flow diagram showing the physiological alterations that occur in congestive heart failure. SNS, sympathetic nervous system; RAAS, renin–angiotensin–aldosterone system; CO, cardiac output; BP, blood pressure; HR, heart rate.

Signs and symptoms

The major signs and symptoms of heart failure are fatigue, exercise intolerance, shortness of breath (dyspnoea) and oedema. Physical activity is typically limited by both fatigue and shortness of breath.

Fatigue results from inadequate oxygen delivery to tissues as a consequence of decreased skeletal muscle perfusion. Skeletal muscle perfusion is impaired by reductions in *cardiac output* (CO) as well as by local factors. These local factors include impaired vasodilatory responses to the metabolic needs of the tissue which are primarily associated with alterations in *nitric oxide* (NO) reproduction. Similar to patients with congestive heart disease (CHD) patients with heart failure have abnormal peripheral blood responses to

pharmacologically (acetylcholine) as well as exercise-induced vasodilation. As a consequence of the reduced oxygen delivery, muscle respiration becomes increasingly anaerobic and thus lactic acid production is enhanced.

The symptoms of *fatigue and exercise intolerance* are not entirely due to the haemodynamic status of patients in heart failure. In addition to abnormal blood flow responses to vasodilators, patients with heart failure have structural and functional abnormalities in their skeletal muscles. These abnormalities include decreased number and size of mitochondria, decreased muscle fibre number and dimension, defects in oxidative and glycolytic enzymes which contribute to the dependence on anaerobic metabolism, excessive early depletion of energy released from phosphate bonds (creatine phosphate and ATP), excessive early intramuscular acidification associated with anaerobic metabolism, defects in beta-oxidation of fats with subsequent increased use of amino acids as substrates and further depletion of skeletal muscle fibre size and number.

The mechanisms responsible for the *dyspnoea* include decreased lung compliance due to pulmonary congestion; increased ventilation associated with the enhanced lactic acid production and possibly underperfusion of respiratory muscles (see Ch. 9.2). Furthermore, abnormalities similar to those in skeletal muscle (described above) have been observed in respiratory muscles. In milder cases of heart failure dyspnoea is only evident on exertion; but with increasing severity of heart failure dyspnoea occurs at rest, whilst lying down (orthopnoea) or in episodes while asleep (paraxysmal nocturnal dyspnoea).

Regardless of the aetiology (congestive, ischaemic or idiopathic) the symptoms of fatigue, exercise intolerance and dyspnoea predominate in chronic stable heart failure, whereas oedema in addition is a characteristic feature of unstable acute heart failure and more severe forms of heart failure.

The most common practical way of classifying the severity of heart failure is according to New York Heart Association (NYHA) functional class. This classification is based on a patient's clinical history describing the symptoms they experience.

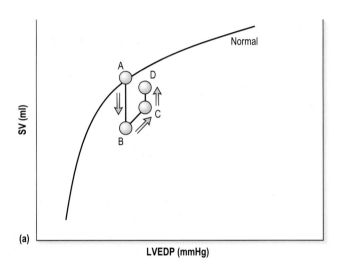

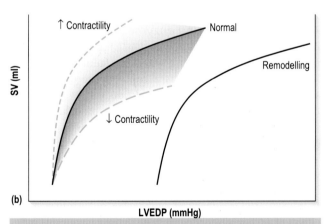

Figure 12.1.6. (a) Diagrammatic representation of Frank–Starling curve showing changes in this relationship due to increases or decreases in contractility or remodelling (dilatation). LVEDP, left ventricular end-diastolic pressure; SV, stroke volume. (b) Diagrammatic representation of changes that occur in the Frank–Starling relationship immediately after an acute ischaemic episode.

Classification of severity of heart failure according to New York Heart Association functional class

Class I. Ordinary physical activity does not cause undue dyspnoea or fatigue (Ordinary physical activity implies activities such as jogging or walking up a hill at mild to moderate intensities, which when preformed at very high intensities can produce dyspnoea even in a normal person. Whereas less than ordinary physical activity refers to activities which would *not*

	normally produce dyspnoea in a normal person.)
Class II.	Comfort is present at rest, but ordinary physical activity results in dyspnoea or fatigue
Class III.	Comfort is present at rest, but less than ordinary physical activity results in dyspnoea or fatigue
Class IV.	Dyspnoea or fatigue may be present at rest and is made worse by any physical effort

Management of patients with heart failure

With respect to the management of patients with heart failure, the pharmacological and non-pharmacological approaches will be discussed briefly. Common surgical treatments have been previously discussed in the coronary heart disease section. Additional surgical procedures are mainly reserved for patients in severe heart failure (for whom exercise rehabilitation is not currently recommended) and hence are not discussed.

The management of congestive heart failure involves (1) the reduction of cardiac workload, including afterload, (2) enhancement of myocardial contractility and (3) control of excessive salt and water retention. In order to achieve these goals both non-pharmacological and pharmacological approaches are used in conjunction.

Non-pharmacological approaches

Part of the management of heart failure involves patient education with respect to dietary and lifestyle modifications which produce beneficial effects on associated signs and symptoms as well as altering the course of the disease thereby improving prognosis. The main advice is to restrict dietary sodium, reduce caloric intake to reduce body weight, avoid smoking and exercise regularly. Although regular exercise does not produce substantial changes in left ventricular function (ejection fraction) or filling pressure (pulmonary capillary wedge pressure), it does improve exercise capacity by reversing the abnormalities observed in skeletal and respiratory muscles. Furthermore, exercise reduces sympathetic tone and increases vagal tone at rest with subsequent decreases in myocardial work (see Ch. 9.1).

Pharmacological approaches

Pharmacological therapy for chronic stable heart failure includes the use of diuretics, digoxin, *angiotensin-converting enzyme* (ACE) inhibitors, angiotensin II receptor antagonists, aldosterone receptor antagonists, beta-adrenergic blocking agents, vasodilators. The benefits, mechanisms of action, common side effects and major contraindications for each of the agents are briefly discussed.

Diuretics

Diuretics are the most commonly prescribed agents for heart failure because of their efficiency in controlling salt and water retention and thus reducing pulmonary and systemic congestion. In association with sodium and water loss due to treatment with some types of diuretics, potassium is excreted and hence may need to be supplemented. Despite their profound benefits on controlling excessive fluid retention, diuretics also activate neurohormonal systems resulting in vasoconstriction. Hence diuretics are always used in combination with an ACE inhibitor and/or a beta-adrenergic blocking agent.

Digoxin

Digoxin is used to provide chronic inotropic (increased myocardial contractility) support for patients in heart failure. The effects of digoxin on myocardial contractility are due to its effects on excitation–contraction coupling. Digoxin inhibits transmembrane sodium and potassium movement by inhibiting Na/K-ATPase. As Na/K-ATPase is coupled to sarcolemmal Na–Ca exchange there is a consequent rise in intracellular calcium concentration which augments myofilament cross-bridge formation and hence contractility. In addition to the effects of digoxin therapy on systolic function (increased ejection fraction), exercise capacity is increased and symptoms of heart failure are reduced. These benefits of digoxin are thought to be related to a decrease in neurohumoral activation of the RAAS and SNS. Consequently digoxin enhances vagal tone and slows down HR and atrioventricular conduction.

Angiotensin-converting enzyme inhibitors

Angiotensin-converting enzyme (ACE) inhibitors have a number of benefits to patients with heart failure. They reduce left ventricular wall stress as a consequence of inhibiting angiotensin II-induced vasoconstriction and by preventing the breakdown of the local vasodilator bradykinin. ACE inhibitor therapy is consequently associated with increased exercise tolerance and decreased symptoms. Importantly by lowering angiotensin II concentrations, ACE inhibitors prevent angiotensin II-mediated cardiac and vascular remodelling and interstitial changes. ACE inhibitors are also reported to decrease the incidence of ventricular arrhythmias. These effects of ACE inhibitors contribute to their favourable influence on the long-term prognosis of chronic heart failure.

Angiotensin II receptor antagonists

Angiotensin II receptor antagonists produce similar effects to the ACE inhibitors. However, there is as yet no data on their long-term benefits in terms of prognosis. Angiotensin II receptor antagonists are generally used only in patients in whom ACE inhibitors are not tolerated because of ACE inhibitor-induced dry cough.

Aldosterone receptor antagonists

Aldosterone receptor antagonists produce sodium diuresis and hence are valuable in preventing fluid retention. Importantly they also block the effects of aldosterone on cardiac and vascular remodelling and on the interstitium. However, a common side effect associated with aldosterone receptor antagonists is the development of gynaecomastia in men often associated with breast pain. Hence these agents are generally only used in women. In addition, long-term benefits have only been shown in a relatively small study. Currently new agents that do not have the side effects of gynaecomastia are under investigation in clinical trials.

Beta-adrenergic blocking agents

The benefits of beta-adrenergic blocking agents are attributed to their blockade of the direct cardiotoxic effects of catecholamines and their suppression of the RAAS. Treatment with beta-adrenergic blockers results in reductions in mortality from congestive heart failure, which is not surprising given that sustained activation of the SNS and elevations in its neurotransmitter noradrenaline (norepinephrine) are implicated in the progression of congestive heart failure. However, these agents must be administered with caution, especially in patients with severe heart failure, as they block the role of the SNS in supporting the failing circulation.

Vasodilators

Although the use of arterial and venous vasodilators is associated with improved haemodynamics, the changes are less favourable than those produced by ACE inhibitors. Furthermore, these agents have not been shown to promote long-term benefits in terms of cardiac remodelling and slowing or halting the progression of the disease. Although useful in acute heart failure, vasodilators are generally not commonly used in the treatment of chronic stable heart failure, unless ACE inhibitors are contraindicated.

Management of patients with heart failure

Non-pharmacological approaches
 Reduce dietary sodium
 Reduce caloric intake
 Cessation of smoking
 Regular physical exercise

Pharmacological treatment
 Diuretics
 Digoxin
 Angiotensin-converting enzyme inhibitors
 Angiotensin II receptor antagonists
 Aldosterone receptor antagonists
 Beta-adrenergic blockers
 Vasodilators

HYPERTENSION

The exact aetiology of hypertension is still uncertain. Approximately 2–5% of patients with hypertension have underlying renal or adrenal disease as the cause of their raised blood pressure (renal hypertension). These individuals are said to have *secondary hypertension*. As this form of hypertension accounts for only a minority of patients with hypertension and the effects of exercise rehabilitation have not been reported, the pathophysiology of secondary hypertension will not be discussed further. However, for the remainder of patients with hypertension (approximately 95%), no clear single identifiable cause is evident. In these patients the condition is termed *primary* or *essential hypertension*. Abnormalities in the physiological mechanisms involved in the regulation of blood pressure are likely to play a major role in the development of essential hypertension. The relative magnitude of the contribution of these inter-related factors may differ between individuals. Examples of such factors are listed in Table 12.1.3. In addition, although not directly causally related, a number of factors are likely to modify the progression of essential hypertension (Table 12.1.4).

Physiological mechanisms involved in blood pressure regulation (Fig. 12.1.7)

The main purpose of normal cardiovascular regulation is to maintain blood pressure and hence blood flow. The

---

Table 12.1.3.   Factors contributing to pathophysiology of essential hypertension

Renin–angiotensin–aldosterone system
Sympathetic nervous system
Obesity
Salt intake
Insulin resistance
Endothelial dysfunction
Genetics
Vasoactive substances

Table 12.1.4.   Factors which modify the progression of essential hypertension

Race – persons of African origin have a worse prognosis than Caucasians
Age of onset – young worse prognosis than old
Gender – males have worse prognosis than females
Smoking
Hypercholesterolaemia
Obesity
Glucose intolerance or diabetes mellitus
Environmental stress
Excessive alcohol consumption

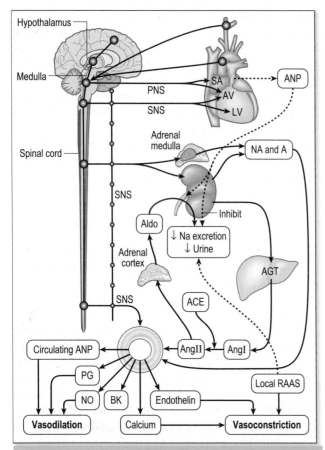

Figure 12.1.7.   **Summary of the systems which interact in order to maintain a normal blood pressure.** ANP, atrial natriuretic peptide; BK, bradykinin; AGT, angiotensinogen; NA, noradrenaline; A, adrenaline; PNS, peripheral nervous system; Aldo, aldosterone; SA, sinoatrial valve; AV, atrioventricular valve; LV, left ventricle; PG, prostaglandin; RAAS, renin–angiotensin–aldosterone system.

frequency of action potentials produced by sensory nerve fibres from the baroreceptors. This altered baroreceptor sensory information travels in the glossopharyngeal (ninth cranial) and the vagus (tenth cranial) nerves to the vasomotor centre located in the medulla oblongata at the base of the brain. An increase in baroreceptor sensory information promotes activation of the *parasympathetic nervous system* (PNS) and inhibits the *sympathetic nervous system* (SNS), whereas a decrease in baroreceptor sensory information will inhibit activity of the PNS and promote activity of the SNS. These events, from the detection of a change in blood pressure by the baroreceptors to alterations in the activity of components of the vasomotor centre, are termed the baroreceptor reflex. Activation of the SNS causes heart rate and myocardial contractility to be enhanced and peripheral vasoconstriction occurs. In addition SNS activity stimulates the release of noradrenaline (norepinephrine) and adrenaline (epinephrine) from the adrenal medulla, which enhances peripheral vasoconstriction and stimulates the release of renin from the kidneys. Furthermore, SNS nerve fibres which synapse on the juxtaglomerular apparatus in the kidney result in an increased secretion of renin. Renin is responsible for the conversion of angiotensinogen (from the liver mainly) to angiotensin I, which is then converted to its active form, angiotensin II, by angiotensin-converting enzyme (ACE). Angiotensin II is a potent vasoconstrictor thereby contributing to the SNS-mediated increase in total peripheral resistance. Factors other than angiotensin II and catecholamines that are important in the regulation of vascular tone include vasoconstrictors such as local RAAS, calcium and endothelin, and the vasodilators *atrial natriuretic peptide* (ANP), nitric oxide (NO) and prostaglandins.

In addition to its vasoactive effects, angiotensin II stimulates the release of aldosterone from the adrenal cortex. Aldosterone is responsible for sodium and water retention by the kidney and thereby the regulation of salt balance, blood volume and blood pressure. Normally when blood pressure is increased, the kidney rapidly excretes sodium and water. This so-called pressure–natriuresis relationship can be altered by factors such as increased renal sensitivity to angiotensin II or catecholamines (noradrenaline and adrenaline).

Pathophysiology of hypertension

All of the mechanisms that are involved in the normal regulation of blood pressure are likely to participate in the pathophysiology of essential hypertension. However, it is unclear as to which control systems are responsible for the initial changes in blood pressure. In the majority of individuals with essential hypertension many of these systems together rather than a single one show abnormal responses. What is known of the pathophysiological role of each of the control systems will be discussed.

maintenance of blood pressure is achieved by regulation of cardiac output and peripheral resistance which in turn are regulated by mechanisms which respond to changes in blood pressure. These mechanisms either respond to changes in blood pressure within seconds (short-term processes) or after a couple of hours (long-term processes). Both of these processes are negative feedback control systems in that they are switched off once blood pressure is returned to its normal levels. The short-term processes are effective over a period of seconds to hours and the long-term processes operate over days to weeks. The short-term processes are neural in origin involving baroreceptors and their connections with the autonomic nervous system. The long-term processes are renal and hormonal.

A sudden change in blood pressure is detected by the carotid and aortic arch baroreceptors, resulting in an alteration in the

Autonomic nervous system

As some individuals with essential hypertension have high plasma concentrations of catecholamines, SNS overactivity was thought to be responsible for the raised total peripheral resistance in these patients. However, there is little evidence to support a *direct* role of noradrenaline or adrenaline in essential hypertension. It is probable that the major role of the SNS in essential hypertension is related to an interaction between the SNS and the RAAS together with sodium and circulating blood volume. It is thought that the SNS perpetuates a high blood pressure by altering the relationship between blood pressure and sodium excretion in the kidney (the pressure–natriuresis relationship – see below). Nevertheless the role of the SNS is still controversial and requires further investigation.

Peripheral resistance

Most patients with essential hypertension have a normal cardiac output but a raised total peripheral resistance. The elevation in peripheral vascular resistance is a consequence of the contraction of smooth muscle in arterioles. Maintenance of smooth muscle contraction for a period of time results in the release of growth factors (most likely mediated by angiotensin II) which induce the proliferation of smooth muscle cells and thus the thickening of arteriolar walls. This in turn leads to an irreversible rise in peripheral vascular resistance. Smooth muscle contraction is maintained by SNS overactivity (see above) as well as increased circulating concentrations of angiotensin II (see below). In addition, increases in intracellular calcium concentrations have been implicated in the augmented contraction of smooth muscle cells. The increase in intracellular calcium has been attributed to an inherited membrane defect, a primary or inherited change in the sodium-ATPases or as a consequence of hormonal and neural factors (see below).

Renin–angiotensin–aldosterone system

The presence of normal renin concentrations in patients with elevated blood pressure is thought to be indicative of abnormalities in the RAAS as one would expect a decreased renin concentration in the presence of an elevated blood pressure. Nevertheless not all persons with essential hypertension have an elevated plasma concentration of renin. Renin values vary substantially with at least 10% of patients having high and 30% having low concentrations. Hence in persons with essential hypertension the circulating RAAS is not thought to be directly responsible for the rise in blood pressure. However, local epicrine (hormones act on adjacent cells) or paracrine (hormones reach cells in the same organ via the extracellular fluid) RAAS is likely to play an important role in essential hypertension. There is evidence that many hypertensive patients fail to respond normally to sodium loads in that their blood pressure increases following intravenous administration of sodium. Such persons are termed salt-sensitive and have been shown to have abnormal pressure–natriuresis curves with decreased sodium excretion relative to normal in response to the same rise in blood pressure. Renal efferent arteriolar constriction subsequent to increased SNS activity and increases in local concentrations of renin and angiotensin II are likely to be responsible for augmenting sodium reabsorption by the kidney. Dietary sodium may also impact on the pressure–natriuresis relationship, particularly in genetically predisposed persons (see below).

Vasoactive substances

Vascular endothelial cells produce a number of potent local vasoactive substances such as the vasodilator nitric oxide (NO) and the vasoconstrictor endothelin.

Nitric oxide

Patients with essential hypertension are reported to have endothelial dysfunction in that nitric oxide (NO) production is impaired. Concentrations of NO can be affected by alterations in the availability of its precursor L-arginine, in activity of the enzyme responsible for its production (endothelial nitric oxide synthase), and in the velocity of its breakdown (enhanced by the presence of reactive oxidative species). In addition, the normal vasodilatory response to endothelial agonists (acetylcholine) is diminished in some patients. In support of a role of NO in essential hypertension, genetic variations in endothelial nitric oxide synthase have been associated with the presence of hypertension and/or an elevation in blood pressure in some populations.

Endothelin

Endothelin is a potent endothelial vasoconstrictor which is known to activate the local RAAS. Hence besides contributing to an increase in peripheral resistance, endothelin is likely to play a role in the abnormal pressure–natriuresis relationship. In support of this role endothelin has been shown to produce a salt-sensitive rise in blood pressure.

Atrial natriuretic peptide

Atrial natriuretic peptide (ANP) is a hormone secreted by the atria of the heart in response to an increased blood volume. The effects of ANP are to increase sodium and water excretion by the kidneys. Possible defects in ANP may cause fluid and sodium retention and thereby essential hypertension.

Bradykinin

Bradykinin (BK) is another endothelial vasodilator. This substance is important in that it is broken down by angiotensin-converting enzyme. Hence one of the benefits of angiotensin-converting enzyme inhibitor therapy is to enhance the concentrations of bradykinin.

Salt intake

In addition to endothelin, there is evidence to suggest that patients with essential hypertension have a genetically determined defect in the ability to extrude sodium from cells. This defect, particularly in the presence of high salt intake, leads to increases in intracellular sodium which are paralleled by increases in intracellular calcium. The latter is likely to increase arteriolar smooth muscle tone. In addition, such individuals are likely to have an altered pressure–natriuresis relationship (see above).

Obesity

A *body mass index* (BMI) >27 is considered obese. Obesity is associated with an increased risk of developing essential hypertension. The mechanisms that link obesity with high blood pressure include insulin resistance, activation of the SNS and RAAS and their effects on the kidney. These effects on the kidney are to increase renal tubular reabsorption, glomerular filtration rate and renal plasma flow. With respect to the RAAS, adipose tissue is also a major site of production of angiotensinogen (primarily produced by the liver). Hence obese persons are likely to have increased concentrations of angiotensinogen with consequent augmentation of the effects of the RAAS.

Genetic factors

Essential hypertension is about twice as common in subjects who have one or two parents with essential hypertension. Evidence from epidemiological studies suggests that genetic factors account for up to 30% of the variation in blood pressure in most populations. Genetic variations in the DNA encoding most of the proteins involved in the regulation of blood pressure (as discussed above) have been linked to either the presence of essential hypertension or elevations in blood pressure. Currently there are many centres worldwide focusing their attentions on determining the genetic basis of essential hypertension and its interactions with or modifications of environmental and other risk factors for essential hypertension.

Other risk factors

Although not directly implicated in the aetiology of essential hypertension, the following factors modify the clinical course of essential hypertension: age, race, gender, smoking, serum cholesterol concentration, glucose intolerance or diabetes mellitus. An adverse prognosis in a person with essential hypertension is indicated by the presence of black race, onset of hypertension at a young age, male gender, smoking, diabetes mellitus, hypercholesterolaemia, obesity and a stressful environment (Table 12.1.4).

Management of patients with essential hypertension

The management of patients with essential hypertension is discussed with reference to the Sixth Report of the Joint National Committee on Prevention, Detection, Evaluation and Treatment of High Blood Pressure (JNCVI) and World Health Organization–International Society of Hypertension (WHO-ISH) guidelines for the management of hypertension. Currently the approach includes non-pharmacological and pharmacological interventions. The choice of approach (Table 12.1.8) depends upon the blood pressure level (severity of essential hypertension) (Table 12.1.5), the presence of associated risk factors (Table 12.1.6) and target organ damage (Table 12.1.7).

The primary goal of treatment for patients with essential hypertension is to reduce blood pressure to normal or optimal levels as well as to achieve a maximum reduction in the risk of cardiovascular morbidity and mortality. To achieve the latter requires treatment of associated diseases as well as lifestyle modifications (non-pharmacological treatments) to reduce cardiovascular risk factors.

Non-pharmacological treatments

Non-pharmacological treatments are used:

- to decrease blood pressure
- to decrease the need for antihypertensive medications
- to maximize the efficacy of antihypertensive medications
- to decrease cardiovascular risk factors
- for prevention of essential hypertension
- for prevention of cardiovascular diseases associated with essential hypertension.

Non-pharmacological treatments for hypertension

Smoking cessation
Weight reduction (decrease caloric intake)
Decrease alcohol consumption (<20–30 ml ethanol for males; <10–20 ml ethanol for females)
Decrease salt intake (<100 mmol/day)
Decrease saturated fat intake (dietary changes)
Increase physical activity
Decrease stress

Weight reduction

In hypertensive individuals who are >10% overweight, reductions in body weight of as little as 5 kg result in decreases in blood pressure. Furthermore, these reductions in body weight produce beneficial effects on insulin resistance, diabetes mellitus, hyperlipidaemia, hypertriglyceridaemia and

Table 12.1.5. Classification of blood pressure level (according to JNCVI)[a]

Category	SBP (mmHg)		DBP (mmHg)
Optimal	<120	and	<80
Normal	<130	and	<85
High normal	130–139	or	85–89
Hypertension[b]			
Stage 1 (mild)	140–159	or	90–99
Stage 2 (moderate)	160–179	or	100–109
Stage 3 (severe)	≥180	or	≥110

[a] Not taking antihypertensive agents and not acutely ill.
[b] Based on an average of two or more readings taken at each of two or more visits.

Table 12.1.6. Major risk factors

Smoking
Hypercholesterolaemia
Hypertriglyceridaemia
Diabetes mellitus
Age (>60 years)
Gender (men or postmenopausal women)
Family history of premature cardiovascular disease
(in females <65 years, in males <55 years)
Excessive alcohol consumption

Table 12.1.7. Target organ damage (TOD)

Heart disease
– left ventricular hypertrophy
– angina
– prior myocardial infarct
– prior need for coronary revascularization procedures
– heart failure
Stroke or transient ischaemic attack
Nephropathy (renal disease)
Peripheral vascular disease
Retinopathy (retinal vascular damage)

left ventricular hypertrophy. The blood pressure lowering effects of weight reduction are enhanced by a simultaneous increase in physical exercise and decreases in sodium and alcohol intake.

Reduction in salt intake

Although there is considerable variation among individuals in their responses to changes in dietary salt intake, the aim should be to achieve an intake of less than 5.8 g (100 mmol) of salt per day. This is best achieved by avoiding added salt, salty foods (especially processed foods) and eating foods cooked directly from natural ingredients.

Dietary changes

In addition to decreased salt intake, changes in diet should include the avoidance of meals high in saturated fats. Furthermore caloric reduction is necessary for weight reduction. Diets high in vegetables, fruits and fibre and low in total and saturated fat are recommended. Furthermore fish (high in omega 3 fatty acids which decrease the risk of cardiovascular diseases) is recommended in preference to chicken or meat.

Stress management

An individual's response to various stresses varies according to their personality type (type A being more stressed than type B). However, besides trying to lower exposure to stress, relaxation, physical activity and psychological measures can improve an individual's ability to cope with stresses.

Physical activity (see Ch. 9.1)

Regular rhythmic exercise such as brisk walking or swimming for 50–60 minutes, 3 to 4 times per week is used to lower blood pressure in borderline essential hypertensives. In addition, such exercise is used as adjunctive therapy in patients with moderate to severe essential hypertension in order to lower blood pressure, maximize efficacy of

Table 12.1.8. Choice of treatment approach

BP (mmHg)	Category	Group A	Group B	Group C
SBP 130–139 DBP 85–89	High normal	Lifestyle modification	Lifestyle modification	Pharmacological treatment[a]
SBP 140–159 DBP 90–99	Stage 1	Lifestyle modification (up to 12 months)	Lifestyle modification (up to 6 months)	Pharmacological treatment[a]
SBP ≥ 160 DBP ≥ 100	Stage 2 and 3	Pharmacological treatment[a]	Pharmacological treatment[a]	Pharmacological treatment[a]

Group A: Presence of risk factors = 0, presence of TOD = 0.
Group B: Presence of risk factors ≥1 not including diabetes mellitus, presence of TOD = 0.
Group C: Presence of risk factors 0 or ≥1 including diabetes mellitus, presence of TOD ≥1.
[a] With pharmacological treatment, lifestyle modification should always be recommended as an adjunctive treatment.

antihypertensive agents and reduce the number of antihypertensive medications required to control blood pressure.

Pharmacological treatments

The general pharmacological approaches to the treatment of essential hypertension are discussed in brief. The six main classes of agents used to lower blood pressure are diuretics, beta-adrenergic blocking agents, calcium channel blockers, ACE inhibitors, angiotensin II antagonists and alpha-adrenergic blockers. Recently aldosterone antagonists have been recommended. The use of antihypertensive agents is governed by the following principles:

- low dose then increased dose if no side effects
- use of low dose drug combinations rather than high dose of one drug to minimize side effects
- change drug class if have no response or adverse effects to first class of agent used
- use of drugs providing 24-hour efficacy.

Pharmacological approach to treatment of hypertension

Diuretic or beta-blocker
(other agents if specifically indicated; for example, ACE inhibitors specifically indicated in hypertensives with diabetes mellitus; calcium antagonists for hypertensives with isolated systolic hypertension)
↓
Increased dose of first drug
OR substitute with another drug of different class
OR add second drug of different class
↓
Substitute second drug
OR add third drug of different class
↓
Add third or fourth drug
OR evaluate further and/or refer

The choice of drug class is influenced by the presence of specific risk factors (Table 12.1.6) and target organ damage (Table 12.1.7) as well as the presence of other diseases.

The mechanisms of action of each of the classes of antihypertensive agents, their side effects and contraindications are briefly discussed and summarized in Tables 12.1.9 and 12.1.10.

Diuretics

This class of agent acts on the renal tubules to affect blood pressure primarily by causing sodium diuresis and depletion of blood volume. In addition, after prolonged use diuretics may reduce peripheral vascular resistance (mechanism currently unknown). The thiazide diuretics are the most frequently used and usually produce their effects on blood

Table 12.1.9. Mechanisms of action of different classes of anti-hypertensive agents

Class of agent	Mechanisms of action
Diuretics	↑ Na excretion ↓ blood volume ↓ total peripheral resistance
Beta-adrenergic blockers	↓ SNS = ↓ myocardial contractility = ↓ renin from JG cells
ACE inhibitors	↓ angiotensin II = ↓ vasoconstriction ↑ bradykinin = ↑ vasodilatation ↓ smooth muscle proliferation = ↓ vascular remodelling ↓ connective tissue synthesis = ↓ vascular remodelling
Angiotensin II receptor antagonists	↓ vasoconstriction ↓ smooth muscle proliferation = ↓ vascular remodelling ↓ connective tissue synthesis = ↓ vascular remodelling
Aldosterone receptor antagonists	↓ sodium and blood volume ↓ connective tissue synthesis = ↓ vascular remodelling
Calcium antagonists	↑ vasodilation
Vasodilators	Direct relaxation of smooth muscle
Central alpha agonists	Direct relaxation of smooth muscle

Table 12.1.10. Major contraindications

Class of agent	Contraindications
Diuretics	Diabetes mellitus Gout
Beta-adrenergic blockers	Bronchospasm (asthma, chronic obstructive pulmonary disease) Diabetes mellitus on hypoglycaemia agents Atrioventricular heart block Severe heart failure
ACE inhibitors and angiotensin II receptor antagonists	Pregnancy Hyperkalaemia Bilateral renal artery stenosis
Aldosterone receptor antagonists	Hyperkalaemia Bilateral renal artery stenosis
Central acting calcium antagonists	Atrioventricular heart block Previous myocardial infarct
Central alpha agonists	Depression

pressure within 3 to 4 days. The most frequent side effects of thiazide diuretics are hypokalaemia due to potassium loss, hyperuricaemia due to uric acid retention and carbohydrate intolerance. Hence plasma potassium concentrations must be monitored and supplemented if necessary. In addition, thiazide diuretics are contraindicated in patients with gout (hyperuricaemia) and insulin resistance or diabetes mellitus. To minimize potassium loss, potassium-sparing diuretics such as spironolactone (aldosterone receptor antagonist), triamterene and amiloride (which both impede sodium reabsorption) can be used.

Beta-adrenergic blocking agents

These agents block beta-adrenergic receptors and thereby block the effects of the sympathetic nervous system on the heart. Consequently cardiac output is reduced and arterial pressure lowered. In addition, these agents block the effects of the SNS on the RAAS in that they block the release of renin from *juxtaglomerular* (JG) cells. These agents are useful in conjunction with diuretics because the latter often cause a rise in plasma renin concentrations. Furthermore, beta-adrenergic blockade counteracts the reflex increase in myocardial contractility associated with vascular smooth muscle relaxing agents (see vasodilators). Beta-adrenergic blockade can aggravate asthma, and hence is contraindicated in susceptible individuals. Cardioselective (beta$_1$-blockers) may be safer than non-selective beta-blockers in patients with bronchospasm. Furthermore, as beta-adrenergic blockers inhibit the SNS response to hypoglycaemia they must be used with caution in patients with diabetes mellitus who are receiving hypoglycaemic therapy. As previously discussed (see management of chronic heart failure), beta-adrenergic blockers must be used with caution in patients with severe heart failure.

Angiotensin-converting enzyme inhibitors

As their name implies, this class of agents inhibit the action of angiotensin-converting enzyme (ACE) thereby reducing the production of the potent vasoconstrictor angiotensin II. In addition, by blocking the action of ACE they prevent the breakdown of the potent vasodilator bradykinin. Hence vasoconstriction is *diminished* and vasodilatation enhanced. In addition to their immediate effects, by reducing the concentration of angiotensin II this class of agent has important effects on vascular remodelling. The long-term benefits of ACE inhibitors are the prevention of smooth muscle proliferation, connective tissue synthesis and hence vascular and cardiac remodelling.

Angiotensin II receptor antagonists

These agents produce similar effects to ACE inhibitors by blocking the receptors for angiotensin II. They are specifically indicated for patients who cannot tolerate ACE inhibitors because they do not produce the ACE inhibitor-induced dry cough.

Aldosterone receptor antagonists

Aldosterone receptor antagonists lower blood pressure by producing a sodium diuresis (in exchange for potassium retention) and hence decreasing blood volume. In addition, they block the effects of aldosterone on connective tissue synthesis and vascular remodelling.

Calcium channel blockers

All calcium channel blockers (cardiac and vascular) inhibit calcium channels in vascular smooth muscle thereby producing potent vasodilator effects. As cardiac calcium channel blockers also inhibit myocardial calcium channels thereby decreasing myocardial contractility and heart rate, they are contraindicated in patients with atrioventricular heart block or left ventricular dysfunction.

Vasodilators

These agents cause relaxation of vascular smooth muscle (e.g. hydralazine) via mechanisms which are independent of the SNS. Their main actions are on the endothelium. However, the efficacy of hydralazine is offset by reflex increases in SNS activity which augments heart rate and cardiac output.

Central alpha agonists

Central alpha agonists reduce blood pressure by directly producing smooth muscle relaxation. These agents, however, commonly cause depression as a side effect.

HYPERTROPHIC CARDIOMYOPATHY

Hypertrophic cardiomyopathy (HCM) is a genetic cardiac disease which has a relatively high frequency of 1 in 500 among the general population. HCM is inherited as a mendelian autosomal dominant trait and is caused by mutations in any one of 10 genes, each of which encode for proteins of the cardiac sarcomere (i.e. components of myosin, actin, troponin or tropomyosin). The physical similarity of these proteins has resulted in the diverse HCM spectrum being regarded as a single disease entity and primary sarcomere disorder. The clinical diagnosis of HCM is established most easily and reliably with two-dimensional echocardiography. HCM is defined as the presence of a hypertrophied (left ventricular wall thickness (LVWT) >12 mm in males, and LVWT >11 mm in females) but non-dilated left ventricular chamber (LVEDD <55 mm) in the absence of another cardiac or systemic disorder which is capable of producing the magnitude of left ventricular hypertrophy that is evident. HCM may be initially suspected because of the presence of a heart murmur, positive family history, new symptoms or abnormal ECG pattern. The mechanisms by which disease-causing mutations cause left ventricular hypertrophy and the HCM disease state are as yet unresolved. The clinical course of HCM can be divided into three subgroups, which progress as indicated below:

- abnormal genotype present but phenotype (clinical manifestation) absent
- no symptoms or mild symptoms of heart failure
  - atrial fibrillation
  - high risk of sudden death

- progressive heart failure symptoms
  - atrial fibrillation
  - high risk of sudden death.

HCM is heterogeneous with respect to presentation and prognosis. In most patients HCM confers little or no disability and hence a normal life expectancy. Indeed overall HCM confers an annual mortality of only about 1%. The majority of patients with HCM (55%) do not demonstrate any of the acknowledged risk factors in this disease and hence it is exceedingly uncommon for such patients to die suddenly. The subset of patients who are at highest risk constitute about 10 to 20% of patients with HCM. Highest risk for sudden death in HCM has been associated with any of the following clinical markers:

- prior cardiac arrest
- spontaneous sustained ventricular tachycardia
- family history of premature HCM related death
- hypotensive blood pressure response to exercise
- extreme left ventricular hypertrophy with left ventricular width ⩾30 mm
- multiple and repetitive or prolonged bursts of non-sustained ventricular tachycardia
- syncope (faint), particularly when exertional or recurrent.

Sudden death occurs most commonly during mild exertion or sedentary activities but is not infrequently related to vigorous physical exertion. Indeed, HCM is the most common cause of cardiovascular sudden death in young people, including trained competitive athletes. As it is an inherited disorder and not an acquired disorder, it is responsible for the majority of sudden deaths in young people (<35 years of age). The often asymptomatic nature of the disease makes it largely unnoticed and hence potentially dangerous. As such the first indication of HCM often comes about when an athlete collapses on the sports playing field. Exercise does not worsen the condition, but can bring about its manifestation, in that symptoms of HCM generally are only apparent when large demands are placed on the heart, for example during physical exertion.

Although healthy competitive athletes also have enlarged hearts (termed the athletic heart), a healthy adolescent athlete's heart can be distinguished from that of an adolescent athlete or non-athlete with HCM. Firstly only a minority of athletic hearts have LVWT >12 mm and secondly in the athlete's heart the left ventricular hypertrophy is most often accompanied by left ventricular chamber enlargement (in HCM the chamber diameter is either normal or reduced). In other words the value of the left ventricular wall thickness to radius ratio remains normal in the athlete's heart (both LVWT and chamber diameter increase), but is increased in persons with HCM (LVWT increases and chamber diameter

is unchanged or reduced). The athletic heart (which develops in response to chronic regular exercise training) regresses fairly rapidly once exercise is ceased. Furthermore, this form of hypertrophy has not been shown to be associated with any clinical cardiovascular abnormalities.

Because of the high risk of sudden death in young athletes associated with HCM, pre-season health screenings including echocardiography are currently routinely performed in athletes in the USA. Subjects with HCM should not be encouraged to exercise unless their condition is clinically stable. For patients with symptoms of heart failure pharmacological intervention (beta-blockers, calcium channel blockers and diuretics) is recommended. Those patients who are at high risk of sudden death (see above), are treated surgically (implantable cardioverter defibrillator). As discussed in Chapter 9.1, currently exercise therapy is only recommended for patients with chronic heart failure which is congestive, ischaemic or idiopathic in origin. Hence, the rehabilitation practitioner is unlikely to encounter patients with diagnosed HCM.

REFERENCES AND FURTHER READING

Beevers G, Lip GYH, O'Brien E (2001) The pathophysiology of hypertension. BMJ 322: 912–916.

Beilin LJ (1994) Non-pharmacological management of hypertension: optimal strategies for reducing cardiovascular risk. J Hypertens 12 (Suppl 10): S71–S81.

DiBianco R (1994) The changing syndrome of heart failure: an annotated review as we approach the 21st century. J Hypertens 12(Suppl 4): S73–S87.

Eagle KA, Haber E, DeSanctis RW, Austen WG (1989) The Practice of Cardiology. Boston: Little, Brown and Company.

Fauci AS, Braunwald E, Isselbacher KJ, et al. (1998) Harrison's Principles of Internal Medicine, 14th edn. New York: McGraw-Hill.

Fox SI (1996) Human Physiology. Dubuque, IA: Times Mirror.

Guidelines Subcommittee of the World Health Organization–International Society of Hypertension (1999) 1999 World Health Organisation-International Society of Hypertension guidelines for the management of hypertension. J Hypertens 17: 151–183.

Hunt SA, Baker DW, Chin MH, et al. (2001) ACC/AHA guidelines for the evaluation and management of chronic heart failure in the adult: executive summary. Circulation 104: 2996–3007.

Leiter LA, Abbott D, Campbell NRC, et al. (1999) Recommendations on obesity and weight loss. CMAJ 160(Suppl 9): S7–S12.

Maron B (2002) Hypertrophic cardiomyopathy. A systematic review. JAMA 287: 1308–1320.

National Institutes of Health (1997) The Sixth Report of the Joint National Committee on Prevention, Detection, Evaluation and Treatment of High Blood Pressure. NIH Publication No. 98-4080.

Sharma S, Maron BJ, Whyte G, et al. (2002) Physiologic limits of left ventricular hypertrophy in elite junior athletes: relevance to differential diagnosis of athlete's heart and hypertrophic cardiomyopathy. J Am Coll Cardiol 40: 1431–1436.

The Circulatory System: Blood and Haemodynamic Disorders

Delva Shamley

HISTOLOGY OF ARTERIES AND VEINS

The vascular system is primarily responsible for the transport of oxygen and nutrients to the tissues and the transport of carbon dioxide and other metabolic waste products from the tissues. It is also involved in temperature regulation and the transport of hormones and cells (e.g. lymphocytes). The vascular system comprises a circuit of vessels ensuring the continuous flow of blood between the heart pump and the tissues of the body. It comprises two systems:

1. The *arterial system* directs blood towards the *capillaries*, which are the main sites for the exchange of gases and metabolites between tissues and blood.
2. The *venous system* returns blood from the capillaries to the heart for re-oxygenation and cleansing.

The vessels of the circulatory system have a common basic structure (Figs 12.2.1 and 12.2.2):

- An inner lining consisting of a single layer of flattened epithelial cells called the *endothelium*. This layer of cells is supported by a basement membrane and thin connective tissue, known as the *tunica intima*. Lying in the connective tissue of the tunica intima are venules, arterioles, capillaries (the blood flow to and from the vessel wall) and components of glands. As vessels get smaller in size (i.e. approaching capillaries) the tunica intima decreases in connective tissue content.
- An intermediate muscular layer, the *tunica media*. This smooth muscle layer is thicker in larger vessels than smaller vessels (generally totally absent from capillaries) and is always thicker in arteries than in veins. When stimulated the smooth muscle layer is responsible for the changes in vessel diameter.
- An outer supporting layer called the *tunica adventitia*. This is a connective tissue layer containing collagen fibres, varying amounts of elastin fibres (greatest in large arteries) and blood vessels. Blood vessels found in the tunica adventitia supply the walls of blood vessels with their own nutrients and are called *vasa vasorum*.

DISORDERS OF THE VENOUS SYSTEM

Chronic venous disease

The clinical spectrum of chronic venous disease (CVD) spans telangiectasis (a vascular lesion formed by dilatation of a group of small superficial blood vessels) and varicose veins through oedema, dermatitis, ulceration and pain. Patients also complain of leg heaviness, aching or night-time calf cramps. Both genetic and environmental conditions favour the development of the disease. CVD is one of the most common diseases of developed nations, affecting as many as 50% of the population in one form or other. A clinical classification scheme has therefore been developed (Table 12.2.1) to allow uniform diagnosis and comparison of patient populations.

CVD can be classified as:

1. congenital – present at birth
2. primary – valvular disorders with no clearly identifiable mechanism of venous dysfunction
3. secondary – usually follows from deep venous thrombosis.

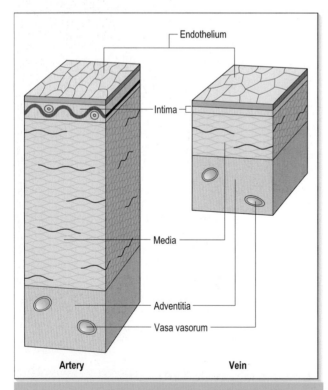

Figure 12.2.1. General structure of the wall of a blood vessel. (Reproduced with permission from Stevens and Lowe, 1996.)

Economic costs of venous ulceration

Annual healthcare costs for venous ulcerations are estimated to be 290 million pounds in the UK, 420 million deutsche marks in Germany, and 1 billion dollars in the USA.

Social costs of venous ulceration

Although more difficult to measure patients have reported fear, social isolation, anger, depression and a negative self-image.

Clinical manifestations are a result of *ambulatory venous hypertension*. This is the body's inability to reduce venous pressure when walking in an upright position. Current knowledge describes valvular reflux, venous obstruction and calf muscle pump dysfunction as the physiological explanations for the maintenance of this high pressure on ambulation.

Primary venous disorders

These include telangiectasis (small superficial veins), reticular varicosities (medium size veins in the connective tissue beneath the epithelium) and varicose veins (large veins in the connective tissue beneath the skin). All have non-functional incompetent valves and valvular reflux appears to be the haemodynamic cause of primary disorders. Valvular reflux itself has two potential causes:

1. Valvular incompetence. Incompetent valves have been shown to develop simultaneously in many different areas of the vein. These may include superficial (telangiectasis), perforating veins (reticular varicosities and deep veins

(varicose veins). When all three levels of veins are involved it is usually associated with skin changes and ulcerations.

2. Vein wall defects. Elastic tissue disruption and reduced elastin content have been shown by some investigators to

Table 12.2.1.   Clinical classification of chronic venous disease

Class 0	No visible or palpable signs of venous disease
Class 1	Telangiectasias or reticular veins
Class 2	Varicose veins
Class 3	Oedema
Class 4	Skin changes ascribed to venous disease (e.g. pigmentation, venous eczema, lipodermatosclerosis)
Class 5	Skin changes, as defined above, with healed ulceration
Class 6	Skin changes, as defined above, with active ulceration

Adapted from the International Consensus Committee on Chronic Venous Disease. Reporting standards in venous disease: An Update. J Vasc Surg 21: 635–645, 1995. Reproduced with permission.

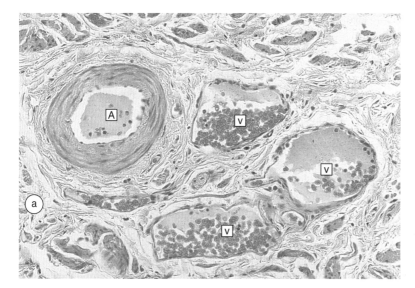

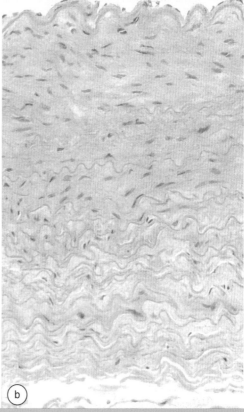

Figure 12.2.2.   Small and large arteries. (a) This photomicrograph shows a small muscular artery (A) cut in transverse section, together with distended thin-walled small veins (V). (b) Micrograph showing a typical large elastic artery (e.g. aorta), at high magnification. The media (M) is composed of alternate layers of pale pink smooth muscle fibres and laminae of wavy intensely pink, elastic tissue. (Reproduced with permission from Biophoto Associates.)

be correlated to refluxing segments of the vein wall. This could lead to weakening and dilation of the vein wall resulting in separation of the valve leaflets and the subsequent reflux of blood on standing.

Two forces act on the venous system which in the presence of the above two morphological changes results in venous dilatation and elongation.

1. *Gravitational force (hydrostatic pressure).* This is the weight of the blood column from the right atrium to the affected vein via incompetent valves.
2. *Muscle pump (hydrodynamic force).* This pressure usually propels blood through open deep valves towards the heart. However, when valves in perforated veins fail, this force is exerted on unsupported subcutaneous veins and venules in the epidermis. Large pressures are therefore exerted on these compromised vessels in a pulsatile manner.

Progression of CVD from mild symptoms to skin changes and ulceration (Fig. 12.2.3) is usually associated with venous volume expansion, increased reflux and progressive ambulatory venous hypertension.

Varicose veins

Varicose veins are distended and have lost their mechanical properties (Fig. 12.2.4). They are characterized by dilatation, tortuosity and elongation. Histological studies have shown patches of vein wall thickening which extend into the media (muscle layer). The thickened area is characterized by the presence of a *neointima* containing smooth muscle cells and increased collagen and elastin fibres. Blood stasis, venous hypertension, hormonal impregnation and changes in shear stress all contribute to the development of varicose veins.

Blood stasis appears to be related to the fact that the smooth muscle cells lose their contractile ability, leading to an increased hydrostatic load (gravitational forces) and venous congestion with increased capillary hydrostatic pressure (Fig. 12.2.5). This leads to fluid exudation in the

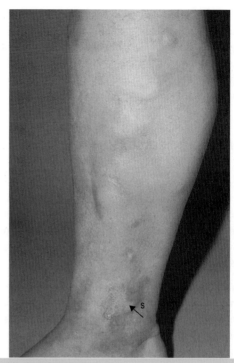

Figure 12.2.4.   Skin changes associated with chronic venous insufficiency. The leg is pigmented around the ankle and the tissue is woody on palpation (lipodermatosclerosis). A healed varicose ulcer (S) is seen above the medial malleolus (arrowed). (Reproduced with permission from Burkitt and Quick, 2001.)

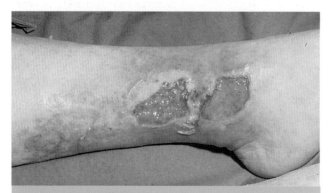

Figure 12.2.3.   Chronic leg ulcers. The characteristic appearance and location of chronic leg ulcers on the medial side of the leg just above the ankle. (Reproduced with permission from Stevens and Lowe, 2000.)

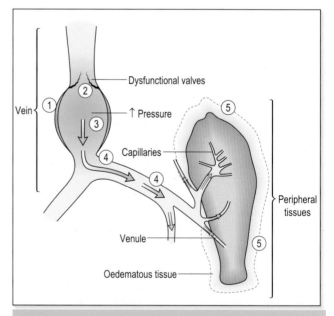

Figure 12.2.5.   Blood stasis on standing. 1, Loss of smooth muscle contraction. 2, Pooling of blood. 3, Increased pressure. 4, Blood reflux towards tissues. 5, Development of oedema.

tissues and the development of oedema. Early in vitro evidence suggests that blood stasis in veins leads to an oxygen deficit across the vein which in turn stimulates an inflammatory response (see Ch. 1 for detail of the inflammatory response). This response is marked by the arrival and adherence of neutrophils to the endothelium. The neutrophils stimulate endothelial cells to release oxygen free radicals and other inflammatory mediators, hydrolases and proteases, all of which may damage the extracellular matrix. These in vitro results are supported by in vivo results showing high levels of neutrophils in CVD patients presenting with blood stasis.

The stasis-induced hypoxia also stimulates the release of growth factors which change a contractile smooth muscle cell into a non-contractile muscle cell capable of synthesizing extracellular matrix. These growth factors include fibroblast growth factor (FGF), platelet growth factor (PGF$_{2\alpha}$) and transforming growth factor (TGF-β). Several growth factors also have chemotactic properties and attract smooth muscle cells into the intima where they continue to lay down extracellular matrix contributing to the thickening of the vein wall.

Indications for surgical intervention for varicose veins

Aesthetic appearance
Ankle hyperpigmentation
Leg heaviness
Aching/Pain
Early onset leg fatigue
Superficial thrombophlebitis
External bleeding
Lipodermatosclerosis
Atrophie blanche
Venous ulcer

Secondary venous disorders

Secondary CVD most commonly occurs following an episode of deep vein thrombosis (DVT) and is known as *post-thrombotic syndrome*. After an episode of acute DVT, patency of the lumen is established in 50–55% of cases within 3–9 months. Recanalization of the lumen involves spontaneous destruction of the thrombus and appears to be dependent on the:

- degree of activated coagulation
- extent to which fibrinolysis (breakdown of collagen) is inhibited by *plasminogen activator inhibitor* (PAI-1).
- level of anticoagulant given to the patient, e.g. warfarin, heparin.

In 33–59% of cases the thrombosis and recanalization process results in valvular damage and reflux. Development of incompetent valves may be due to:

- the rate of recanalization – patients experiencing earlier recanalization have a lower incidence of valvular incompetence
- the number of recurrent episodes of thrombosis
- persistent proximal obstruction: this may also be responsible for the development of reflux in uninvolved segments of the vein.

Both the extent of the reflux due to incompetent valves and the number of segments involved determine the clinical presentation of the syndrome.

Post-thrombotic skin changes (including ulceration) are commonly associated with:

- persistent obstruction of the popliteal vein
- reflux in deep veins, particularly popliteal and posterior tibial
- superficial venous reflux whether associated with deep vein thrombus or not.

PERIPHERAL ARTERIAL DISEASE (PAD)

Peripheral arterial disease most commonly results from atherosclerosis of the distal aorta or arteries of the pelvis or lower limbs. PAD has traditionally been considered as an ageing process but more recently identification of the disease in young adults (second decade) has challenged this theory. For a number of reasons (including lack of reporting by patients and lack of diagnosis by doctors) it is generally considered that the incidence and prevalence of this disease are underestimated. However, a number of studies suggest that the disease increases from 2/1000/year at the age of 30 years, to 6/1000/year at age 60 and 7/1000/year at age 70 and over, and occurs in: 0–2% at age <40, 0.5–2.5% at age 50, 1–4.5% at age 60 and 2–9% at age 70. The disease is less prevalent in Indo-Asians and Afro-Caribbeans than in Caucasians in spite of a higher incidence of the classical risk factors.

The presence of PAD is associated with the presence of coronary artery disease and cardiovascular disease (see Ch. 12.1). Patients with PAD therefore have a high risk of heart attack or stroke, raising the importance of early detection methods. Knowledge of the underlying pathophysiological mechanisms is currently the subject of intense research activity. Most notably for rehabilitation, recent studies have explored the effect of chronic ischaemia due to arterial insufficiency on skeletal muscles of patients with PAD.

Key risk factors for PAD

- Male gender (recent evidence has raised some doubts about this factor)
- Ageing

- Family history
- Diabetes
- Smoking
- High levels of fibrinogen
- Abnormal lipid profile
- Hypertension.

Pathogenesis of atherosclerosis

Atherosclerosis of arteries occurs in many sites in the body. In the lower limbs atherosclerotic plaques occur most commonly in the proximal portion of the arteries, at bifurcations and sites of atherogenesis.

Atherosclerotic changes in the distal abdominal aorta are greatest and appear to precede those in the coronary arteries.

Damage to the endothelial surface can be caused by:

1. mechanical forces (e.g. hypertension)
2. metabolic factors (e.g. hyperlipidaemia, diabetes)
3. immune response
4. inflammatory response.

The cellular mechanisms thought to lead to plaque formation on the endothelium appear to be triggered by the generation of free oxygen radicals during the above processes resulting in:

1. increased endothelial permeability
2. stimulation of cytokine expression
3. stimulation of adhesion molecule expression, e.g. selectins, which facilitates the binding of monocytes and leucocytes to the endothelium
4. migration of activated monocytes into the subendothelial connective tissue and release of chemokines which attract macrophages into the intima; macrophages also release a tissue factor which stimulates clot formation in plaques and their destabilization from the endothelial wall
5. platelet adherence to the plaque and release of thrombogenic factors, e.g. thrombin, serotonin
6. release of platelet-derived growth factor which is partly responsible for the growth of the smooth muscle in the wall of the artery, creating fibrous plaques.

These mechanisms result in the focal accumulation of lipids, carbohydrates, blood and blood products, fibrous

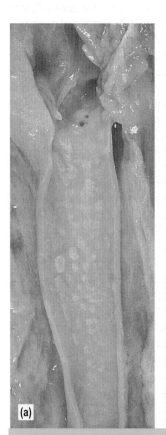 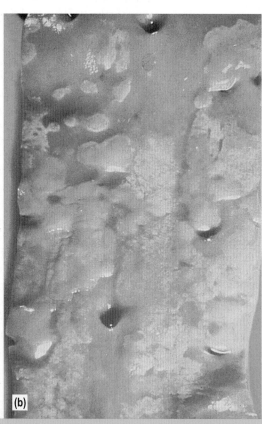 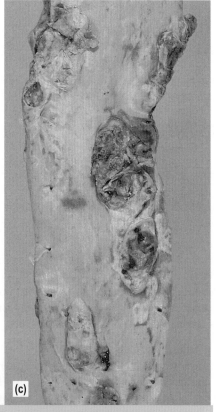

Figure 12.2.6.   Lesions of atherosclerosis. (a) Multiple fatty streaks in the carotid artery of a 39-year-old man. (b) Large fibrolipid plaques in the abdominal aorta of a 64-year-old man with extensive atherosclerosis. (c) Complicated aortic atherosclerosis in a 73-year-old woman. (Reproduced with permission from Underwood, 2000.)

tissue, calcium deposits and changes in the media (muscle layer) of the artery. Atherosclerotic plaques are of two major types:

1. characterized by prominent proliferation of cells with small accumulation of lipids
2. characterized by mostly intracellular and extracellular lipid accumulation and a small amount of cellular proliferation.

Patients with PAD typically have multiple atherosclerotic lesions often in different vessels (Figs 12.2.6 and 12.2.7). Smokers have more extensive, raised lesions than non-smokers and women have a greater number of fatty streaks in the abdominal aorta than men but not in the coronary arteries.

Haemodynamics of PAD

The clinical manifestations of PAD result from the reduction of blood flow to the limbs. The main factor contributing to the altered haemodynamics (turbulence) is the extent of arterial stenosis. The degree to which normal laminar blood flow in arteries becomes turbulent depends on:

- the length of the stenosis
- peripheral resistance
- the extent to which collateral blood flow is being utilized to compensate for the stenotic vessel.

At rest a patient may therefore be able to maintain normal flow in the presence of a stenosis by reducing peripheral resistance (peripheral vasodilation), rendering the effect of the stenosis negligible. In fact stenosis only becomes notable at rest with a reduction in arterial diameter of >80%. During exercise, however, there is a much larger pressure drop over the stenotic area and the body's ability to compensate may be compromised by inadequate vascular bed reserve, vasodilatory potential and development of collateral flow. In spite of the normal physiological response of peripheral vasodilation during exercise, studies have shown a drop in arterial blood index (ABI = blood gas levels) in patients with PAD, indicating, among other things, an inadequate collateral flow.

The effect of PAD on skeletal muscle

The ability to carry out exercises in the presence of PAD depends very much on the degree to which revascularization (regrowth of vessels) occurs. There are a number of metabolic indicators which provide information on the extent of muscle damage and the subsequent ability to carry out exercises. For example, ischaemia associated with atherosclerosis has the following affects on skeletal muscle:

1. Interrupted oxidative metabolism with the accumulation of lactate and intermediates of oxidative metabolism such as acylcarnitines. Accumulation of acylcarnitines has been shown to be a better indicator of exercise performance than ABI in patients with PAD.
2. Damage to mitochondrial DNA (4977-dp deletion) of skeletal muscle which has been found in unaffected limbs as well. The theory is that PAD might accelerate mitochondrial mutations in general.
3. Distal denervation which has been found in association with the loss of type II fibres. Type II fibres also have large numbers of mitochondria and may therefore be subjected to both the denervation and DNA depletion effects.

Exercise rehabilitation of patients with PAD (including patients presenting with claudication) should include walking, as walking is able to reverse some of these effects and improve blood flow to the lower limbs.

Key clinical points

- PAD is associated with a high risk of cardiovascular morbidity and mortality.

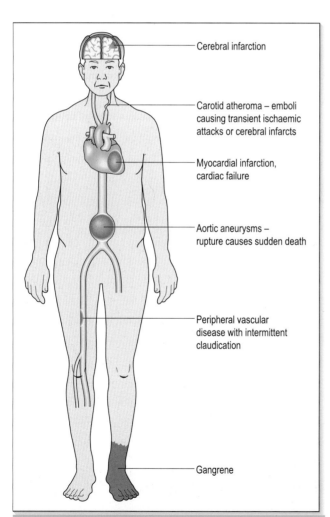

Figure 12.2.7.   The complications of atherosclerosis. (Reproduced with permission from Underwood, 2000.)

Labels in figure:
- Cerebral infarction
- Carotid atheroma – emboli causing transient ischaemic attacks or cerebral infarcts
- Myocardial infarction, cardiac failure
- Aortic aneurysms – rupture causes sudden death
- Peripheral vascular disease with intermittent claudication
- Gangrene

- Symptoms of PAD include intermittent claudication, leg cramps and tiredness in the legs. These symptoms may be aggravated by prolonged periods of sitting and by exercise or exertion and relieved by rest. When sitting the patient bends the hips and knees, temporarily occluding the involved vessel/s.

- During an ABI treadmill test, the release of nitric oxide causes vasodilation distal to the stenosis. However, the occlusion prevents an increase in blood flow so the pressure distal to the stenosis declines (ABI declines). This effect is seen typically in the case of inadequate collateral flow.

- Patients presenting with claudication also show evidence of skeletal muscle weakness and metabolic abnormalities.

- An exercise programme should be a part of every PAD patient's management.

- All patients with PAD whether symptomatic or not should be on anti-platelet therapy, e.g. aspirin.

Exercise for intermittent claudication

Current evidence suggests a 1 hour session 3×/week.
Using a treadmill, the patient walks to near maximal pain, stops long enough to relieve pain and then walks to near maximal pain again.

REFERENCES AND FURTHER READING

Abenhaim L, Kurz X (1997) The VEINES study: an international cohort study on chronic venous disorders of the leg. VEINES Group. Angiology 48: 59–66.

Araki CT, Back TL, Padberg FT, et al. (1994) The significance of calf muscle pump in venous ulceration. J Vasc Surg 20: 872–877.

Burkitt HG, Quick CRG (2001) Essential Surgery. Edinburgh: Churchill Livingstone.

Labropaulos N, Giannoukas AD, Nicolaides AN, et al. (1996) The role of venous reflux and calf muscle pump function in non-thrombotic chronic venous insufficiency. Correlation with signs and symptoms. Arch Surg 131: 403–406.

Meissner MH, Caps MT, Zierler BK, et al. (1998) Determinants of chronic venous disease after acute deep venous thrombosis. J Vasc Surg 28: 826–833.

Michiels C, Bouaziz N, Remacle J (2002) Role of the endothelium and blood stasis in the appearance of varicose veins. Int Angiol 21(1): 1–8.

Stevens A, Lowe J (1996) Human Histology. St Louis: Mosby.

Stevens A, Lowe J (2000) Pathology. St Louis: Mosby.

Tran NT, Meissner MH (2002) The epidemiology, pathophysiology and natural history of chronic venous disease. Semin Vasc Surg 15(1): 5–12.

Travers JP, Brookes CE, Evans J, et al. (1996) Assessment of wall structure and composition of varicose veins with reference to collagen, elastin and smooth muscle content. Eur J Vasc Endovasc Surg 11: 230–237.

Underwood JCE (2000) General and Systematic Pathology. Edinburgh: Churchill Livingstone.

Venturi M, Bonavina L, Annoni F, et al. (1996) Biochemical assay of collagen and elastin in normal and varicose veins. J Surg Res 60: 245–248.

The Respiratory System

13

Alex Hough

INTRODUCTION

Lung diseases and their effects on patients do not attract a high profile because their outcomes are not easy to monitor, they do not enjoy media attention and their association with smoking seems to limit support from public and professionals.

It would be convenient to divide lung diseases into those of airways and those of parenchyma, thus identifying them according to the functions of ventilation and gas exchange, but the body refuses to be neatly classified, and conditions such as chronic obstructive pulmonary disease (COPD) straddle the fence. Lung disorders are usually divided into obstructive and restrictive disease, plus those that fit neither or both categories.

Obstructive airway disease increases airflow resistance and the work of breathing, as indicated by decreased peak expiratory flow rates. Causes are:

- reversible factors, e.g. inflammation, bronchospasm, mucus plugging
- irreversible factors, e.g. fibrotic airway walls or floppy airways due to loss of the elastic recoil that normally supports them (Fig. 13.1)
- localized lesions, e.g. upper airway tumour or foreign body.

CHRONIC OBSTRUCTIVE PULMONARY DISEASE

Chronic bronchitis and emphysema usually occur together as COPD, with some patients having a preponderance of one or other disease entity. Asthma can overlap with COPD (Fig. 13.2) but is traditionally classified separately even though it is a chronic obstructive disease of the airways.

The natural history of COPD spans 20–50 years, but the disease is asymptomatic at first because changes in small airways barely affect total airways resistance. A morning cough is tolerable and considered normal amongst smokers, and patients may not seek medical advice until symptoms become troublesome, especially shortness of breath on exertion, which does not emerge until forced expiratory volume in 1 second (FEV_1) has declined to roughly half normal. Shortness of breath is a symptom associated with a variety of respiratory and other disorders such as heart disease, anaemia or pulmonary embolus, and lung function tests are necessary to confirm COPD (Fig. 13.3 and Fig. 13.4).

COPD is a slowly progressive disease characterized by fixed airways obstruction (FEV_1 <80% predicted, and FEV_1/forced vital capacity (FVC) <70%). It is classified as:

- mild – FEV_1 <80% predicted, smoker's cough, little or no breathlessness

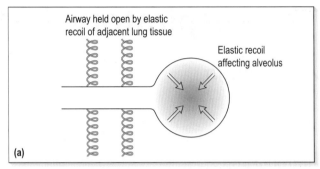

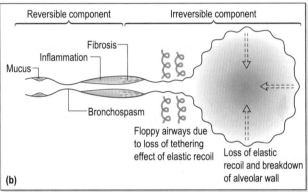

Figure 13.1.   Mechanism of airways obstruction: (a) normal; (b) COPD.

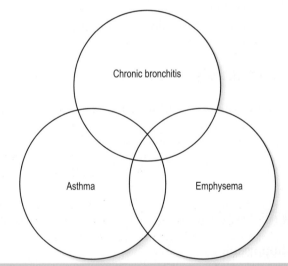

Figure 13.2.   Relationship between the commonest obstructive lung diseases.

- moderate – FEV_1 <60% predicted, breathless on moderate exertion
- severe – FEV_1 <40% predicted, breathless at rest, hyperinflation, peripheral oedema.

Most airways obstruction is irreversible, but medication may lead to some reversibility.

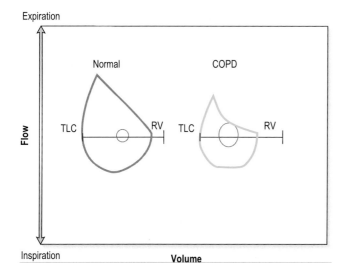

Figure 13.3.   Flow-volume loop on spirometry in COPD compared with a normal flow-volume loop. The normal individual performs a full inspiration, followed by a linear expiration pattern. In COPD, by comparison, the expiratory part of the curve has a characteristic concave appearance, representing the effect of small airway obstruction during the forced expiratory manoeuvre. TLC, total lung capacity (full inspiration); RV, residual volume (at full expiration). (Reproduced with permission from Forbes and Jackson, 2002.)

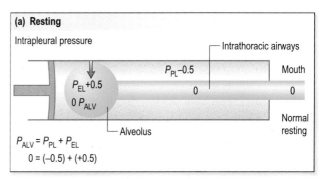

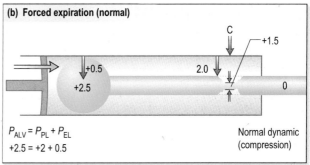

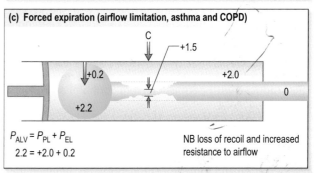

Figure 13.4.   Diagrams showing ventilatory forces. (a) During resting at functional residual capacity. (b) During forced expiration in normal subjects. (c) During forced expiration in a patient with COPD. The respiratory system is represented as a piston with a single alveolus and the collapsible part of the airways within the piston (see text). C, compression point; P_{ALV}, alveolar pressure; P_{EL}, elastic recoil pressure; P_{PL}, pleural pressure. (Reproduced with permission from Kumar and Clark, 2002.)

COPD is laden with gloomy statistics:

- It is the third commonest cause of certified illness in the UK.
- It is projected to be the fourth leading cause of death worldwide by 2020.
- It is reaching 'epidemic proportions' in the Third World as multinational companies offload their stocks of tobacco.
- Five-year mortality is 55%, which is equivalent to breast cancer.
- It is common in elderly people but often underdiagnosed and undertreated, tending to be met with therapeutic nihilism because of the widespread view that it is self-inflicted.
- It boasts 89 symptoms.
- It is largely preventable.

Causes

Not all smokers develop COPD, but smoking is the major cause. Other contributors are poverty, pollution, occupation, housing, climate, nutrition, childhood respiratory illness, in utero exposure to smoking or malnourishment and a genetic risk factor which augments susceptibility to COPD with smoking.

Pathophysiology

Cigarette smoke stimulates epithelial cells (in chronic bronchitis) and alveolar macrophages (in emphysema) to release inflammatory mediators which initiate the damage.

Chronic bronchitis

Chronic bronchitis is a disease of the airways. It is characterized by excess mucus secretion and a productive cough. The cough is called a smokers' cough in the early stages, but once mucus production has been excessive for 3 months a year over 2 years, this becomes the inadequate but traditional definition of chronic bronchitis.

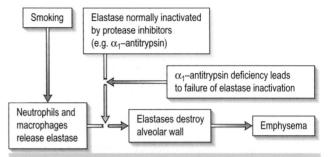

Figure 13.6.   Pathogenesis of emphysema. Normally, proteases secreted by inflammatory cells are inactivated by extracellular proteases, particularly alpha$_1$-antitrypsin. If proteases are not inactivated they can destroy lung tissue. Emphysema is caused by imbalance in the activity of proteases and protease inhibitors. Smoking increases release of proteases. Congenital lack of protease inhibitors is an important cause of excess protease activity. (Reproduced with permission from Stevens and Lowe, 2000.)

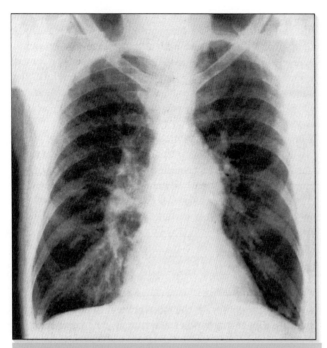

Figure 13.5.   Severe chronic bronchitis with marked hypoxaemia and pulmonary hypertension. In keeping with airways obstruction the lungs are of large volume. The main pulmonary artery (see below the aortic knuckle) is massively enlarged, as are the branches of the left and right pulmonary arteries. (Reproduced with permission from Souhami and Moxham, 2002.)

Repeated inhalation of tobacco smoke irritates the sensitive lining of the airways, leading to inflammation, mucus hypersecretion and sometimes bronchospasm. *Inflammation* is the key process. It causes narrowing first in the distal small airways and then the proximal large airways. Chronic inflammation leads to fibrotic changes and scarring. *Mucus hypersecretion* is associated with rampant increase in the size and number of mucus-secreting goblet cells. Excess mucus causes little overall airways obstruction and does not appear to affect mortality, but, along with the damaged epithelium, provides a medium for bacterial adherence and is associated with lung function decline. Breathlessness is a more troublesome symptom for the patient and is caused by airway narrowing, hyperinflation (Fig. 13.5), inefficient breathing, muscle weakness and hypermetabolism. *Bronchospasm*, when present, is thought to be caused by acetylcholine release due to inflammatory stimulation of the parasympathetic nervous system.

Emphysema

Emphysema usually occurs with chronic bronchitis and shares a similar aetiology, but is primarily a disease of alveoli and smallest airways, with secondary effects on other airways. Normally, emphysema is caused by inflammatory damage to alveoli from smoking. Occasionally, a genetic condition called alpha$_1$-antitrypsin deficiency (Fig. 13.6) occurs in white Europeans with an incidence similar to cystic fibrosis,

leading to a diagnosis of primary emphysema in the third to fifth decade of life.

Protein breakdown is the villain of emphysema, leading to erosion of alveolar septa, dilation of distal airspaces and destruction of elastic fibres. The walls of the terminal bronchi are normally supported by radial traction exerted by alveolar septa, but loss of elastic tissue means that during expiration, compressive forces are not opposed by radial traction, and the floppy airways collapse.

Types of emphysema are described and may coexist. Centrilobular emphysema affects mainly the respiratory bronchioles. Panlobular/panacinar emphysema affects the alveoli.

The obstructed airways of emphysema lead to hyperinflation (Fig. 13.7) by the following mechanisms:

1. Passive hyperinflation is caused by reduced elastic recoil, which allows the airways to collapse on expiration, causing gas trapping.
2. Dynamic hyperinflation is caused by the patient having to actively sustain inspiratory muscle contraction in order to hold open the airways. This unfortunate but necessary process is achieved at the cost of excess work of breathing (WOB), a barrel chest, reduced diaphragmatic contribution to breathing and a lung volume that can exceed the predicted total lung capacity.
3. Excess pressure also contributes to hyperinflation. Airways obstruction and reduced expiratory flow prevent expired air being fully expelled before the next inspiration starts, leading to positive pressure in the chest known as intrinsic positive end-expiratory pressure (PEEP) (Fig. 13.8), especially during exacerbations or with rapid breathing. The lungs are prevented from emptying to their usual relaxed volume between inflations by an average positive pressure of 2 cmH$_2$O. This imposes an extra threshold load at the start of inspiration because the

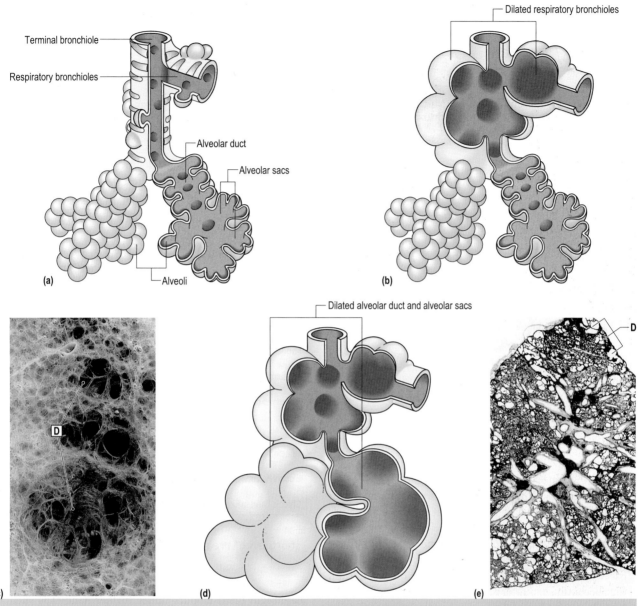

Figure 13.7. Generalized emphysema. (a) Normal distal lung acinus. (b) Centriacinar emphysema. (c) Centriacinar emphysema. (d) Panacinar emphysema. (e) Panacinar emphysema (Gough-Wentworth section). The normal lung acinus distal to the terminal bronchiole consists of respiratory bronchioles, alveolar ducts and terminal acini. In centriacinar emphysema, there is dilatation of the respiratory bronchioles at the centre of the acinus (b). This is seen in a very high power macroscopic photograph (c) of a portion of affected lung, in which the dilated air spaces (D) are surrounded by normal-sized alveoli. In panacinar emphysema (d), there is dilatation of the terminal alveoli and alveolar ducts, which later affects respiratory bronchioles, thereby affecting the whole acinus. The extent of this process in a whole lung can be seen in (e), which is a Gough-Wentworth preparation made by taking a slice, 1 mm thick, through a whole lung and mounting it on paper. The dilated air spaces (D) caused by emphysema are evident in all lobes. (Reproduced with permission from Stevens and Lowe, 2000.)

inspiratory muscles have to overcome this positive pressure before inspiration can begin. It also hinders cardiac output and impairs perfusion to the labouring inspiratory muscles. Stabilization occurs at volumes and pressures that are higher than normal, which reduces lung compliance. The distended alveoli require a greater than normal pressure in order to inflate.

Excess WOB is required to:

- overcome the resistance of obstructed airways
- assist expiration, which becomes active rather than passive when air has to be forced out through narrow airways, and which tends to increase intrinsic PEEP with the positive pressure created

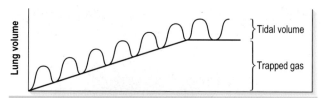

Figure 13.8. Development of intrinsic PEEP. The sloping line indicates functional residual capacity.

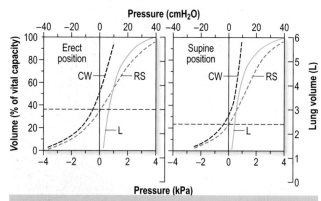

Figure 13.9. Pressure volume curve describing compliance of lung (L), chestwall (CW) and total respiratory system (RS). (Reproduced with permission from Sykes, 1999.)

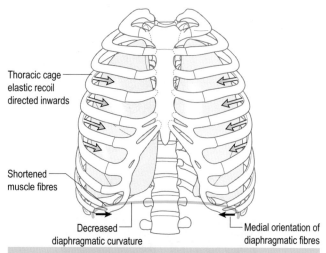

Figure 13.10. The detrimental effects of hyperinflation on the mechanics of breathing.

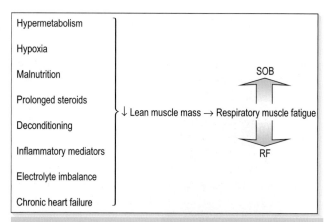

Figure 13.11. Muscle weakness in COPD. SOB, shortness of breath; RF, respiratory failure.

- sustain inspiratory muscle action throughout the respiratory cycle so that high lung volumes are maintained, with alveoli being opened at a high point on the compliance curve (Fig. 13.9)
- compensate for the altered geometry and interaction of the respiratory muscles, the flat diaphragm having to work paradoxically by pulling in the lower ribs on inspiration, thus becoming expiratory in action (Hoover's sign)
- compensate for loss of the bucket handle action of the ribs (Fig. 13.10)
- compensate for reversed action of rib cage recoil, which in the hyperinflated chest is directed inwards rather than outwards, thus resisting instead of assisting inspiration (Fig. 13.10)
- overcome the threshold resistance at the start of inspiration caused by intrinsic PEEP.

Some patients can only inhale by lifting up their entire rigid rib cage with their accessory muscles. These accessory muscles therefore have a dual role when unsupported arm activities are required. Excess use of accessory muscles increases the sensation of breathlessness because these muscles are richly supplied with muscle spindles and tendon organs to increase afferent feedback. Normal muscle is able to respond to increased load by hypertrophy, but an emphysematous

diaphragm often labours under further handicaps such as malnutrition, and diaphragmatic weakness is common.

Malnourishment, caused by excess energy demand and reduced energy supply, has been reported in 20–35% of stable patients and up to 70% of acute patients with COPD, mainly those with emphysema. This leads to cannibalism of the respiratory muscles for their protein, accelerating the process of emphysema and causing a direct association of malnutrition with mortality. COPD is more likely to develop in underweight men.

Malnutrition is one of a multitude of factors which weakens muscles. This leads to breathlessness (Fig. 13.11) and leg fatigue, which for some patients can be a greater problem than breathlessness in limiting exercise tolerance. The energy expenditure of food digestion and assimilation aggravates hypoxia, and hypoxia aggravates inflammation, which itself is related to weight loss. People with emphysematous disease

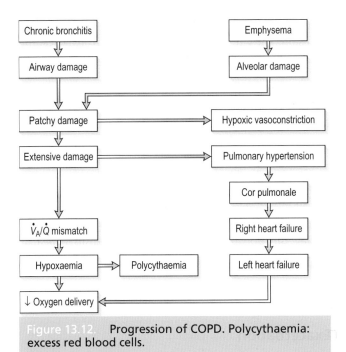

Figure 13.12. Progression of COPD. Polycythaemia: excess red blood cells.

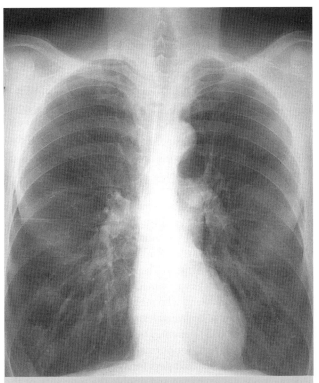

Figure 13.13. Cor pulmonale in a patient with COPD. Both pulmonary arteries are enlarged, and there is marked peripheral pruning of the pulmonary vessels. There is also a small pleural effusion on the right in the horizontal fissure. (Reproduced with permission from Forbes and Jackson, 2002.)

show more than twice the oxygen cost of breathing than those with chronic bronchitis.

Chronic bronchitis and emphysema

The gradual airway narrowing of chronic bronchitis, augmented by the floppy airways of emphysema, leads to uneven distribution of ventilation (Fig. 13.4). Damaged alveoli further hinder gas exchange, and anaerobic metabolism develops. The inexorable downhill path of advanced COPD is illustrated in Figure 13.12. Chronic hypoxia leads to compensatory proliferation of red cells, known as polycythaemia. This increases the oxygen-carrying capacity of blood at first, but once the packed cell volume reaches 55%, the thickened blood impairs oxygen delivery, burdens the heart, augments pulmonary hypertension and causes headaches. If the disadvantages of polycythaemia outweigh the advantages, haematocrit can be reduced by multiple venesections (blood-letting), exchange transfusion or haemodilution. Well-managed long-term oxygen therapy can stabilize or reverse polycythaemia.

Capillary destruction and widespread hypoxic pulmonary vasoconstriction further augment pulmonary hypertension. This increases the load against which the right ventricle must pump, leading to hypertrophy and dilation of the right ventricular wall, a condition known as cor pulmonale (Fig. 13.13). Once nocturnal oxygen saturation drops below 90%, right heart failure develops. Systemic blood pressure rises in order to overcome the increased right atrial pressure and maintain cardiac output. This process eventually strains the left ventricle and leads to left heart failure. Meanwhile lung damage continues (Plate IV; see plate section p xi), and death is usually due to inadequate gas exchange rather than cardiac involvement.

Once hyperinflation develops, this becomes a major cause of symptoms. The extra energy expenditure of breathing inefficiently, accompanied by the hypermetabolism of inflammation, is accompanied by reduced physical activity. Fatigue is widespread and sleep of poor quality.

In advanced disease, depression is 2.5 times higher than normal and is often undetected, possibly because fatigue and insomnia may be attributed to the disease itself.

Objectively, there is a rich tapestry of signs such as laboured breathing, a plethoric or cyanotic appearance, weight loss and/or oedema, barrel chest, forced expiration with pursed lip breathing, and prolonged expiration with an I:E ratio of 1:3 or 1:4. Soft tissue recession and other signs of laboured breathing are evident due to inspiratory effort and malnutrition. Patients may lean forward on their elbows to force the diaphragm into a more efficient dome shape and stabilize the shoulder girdle for optimum accessory muscle action. Auscultation demonstrates the crackles of chronic bronchitis or the quiet breath sounds of emphysema.

Gas exchange is preserved in the early stages, $\dot{V}_A/\dot{Q}$ match being maintained by hypoxic vasoconstriction and collateral ventilation. However, hypoxaemia gradually takes over, with nocturnal oxygen desaturation playing a damaging role: a third of patients who are not hypoxaemic when awake are hypoxaemic when asleep, and 90% of these show pulmonary hypertension despite no specific signs or symptoms, underscoring the importance of accurate oxygen therapy. FEV_1 decline accompanies disease progression and once it is below 1 litre, activities of daily living are impaired and 5-year survival is 50%. If hypoxaemia is out of proportion to FEV_1, sleep apnoea may also be present. Hypercapnia is a sign of advanced disease but can be tolerated for many months in the chronic state without affecting the central nervous system or destabilizing pH, so long as oxygenation is maintained. However, patients do not have to retain CO_2 to have severe airflow obstruction. The variation in blood gas response to COPD is represented by the spectrum of the 'pink puffer' (PP) patient, who maintains near-normal blood gases at the expense of breathlessness and weight loss, and the 'blue bloater' (BB) patient. The BB patient is less breathless, abandons the fight for normal blood gases, suffers more nocturnal hypoxaemia and pays for symptomatic relief with oedema, poor gas exchange and double the mortality of the PP patient.

It was originally thought that repeated hypoventilation in BB patients desensitized their chemoreceptors to hypercapnia so that they became dependent on low oxygen tension as a stimulus to breathe. However, there is no correlation of hypercapnia with ventilatory drive, and the purpose of hypoventilation may be to preserve the respiratory muscles by 'choosing' to rest them. This minimizing of breathlessness and fatigue has led to BB patients being considered physiologically wise.

The relevance to rehabilitation of the PP/BB spectrum is that PP patients in particular respond to breathlessness management techniques and tend to show the following characteristics:

- anxiety and physical tension
- tendency to desaturate on exercise
- counterproductive tendency to rush at activities.

Related pathologies

Osteoporosis is a significant problem in advanced COPD and should not await fracture for diagnosis. Contributing factors include malnutrition, smoking, steroids and inactivity. Other disorders associated with COPD are vascular disease and diabetes, which occur in 40% of patients.

The appearance of peripheral oedema is a turning point in the progression of COPD, indicating a 5-year survival of less than 50%. Oedema in COPD is caused by impaired renal perfusion. The gut lining is also sensitive to hypoxia, leading to the association of COPD with peptic ulceration. Oedema may also be associated with heart failure because half of all COPD patients aged over 50 have cardiovascular disorders due to the common aetiology of smoking.

Respiratory function tests are useful indicators of obstruction but relate weakly to breathlessness or functional impairment. However, once FEV_1 falls below 1 litre, most daily activities are affected. Peak flow is of some relevance but it measures airflow in early exhalation, which only reflects large airway function. Low gas transfer is a sensitive test for emphysema and distinguishes it from chronic bronchitis.

Exacerbation

Worsening symptoms over 48 hours indicate an exacerbation, which occurs on average one to four times a year, contributes to decline in lung function and leaves survivors with a reduced quality of life. Infection is a common cause, especially when patients are chronically colonized with multiple organisms, which may differ in the upper and lower airways. Viral infection is associated with 56% of exacerbations in hospitalized patients. Other causes are bacterial infection, air pollution, panic attacks and cold temperature.

Exacerbation causes increased airflow obstruction, hyperinflation, breathlessness and sometimes fever. A quarter of patients produce mucopurulent or purulent sputum, and mucus clearance is hampered by cilia rendered inefficient by damaged epithelium, airway collapse and abnormal hydration. Airflow obstruction requires recruitment of expiratory muscles to support ventilation, which compromises flow further by inducing airway collapse. Hospital mortality during exacerbations is 10%, or 25% if hypercapnic respiratory failure develops, and 40% die in the following year.

Physiological effects of medical management

Recommended treatment for each stage of severity is detailed in the British Thoracic Society Guidelines. The pathological process is irreversible, but the following have been found beneficial:

- Smoking cessation, which slows the damage and is the most important intervention, without which treatment is like running a bath without the plug.
- Oxygen therapy, which can reduce hypoxaemia and some of its effects such as oedema.

- Food supplementation, which improves pulmonary function and exercise capacity.
- Drug therapy (Chap. 15), which can ease symptoms.

Long-term oxygen reduces mortality for patients with persistent hypoxaemia at Pao_2 <8 kPa (60 mmHg), especially if they desaturate at night. Simple nutritional advice such as eating apples has been associated with fewer exacerbations. Bronchodilators reduce airflow obstruction in two-thirds of patients with chronic disease, thereby reducing hyperinflation and possibly breathlessness, but should be used only 'as required' because continuous use can worsen lung function, and if they are prescribed regularly, patients consume twice as much as when prescribed as required. A quarter of patients respond to theophylline. Anticholinergics can ease bronchospasm, dry secretions, reduce nocturnal desaturations and improve sleep. However, combination therapy with different classes of bronchodilator may be the most beneficial approach.

Steroids have been advised for exacerbations, but the inflammatory process in COPD is relatively resistant to steroids and in the chronic state steroids reduce airways obstruction in only 10% of patients. A short course is often as beneficial as a long one, and continued use is associated with myopathy.

Drug assessment should include quality of life scores and peak flow monitoring with sequential testing of different bronchodilators, steroids, combinations and delivery systems. Short-term reversibility studies should not be substituted for long-term assessment. Inhalers are indicated for acute and chronic disease unless nebulizers are objectively more effective.

Additional drugs used to manage COPD include:

- mucolytics, which are associated with reduced exacerbations
- drugs for breathlessness
- the hypnotic drug zolpidem, which may help COPD patients with disturbed sleep without affecting oxygenation or ventilation
- diuretics, which are widely used but may worsen hypercapnia.

In stable disease, quality of life is primarily affected by breathlessness, exercise limitation and the interaction of depression and fatigue. Depression relates to treatment failure and mortality is directly related to ability to cope, which may explain why education has been found to pay for itself nearly 5 times over. Pulmonary rehabilitation comprises education and exercise training (Chapter 9.2) and is the most

appropriate form of physiotherapy. For severe disease, non-invasive ventilation at home may help to unload the respiratory muscles and improve blood gases.

ASTHMA

Asthma is more common, more serious and more manageable than is generally thought. It shows the following trends:

- Asthma affects 5% of adults and 10–15% of children in the UK, its prevalence doubling over the final 2–3 decades of the twentieth century.
- It kills about 1600 adults and 20 children a year in the UK.
- Some GP practices treat less than half of their asthmatics, and up to half of those treated take only half their prescribed medication.
- Up to 86% of asthma deaths are considered preventable.

Age and gender vary. Asthma is more frequent in advanced age than in adults, but is often overlooked in this age range because of its association with younger people. Adolescence is a period when asthma may remit or may become more difficult to manage, and is the time when the male preponderance of childhood gives way to the female preponderance of adulthood.

Asthma is a chronic inflammatory condition of the airways, characterized by undue responsiveness to stimuli that are normally innocuous, a mechanism known as hyperreactivity (see Ch. 2). Airway narrowing usually reverses spontaneously or with treatment. The disease is distinguished by the variability and reversibility of its presentation, which makes evaluation of severity difficult, especially as the symptoms of wheeze, breathlessness and cough are general respiratory complaints. Asthma shares with COPD the pathology of small airways obstruction, and in elderly people it is sometimes difficult to distinguish between the two, but the differences are shown in Table 13.1 and in Figure 13.14.

Diagnosis is made from a history of recurrent attacks, then confirmed by respiratory function tests. If the peak expiratory flow ('peak flow') varies by more than 15%, either diurnally, after exercise, or after bronchodilator treatment, the patient is considered to have asthma. This should be confirmed by a 15% increase in FEV_1 after a 14-day trial of prednisolone. Induced sputum can also be diagnostic.

Causes

Allergy is a cause of asthma in 50% of patients, varying from 80% in childhood to 20% after middle age. Sensitization can begin in utero, especially if the fetus has a gene which causes atopy. Atopic people are those prone to allergy, as identified by a positive skin prick test. This can be modified subsequently by diet, allergens or infection. Allergens may initiate sensitization, enhance the allergic response or induce attacks.

Table 13.1. Distinguishing features of asthma and COPD

	Asthma	COPD
Smoking history	Not necessarily	Usually
May start in childhood	Yes	No
Onset	Variable	Slow
Atopy	50%	No
Timing of symptoms	Episodic, diurnal, seasonal	Minor fluctuations only
Provocation of symptoms	Weak stimulus, e.g. cold air	Strong stimulus, e.g. infection
Cough at night	Patient wakes coughing	Wakes then coughs
Bronchodilator response	Yes	Sometimes
Steroid response	Yes	Sometimes

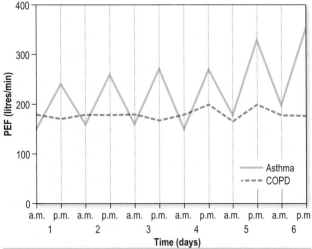

Figure 13.14. 'Morning dipping'. Serial recordings of peak expiratory flow (PEF) in patients with COPD and asthma. Note sharp overnight fall (morning dip) and subsequent rise during the day in patients with asthma, which does not occur in patients with COPD. (Reproduced with permission from Haslett et al., 2002.)

A 'hygiene theory' suggests that infections in early childhood, when the immune system is developing, protect against allergy. Antibiotics in the first 2 years of life limit this protection, possibly because they devour friendly gut flora which normally help educate the developing immune system. However, the hygiene theory is not always accepted, and viral infection in particular can cause asthma, either gradually or explosively. Viruses share with passive smoking a tendency to damage epithelium and make it more sensitive to allergens.

Contributing factors to the development of asthma include:

- the faeces of house-dust mite, tiny creatures who consume the dead skin of humans while multiplying in their bedding
- damp homes, which favour house-dust mite

- anxiety, which also influences symptom perception and management
- poverty
- tobacco smoke absorbed in utero, and later a history of a stressful birth, parents who smoke, anxious parents or lack of breastfeeding
- pollution such as oxidants, especially when air is stagnant
- poor diet, particularly lack of antioxidants such as vitamin C
- immediate or delayed food intolerance.

Pathophysiology

Three phases of response take place (Fig. 13.15):

1. *Sensitization* stage, which occurs in atopic people: exposure to allergens in fetal or early life stimulates production of excess immunoglobulin-E (IgE) antibodies in the serum. IgE becomes fixed to mast cells, which then react to antigens by releasing bronchoconstrictor mediators such as histamine. Serum IgE is five times greater in people with asthma than in those without. Once allergic asthma has developed, removal from the allergen, if delayed, does not always prevent continuing asthma.
2. *Hyperreactive* stage, which occurs with or without an allergic component: continued exposure to allergens, or response to other stimuli, leads to mast cell degranulation and release of inflammatory cytokines such as interleukins and eosinophils, bronchoconstrictor mediators such as histamine, and extra mucus. Chronic low-grade inflammation damages the surface epithelial layer, causing hyperreactivity of bronchial smooth muscles.
3. Bronchoconstrictor mediators and hyperreactive bronchial smooth muscles lead to exaggerated bronchoconstriction, i.e. *bronchospasm*, intermittently in response to a variety of stimuli.

The stimulus which can trigger an asthma attack may or may not be related to the original cause, e.g:

- foods such as dairy products, eggs, wheat, peanuts, fish, citrus fruits, additives, alcohol, cola or other acidic drinks
- environmental allergens such as warm-blooded pets or pollen
- other environmental irritants such as car exhaust, pesticides, active or passive smoking
- weather, especially change in temperature, or thunderstorms, which sweep up pollutants
- wine, orange juice or other drinks that contain sulphites
- certain drugs such as timolol (used for glaucoma), beta-blockers or aspirin
- anxiety, depression, frustrated expression of emotion and/or hyperventilation
- chest infection
- exercise without warm-up.

Impaired mucociliary transport continues after an exacerbation for longer than airflow obstruction, although this can be

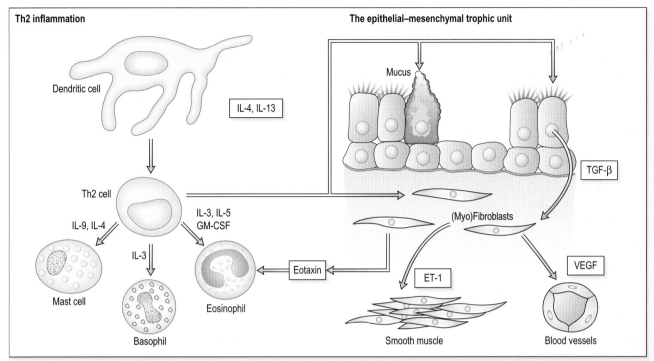

Figure 13.15. Pathogenesis of asthma. Antigen-presenting cells (dendritic cell) activate Th2 T-cells causing them to release cytokines which attract mast cells and eosinophils. IL-9 and IL-4 activate mast cells to release LTC$_4$, PGD$_2$ and histamine which act on smooth muscle and blood vessels. IL-3, IL-5 and GM-CSF attract eosinophils; these are also attracted by chemokines which act on type 3 C-C chemokine receptors (CCR-3, e.g. eotaxin, RANTES, MCP-1, -3 and -4). Activated eosinophils release LTC$_4$, MBP, ECP and peroxidase (EPX) which are toxic to epithelial cells. IL-4 and IL-13 produced by activated T-cells maintain the allergic reaction and cause mucus secretion and smooth muscle contraction. IL, interleukin; GM-CSF, granulocyte and macrophage colony-stimulating factor; RANTES, regulated upon activation, normal T-cell expressed and secreted; MBP, major basic protein; ECP, eosinophilic cationic protein; LTC$_4$, leukotriene C$_4$; MCP, monocytic chemoattractant protein; PGD$_2$, prostaglandin D$_2$; TGF-β, transforming growth factor-β; VEGF; vascular endothelial growth factor; ET-1, endothelin-1. (Reproduced with permission from Kumar and Clark, 2002.)

attenuated by sodium cromoglicate. Secretions are thicker and more difficult to clear than with other obstructive diseases.

Airflow obstruction in asthma is caused by inflammatory oedema and, in the acute phase, by bronchospasm and sometimes mucus plugging (Fig. 13.16). Persistent inflammation leads to fibrosis, causing further airflow obstruction and irreversibility. Heightened vascularity of submucosa is thought to impair nutrition, temperature regulation and humidification of the airway wall, and subsequent remodelling may hinder removal of inflammatory mediators.

The mechanism of asthma is thought to be localized because asthmatic recipients of transplanted normal lungs lose their asthma, while people who receive asthmatic lungs develop the disease.

Associated factors such as postnasal drip or gastro-oesophageal reflux (GOR) may be present, and need to be treated. GOR has been found in 62% of patients with stable asthma, even in the absence of oesophageal symptoms, and treatment of the reflux may improve asthma control. Asthma symptoms may occur at night, after meals, on lying down or after exercise. GOR may be cause or effect: it may cause asthma

by micro-aspiration of acid into the upper airway, or the asthma may be causing GOR by:

- prolonged coughing and wheezing causing excess intra-abdominal pressure
- bronchodilators causing lower oesophageal relaxation
- steroids increasing oesophageal acid.

Throat symptoms in someone with asthma may indicate GOR or hyperventilation syndrome.

For children, a useful screening tool is a free-running test in which spirometry is performed before and after an 8-minute outdoor run during which the pulse must exceed 170 for at least 6 minutes. A fall in FEV$_1$ of 10% or more, taken at 5, 10, 15 and 20 minutes post-exercise compared to pre-run, is indicative of asthma. From age 3 to adulthood, reversibility of FEV$_1$ following bronchodilators is diagnostic of asthma. Preschool children require tests without forced expiration.

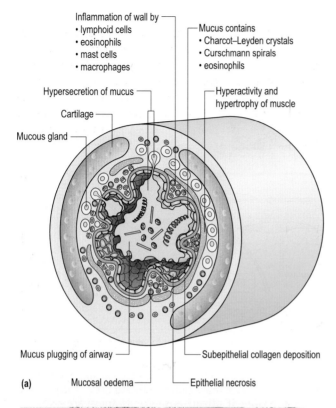

Inflammation of wall by
• lymphoid cells
• eosinophils
• mast cells
• macrophages

Mucus contains
• Charcot–Leyden crystals
• Curschmann spirals
• eosinophils

Hypersecretion of mucus

Hyperactivity and hypertrophy of muscle

Cartilage

Mucous gland

Mucus plugging of airway

Subepithelial collagen deposition

(a)   Mucosal oedema   Epithelial necrosis

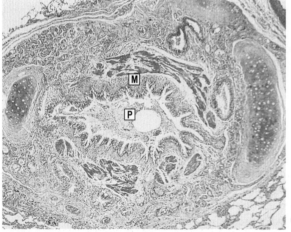

(b)

Figure 13.16. Structural changes in asthma. The main events that take place in the airways in asthma are shown diagrammatically (a) and histologically (b). There is bronchoconstriction due to increased responsiveness of bronchial smooth muscle (M); hypersecretion of mucus leading to plugging of airways (P); mucosal oedema leading to narrowing of airways; extravasation of plasma in submucosal tissues due to leakage from vessels; infiltration of bronchial mucosa by eosinophils, mast cells, lymphoid cells and macrophages; focal necrosis of airway epithelium; deposition of collagen beneath bronchial epithelium in long-standing cases. Sputum contains Charcot–Leyden crystals (derived from eosinophil granules) and Curschmann spirals (composed of mucus plugs from small airways). (Reproduced with permission from Stevens and Lowe, 2000.)

Classification and physiology of clinical features

Allergic asthma, known as *extrinsic*, usually occurs in early life. *Intrinsic* asthma develops in adulthood, shows normal IgE levels, and is more fulminant and less responsive to treatment. Classic features are wheeze, breathlessness, chest tightness and cough, particularly at night or in the early morning.

Mild chronic asthma

This manifests as an intermittent dry cough, often at night, or a morning wheeze once or twice a week. Peak flow varies by less than 25%. Even when asymptomatic, peripheral airflow resistance can be five times normal and severe attacks are possible. Deconditioning is common because of aversion to breathlessness.

Severe chronic asthma

This means frequent exacerbations and symptoms that affect quality of life. Psychosocial factors play a prominent role. Peak flow varies by more than 25%, and daily anti-inflammatory drugs are required.

Brittle asthma

One in 2500 asthmatics have severe and unstable chronic brittle asthma, a form which shows greatly fluctuating peak flows day and night, persistent symptoms despite multiple medications, and unpredictable dips in lung function. They need investigation for food intolerance and individual arrangements for direct hospitalization when needed.

Acute asthma

This reflects failure of preventive management and/or exposure to a relevant stimulus. Work of breathing is increased by airflow resistance up to 15 times normal, caused by bronchospasm of large airways and oedema of small airways. Resistance may be further increased by mucus plugging and breathing made inefficient by hyperinflation, and patients feel as if they are breathing through a narrow straw. $\dot{V}_A/\dot{Q}$ mismatch reduces Pao_2, and rapid breathing reduces $Paco_2$. There is chest tightness and sometimes chest pain, which is benign and self-limiting but may cause diagnostic confusion and patient anxiety. Objectively a wheeze can be heard, often without a stethoscope.

Monitoring by oximetry is usually adequate, but blood gases are required if Sao_2 (oxygen saturation in arterial blood) falls below 92% or peak flow drops below 30% predicted.

Severe acute asthma

This usually develops slowly, sometimes after several weeks of wheezing. Deterioration can be deceptive and even paradoxical: subjectively, there may be a blunted perception of dyspnoea and denial, and objectively, the patient may appear less distressed (but more drowsy) if the condition becomes

Table 13.2. Some features of acute asthma

	Severe	Life-threatening
Pa_{O_2}	↓	<8 kPa (60 mmHg)
Respiratory rate	>25	↓
Pa_{CO_2}	↓	>5 kPa (36 mmHg)
Pulse	>110	↓
Blood pressure	↑	↓
Pulmonary function	<50% predicted	<33% or unrecordable
Speech	Difficult	Impossible
Auscultation	Wheeze	Silent
Colour		Any change
Consciousness		Any change

severe. Medical help should be sought immediately if the patient shows the signs in Table 13.2 or the following:

- pallor or sweating
- peak flow <50% predicted, or <200 l/min
- ↓ response to bronchodilator
- as fatigue progresses, decreased respiratory effort and retention of Pa_{CO_2}, which is associated with FEV_1 <20% predicted
- silent chest on auscultation if airflow is too slow to oscillate the airways, and loss of wheeze
- hypotension, as venous return is impaired by the hyperinflated chest
- cyanosis or altered consciousness, which only occurs in 1% of cases but indicates grave illness.

If Pa_{CO_2} rises over 6.7 kPa (50 mmHg), intensive care is required. Hypoxia, dehydration, acidosis and hypokalaemia render the patient vulnerable to arrhythmias and cardiac arrest.

Very breathless patients cannot produce reliable peak flow or spirometry readings, and for those too breathless to speak, the manoeuvre can exacerbate bronchospasm.

Mucus plugging is invariably found in fatal asthma. Sudden deaths have been reported without exacerbation of airflow obstruction, in which case depressed mood and impaired respiratory drive have been implicated. Factors associated with preventable asthma deaths are thought to be behavioural rather than pharmacotherapeutic.

Status asthmaticus

This term is sometimes used interchangeably with severe acute asthma, but specifically describes an asthma attack prolonged over 24 hours, leading to dehydration, due to inability to drink and extra fluid loss from the respiratory tract, and exhaustion.

Asphyxic asthma

Otherwise known as 'catastrophic asthma', this attack leads to respiratory arrest within hours, or occasionally within minutes.

Exercise-induced asthma

Considered a sign of poorly controlled asthma, this is nevertheless present in 80% of asthma sufferers, and in some is the only manifestation of the disease. Hyperventilation during exercise, especially in cold weather, causes evaporation of airway surface liquid, hyperosmolality and heat loss, leading to bronchospasm. Bronchospasm occurs during or up to 10 minutes after exertion and recovery is usually complete 30 minutes later (Fig. 13.17). Preventive measures include

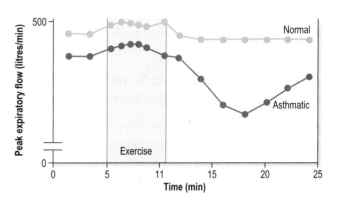

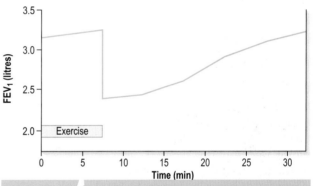

Figure 13.17. (a) Peak expiratory flow (PEF) responses to an exercise test. In normal and asthmatic patients there is a small degree of bronchodilatation during exercise, but in asthmatic patients this initial bronchodilatation is followed by bronchoconstriction, reaching its maximum 5–10 minutes after the end of exercise. A 15% drop from baseline levels of PEF is considered a positive test, and the fall in PEF can be rapidly reversed with an inhaled bronchodilator. Exercise-induced asthma is a particularly common problem in childhood. (Reproduced with permission from Forbes and Jackson, 2002.) (b) Exercise-induced asthma. Serial recordings of forced expiratory volume in 1 second (FEV_1) in a patient with bronchial asthma before and after 6 minutes of strenuous exercise. Note initial slight rise on completion of exercise, followed by sudden fall and gradual recovery. Adequate warm-up exercise or pre-treatment with a β_2-adrenoceptor agonist, nedocromil sodium or a leukotriene antagonist (e.g. montelukast sodium) often protects against exercise-induced symptoms. (Reproduced with permission from Haslett et al. 2002.)

training to improve physical fitness, warm-up and cool-down periods, a scarf over the mouth on cold days to warm the inspired air, and a cromone or bronchodilator before exercise if found beneficial. Routine unnecessary bronchodilators can worsen exercise-induced bronchospasm.

Nocturnal asthma

Nocturnal worsening of airway obstruction may be a distinct entity or a manifestation of more severe asthma. The term 'nocturnal asthma' is used loosely, but accurately applies only to those who suffer at night and are symptom-free in the day. It causes fatigue and interferes with sexual activity, and has been associated with gastro-oesophageal reflux and obesity. It occurs in 80% of people with asthma, mostly during REM sleep.

Nocturnal asthma is diagnosed by a morning dip in peak flow of over 20% compared to the previous evening. Possible trigger factors are an exaggerated bronchial response to cold bedrooms, reduced lung volume in supine, allergens in bedding, GOR due to reduced lower oesophageal sphincter tone, or hormonal circadian oscillations in airway patency. Airways are narrowest at about 4 a.m.

Once avoidable factors are removed, treatment consists of a slow-release bronchodilator, and if nocturnal attacks are recurrent, anti-inflammatory drugs, preferably not steroids in the first instance. If triggered by snoring, a sleep study may identify sleep apnoea.

Occupational asthma

Between 5% and 10% of asthma in young adults may be attributable to substances encountered at work, though this may not become apparent for weeks or years. Symptoms usually worsen during the week and ease at weekends, but several work-free days may be needed before improvement is apparent. It is usually diagnosed by a fall in FEV_1 of >20% over the working day or week.

Aspirin-induced asthma

Aspirin intolerance occurs in about 10% of people with asthma, who react within hours of ingesting aspirin or other non-steroidal anti-inflammatory drug, developing an acute attack superimposed on a background of chronic severe asthma. Many do not realize that aspirin triggers their attack. Suspicions are raised if questioning reveals rhinitis or cumulative lifelong analgesic consumption.

Premenstrual asthma

This presents as particularly severe monthly asthma attacks during the 5–10 days leading up to menstruation, and can be demonstrated in 40% of asthmatic females. It may be associated with endometriosis affecting the pleura. Long-acting bronchodilators before menstruation may ease the attack.

Difficult asthma

People who have symptoms that do not match up or respond to medication are sometimes described as having difficult asthma, especially if psychosocial factors are evident. This may be because the patient does not actually have asthma. The commonest misdiagnosis is hyperventilation syndrome.

Education and prevention

Self-management is the essence of asthma management, and is at least as effective as primary care. People with asthma benefit from pulmonary rehabilitation (Ch. 9.2), including education, exercise training, breathing techniques and relaxation. Prevention by education is central because the characteristics of asthma discourage patients from adhering to treatment: it is a chronic condition with long periods of remission, and drug regimes may not show immediate benefit. Patients tend to underestimate symptoms and most do not monitor peak flow during an exacerbation or call an ambulance during a life-threatening attack. Following life-threatening acute asthma, a 40% incidence of denial and fear has been identified. Comprehensive preventive measures have shown:

- freedom from symptoms for most people with stable disease
- 73% reduction in acute admissions
- ↓ medication use and ↑ quality of life
- the potential to reduce asthma deaths to zero.

Self-management by drugs is based on identifying the individual best peak flow and adjusting medication if it falls below this. Optimal readings are identified by measuring PEF within 30 minutes of waking and in the evening, and adjusting bronchodilators until best values are achieved. If this is less than 80% predicted for sex, age and height, a 2-week course of anti-inflammatory drugs, followed sometimes by 2 weeks of bronchodilators, are needed to find the maximum PEF. If a nebulizer is used, an initial period of saline reduces the placebo effect of the test. Thereafter, PEF readings should be taken twice daily for people with chronic asthma and four times a day for those with severe chronic asthma, using charts from asthma organizations or drug manufacturers. The following action is then advised:

- PEF >80% of optimal: continue routine treatment
- PEF 50–80% of optimal: start pre-planned drug regime, e.g. extra bronchodilator and steroid inhalers, and/or oral steroids
- PEF <50% of optimal: start self-treatment and seek urgent medical attention.

Stepwise use of drugs in chronic asthma with increasing severity of disease (British Thoracic Society, 2003 guidelines)

Step 1. Mild intermittent asthma – short-acting bronchodilator as required
Step 2. Regular preventive drugs – add inhaled anti-inflammatory drug
Step 3. Add-on drugs – add long-acting bronchodilator ± increase steroid ± add other drug(s)
Step 4. Persistent poor control – increase steroid ± add other drug(s)
Step 5. Need for continuous or frequent steroids – oral steroids, high-dose inhaled steroid

If 'as required' bronchodilators (step 1) are needed more than once a day, taken appropriately, patients move to step 2. Patients who are still symptomatic move through the steps until symptoms are controlled.

Table 13.3.   Conditions associated with bronchiectasis

Infective: bacterial, viral, fungal
Congenital: cystic fibrosis, primary ciliary dyskinesia
Inflammatory: rheumatoid disease, inflammatory bowel disease
Predisposing: immune deficiency, foreign body aspiration, sinusitis

BRONCHIECTASIS

Bronchiectasis belongs to the family of chronic obstructive lung diseases, airflow obstruction being caused by permanent distortion and dilation of the airway walls. This 'orphan disease' is less common than COPD or asthma, suffers an unknown incidence and is often missed as a diagnosis.

Bronchiectasis is not a final diagnosis so much as a common pathway of several acquired or congenital conditions predisposing to persistent lung infection. Causes may be multiple or unknown, but associated factors are shown in Table 13.3.

Bronchiectasis has been found in a third of people with rheumatoid arthritis, in which case the joint pain may respond to antibiotics given for the bronchiectasis. Bronchiectasis is diminishing in countries where living standards are rising and children are vaccinated against diseases such as whooping cough and measles.

Pathophysiology

Inflammatory damage to the bronchial wall may be focal or diffuse, the latter often accompanied by sinusitis or other disorder. The warm moist environment of the lung combines with excess mucus to set up a vicious cycle of infection, inflammation and further obstruction (Fig. 13.18). Thick mucus sits heavily on the tender cilia and causes further damage. An over-exuberant immune response to the colonizing microbes releases toxic inflammatory chemicals, particularly neutrophils, which chew up lung tissue. Persistent inflammation leads to fibrosis and sometimes sets off bronchospasm, which augments the cycle. Abscesses may develop.

Pseudomonas aeruginosa is a particularly virulent bug, and if isolated in the sputum, tends to displace other organisms and lead to accelerated decline in pulmonary function.

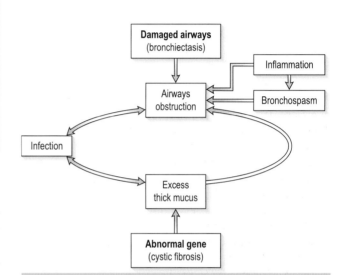

Figure 13.18.   Vicious cycle that augments the processes of cystic fibrosis and bronchiectasis. CF is progressive, whereas the course of bronchiectasis varies according to cause and management.

Anatomic disorganization is greatest if the disease starts in early childhood before the lungs are fully developed. Progressive destruction occurs in anything between 3% and 48% of patients, depending partly on medical and physiotherapy intervention to preserve the airways. Advanced disease may bring pulmonary hypertension and cor pulmonale.

Physiology of clinical features

Voluminous quantities of sputum are produced despite inefficient clearance mechanisms caused by corrugated airways and damaged cilia. Acute infection can erode the airways and cause haemoptysis, which itself leaves the airways more vulnerable to infection, and some physicians recommend prophylactic antibiotics at this time. Secretions and collapsing airways on expiration create coarse wheezes and crackles.

Other features are fatigue, due to persistent cough and recurrent infection, loss of appetite, dyspnoea and occasionally finger clubbing. Pleuritic pain occurs in 50% of patients, reflecting distal pneumonitis adjacent to the sensitive pleural surface. Breathlessness and reduced exercise tolerance predispose to depression or anxiety.

Table 13.4. Distinguishing features of bronchiectasis and COPD

	Bronchiectasis	COPD
Age	Varied	Older
Smoking history	Not necessarily	Usually
Auscultation	Noisy, may be localized	Diffuse crackles
Sputum	Excessive, often thick and green	Moderate
Haemoptysis	Sometimes	No
Finger clubbing	Sometimes	No
X-ray	Specific	Variable

Tests

Spirometry usually shows airway obstruction and bronchiectasis may be misdiagnosed as COPD. Table 13.4 clarifies the distinction.

Periodic sputum culture is needed to identify micro-organisms, which colonize the distal airways of 60% of patients in the chronic state. X-rays may show chronic increased markings caused by infiltrates or scarring. Parallel tramlines represent thickened airway walls, and 1 cm 'bunch of grapes' ring shadows represent groups of dilated airways seen in cross-section. Neglected disease shows 'glove finger shadows' which are dilated bronchi full of thick secretions, and the ring shadows may have fluid levels. A normal X-ray does not exclude the diagnosis, and high-resolution CT scanning or xenon scan is more sensitive. A bronchogram outlines the dilated airways but is rarely performed now.

Physiological effects of medical treatment

Liberal use of antibiotics helps control infection, usually by organism-specific rather than continuous prescription. Patients are given a store of antibiotics to be taken at the first sign of colour change in their sputum. For patients who deteriorate every winter, regular oral antibiotics can be taken in the cold months. The intravenous and inhaled route can also be used.

Antibiotics do not control the persistent inflammation which may be progressively destroying the airways, but inhaled steroids can assist this and reduce the volume of sputum. Another drug which may decrease sputum volume or improve mucociliary clearance is erythromycin, and dry powder mannitol bronchodilators are used if there is demonstrable hyperreactivity. Sometimes the cause of the disorder might be treatable, e.g. topical steroids for rhinosinusitis to prevent mucus sliding from the back of the nose into the lung.

If medical treatment is unsuccessful or symptoms such as pain intractable, surgical resection of non-perfused lung may be indicated for localized disease. Outcomes are usually positive when complete resection of the disease is achieved. Limited surgery may be indicated in non-localized bilateral bronchiectasis with cystic and functionless areas. Occasionally transplantation is possible in late-stage disease.

CYSTIC FIBROSIS

Cystic fibrosis (CF) is no longer a disease of childhood. Survival to adulthood is the norm. This obstructive airways disease is caused by a chronic progressive disorder of the exocrine glands. It is the commonest lethal inherited disease among white people, acquired as an autosomal recessive disorder. The gene is carried by one in 25 Caucasians and comes to life when inherited from both parents. Two carriers have a one-in-four chance of having an affected baby and a one-in-two chance that their baby will be a carrier.

The rogue gene has been identified, and prenatal diagnosis and organ transplantation are available, but improved survival is mainly because of attention to detail in conventional treatment, i.e. antibiotics, physiotherapy and nutrition. However, the disease is still eventually fatal and treatment is aimed primarily at improving quality of life.

Pathophysiology

In most cells the gene encoding CF is dormant, but in epithelial cells it is switched on. This impairs ion and water transport across epithelial surfaces of the body, causing obstruction of various body lumens. In the gut, pancreatic insufficiency leads to malabsorption and intolerance of fat. In the male reproductive system, blockage causes infertility in 98% of patients. In the lungs, sodium and chloride ions cannot escape from the epithelial cells into the airways (Fig. 13.19) in order to maintain salinity of mucus. Inflammatory mediators such as neutrophils release DNA, whose strands bind together and thicken secretions, encouraging bacterial adherence.

The respiratory component determines the quality of life and is the usual cause of death. The lungs are structurally normal at birth, but inflammatory changes are evident as early as 4 weeks of age and intractable infection soon becomes established, even when the patient is clinically well, leading to progressive damage by a smouldering course of bacterial colonization punctuated by exacerbations. Viruses and fungi play a role, and long-term antibiotics predispose the lungs to *Aspergillus* colonization.

The range of bacteria is curiously restricted. *Staphylococcus aureus* causes significant harm. *Pseudomonas aeruginosa* is the commonest bacterium and is associated with progressive decline in pulmonary function, although vaccination affords some protection. *Burkholderia cepacia*, the organism responsible for onion rot, is particularly feared; some strains are untreatable and reduce lifespan by an average 10 years, with 20% of patients developing fatal fulminant pneumonia. Preventive measures against *B. cepacia* include segregation of patients with and without *B. cepacia*, at great personal cost for those who have previously socialized freely. Even sibling separation is tolerated by some families. Respiratory equipment and treatment locations are segregated, and healthcare personnel must wash their hands in an antiseptic such as Hibiscrub.

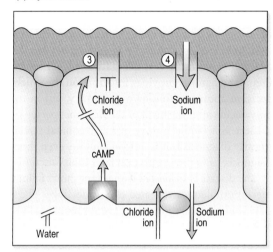

(a) Normal   (b) Cystic fibrosis

β$_2$-adrenoceptor

Figure 13.19. Cystic fibrosis: basic defect in the pulmonary epithelium. (a) The CF gene codes for a chloride channel (1) in the apical (luminal) membrane of epithelial cells in the conducting airways. This channel is normally controlled by cyclic adenosine monophosphate (cAMP) and indirectly by β-adrenoceptor stimulation. It is one of several apical ion channels which together control the quantity and solute content of airway-lining fluid. Normal channels appear to inhibit the adjacent epithelial sodium channels (2). (b) In CF, one of many CF gene defects causes absence or defective function of this chloride channel (3). This leads to reduced chloride secretion and loss of inhibition of sodium channels with excessive sodium resorption (4) and dehydration of the airway lining. The resulting abnormal airway-lining fluid is believed to predispose to infection by mechanisms which are not fully understood. (Reproduced with permission from Haslett et al., 2002.)

Malnutrition may contribute to impaired respiratory defence. Resting energy expenditure is 20% higher than normal in adults, half of it caused by the inefficiency of breathing with hyperinflated lungs. Pneumothorax occurs in up to 10% of children and 20% of adults, due to rupture of a sub-pleural bleb or bulla.

Longer-term survival has given rise to new difficulties. Pancreatic and biliary damage can cause diabetes and cirrhosis, vasculitis can affect joints, skin and brain, bronchial artery hypertrophy may lead to pulmonary haemorrhage, and excessive coughing has led to over a third of female patients developing stress incontinence. A six-fold increase in the incidence of gut cancer may be related to survival of an older population and/or gastro-oesophageal reflux.

Clinical features

Incessant coughing, small stature, delayed puberty, flatus, increasing breathlessness and unrelenting weariness. If chest pain occurs, it may be due to pleural inflammation, muscle strain from coughing or pneumothorax. Normal conception is not feasible for most males, but sexual function is not affected, and fatherhood is possible artificially. Women can have children, and optimum nutrition and respiratory care

are required prior to pregnancy to prevent hypoxia damaging the fetus.

By the age of 3 months, 50% of babies have respiratory symptoms. Later, wheezes are heard on auscultation as a bronchiolitis-like process develops in the small airways, then widespread crackles. If there is hepatomegaly, diaphragmatic function is impaired. The radiograph is normal at first, then shows patchy opacities in the apical regions, then signs of widespread bronchiectasis, emphysema and finally cor pulmonale.

Growth may be stunted because of energy imbalance, energy supply being reduced by malabsorption and anorexia, and energy demand increased by excess WOB and recurrent pulmonary sepsis. Weight loss is a risk if malabsorption is uncontrolled or diabetes develops, but good nutrition means that the patient should not be malnourished except in the terminal phase or if the liver is involved.

In the later stages, FEV_1 declines, Pa_{O_2} falls and eventually Pa_{CO_2} rises. The inexorable deterioration is anticipated by patients, who each respond in their individual way. They often form strong attachments to each other, which provide comradeship but can be devastating when one dies.

Diagnostic tests

Screening is possible at three stages. Carrier screening helps when making decisions about reproduction, and if two carriers want to have a child, they can be offered in vitro fertilization, genetic screening and implantation of a healthy embryo. Prenatal diagnosis provides information on which to base a decision about continuing a pregnancy, but in the UK this only occurs after the birth of the first unexpected CF child or if there is a family history of CF. Neonatal screening leads to early diagnosis but is not yet routine, even though timely diagnosis has a direct effect on later lung function.

The disease is suspected if an infant shows failure to thrive, meconium ileus or repeated chest infections. The skin tastes salty, and confirmation is by a test for abnormally salty sweat at 6 weeks. X-ray findings are absent in the early stages. When present they are non-specific, showing signs of bronchiectasis and then emphysema. High resolution CT scans are more sensitive and can indicate the extent of disease. A yearly glucose tolerance test is required from age 10.

> The drug rhDNase (recombinant human deoxyribonuclease) contains a clone of the gene responsible for breaking down DNA, and when given as an aerosol can decrease sputum viscosity, lessen intractable atelectasis and may influence disease progression. It benefits 50% of patients but nearly doubles the cost of their care, with some of the cost being offset by reduced infectious episodes. Sometimes the drug causes deterioration due to overliquification of secretions so that mucociliary clearance becomes very difficult to achieve.

PRIMARY CILIARY DYSKINESIA

Primary ciliary dyskinesia (PCD) is a recessively inherited group of disorders affecting one in 20 000 people. Immotility or abnormal motility of cilia leads to uncoordinated ciliary action and excess secretions, as if an escalator is malfunctioning in rush hour. The result is recurrent infection of ears, sinuses and lungs. In 50% of patients , the X-ray shows dextrocardia and a middle lobe on the left, indicating Kartagener syndrome, which includes additional features of subfertility (due to dyskinetic cilia in fallopian tubes or on sperm tails) and situs inversus (mirror image of internal organs), suggesting a link between cilia and establishment of the body's axis in early development.

Clinical signs may be evident as early as the first year of life, but diagnosis tends to be late or inaccurate because the syndrome is not common, and it shares similarities with bronchiectasis and CF. PCD is suspected in children with a perpetually runny nose, glue ear, chronic sinusitis and frequent chest infections.

If detected, PCD should not be a progressive disorder so long as the twin pillars of selective antibiotics and regular physiotherapy are utilized to prevent the onset of bronchiectasis. Left untreated, there may be progression to pulmonary hypertension and eventual cor pulmonale. Some patients benefit from rhDNase drugs but β_2-agonists can cause deterioration, so both should be monitored objectively. Ear grommets are contraindicated because of subsequent ear discharge.

ALLERGIC BRONCHOPULMONARY ASPERGILLOSIS

The *Aspergillus* fungus lives in the soil, is ubiquitous, and inhalation is common. Infection is rare in immunologically competent people, but occurs in 10% of people with CF and sometimes in cavitating lung diseases such as tuberculosis. This leads to aspergillosis, an inflammatory disease manifesting mainly in the lungs as allergic bronchopulmonary aspergillosis.

Patients present with malaise, weight loss, breathlessness, fever, haemoptysis and a cough productive of brown rubbery mucus casts sometimes in the shape of the bronchial tree. X-ray signs are cavitating lesions containing white fungus balls. The disorder may continue for years with episodes of pulmonary infiltration and wheezing, sometimes leading to fibrosis and cor pulmonale.

Diagnosis is by bronchoscopy or CT scan. Treatment is by inhaled steroids to help prevent the development of a form of bronchiectasis which tends to affect the upper lobes. Antifungal agents can be delivered bronchoscopically or percutaneously. Surgical resection may be required.

ACKNOWLEDGEMENT

Parts of this chapter (including Figs 13.1, 13.2, 13.8, 13.9, 13.12, 13.18) are reproduced with the permission of Nelson Thornes from *Physiotherapy in Respiratory Care*, 3rd edition, by Alexandra Hough – ISBN 0 7487 4037 6 (2001).

REFERENCES AND FURTHER READING

COPD

Barnes PJ (1995) Chronic obstructive pulmonary disease. Update, 51: 91–97.

Baughman RP, Lower EE, de Bois RM (2003) Sarcoidosis. Lancet 361: 1111–1118.

Benditt JO (2000) Adverse effects of low-flow oxygen therapy. Respir Care 45(1): 54–61.

Bienenstock J (2002) Stress and asthma: the plot thickens. Am J Respir Crit Care Med 165: 1034–1035.

Debigare R, Cote CH, Maltais F (2001) Peripheral muscle wasting in chronic obstructive pulmonary disease: clinical relevance and mechanisms. Am J Respir Crit Care Med 164: 1712–1717.

Fehrenbach C (1998) Chronic obstructive pulmonary disease. Prof Nurse 13: 771–777.

Forbes CD, Jackson WF (2002) Color Atlas and Text of Clinical Medicine. St Louis: Mosby.

Gibson GJ (1996) Pulmonary hyperinflation. Eur Respir J 9: 2640–2649.

Kumar P, Clark M (2002) Clinical Medicine. London: Saunders.

Souhami RL, Moxham J (2002) Textbook of Medicine. Edinburgh: Churchill Livingstone.

Stevens A, Lowe J (2000) Edinburgh: Mosby.

Sykes K (1999) Respiratory Support. London: BMJ Publishing.

Underwood JCE (2000) General and Systematic Pathology. Edinburgh: Churchill Livingstone.

Asthma

British Thoracic Society (1993) Guidelines for management of asthma: a summary. BMJ 306: 776–782.

Demeter SL (1986) Hyperventilation syndrome and asthma. Am J Med 81: 89–94.

Ducharme FM, Hicks GC (2001) Anti-leukotriene agents compared to inhaled corticosteroids in the management of recurrent and/or chronic asthma (Cochrane review) The Cochrane Library Issue 3.

Goldberg BJ, Kaplan MS (2000) Non-asthmatic respiratory symptomatology. Curr Opin Pulmon Med 6: 26–30.

Haslett C, Chilvers ER, Boon NA, et al. (2002) Davidson's Principles and Practice of Medicine. Edinburgh: Churchill Livingstone.

Kilpelainen M, Koskenvuo M, Helenius H, Terho E (2001) Home dampness, current allergic diseases, and respiratory infections among young adults. Thorax 56: 462–467.

Koopman LP, Brunekreef B, de Jongste JC, Neijens HJ (2001) Respiratory infections in infants: interaction of parental allergy, child care, and siblings – the PIAMA study. Pediatrics 108: 943.

Little S, Thomson NC (2003) Asthma management. Update (www.DoctorUpdate.net).

Luce PJ (1996) Asthma in the elderly. Br J Hosp Med 55: 118–124.

Cystic fibrosis

Aspin AJ (1991) Psychological consequences of cystic fibrosis in adults. Br J Hosp Med 45: 368–371.

Britto MT, Kotagal UR, Homung RW, et al. (2002) Impact of recent pulmonary exacerbations on quality of life in patients with cystic fibrosis. Chest 121: 64–72.

Chilvers MA, O'Callaghan C (2000) Local mucociliary defence mechanisms. Paediat Respir Rev 1: 27–34.

Conway SP, Watson A (1997) Nebulised bronchodilators, corticosteroids, and rhDNase in adult patients with cystic fibrosis. Thorax 52 (Suppl 2): S64–S68.

Conway SP, Morton AM, Oldroyd B, et al. (2000) Osteoporosis and osteopenia in adults and adolescents with cystic fibrosis: prevalence and associated factors. Thorax 55: 798–804.

Dakin CJ, Numa AH, Wang HE et al. (2002) Inflammation, infection, and pulmonary function in infants and young children with cystic fibrosis. Am J Respir Crit Care Med 165: 904–910.

Davies J, Trindade MT, Wallis C, et al. (1997) Retrospective review of the effects of rhDNase in children with cystic fibrosis. Pediatr Pulmonol 23: 243–248.

Davis PB, Drumm M, Konstan MW (1996) Cystic fibrosis. Am J Respir Crit Care Med 154: 1229–1256.

Hankard R, Munck A, Navarro J (2002) Nutrition and growth in cystic fibrosis. Horm Res 58(Suppl 1): 16–20.

Hausler M, Meilicke R, Biesterfield S, et al. (2000) Bronchiolitis obliterans organizing pneumonia: a distinct pulmonary complication in cystic fibrosis. Respiration 67(3).

Ionescu AA, Nixon LS, Luzio S, et al. (2002) Pulmonary function, body composition, and protein catabolism in adults with cystic fibrosis. Am J Respir Crit Care Med 165: 495–500.

Orr A, McVean RJ, Webb AK, Dodd ME (2001) Questionnaire survey of urinary incontinence in women with cystic fibrosis. BMJ 322: 1521 (23 June). Bmj.com.

Parker AE, Young CS (1991) The physiotherapy management of cystic fibrosis in children. Physiotherapy 77: 584–586.

Parmar JS, Howell T, Kelly J, Bilton D (2002) Profound adrenal suppression secondary to treatment with low dose inhaled steroids and itraconazole in allergic bronchopulmonary aspergillosis in cystic fibrosis. Thorax 57: 749–750.

Reid DW, Wither NJ, Francis L, et al. (2002) Iron deficiency in cystic fibrosis: relationship to lung disease severity and chronic *Pseudomonas aeruginosa* infection. Chest 121: 48–54.

Wills PJ, Hall RL, Chan W, Cole PJ (1997) Sodium chloride increases the ciliary transportability of cystic fibrosis and bronchiectasis sputum on the mucus-depleted bovine trachea. Rapid Publication 99(1): 9–13.

Infections and miscellaneous

Helen M, Sorenson MA (2000) Managing secretions in dying patients. Respir Care 45(11): 1355–1364.

Henderson A (1994) Chronic respiratory failure. Practitioner 238: 345–350.

Niederman MS, Ahmed QAA (2002) Community-acquired pneumonia in elderly patients. Clin Geriatr Med 19: 101–120.

Partridge MR (1996) Self-management plans (asthma). Br J Ther Rehab 3: 271–275.

Peek GJ, Morcos S, Cooper G (2000) The pleural cavity. BMJ 320: 1318–1321.

Sevransky JE, Haponik EF (2002) Respiratory failure in elderly patients. Clin Geriatr Med 19 (2003): 205–224.

Thickett KM, Kumararatne DS, Banerjee AK, et al. (2002) Common variable immune deficiency: respiratory manifestations, pulmonary function and high-resolution CT scan findings. Q J Med 95: 655–662.

The Urinary System: The Renal System

Lukas Foggensteiner

INTRODUCTION

The kidneys and urinary tracts constitute a complex yet elegant system for the excretion of soluble waste products from the body. The kidneys process blood to remove water, salts and other molecules to generate urine. This process is highly regulated and responsive to physiological need, as will be appreciated by anybody deprived of water whose kidneys will avidly conserve water, or who has a high salt intake whose kidneys will excrete surplus salt. The result is that even with dramatic differences in dietary and fluid intake, individuals will maintain within very narrow limits, the body water and electrolyte concentrations necessary for life. Fortunately the kidneys are physiologically robust and have considerable reserve capacity but when renal disease does occur it can have devastating consequences, as we shall discuss. Urine generated by the kidneys is stored in the bladder to be voluntarily voided. The renal tracts including the ureters, bladder, prostate and urethra facilitate this process. Disorders of the urinary tracts, which include urinary infections, obstruction to urine flow and incontinence, are more common than renal disease and will also be considered.

BASIC RENAL PHYSIOLOGY AND ANATOMY

The two kidneys lie on the posterior abdominal wall behind the peritoneal cavity. Adult kidneys typically weigh approximately 150 g each and measure 10–12 cm from pole to pole. A single artery and vein entering at the hilum connects each organ to the aorta and vena cava below the crus of the diaphragm (Fig. 14.1.1). If the kidney is bisected from top to bottom the two major regions that can be identified are the cortex and the medulla. The medulla is further divided into multiple cone-shaped masses of tissue called the renal pyramids. The apex of each pyramid projects into the renal pelvis to form the renal papillae. The intrarenal portion of the renal pelvis is thus divided into calices which converge to form the extrarenal pelvis. This in turn converges into the ureter, which follows a retroperitoneal course to the bladder.

The nephron

Each kidney in the human is made up of about 1 million nephrons. Each nephron consists of a glomerulus in which urinary filtrate is generated, and a tubule which processes the filtrate by active excretion and absorption. Filtrate passes through the nephron into the collecting ducts, which converge at the papillae to discharge urine into the renal pelvis (Fig. 14.1.2). The nephrons are all almost identical and can therefore be considered as the functional unit of the kidneys.

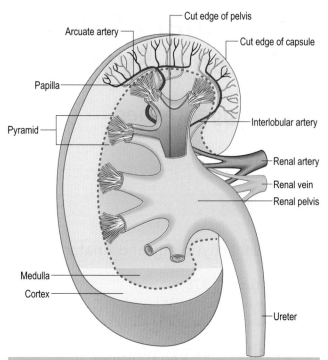

Figure 14.1.1. Anatomy of the kidney. (Reproduced with permission from Davies et al., 2001.)

The glomerulus and glomerular filtration

The glomerulus is a highly specialized structure consisting of a capillary network or 'tuft' supported by podocytes and mesangial cells, and encased in Bowman's capsule (Fig. 14.1.3). Each glomerulus has a single afferent and efferent capillary taking blood into and out of the glomerulus respectively. The capillaries within the glomerulus are unusual in that they are highly permeable to water, electrolytes and small proteins but largely impermeable to albumin and other large proteins. This selectivity is due to the three layers constituting the capillary wall. These are the vascular endothelial cells, the glomerular basement membrane (GBM) and the podocytes. The endothelial cells of the glomerulus differ from those in other capillary beds because they are perforated by thousands of fenestrae or pores which render them highly permeable to water, electrolytes and proteins. The endothelial cells rest upon the GBM, which consists of a matrix of collagen and proteoglycan. Within this matrix there are spaces through which can filter water and electrolytes but not larger plasma proteins. This is a function of both the size of the spaces within the GBM and the negative charge on the proteoglycans which repel positively charged plasma proteins. The capillaries and GBM are surrounded by a unique type of epithelial cell, the podocyte. These cells are not continuous but rather support the capillary loops by a network of interdigitating foot processes. These foot processes are separated by small gaps called slit pores which offer further selectivity to the filtration process by virtue of

(a)

(b)

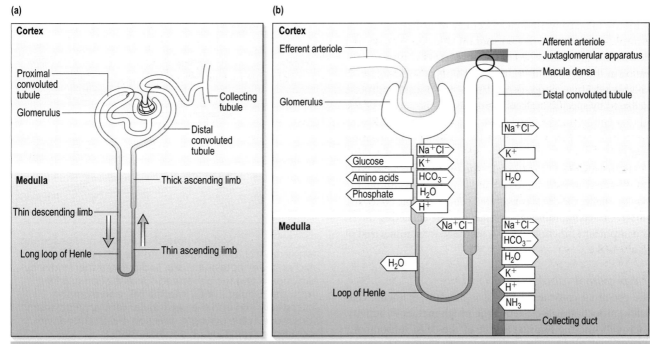

Figure 14.1.2. (a) Components of the nephron. (b) Major functions of different parts of the nephron. (Reproduced with permission from Kumar and Clark, 2002.)

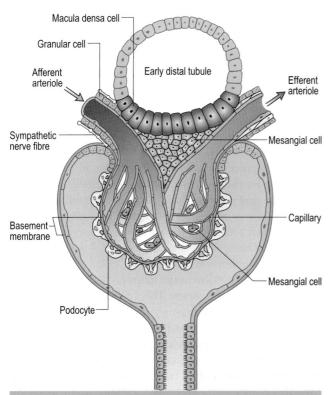

Figure 14.1.3. Structure of the glomerulus. (Reproduced with permission from Davies et al., 2001.)

their size and negative charge. The capillary wall is therefore permeable to water and electrolytes but virtually impermeable to proteins of over 64 kDa in molecular mass including albumin. Filtrate is generated by the movement of water and solute across the capillary wall in response to the hydrostatic and colloid pressure gradient between the capillary lumen and Bowman's space while proteins and cells are retained in the circulation. The integrity of this filtration surface is essential to the functioning of the kidney, and disease processes which impair its function can lead to renal disease, as we shall see.

A substantial quantity of glomerular filtrate is generated daily. Renal blood flow typically represents 20% of cardiac output and 20% of renal plasma flow is filtered, resulting in a glomerular filtration rate (GFR) of 125 ml/min or 180 l/day in an average adult.

The renal tubules and processing of the glomerular filtrate

Filtrate generated in the glomerulus passes through a series of tubules during which its composition and concentration are modified by the tubular epithelial cells. Substances may be reabsorbed from the filtrate into the blood or excreted into the filtrate from the blood and it is the balance of the three processes of filtration, tubular reabsorption and tubular excretion which determine the final composition of the urine. Quantitatively tubular reabsorption is more important than excretion, however, and it is this process that allows 180 l/day of filtrate to be converted into 1–2 l/day of urine output. For example, over 99% of filtered sodium chloride, glucose and bicarbonate are reabsorbed by the tubules. In contrast to filtration at the glomerulus, tubular handling of some solutes is a highly selective energy-dependant active transport process mediated by specific molecular 'pumps' on the surface of the tubular epithelial cells. Passive movement of water and some electrolytes can then occur across the resulting concentration gradients.

Anatomically and functionally the tubules can be divided into discrete segments, the proximal convoluted tubule, the loop of Henle, the distal convoluted tubule and the collecting tubule. Collecting tubules converge into the collecting ducts. The important functions of each segment are summarized in Figure 14.1.2.

The proximal tubule

The proximal convoluted tubule is lined by epithelial cells rich in mitochondria, reflecting their high metabolic activity. Microvilli line the luminal aspect of the cells, substantially increasing the surface area in contact with filtrate. The proximal tubule is the main site of sodium, chloride and water reabsorption. Sodium reabsorption is mediated by sodium-potassium ATPase on the basolateral cell surface that transports sodium ions out of the cell in exchange for potassium ions at the expense of hydrolysing ATP. This pump maintains a low intracellular sodium concentration, facilitating the diffusion of sodium ions into the cell from the tubular lumen along the resulting sodium concentration gradient (Fig. 14.1.4). A passive transport mechanism is responsible for the movement of chloride and water, which follow the movement of sodium ions due to the resulting electrochemical gradient generated. This gradient also enables sodium co-transporters on the apical cell surface to transport glucose, amino acids and other molecules from the filtrate into the cell. Counter-transport mechanisms reabsorb sodium while excreting other molecules, notably hydrogen ions, into the filtrate. The proximal tubule is responsible for the absorption of 65% of filtered sodium chloride and water and virtually all of the filtered glucose and amino acids. It is an important site for the excretion of many molecules including hydrogen ions, bile salts, oxalate, catecholamines and drugs.

The loop of Henle

The loop of Henle can be functionally and morphologically divided into three segments, the descending thin segment, the ascending thin segment and the thick ascending segment. The descending part of the thin segment is lined by flat epithelial cells. It is high permeable to water, urea and most electrolytes. Both thin and thick ascending parts of the loop of Henle are impermeable to water but the thick ascending segment is capable of active reabsorption of sodium, chloride, potassium and other ions including calcium, magnesium and bicarbonate.

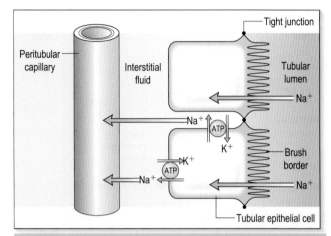

Figure 14.1.4. Sodium/potassium ATPase pumps sodium ions from the tubular lumen into the interstitial fluid in exchange for potassium ions. Sodium ions then move by diffusion along the generated concentration gradient from the tubular lumen into the cell, and from the interstitial fluid into the peritubular capillary. Potassium ions move in the opposite direction. (Reproduced with permission from Guyton and Hall, 1995.)

The impermeability of the ascending segment of the loop is a critical feature of the countercurrent multiplier system in the loop of Henle for producing a hyperosmotic renal medulla (Fig. 14.1.5). This well-described process is required to concentrate the urine and is generated as follows. Sodium and chloride ions are actively pumped from the filtrate of the thick ascending limb into the interstitium, which becomes hypertonic. Water, however, cannot follow the sodium and chloride because the ascending limb is impermeable to water. Water therefore moves from the filtrate in the descending limb into the interstitium, rendering the filtrate in the descending limb hypertonic. This filtrate, on reaching the ascending limb, presents a higher concentration of sodium chloride to be transported back into the interstitium. This continuous process gradually traps solutes in the medulla and multiplies the concentration gradient established by the active pumping of ions out of the thick ascending loop of Henle, eventually raising the interstitial medullary osmolarity to between 1200 and 14 000 mOsm/l. To prevent this gradient simply being washed away by blood flow through the tissues, the capillaries of the medulla, called the vasa recta, are anatomically similar to the loops of Henle, dipping into the medulla from the cortex. This enables a countercurrent mechanism to preserve the high medullary osmolality.

Another mechanism contributes to the concentration gradient. The collecting duct is largely impermeable to urea, one of the products of protein metabolism. The medullary portion of the collecting duct is, however, highly permeable to urea. As a consequence urea is concentrated in the urine but some diffusion of urea into the medullary interstitium does occur through the medullary collecting duct into the

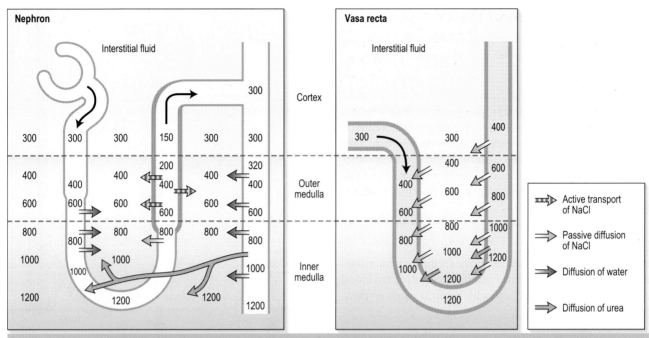

Figure 14.1.5.   Generation of the medullary concentration gradient. (Reproduced with permission from Rang et al., 2003.)

medullary interstitium, contributing to the high medullary concentration gradient.

It is the medullary concentration gradient that enables concentrated urine to be generated as discussed below.

The distal convoluted tubule

Although the early distal convoluted tubule reabsorbs sodium, chloride and potassium, the late distal tubule contains two specialized cell types with different functions. The intercalated cells avidly secrete hydrogen ions and reabsorb bicarbonate and are important for the regulation of acid–base balance as discussed later. The principal cells, which constitute the majority of the cells of the late distal convoluted tubule, reabsorb sodium and excrete potassium. This is therefore the main site for the regulation of potassium homeostasis. Potassium excretion is regulated both by a direct effect of extracellular potassium on the sodium-potassium ATPase and via aldosterone, which stimulates this pump causing sodium retention and potassium excretion. Acidosis inhibits potassium excretion, which is why an alkali such as sodium bicarbonate is a useful treatment of hyperkalaemia.

Collecting ducts

The collecting ducts are the final site for the processing of urine and are important in determining the final urinary composition. Urine entering the collecting duct is hypotonic with an osmolality of around 100 mOsm/l. Urine leaving the collecting duct may, however, be concentrated to 1200 mOsm/l. The final urine concentration is determined by the circulating levels of antidiuretic hormone (ADH) and the medullary concentration gradient described above. This occurs as follows. The collecting duct epithelial monolayer is highly impermeable to water in the absence of ADH, in which case the urine remains dilute. In the presence of ADH, however, water channels called aquaporins open, allowing water to pass from the urine into the renal medulla, driven by the high osmolality of the medullary interstitium. The result is concentrated urine. ADH, a peptide hormone secreted by the pituitary gland, is in turn regulated by the serum osmolality. When the serum osmolality rises, ADH is secreted and water is therefore retained, causing the serum osmolality to fall. The reverse process occurs when serum osmolality falls.

Acid–base balance

Peripheral blood hydrogen ion concentration is maintained within narrow limits by the chemical acid–base buffer systems of the body fluids, the respiratory excretion of carbon dioxide and the renal excretion of hydrogen ions or bicarbonate. The kidneys are capable of producing urine with a pH of 4.5–8, representing a 3000-fold difference in hydrogen ion concentration. This constitutes the main mechanism for the long-term maintenance of acid–base homeostasis. The pH of urine is determined largely by the tubular secretion of hydrogen ions and the reabsorption of filtered bicarbonate in a process regulated by plasma hydrogen ion concentration. Renal disease often results in a metabolic acidosis when the kidney's ability to excrete hydrogen ions becomes impaired.

Endocrine functions of the kidney

As well as functioning to remove soluble waste from the body, the kidneys have a number of endocrine functions.

Vitamin D metabolism

Renal tissue contains the enzyme 1-α-hydroxylase which hydroxylates cholecalciferol to 1-α-hydroxycholecalciferol. This is the precursor to the metabolically active form of vitamin D, 1,25-dihydroxycholecalciferol. Renal disease is therefore associated with a deficiency in active vitamin D and this contributes to the disturbed calcium and phosphate balance seen in renal failure.

Erythropoietin

Renal tissue contains cells that secrete erythropoietin, a hormone that stimulates the bone marrow to produce red blood cells. Renal failure is associated with anaemia when erythropoietin levels decline.

The renin–angiotensin system

The renin–angiotensin system (RAS) is an important mechanism for the regulation of renal blood flow and systemic blood pressure (see also Ch. 12). Additionally numerous other consequences of RAS activation have been identified. The system is summarized in Figure 14.1.6. The enzyme renin is synthesized and secreted by a specialized cell type of the kidney located in the walls of the afferent arterioles immediately proximal to the glomeruli. These cells, called *juxtaglomerular cells*, are modified smooth muscle cells which respond to a reduction in blood pressure by releasing renin into the systemic circulation. This catalyses the cleavage of the 10-amino-acid peptide angiotensin I from the protein angiotensinogen. Angiotensin I is in turn converted to the 8-amino-acid peptide angiotensin II by angiotensin-converting enzyme (ACE) located in the vascular bed of the lung. Angiotensin II is an extremely powerful systemic vasoconstrictor which acts to raise the blood pressure by acting on angiotensin receptors. Within the kidney angiotensin II causes constriction of the efferent glomerular arteriole, reducing blood flow within the glomerular capillaries. Angiotensin II also acts on the adrenal cortex to stimulate the release of aldosterone which promotes sodium retention at the distal convoluted tubule. Many other consequences of RAS activation have been identified including effects of angiotensin II on cardiac and vascular hypertrophy. Drugs that block the RAS, namely ACE inhibitors and angiotensin receptor blockers, cause a selective dilation of the efferent glomerular arteriole. This results in a fall in transglomerular filtration pressure. It has been postulated that elevated glomerular pressure accelerates the decline in renal function seen in renal diseases, particularly diabetes, and this may explain why RAS blocking agents are beneficial in such

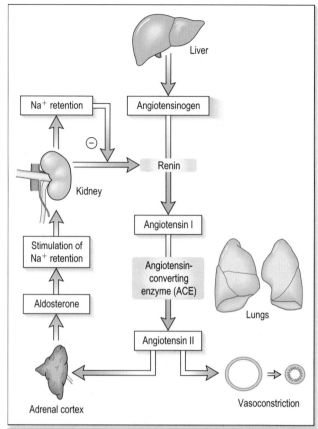

Figure 14.1.6.   The renin and angiotensin system. (Reproduced with permission from Page et al., 2002.)

conditions. These agents have therefore become very important in the management of renal impairment, proteinuria and hypertension.

THE PATIENT WITH RENAL DISEASE

Presentation

The presentation of the patient with renal disease will depend on the underlying diagnosis and the rate at which renal function is declining. The term 'renal failure' implies a declining GFR, and end-stage renal failure a GFR that is no longer sufficient to sustain life. Patients may suffer a precipitous decline in renal function over a few days or a very slow decline in renal function over many years, causing what is referred to clinically as acute or chronic renal failure. The symptoms of chronic renal failure are insidious and include lethargy, anorexia, weight loss and polyuria. Together these symptoms are sometimes called uraemia, although it should be noted that it is not the elevated urea concentration itself that is responsible but other unidentified 'uraemic toxins' which accumulate in the blood.

Symptoms of chronic renal failure

- Anorexia and weight loss
- Fatigue and malaise
- Vomiting
- Pruritus
- Breathlessness
- Polyuria and polydipsia
- Peripheral oedema
- Altered mental state

Typically the cause of these symptoms is only revealed when the serum creatinine is measured and found to be elevated. Acute renal failure may present more dramatically with pulmonary oedema, severe metabolic acidosis, coma or sudden death. Patients with nephrotic syndrome may describe peripheral oedema and frothy urine due to the high urinary protein concentrations. Patients also often come to medical attention before they develop symptoms, for example if proteinuria or haematuria is detected at a routine medical examination, if blood tests performed for other reasons reveal renal impairment or if they present with a family history of renal disease.

Clinical features of renal failure

Renal failure has widespread systemic consequences and patients may exhibit many clinical and biochemical abnormalities.

In advanced renal failure the kidney's capacity to excrete waste products may lead to an accumulation of certain solutes in the blood. These include potassium, hydrogen ions, phosphate and urate as well as urea and an unknown number of unidentified uraemic toxins. Hyperkalaemia (elevated serum potassium) is asymptomatic but may lead to cardiac arrhythmias culminating in ventricular fibrillation and death. Metabolic acidosis is a consequence of the failing kidney's inability to excrete hydrogen ions. The physiological response to a metabolic acidosis is to increase the respiratory rate and thus 'blow off' more carbon dioxide. This can cause a sensation of breathlessness. When severe, a deep sighing pattern of breathing known as Kussmaul's respiration is seen. Elevated phosphate levels are associated with itching of the skin and conjunctiva. Furthermore calcium and phosphate may precipitate in the vasculature as calcium phosphate, contributing to vascular disease. Elevated serum urate levels may give rise to gout, a very common problem in patients with renal disease. Serum urea concentration may be markedly elevated in advanced renal failure but is not directly responsible for the altered conscious level, faint yellow tinge to the skin and nausea and vomiting which are

described as uraemia. These symptoms are presumed to be due to as yet unidentified substances.

As renal function deteriorates the capacity of the kidney to concentrate the urine may become impaired, leading to polyuria and compensatory polydipsia. Patients often notice this at night (nocturia). As renal function declines further, urine output falls and patients may accumulate salt and water. This can lead to hypertension, weight gain and peripheral oedema. Fluid may eventually accumulate in the lungs (pulmonary oedema) causing breathlessness and respiratory failure.

Malnutrition is a common feature of longstanding renal disease. Its cause is unclear but it is likely that both the anorexia and metabolic disturbance seen in renal failure play a part. Weight loss may be reported but this is often disguised by accumulating fluid. Anthropometric measurements usually reveal features of malnutrition and patients may have muscle wasting severe enough to cause clinically evident weakness. Biochemical markers of malnutrition include vitamin B_{12}, folate, ferritin and serum albumin all of which may be deranged. The degree of malnutrition at presentation has been found to be an important prognostic factor for patient survival.

Failure of the kidney to produce erythropoietin leads to anaemia which contributes to the symptoms of fatigue that patients experience. Failure to hydroxylate cholecalciferol results in a deficiency in active vitamin D causing hypocalcaemia. This stimulates the parathyroid glands to produce parathyroid hormone (PTH), which acts on the skeleton to release calcium. Longstanding hyperparathyroidism may lead to bone and joint pains.

There are many other clinical and biochemical abnormalities in patients with renal failure often of uncertain and complex aetiology. For example, there is an accelerated rate of vascular disease in renal failure which may relate to hypertension, hyperlipidaemia and vascular calcification. Many of these problems are not resolved by renal replacement therapy and become significant in patients on dialysis. They are further considered in the section on dialysis.

Clinical and physiological features of renal failure

- Disturbed fluid balance
- Electrolyte disturbances
- Metabolic acidosis
- Anaemia
- Hypocalcaemia and hyperphosphataemia
- Secondary hyperparathyroidism
- Peripheral neuropathy
- Hyperlipidaemia
- Malnutrition
- Accelerated vascular disease
- Hypertension
- Amenorrhoea

Table 14.1.1. Measures of renal function

Measure	Normal value	Significance
Serum sodium	134–146 mmol/l	May be elevated or low in renal disease
Serum potassium	3.4–5.2 mmol/l	Elevated in advanced renal disease
Serum urea	3.4–7.6 mmol/l	Rises as GFR declines
Serum creatinine	<125 μmol/l	Rises as GFR declines
Serum bicarbonate	22–36 mmol/l	Falls as metabolic acidosis develops
Serum calcium	2.1–2.6 mmol/l	Falls as GFR declines
Serum phosphate	0.8–1.2 mmol/l	Rises as GFR declines

Evaluation of the patient with renal disease

A comprehensive clinical history from patients presenting with renal disease is important and may reveal a family history of an inherited renal disorder or the presence of other conditions associated with renal failure such as diabetes mellitus. A thorough clinical examination is mandatory and may reveal the cause for the renal failure, for example when large polycystic kidneys are palpable. Usually, however, the diagnosis of renal disease depends on one or more of the following investigations.

Examination of the urine

The urine must always be tested by dipstick analysis for the presence of blood and protein.

Haematuria

Modern urine dipsticks are highly sensitive for the presence of haemoglobin in the urine. When haemoglobin is detectable but not visible to the naked eye this is referred to as microscopic haematuria whereas macroscopic haematuria implies the visible presence of blood. Haematuria may originate anywhere in the renal tracts from the kidneys to the urethra and must be investigated. Urine microscopy may reveal the presence of red cell casts. These are agglomerations of red cells in a cylindrical shape and are formed when red cells leak through the glomerulus into the tubular fluid. Here they stick together within the tubular lumen adopting the characteristic shape. The presence of red cell casts always indicates the presence of glomerular disease. Other causes of haematuria include renal and bladder tumours and these must be excluded.

Proteinuria

Normal urinary protein excretion is less than 150 mg/day. Many renal diseases give rise to elevated urinary protein called proteinuria. Urine dipstick analysis is a useful screening test for proteinuria and if positive should be followed by a 24-hour urine collection and laboratory measurement of protein excretion.

Pyuria

The presence of white blood cells in the urine may represent infection of the renal tract or inflammation within the kidney and is best detected by urine microscopy. White blood cells may also form casts in the same way as red blood cells.

Crystals

If substances in the urine are present in concentrations exceeding their solubility product they may precipitate to form crystals. These may be seen by microscopy of the urine. Crystals commonly encountered include calcium oxalate, urate and cysteine.

Assessment of renal function

The function of the kidneys is diverse and there are therefore a number of measurable parameters that may reflect renal disease. The concentrations of salts and other molecules in the blood are frequently perturbed in renal disease and the most commonly measured are the serum electrolytes, bicarbonate, urea (blood urea nitrogen or BUN) and creatinine concentrations (Table 14.1.1).

Urea, which is the main nitrogenous by-product of protein metabolism, rises in renal failure in an unpredictable fashion. Creatinine is a molecule present in low concentrations in serum which is a more useful reflection of the GFR. As the GFR declines the creatinine concentration rises due to the reduced renal clearance of the molecule. A more precise estimate of GFR can be obtained by using the Cockroft–Gault formula, which corrects for patient age and weight.

Estimated GFR = (140 − age in years) × weight in kg/serum creatinine in μmol/l in ml/min

The urinary clearance of creatinine is similar to the GFR and can be measured. This requires a 24-hour urine collection as well as a measure of serum creatinine. The result, expressed in ml/min, is a good approximation of the GFR but an accurate 24-urine collection is surprisingly difficult to perform. A more precise measure of the GFR can be obtained by measuring the urinary clearance of ^{51}Cr-labelled ethylenediaminetetra-acetic acid (EDTA) by scintigraphic means.

Measurement of renal function

- Serum creatinine
- Cockroft–Gault formula
- 24-h creatinine clearance
- ^{51}Cr EDTA clearance

Radiological assessment of the kidneys

The two kidneys appear as shadows on a plain abdominal X-ray but apart from revealing the presence of stones this is of limited use. The intravenous pyelogram involves the intravenous administration of a contrast media which is excreted by the kidneys. This allows the kidneys and renal tracts to be visualized by plain radiography and gives some information about renal anatomy and the presence of renal or ureteric stones. Renal ultrasound, however, has now become the imaging modality of choice for renal assessment. It is completely non-invasive and safe and will reveal the size of the kidneys and pelvi-caliceal system, the presence of stones or renal masses and permit evaluation of renal blood flow. Computed tomography (CT) and magnetic resonance imaging (MRI) also have a role in renal imaging in certain circumstances. Methods in which radiolabelled substances such as diethylenetriaminepentaacetate (DTPA) are administered intravenously and their renal excretion monitored scintigraphically can also give information about renal function and blood flow.

Immunological tests in renal disease

Renal disease may be caused by autoimmune inflammatory conditions such as systemic lupus erythematosus (SLE) or vasculitis as discussed below. Many of these conditions are associated with the presence of characteristic autoantibodies in the blood and these can be measured. In SLE, for example, antinuclear antibodies or more specifically anti-double-stranded DNA antibodies are usually detectable.

Renal biopsy

The presence of renal impairment with no apparent cause may be an indication to perform a renal biopsy. This procedure involves visualizing the kidneys by ultrasound and passing a biopsy needle through the skin into the lower pole of either kidney to obtain a small sample of tissue for histological examination. The tissue is usually subjected to conventional light microscopy following staining, immunofluorescence microscopy and electron microscopy. In the majority of cases this enables the histopathologist to determine the nature of the renal disease present. Renal biopsy is not without risk, however, and significant bleeding may occur in up to 1% of cases. This risk is elevated and biopsy may not be possible if the kidneys are small and scarred.

Table 14.1.2. Causes of ESRF in England and Wales, 2001

Diagnosis	Age <65 (%)	Age >65 (%)
Aetiology uncertain	16	24
Glomerulonephritis	14	6
Diabetes	19	13
Polycystic kidney	10	2
Pyelonephritis	8	7
Renal vascular disease	2	10
Hypertension	4	5
Other	13	12
Diagnosis not recorded	15	20

CAUSES OF RENAL DISEASE

The causes of end-stage renal failure (ESRF) in the UK in 2001 are listed in Table 14.1.2.

In a large proportion of patients no definitive diagnosis can be made because the kidneys are small and atrophic. Such patients, who are frequently elderly, may have had a glomerulonephritis, hypertensive nephropathy or renovascular disease.

Acute tubular necrosis

Any condition which results in a sudden reduction in blood pressure and hence renal perfusion pressure can result in acute tubule damage. This is usually but inaccurately referred to as acute tubular necrosis (ATN). The reason this appellation is inappropriate is that the damaged tubular cells usually recover. A typical scenario in which ATN is seen is the patient with severe blood loss following trauma or surgery or the patient who has a severe systemic infection. Acute renal failure may develop and renal biopsy will reveal highly abnormal renal tubular epithelial cells some of which may detach and slough into the tubule. Fortunately the capacity of these cells to regenerate is good and most patients will recover renal function in weeks or months. ATN is therefore not a common cause of long-term renal failure.

Glomerulonephritis

The renal glomeruli are unique structures consisting of a tuft of highly specialized capillaries, mesangial cells and podocytes within a capsule lined by epithelial cells (Fig. 14.1.3). These tufts are susceptible to a variety of insults which can give rise to inflammation and glomerular damage. These are collectively known as glomerulonephritis. The classification of glomerulonephritis remains based on the histological appearance of the damaged glomerulus rather than on the underlying pathological process. This can lead to confusion as different mechanisms appear to give rise to a similar pattern of glomerular damage. A thorough review of glomerulonephritis and its treatment is beyond the scope of this chapter but the more common forms are outlined in Table 14.1.3. Glomerulonephritis is sometimes associated with extrarenal manifestations of the condition. For example, in IgA nephropathy the skin and bowel can exhibit the same histological IgA deposition. Another group of conditions that are frequently systemic with renal involvement are those in which inflammation of the blood vessels, called vasculitis, is seen. These include Wegener's granulomatosis and microscopic polyangiitis. Such conditions may give rise to very rapidly progressive glomerulonephritis causing renal failure, accompanied by evidence of vascular damage elsewhere such as in the lungs, skin, nerves and joints. Another systemic autoimmune disease frequently complicated by renal involvement is systemic lupus erythematosus (SLE). This condition, which usually affects young women, most commonly causes joint pains and rashes. Several patterns of glomerulonephritis can also occur, however, and renal failure may supervene. Vasculitis and SLE are among the few causes of glomerulonephritis that respond dramatically to treatment with immunosuppressive therapies.

Diabetes

Both type 1 and type 2 diabetes can be complicated by disease of the small blood vessels which can affect many organs including the eyes, nerves, peripheries and the glomerular capillaries (see Ch. 4 for details). Diabetic nephropathy is characterized initially by the development of proteinuria and subsequently renal impairment which can progress to end-stage renal failure. The prevalence of type 1 diabetes has remained static in the population at around 0.3–0.4% but the prevalence of type 2 diabetes has been rising relentlessly. At least 5% of Americans and 3% of Britons are now type 2 diabetic and this is reflected in the increasing numbers of diabetics on dialysis programmes.

In certain ethnic communities such as Asians in the UK, the prevalence of type 2 diabetes is greater still. Approximately 20% of type 2 diabetics develop renal involvement of which 2–3% progress to end stage. In the UK about 20% of patients on dialysis are diabetic but in the USA the figure has reached 50%. Diabetes is now thus the commonest single cause of renal failure in the West. Such patients pose an enormous burden to healthcare systems due to the considerable co-morbidity experienced by diabetics in renal failure, particular in the form of ischaemic heart disease and peripheral vascular disease. Fortunately significant progress has been made over the last few decades in retarding the progression of diabetic nephropathy. This involves identifying patients with early diabetic nephropathy by screening for the presence of small concentrations of albumin in the urine (microalbuminuria). Such patients are usually hypertensive and this should be aggressively treated as lowering the blood pressure has been shown to dramatically slow the progression of renal disease. The preferred agents to treat hypertension are those that block the renin–angiotensin system, namely ACE inhibitors or angiotensin receptor blockers. These agents appear to offer more renal protection than other antihypertensives for reasons discussed previously. Improved diabetic control, weight loss, cholesterol-lowering drugs and smoking cessation regimes are other important factors in the management of these patients.

Hypertension

The kidneys are extremely important in the long-term regulation of blood pressure due to their role in volume homeostasis and the activity of the renin–angiotensin system. It is therefore

Table 14.1.3.   Glomerulonephritis

Type of glomerulonephritis	Clinical features	Causes/association
IgA nephropathy	Slowly progressive renal failure Haematuria following upper respiratory tract failure	Idiopathic
Minimal change glomerulonephritis	Nephrotic syndrome Normal renal function Most common in children	Idiopathic
Membranous glomerulonephritis	Nephrotic syndrome and/or slowly progressive renal failure	Idiopathic Infection Malignancy SLE
Focal and segmental glomerulosclerosis (FSGS)	Nephrotic syndrome and/or slowly progressive renal failure	Idiopathic Hereditary
Mesangiocapillary glomerulonephritis	Slowly progressive renal failure	Infection Autoimmune disease Complement deficiency Malignancy
Rapidly progressive glomerulonephritis	Acute renal failure Systemic features of vasculitis	Vasculitis including Wegener's granulomatosis and microscopic polyangiitis

not unexpected that renal disease is frequently complicated by hypertension. Hypertension from any cause may, however, also cause renal impairment and ultimately end-stage renal disease. This phenomenon, known as hypertensive nephropathy, is due hypertension-induced sclerosis of the renal vasculature. This has become a common cause of renal failure, particularly in the black community who have a higher than average risk of hypertension. It is frequently the case that patients present with advanced renal impairment and hypertension in which it is unclear whether the high blood pressure is the cause or a consequence of the renal disease. In either case there is little doubt that aggressive treatment of the hypertension will slow the progression of the renal impairment and such treatment forms the cornerstone of management in these patients. The use of ACE inhibitors and angiotensin receptor blockers should be considered in all patients with renal impairment for reasons discussed above with the exception of those with renovascular disease (see below).

Renovascular disease

Atherosclerotic vascular disease is the commonest cause of death in the Western world and commonly affects large and medium-sized arteries including the coronary and cerebral arteries and the peripheral vasculature. The renal arteries and their branches are frequently also involved and may impair the perfusion of the kidneys. This can lead to renal ischaemia and renal impairment. Ischaemic kidneys respond by releasing renin, causing a rise in systemic blood pressure which tends to restore renal perfusion. Renovascular disease can therefore result in renal impairment and/or hypertension. This is becoming an increasingly common problem as the population ages. Management includes addressing risk factors for atherosclerotic disease such as hypercholesterolaemia and smoking, treating hypertension and dilating stenosed renal vessels by angiographic means. Agents that block the renin–angiotensin system should be used with caution in this setting as dilating the efferent glomerular capillary can result in a precipitous drop in glomerular blood flow in such patients which can precipitate acute renal failure.

Genetic renal diseases

The development and progression of many renal diseases including diabetes, SLE and vasculitis are influenced by multiple genetic factors. There is, however, a group of renal diseases which have a clear Mendelian pattern of inheritance and are caused by defects in a single gene. The commonest single gene disorders causing renal disease are summarized in Table 14.1.4.

By far the commonest of these is autosomal dominant polycystic kidney disease. This has a prevalence of 1:1000 in the population and is responsible for up to 10% of cases of end-stage renal failure in the West. The disease is characterized by the progressive development of renal and hepatic cysts throughout the patient's life. The renal cysts eventually compress the surrounding normal renal tissue causing renal impairment. Patients frequently complain of lower back pain, macroscopic haematuria and recurrent urinary tract infections. End-stage renal failure typically develops in middle age. At present there is no specific treatment for this condition. A rarer autosomal recessive form of polycystic kidney disease has a more severe phenotype and generally causes death in affected infants.

Alport's syndrome is also common, affecting 1:5000 of the population. This condition gives rise to deafness and renal failure. The most frequent pattern of inheritance is X-linked, with males developing the renal failure and deafness and females only microscopic haematuria.

Vesico-ureteric reflux (VUR) is a condition in which urine can be demonstrated to reflux from the bladder into the ureters on micturition. The resulting failure to void completely results in recurrent urinary tract infections which involve the kidney and may cause renal scarring and ultimately renal impairment. The disease behaves as a single gene disorder with a dominant pattern of inheritance but with variable penetrance. It is thought that approximately 0.15% of the population have the defective gene of which 50% develop clinical evidence of VUR.

Infection

Human urine is usually sterile. In a proportion of asymptomatic subjects, however, bacteria can be cultured from the

Table 14.1.4.   Single gene disorders causing renal disease

Disease	Mode of inheritance	Gene
Autosomal dominant polycystic kidney disease	Autosomal dominant	PKD1 gene or PKD2 gene
Autosomal recessive polycystic kidney disease	Autosomal recessive	Fibrocystin gene
Alport's syndrome	Autosomal dominant, Autosomal recessive or X-linked dominant	Type IV collagen genes
Vesico-ureteric reflux	Autosomal dominant with variable penetrance	Unknown

urine. This phenomenon, known as asymptomatic bacteriuria, is much more common in women, presumably because of the shorter urethra permitting the retrograde migration of bacteria from the perineum. Symptomatic urinary infections usually only involve the bladder and cystitis is a very common presentation in general practice, again almost exclusively in women. Rarely infection can ascend the ureters into the kidneys resulting in pyelonephritis, particularly if VUR is present. Patients may complain of back or loin pain and are usually febrile and unwell. This is regarded as a medical emergency and should be urgently treated in hospital with intravenous antibiotics. Recurrent pyelonephritis can result in renal scarring and ultimately renal failure.

Obstruction

Obstruction to the flow of urine can occur anywhere in the urinary tract from the renal pelvis to the urethra. If obstruction affects both kidneys renal failure will develop. Slowly progressive obstruction may present with advanced renal failure but patients with more acute obstruction may complain of lower back pain. The diagnosis is usually made on renal ultrasound which reveals a dilated renal pelvis (hydronephrosis). The commonest cause by far is bladder outflow obstruction caused by benign prostatic hypertrophy or carcinoma in males, in which case the bladder is also distended. Other causes include bladder tumours which obstruct the ureteric orifices, urethral strictures or posterior urethral valves, retroperitoneal fibrosis or malignancy involving the ureters, or strictures at the pelvi-ureteric junction. Renal stones also occasionally obstruct one or both ureters. The management is to relieve the obstruction. In the case of bladder outflow obstruction this may simply involve passing a urethral catheter. In other situations a percutaneous nephrostomy tube may be required prior to the surgical correction of the underlying cause. This involves passing a tube through the skin into the kidney via which urine can drain, bypassing the obstruction.

Urinary stone disease

The urine is an aqueous solution containing calcium, oxalate, magnesium, phosphate and many other poorly soluble substances which may precipitate to form solid crystals. When these crystals aggregate into large enough masses they are described as stones. This can occur in the kidneys or the bladder and is referred to as urolithiasis (Fig. 14.1.7). Symptomatic urolithiasis is relatively common, with an annual incidence in UK general practice of 7 per 10 000 increasing to 21 per 10 000 in men aged 45–60 years. Typical features of urolithiasis are loin pain, intermittent renal colic caused by small stones passing down a ureter, recurrent urinary tract infections, macroscopic or microscopic haematuria, proteinuria and occasionally renal impairment. The

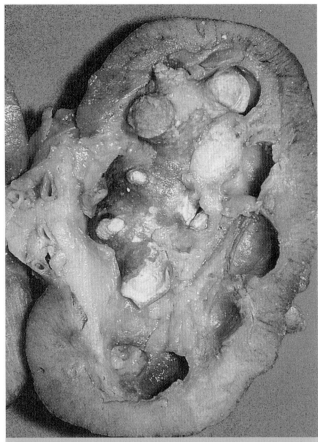

Figure 14.1.7.   A staghorn calculus within the kidney. (Reproduced with permission from Underwood, 2000.)

main risk factor for the development of stones is the urine calcium concentration. People who live in hot climates and those with a limited fluid intake will produce concentrated urine predisposing to the precipitation of calcium salts. Urine calcium concentrations may, however, be elevated in the absence of the above factors in patients with idiopathic hypercalciuria. This is presumed to be due to a genetic factor altering the renal tubular capacity to handle calcium. Other causes of stones include elevated serum uric acid levels which can cause gout and uric acid stones, urinary tract infection which predisposes to magnesium ammonium phosphate stones, and hereditary cystinuria which results in cystine stones.

Common renal stones

- Calcium oxalate
- Magnesium ammonium phosphate
- Uric acid
- Cystine

The initial management of all renal stone disease is to reduce the concentration of the offending salt in the urine. This can often be achieved by increasing fluid intake. Pharmacological means of reducing urinary calcium excretion and increasing stone solubility can also be employed. Large or problematic stones may need to be managed surgically by endoscopic or percutaneous lithotomy. An alternative is extracorporeal shock wave lithotripsy, which involves the non-invasive use of ultrasound to shatter stones allowing the fragments to be passed.

Other causes of renal disease

Many other causes of renal impairment and end-stage renal disease have been described. The diverse nature of renal disease illustrates the vulnerability of the kidney to a wide range of disease processes.

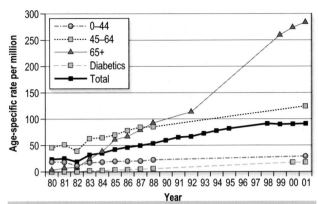

Figure 14.1.8.   Patients accepted for renal replacement therapy in the UK, expressed in patients per million per year. Source: UK Renal Registry.

Rarer causes of renal failure

- Metabolic diseases, e.g. cystinosis
- Amyloidosis
- Multiple myeloma
- Drug toxicity, e.g. gentamicin
- Interstitial nephritis
- Heavy metal poisoning, e.g. lead poisoning
- Rhabdomyolysis due to muscle injury
- Haemolytic uraemic syndrome
- Hepatorenal syndrome seen in liver failure
- Eclampsia and pre-eclampsia

END-STAGE RENAL DISEASE

The incidence and prevalence of end-stage renal disease in the Western world has been steadily rising over the last few decades. This is partly due to an increased awareness and recognition of renal disease, an ageing population and the increased prevalence of type 2 diabetes. In the UK there are now around 30 000 patients with end-stage renal disease, representing approximately 550 patients per million of the population, and about 100 new patients per million commence dialysis each year. The USA, however, reports a prevalence of end-stage renal disease of 1217 per million with 317 patients starting dialysis per million per year. There are also important differences in the epidemiology of renal disease between populations, with black Americans being 3–4 times as likely to develop renal failure as their white counterparts, and British Asians some 3–5 times as likely to develop renal failure as white Britons. These differences probably reflect the higher incidence of hypertension and diabetes in these communities as well as other as yet undefined genetic differences.

Both the incidence and prevalence of renal failure continue to rise throughout the world, particularly in the elderly, and the growth in the UK dialysis population over the last 20 years has been largely in the over-65 age group (Fig. 14.1.8).

Renal replacement therapy

When end-stage renal failure develops the patient will die without renal support. This can be offered in the form of dialysis therapy or renal transplantation. The term dialysis refers to the replacement of native renal function with an artificial means of clearing the blood of soluble waste products. Two types of dialysis are available, haemodialysis and peritoneal dialysis (PD). Ideally the choice of dialysis modality should be left to the individual. In practice clinical necessity and local availability may determine which modality is employed. In the UK about 60% of dialysis patients are maintained on haemodialysis and 40% on PD.

Haemodialysis

Haemodialysis is a process in which blood is drawn from the patient and passed through an apparatus where it comes into contact with a semi-permeable dialysis membrane. This membrane separates the blood from a buffered aqueous solution referred to as the dialysate. Molecules in the blood will pass by diffusion across the dialysis membrane into the dialysate. Molecules in the dialysate will also diffuse into the blood but as the dialysate contains no urea or other waste products, to start with, the net movement of such molecules will be from blood to dialysate. The composition of the dialysate is carefully controlled so that excessive amounts of sodium, calcium and other salts are not lost. If there is a hydrostatic pressure gradient across the dialysis membrane a second process will occur, namely convection. This is the movement of water across the membrane driven by a pressure difference. Water crossing the membrane in this way will carry solute with it and this is referred to as convective

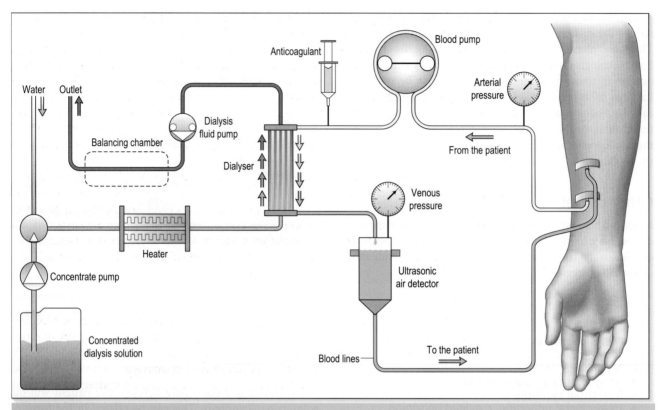

Figure 14.1.9.   **A typical dialysis circuit.**

transport. The most important component of the dialysis system is the dialysis membrane. The characteristics of this membrane will largely determine the rate of diffusion and convection that occurs. The membrane should allow the easy passage of water, salts and uraemic toxins but must retain large plasma proteins.

The modern haemodialysis machine consists of a blood pump which moves blood from the access site, through the dialyser and back to the patient (Fig. 14.1.9). Another pump passes the dialysate through the dialyser. A series of failsafe devices and bubble traps ensure that accidental blood loss or air introduction does not occur. Historically the dialysis membrane was a flat sheet or tube but modern membranes consist of small hollow fibres encased in a plastic cartridge. These occupy little space but have a large dialysis surface area. Generally they are used once then disposed of.

Access to the circulation can be via a vascular catheter but these may become infected with serious consequences. Long-term vascular access is therefore achieved by forming an arterio-venous fistula, usually on the forearm. This involves the surgical anastamosis of an artery with an adjacent vein. The vein, exposed to arterial pressures, dilates and thickens. Needles can then easily be passed into these vessels to withdraw and return blood. In fact the development of these fistulas represented a huge breakthrough in haemodialysis, permitting patients to remain on dialysis treatment for many years.

In practice patients will require a minimum of three sessions of haemodialysis per week each lasting from 3 to 5 hours. Most patients attend a dialysis unit for their treatment but haemodialysis can be undertaken by patients in their own homes, considerably increasing the flexibility and convenience of this treatment modality. Many other variations of haemodialysis exist, including continuous haemodialfiltration, overnight haemodialysis and daily haemodialysis.

Peritoneal dialysis

Peritoneal dialysis (PD) offers an alternative to haemodialysis and is widely practised in the UK but less so in other Western countries. This form of dialysis utilizes the peritoneal membrane as the dialysis surface. The peritoneal membrane is an epithelial cell monolayer lining the abdominal cavity forming an enclosed space which normally contains only a small amount of fluid. The peritoneal cavity can, however, accommodate several litres of fluid. In peritoneal dialysis a buffered dialysis fluid is instilled into the peritoneal cavity through a latex tube in the abdominal wall. The fluid is left to dwell for several hours during which diffusion of solute between the blood in the capillaries lining the peritoneal membrane, and the dialysate occurs. Additionally if the dialysate has an osmolality higher than that of serum, water and with it solute will be drawn across the membrane in a convective process. The original form of PD required the patient to manually perform the fluid exchanges in a process called continuous ambulatory peritoneal dialysis (CAPD). Typically four exchanges of two litres of dialysate per day are required in order to achieve satisfactory clearance of uraemic toxins and water. More recently an automated form of PD (APD) has become available. This is performed during the night by a machine which mechanically controls the movement of dialysate into and out of the peritoneum, leaving patients free of dialysis during the day. As with haemodialysis, the composition of the dialysate is carefully controlled. Dialysate solutions of varying osmolalities are available enabling the user to control the amount of water removed at each exchange.

The advantages of PD over haemodialysis are that it liberates patients from the need to attend a dialysis unit and gives the individual some control over the organization of their day. Patients may also travel by simply taking supplies of fluid or arranging delivery at their destination with the supplier. The drawbacks are that patients need to be motivated, well trained, compliant and able to carry out the dialysis adequately. Furthermore, dialysis needs to be performed on a daily basis. Complications of PD include infection of the peritoneal cavity, usually caused by contamination of the catheter tip during handling.

Complications of dialysis

Unfortunately dialysis treatment is not a complete substitute for native renal function. The sophistication of the kidney in selectively removing waste products cannot be matched by the relatively crude means available at present and this is well illustrated by the accumulation of β-2 *microglobulin* in dialysis patients. This protein is normally selectively cleared by the kidney but is poorly removed by both haemodialysis and PD and therefore plasma levels of β-2 microglobulin are substantially elevated in dialysis patients. The protein is deposited in a characteristic pattern in which the protein molecules adopt a β-pleated sheet tertiary structure known as amyloid (starch-like substance that destroys local tissue). These highly insoluble deposits accumulate in joints and other tissues and frequently give rise to arthritis and nerve entrapment. Carpal tunnel syndrome is particularly common and is seen in a large proportion of longstanding dialysis patients.

Dialysis is also no substitute for the endocrine functions of the kidneys. Erythropoietin deficiency results in anaemia which can be disabling, particularly for young and active patients. Fortunately there are now several recombinant human erythropoietin preparations available for intravenous or subcutaneous administration which will raise the haemoglobin significantly in the majority of subjects. The deficiency in 1,25-dihydroxycholecalciferol (the metabolically active vitamin D discussed previously) contributes to the bone disease seen in dialysis patients. The low vitamin D levels result in hypocalcaemia which in turn leads to stimulation of the parathyroid glands to release parathyroid hormone

(PTH). The PTH causes localized bone lesions (osteitis fibrosa cystica) which may be associated with disabling bone pain or pathological fractures. Other factors contributing to the bone disease include the poor clearance of phosphate by dialysis and the chronic acidosis seen in dialysis patients. Treatment for renal bone disease includes vitamin D supplements in the form of 1-α-hydroxycholecalciferol, oral calcium carbonate to bind phosphate in the gut and prevent its absorption and occasionally surgical removal of the parathyroid glands.

Even with the best treatment available today the morbidity and mortality associated with dialysis is substantially elevated compared to the general population. In particular, patients develop accelerated cardiovascular disease as well as an increased incidence of infection. These two factors largely account for the increased risk of illness and death in this population group.

Renal transplantation

Renal transplantation is the preferred treatment of renal failure. Compared to patients on dialysis, renal transplant recipients live longer with fewer illnesses and with a better quality of life. Because the renal transplant is a normal human kidney many of the inadequacies and complications of dialysis are overcome. Ideally therefore transplantation should replace dialysis in suitable patients. Unfortunately, however, the demand for transplants substantially exceeds the supply of donor organs. In the UK, for example, there were in 2001 around 5000 patients on the kidney transplant waiting list but only 1743 renal transplants were performed.

Organs for renal transplantation can be obtained from subjects suffering brain stem or cardiovascular death typically due to head injury or cerebrovascular accident (cadaveric donors), or from living persons who elect to donate one of their kidneys (living donors). Living donors are usually relatives of the recipient. The availability of cadaveric donors has remained static over the last few decades and may in fact be declining due to road safety legislation. This has led to an effort to increase the living related transplant programme as the only means of increasing transplant numbers. In the UK in 2001, 21% of renal transplants were from living donors, representing a substantial increase over previous years.

The genetic matching of donor organs with recipients has received much attention during the development of transplantation. Early on it was realized that the donor and recipient must be of compatible ABO blood group. Blood group incompatible transplants are immediately rejected by the recipient immune system due to the presence of ABO antibodies in the recipient circulation. Matching at other genetic loci, however, only results in modest improvement in transplant outcomes. Currently practice is to match cadaveric transplants at three HLA loci, namely A, B and Dr (see Ch. 2). This involves a matching scheme where recipient data is stored centrally and cadaveric kidneys are distributed nationally according to the most favourable match. The value of this strategy with improving immunosuppression has, however, been questioned, particularly as it disadvantages rarer genotypes in the population. Living related transplants cannot of course be deliberately matched and only ABO compatibility is required.

Immunosuppression is essential in renal transplantation with the exception of transplantation between identical twins. Even the best-matched kidneys will be rejected within days unless the recipient immune system is prevented from responding to the presence of foreign tissue. Immunosuppression regimes have improved enormously over the last three decades and these developments have largely been responsible for the improvement in transplant outcomes seen. Standard immunosuppression now consists of corticosteroids, azathioprine and ciclosporin although many newer drugs are now also widely used. In addition, monoclonal antibodies directed against specific components of the immune system have been developed. Unfortunately immunosuppression is required for the life of the transplant as immunological tolerance (the immunological acceptance of the donor organ by the recipient) does not develop. Side effects of the immunosuppressive drugs are therefore very important. Long-term steroids may cause osteoporosis, myopathy, weight gain and thinning of the skin. Ciclosporin can cause hirsutism, gingival hyperplasia and paradoxically renal impairment, and azathioprine can cause bone marrow suppression.

Renal transplant outcomes are now very good and have been improving steadily. Around 90% of recipients will have a functioning transplant after one year and 85% after 5 years. Living related transplants have a slightly better outcome than cadaveric transplants.

Unfortunately not all patients are suitable for transplantation. Contraindications include significant cardiovascular disease, urological abnormalities and anticipated poor compliance with medications. There is no defined age limit for recipients but few patients with renal failure over the age of 70 prove suitable and it is this group whose numbers are expanding most.

UROLOGICAL TUMOURS

Malignancy can affect the kidneys, ureters, bladder, prostate and urethra.

Prostate cancer

By far the commonest urological malignancy is prostate cancer. Histological evidence of prostate cancer can be found in over 50% of men over 50 years old but fortunately the prevalence of clinically significant cancer is much less. Nevertheless prostate cancer ranks as the sixth commonest cause of death

in men in the USA. The condition may be detected incidentally or may present with localized symptoms of difficulty, frequency or urgency of micturition. Less commonly patients present with bone pain due to metastatic disease, bladder outflow obstruction or renal failure. The diagnosis can be definitively made by prostatic biopsy but an elevated prostate-specific antigen in the circulation or a hard and irregular prostate on rectal examination are highly suggestive.

The treatment of prostate cancer is controversial because the majority of these malignancies do not progress to become clinically significant. For localized disease a number of treatment options are available including 'watchful waiting' in which regular surveillance of known tumours is undertaken, surgical prostatectomy or radiotherapy. Disease which has spread beyond the prostate is usually treated with hormone therapy. This is based on the observation that androgens accelerate and oestrogens retard the progression of the tumours. Historically a reduction in androgen exposure was achieved by total orchidectomy and oestrogens were administered in the form of diethylstilbestrol. Newer pharmacological means of achieving androgen blockade have superseded orchidectomy, and oestrogen stimulation with luteinizing hormone releasing hormone analogues has now replaced diethylstilbestrol. The management of prostate malignancy remains controversial and poses a challenge to urologists. The prognosis of the cancer depends on its stage, although even advanced tumours may grow very slowly, particularly in the elderly.

Renal tumours

Adenocarcinomas

Renal tumours of the adult are almost always renal adenocarcinomas derived from renal tubular epithelial cells. The term hypernephroma describes the same entity but has fallen out of use. Renal adenocarcinomas are more common in the elderly and affect males more frequently than females. At presentation 10% of patients have bilateral disease. Patients may present with macroscopic haematuria, loin pain and a palpable mass in the kidney. Frequently patients describe systemic symptoms such as malaise and weight loss and may have an intermittent fever associated with a raised erythrocyte sedimentation rate (ESR) or serum C-reactive protein (CRP) level. Hypertension is present in 20–40% and is due to renin release by the tumour in some cases. A small percentage of renal masses are due to other tumour types including oncocytomas, angiomyolipomas, leiomyosarcomas or non-malignant inflammatory masses in chronically infected kidneys. Renal adenocarcinomas spread lymphatically and haematologically as well as by direct invasion of surrounding structures. The haematological dissemination of the tumour accounts for the many unusual metastatic sites described. Most commonly there is spread up the inferior vena cava in the lungs, liver, bone adrenal gland or opposite kidney. Approximately one-third of patients will have metastases at the time of presentation. The diagnosis of renal adenocarcinomas is made clinically and radiologically. Renal ultrasound or intravenous urogram (IVU) are frequently used, followed by CT, angiography or MRI to assess more precisely the size and local spread of tumours. In patients with renal tumours imaging of the chest is also performed to identify pulmonary metastases.

The treatment of renal tumours is largely surgical by either radical or partial nephrectomy. Partial nephrectomy is generally reserved for patients with small tumours or those with single kidneys who would otherwise require dialysis treatment with all its attendant complications. Radiotherapy and chemotherapy have limited roles in renal tumours. The prognosis depends on the stage of the tumour at presentation. Localized malignancy is frequently cured by surgery whereas the prognosis for more advanced tumours can be bleak.

Wilms tumour

Wilms tumour is the commonest urogenital malignancy of children, occurring in about 8 per million of the under-15 population per year. It is an embryonal neoplasm consisting histologically of varying proportions of blastema, stroma and epithelium. Although most cases are sporadic, familial cases of Wilms tumour occur. Furthermore various congenital abnormalities including genitourinary anomalies, aniridia (absent iris) and mental retardation are associated with the condition. Subjects with all three of these abnormalities usually have a deletion on the short arm of chromosome 11 and have a 50% risk of developing Wilms tumour. These observations led to the identification of the WT-1 gene on chromosome 11. Although the genetics of Wilms tumour has proved complex, it is now known that mutations in WT-1 predispose to the development of the disease. These mutations may be germ-line (present at birth) or acquired, and must be present in both alleles of the gene within a single cell for the tumour to develop.

Clinically the tumour most often presents with an abdominal mass. Metastases, usually to the lungs, may also be present. As with adenocarcinomas in adults the diagnosis is made radiologically. The treatment options include surgery, chemotherapy and radiotherapy. The prognosis depends on the exact histological type of the tumour as well as the stage.

Bladder cancer

The bladder is lined with a specialized transition cell epithelium that can give rise to malignancy. The incidence of bladder cancer increases with age and it is more common in men than in women. The aetiology of bladder cancer is complex but a number of factors have been identified. Environmental exposure to aniline dye as a cause of bladder cancer allowed one of the first successful interventions by occupational medicine. Other environmental factors have been identified as increasing risk including cigarette smoke and infection with *Schistosoma haematobium*. Genetic factors are also important and a number of genetic polymorphisms have been identified which increase risk.

Clinically bladder cancer may present with the incidental finding of microscopic haematuria, the presence of macroscopic haematuria or more uncommonly with symptoms of bladder irritation. The diagnosis is made by cystoscopy when the bladder wall is visualized. Transurethral resection of the tumour may then be performed to the depth of the bladder muscle to allow histological staging to be performed. Subsequent investigation and management is determined by the histological stage. Patients with superficial lesions are managed by regular endoscopic surveillance and resection. Additional intravesical chemotherapy is being increasingly used in this group of patients. More advanced tumours require more radical surgery, radiotherapy or chemotherapy.

REFERENCES AND FURTHER READING

Ansell D, Feest T, Byrne C (2002) Renal Registry Report 2002. UK Renal Registry.

Bradley J, Smith K (1998) Diagnostic Tests in Nephrology. Philadelphia: Lippincott Williams & Wilkins.

Campbell MF, Walsh PC, Retic AB (2002) Campbell's Urology. London: Saunders.

Danovitch GM (2001) Handbook of Kidney Transplantation. Philadelphia: Lippincott Williams & Wilkins.

Davidson AM, Cameron JS, Grunfeld J-P, et al. (1998) Oxford Textbook of Clinical Nephrology. Oxford: Oxford University Press.

Davies A, Blakeley AGH, Kidd C (2001) Textbook of Medical Physiology. Edinburgh: Churchill Livingstone.

Foggensteiner L, Mulroy S, Firth J (2001) Management of diabetic nephropathy. J R Soc Med, 94(5): 210–217.

Guyton RC, Hall EH (1995) Textbook of Medical Physiology, 9th edn. Philadelphia: Saunders.

Kumar P, Clark M (2002) Clinical Medicine. London: Saunders.

Page C, Curtis M, Sutter MC (2002) Integrated Pharmacology, 2nd edn. Edinburgh: Mosby.

Rang HP, Dale MM, Ritter JM, Moore P (2003) Pharmacology, 5th edn. Edinburgh: Churchill Livingstone.

Underwood JCE (2000) General and Systematic Pathology. Edinburgh: Churchill Livingstone.

The Urinary System: The Overactive Bladder

Jacek L. Mostwin

Overactive bladder (OAB) is the most common term currently used in clinical medicine to describe a complex of lower urinary tract symptoms (LUTS) with or without incontinence but most commonly consisting of urgency, frequency, nocturia, troublesome or incomplete emptying, and, occasionally, pain. With the exception of pain and incontinence, these symptoms are often found together; thus, the term LUTS has come to replace previous terms, such as *urgency frequency syndrome*, *urethral syndrome* and *prostatism*.

OAB encompasses many previously used diagnostic and descriptive terms that remain in clinical use but are gradually being subsumed under the newer term OAB. These other terms include *neurogenic bladder*, *neuropathic bladder*, *unstable bladder* and *uninhibited bladder*. The newer term permits easier concentration on the bothersome aspect of LUTS without requiring a specific reference to cause.

The term OAB implies but does not actually identify specific causes or disease entities. It does not:

- distinguish incontinent patients from those who are not incontinent
- distinguish women with stress urinary incontinence from those who have incontinence for other reasons
- distinguish between intrinsic sphincter deficiency and other causes of stress urinary incontinence
- distinguish between patients who have LUTS with clearly defined origins from those who have LUTS with no apparent origin and who may be classified as having an idiopathic condition.

The term OAB is descriptive, not diagnostic. It describes the experience of patients who have LUTS with or without incontinence and with or without neurological disease or injury. It does not distinguish patients with LUTS who have demonstrable findings on cystometry (such as unstable contractions or hypersensitivity) from those who have normal cystometric findings. It does not address causes or varieties of incontinence.

OAB is a convenient clinical term because LUTS are common and ubiquitous. They are seen in association with many different urinary tract conditions, including urinary infection and inflammation, stones, foreign bodies and, occasionally, neoplasm. These particular conditions are listed for the sake of completeness, but they will not be discussed further in this chapter. These conditions are usually excluded in the evaluation of the patient with OAB symptoms, and OAB is more commonly associated with neuro-urological conditions.

The term OAB is convenient because it allows non-specialists to consider the many and varied types of incontinence and voiding dysfunction as a single kind of condition. Experts, such as neuro-urologists, urogynaecologists, and some paediatric urologists, can also use the term to focus on the symptoms reported by patients as being most bothersome, while remaining mindful of the numerous disease conditions that cause them. To summarize, LUTS has replaced former terms describing symptoms of the lower urinary tract, and OAB has replaced terms that formerly implied specific symptom origins.

GENERALLY ACCEPTED CAUSES OF OVERACTIVE BLADDER

Neurological illness and injury

Neurological illness and injury are well-known causes of voiding dysfunction, OAB symptoms and overactive detrusor activity. Descriptions of the varieties of voiding dysfunction in different kinds of illnesses, such as multiple sclerosis, stroke, diabetes, Alzheimer's disease, spinal stenosis, spinal cord injury or myelodysplasia, are familiar to clinicians in the field.

These conditions often require assessment and possible intervention by a clinician familiar with urodynamic testing and the spectrum of disorders. They require an understanding of changes in bladder tone and stability produced by the various disorders, the relation of bladder function to coordinated sphincter function, and the effect of bladder dysfunction on renal function.

Early experience with bladder activity in neurological illness and injury was mostly with spinal cord injury patients in England after World War II and in the United States after the Korean War. Many of these patients had limited, abnormal, or absent sensation associated with bladder activity. Simple cystometry was used as a rough measurement of bladder contractility and tone. Patients who experienced urgency, frequency or troublesome voiding symptoms often had abnormal findings on cystometry, such as hypertonicity or hyperreflexia. These motor abnormalities came to be associated with the symptoms and, by association, were thought to cause the symptoms. A similar interpretation was made about LUTS in men with bladder outlet obstruction.

Increasing knowledge of the changes that take place in neuroanatomic pathways and pharmacological mechanisms in various disease and injury conditions is increasing the possibilities for therapeutic intervention. It is known that suprapontine areas can exert an inhibitory influence on the pontine micturition centre (Figs 14.2.1 and 14.2.2). Damage to these areas by stroke or Alzheimer's disease can reduce this inhibitory action. In animal models of stroke and Parkinson's disease, glutamatergic and dopaminergic pathways have been found to modulate micturition activity.

Suprasacral spinal cord injury disrupts voluntary and suprasacral modulation of micturition, leading to spinal reflex-mediated micturition. These abnormalities may be associated with loss or changes in sensation of micturition events and a change in sphincter coordination. An important neuropharmacological finding has been the change in afferent activity

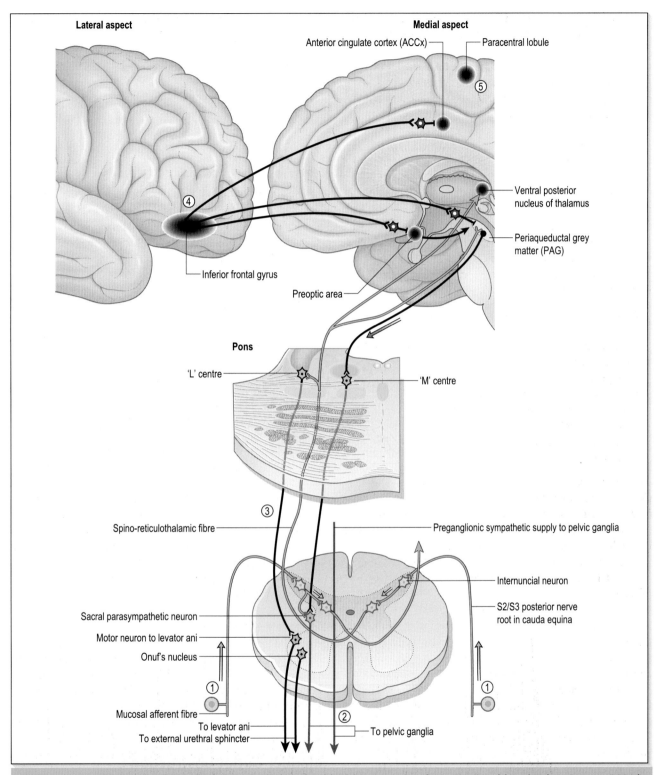

Figure 14.2.1.   Higher level bladder controls. (Reproduced with permission from FitzGerald and Folan-Curran, 2001.)

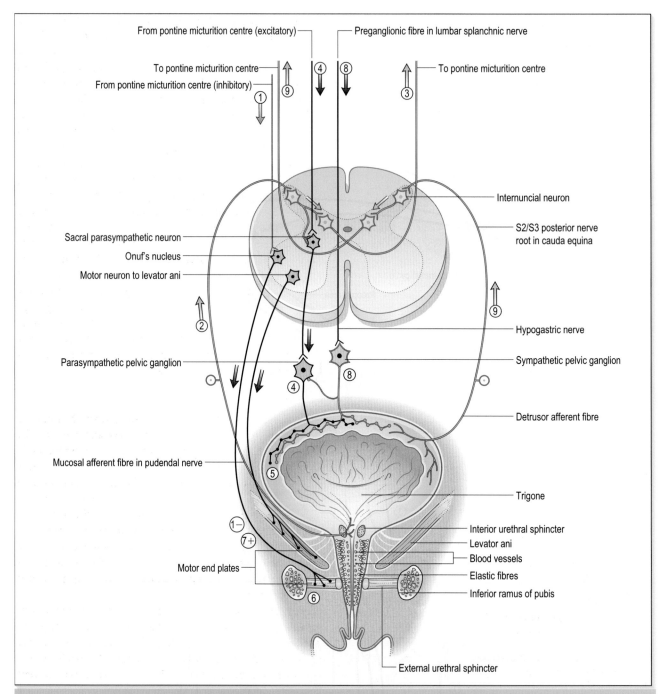

From pontine micturition centre (excitatory)

Preganglionic fibre in lumbar splanchnic nerve

To pontine micturition centre

From pontine micturition centre (inhibitory)

To pontine micturition centre

Internuncial neuron

S2/S3 posterior nerve root in cauda equina

Sacral parasympathetic neuron

Onuf's nucleus

Motor neuron to levator ani

Hypogastric nerve

Parasympathetic pelvic ganglion

Sympathetic pelvic ganglion

Detrusor afferent fibre

Mucosal afferent fibre in pudendal nerve

Trigone

Interior urethral sphincter

Levator ani

Blood vessels

Elastic fibres

Inferior ramus of pubis

Motor end plates

External urethral sphincter

Figure 14.2.2.   Lower level bladder controls. (Reproduced with permission from FitzGerald and Folan-Curran, 2001.)

from myelinated A-afferents to unmyelinated C-afferents, which do not respond to bladder distension. C-fibre bladder afferents show a change in electrical excitability. C-afferents are capsaicin sensitive, a finding that has led to treating bladder overactivity in spinal injury and multiple sclerosis. The favourable results suggest that overactivity may be mediated by capsaicin-sensitive C-afferents.

Bladder outlet obstruction

Bladder outlet obstruction is caused by prostatic enlargement, bladder neck dysfunction, posterior urethral valves, uncoordinated sphincter activity (Fig. 14.2.3) (as seen in spinal injury, myelodysplasia, and Hinman syndrome), and iatrogenic obstruction (e.g. after surgery for stress incontinence). Bladder outlet obstruction in association with

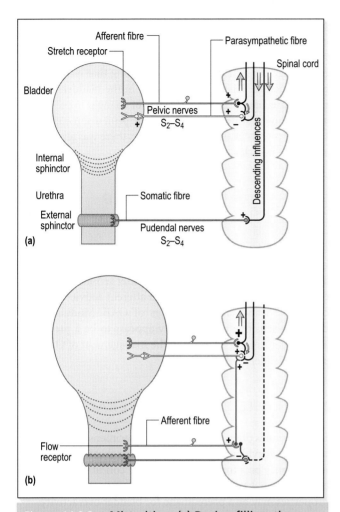

Figure 14.2.3.   Micturition. (a) During filling, the descending inhibitory influence on the parasympathetic supply to the detrusor muscle and the descending excitatory influence on the somatic supply to the external sphincter *inhibit* micturition (− and + signs indicate inhibitory and excitatory influences respectively). (b) During emptying, *activation* of the parasympathetic supply to the detrusor muscle causes its contraction, and *removal* of the tonic excitatory influence on the somatic supply to the external sphincter causes its opening. Emptying of the bladder is facilitated by the input from the flow receptors in the urethra, which reinforces the contraction of the detrusor muscle and the relaxation of the external sphincter. (Reproduced with permission from Davies et al., 2001.)

prostatic disease was the first condition other than neurological injury or illness that was found to be associated with unstable detrusor contractions during filling cystometry. The association of these findings with LUTS common in men with prostatic outlet obstruction led to the impression that LUTS were the symptomatic correlate of bladder instability. Relief of unstable contractions and improvement in LUTS in men after prostatectomy further reinforced the impression that bladder instability and LUTS were causally related.

Experimental outlet obstruction in animal models grew out of these clinical observations. Experimentally produced bladder outlet obstruction was the primary source of bladder tissue used to study histological, pharmacological and physiological changes in a search for underlying mechanisms. With rare exception, because of their subjective nature, LUTS could not be studied in experimental animals. It was generally assumed that understanding pathophysiological mechanisms would lead to improved treatment directed at the muscle itself and, therefore, would lead to improvement in OAB symptoms. Subsequent clinical studies in humans, however, have not shown a strong causal relation between LUTS and bladder outlet obstruction. Clinical studies have emphasized the ubiquity of LUTS in women and the general relation of LUTS to ageing. Therefore, although uncertainty exists about the exact interrelation of LUTS, bladder outlet obstruction and OAB, it is fair to say that, in experimental situations, bladder outlet obstruction gives rise to instability and abnormalities in the bladder that may cause OAB symptoms and abnormal cystometric behaviour. Basic scientific research into causes of bladder dysfunction in bladder outlet obstruction has focused on changes in bladder muscle, bladder innervation and voiding reflexes.

Bladder muscle in obstruction

The obstructed bladder increases in weight, and histological examination shows myocyte hypertrophy and hyperplasia, increased collagen deposition, and a loss of parasympathetic nerve terminals. Pharmacological studies of muscle strips from the experimentally obstructed bladders of animals have shown that the muscle behaves in a manner consistent with denervation supersensitivity: the response to cholinergic stimulation increases, whereas the response to nerve stimulation decreases. It has been shown that arterial blood flow and tissue oxygen levels decrease during bladder muscle contraction in animal models, suggesting that denervation may be caused by ischaemic damage.

Studies of muscle contraction have shown loss of efficiency in contraction and reduced maintenance of energy required for contraction. Electrophysiological studies have shown that hypertrophied muscle cells may be less electrically stable than normal cells and may have disordered patterns of current spread. These findings would support experimental observations that the hypertrophied bladder contracts with a lower threshold of stimulation, and its contractions may be weaker and less sustained than those of the normal bladder.

Bladder innervation and voiding reflexes in obstruction

Bladder outlet obstruction affects sensory and motor aspects of voiding reflexes. In a rat model of bladder outlet obstruction, there is hypertrophy of bladder afferent and efferent neurons accompanying increased reflex micturition activity and cystometric signs of bladder overactivity. Nerve growth factor has been found to increase in the experimentally obstructed bladders of rats, suggesting an explanation for the increases in afferents.

OVERACTIVE BLADDER SYMPTOMS IN WOMEN

The findings of OAB symptoms in women with stress incontinence have increased uncertainty about the causal relation of OAB and LUTS to bladder outlet obstruction. Women with genuine stress urinary incontinence, intrinsic sphincter deficiency, or a combination of both may complain of LUTS. Some show unstable contractions on filling cystometry. Many of these patients will be in the diagnostic category of mixed incontinence. Many may experience resolution of LUTS after successful stress incontinence surgery, thereby suggesting a causal relation in this group. A possible explanation is that urine entering a weak, poorly coapted, or poorly supported proximal urethra may trigger a micturition reflex, an explanation supported by earlier experiments of F.J.F. Barrington in the 1930s and 1940s.

The finding that urethral sphincter muscle mass decreases in ageing women may well be extrapolated to men, although men have not yet been studied. Decreasing sphincter function in women may contribute to intrinsic sphincter deficiency.

- Dulox-etine is a serotonin and noradrenaline (norepinephrine) reuptake inhibitor that has been shown to increase striated sphincter activity in animal models. It is currently undergoing clinical trials and is expected to be available for the treatment of stress incontinence in women in the near future.
- Recent experience with sacral cord stimulation using the Interstim device (Medtronic, Minneapolis, MN) has suggested that modulation of the striated urethral sphincter may reduce LUTS and successfully treat OAB with associated incontinence.

Further investigation into the contributions of somatosensory sphincter activity to bladder control and overactivity may open up new ways of looking at the relation of LUTS and OAB.

DETRUSOR HYPERACTIVITY AND IMPAIRED CONTRACTILITY IN ELDERLY PATIENTS

LUTS and OAB findings are common in both elderly men and women. Sixty per cent of institutionalized elderly men and women show evidence of bladder overactivity. A specific entity, detrusor hyperactivity and impaired contractility in elderly patients, has been described. In this condition, symptoms and cystometric evidence of bladder overactivity are found together with incomplete emptying that is not caused by obstruction. Histological changes in the bladders of ageing humans have provided evidence of changes in cell-to-cell connections manifested by increased protrusion junctions. In patients with impaired contractility, there was also degeneration of muscle cells and nerve axons.

HYPERSENSITIVITY-INDUCED OVERACTIVITY

Unmyelinated, capsaicin-sensitive C-afferents have been found in the human bladder. These C-afferents are thought to mediate pain and may also contribute to other sensations of bladder fullness and urgency. Increased afferent activity may well cause LUTS and clinical findings of OAB. Modulation of capsaicin-sensitive nerve activity appears to be a promising area for clinical intervention in the management of OAB and painful bladder symptoms.

IDIOPATHIC BLADDER OVERACTIVITY

Denervation is often found in biopsy specimens from humans with clinical evidence of OAB, suggesting that muscle abnormalities may be a frequent cause of the condition. It has also been suggested that some sort of change in smooth muscle properties may be a prerequisite for bladder overactivity.

POSSIBLE FUTURE RESEARCH DIRECTIONS FOR UNDERSTANDING CAUSES OF OVERACTIVE BLADDER

The ubiquity of LUTS might suggest that they are caused by similar mechanisms and, theoretically at least, would be amenable to a single form of effective therapy. Conversely, the limited kinds and number of LUTS and the limited representation of lower urinary tract structures in the central nervous system may mean that several different causes produce similar symptoms, but these are not amenable to a single form of effective therapy. There is a problem in that LUTS and OAB appear in neurologically healthy and neurologically impaired individuals. Much of our earlier understanding about OAB came from the study of the latter, but much of our activity is now directed at the former.

At this time, it is difficult to consolidate all knowledge about bladder overactivity and LUTS into a single theory. There are simply too many observations that do not easily fit together. For example, men with bladder outlet obstruction and women with genuine stress urinary incontinence may have similar

LUTS. It is tempting to conclude, as in elderly patients, that both OAB and LUTS are independent of sex, yet LUTS and OAB in men resolve after successful treatment, as do the symptoms of women with genuine stress urinary incontinence after successful treatment. Work with animal models supports these clinical observations: the micturition reflex can be elicited by running water through the proximal urethra, and experimentally creating bladder outlet obstruction can induce bladder overactivity.

It has also been difficult to integrate experimental results on changes in bladder muscle with changes seen in afferent nerve activity after bladder outlet obstruction. Although these changes may well occur concurrently in humans and other animals, it is not clear how to integrate our knowledge about them.

ACKNOWLEDGEMENT

This chapter is reproduced (in modified form) from Mostwin (2002) with permission of Elsevier.

REFERENCES AND FURTHER READING

Ashton-Mille RJA, Howard D, DeLancey JO (2000) The functional anatomy of the female pelvic floor and stress continence control system. Scand J Urol Nephrol Suppl 207: 1–7.

Brading AF (1997) A myogenic basis for the overactive bladder. Urology 50 (suppl 6A) 57–67.

Davies A, Blakeley AGH, Kidd C (2001) Human Physiology. Edinburgh: Churchill Livingstone.

de la Rosette JJ, Witjes WP, Schafer W, et al. (1998) Relationships between lower urinary tract symptoms and bladder outlet obstruction: results from the ICS. Neurourol Urodyn 17: 99–108.

Elbadawi A, Hailemariam S, Yalla SV, et al. (1997) Structural basis of geriatric voiding dysfunction. VII: Prospective ultrastructural/urodynamic evaluation of its natural evolution. J Urol 157: 1814–1822.

FitzGerald MJT, Folan-Curran J (2001) Clinical Neuroanatomy and Related Neuroscience. Philadelphia: Saunders.

Greenland J, Brading A (2001) The effect of bladder outflow obstruction on detrusor blood flow changes during the voiding cycle in conscious pigs. J Urol 165: 245–248.

Janknegt RA, Hassouna MM, Siegel SW, et al. (2001) Long-term effectiveness of sacral nerve stimulation for refractory urge incontinence. Eur Urol 39: 101–106.

Mills IW, Greenland JE, McMurray G, et al. (2000) Studies of the pathophysiology of idiopathic detrusor instability: the physiological properties of the detrusor smooth muscle and its pattern of innervation. J Urol 163: 646–651.

Pitsikas N (2000) Duloxetine Eli Lilly & Co. Curr Opin Investig Drugs 1: 116–121.

Mostwin JL (2002) Pathophysiology: the varieties of bladder overactivity. Urology 60 (5: Suppl 1): 22–26.

Saito M, Yokoi K, Ohmura M, et al. (1997) Effects of partial outflow obstruction on bladder contractility and blood flow to the detrusor: comparison between mild and severe obstruction. Urol Int 59: 226–230.

PHARMACOLOGY

Section 5

PHARMACOLOGY

Section

15 Normal Drug Action 405
16.1 Drug Toxicity and Overdose 428
16.2 Drug Abuse and Dependence 435

Normal Drug Action

Leif Rune Skymoen

DRUGS USED IN BONE DISORDERS

Bone loss (resorption) and formation is a continous process throughout life. In osteoporosis, the equilibrium between resorption and formation is disturbed, resulting in an excessive bone loss (see Ch. 7 for details). This results in an increased risk of fractures and bone compression, causing significant morbidity and loss of independence for those affected. The causes of osteoporosis may range from postmenopausal loss of endogenous oestrogen production, to dietary insufficiencies and drug side effects. Osteoporosis therapy aims at early diagnosis and prevention of fractures.

In osteomalacia and rickets, inadequate bone mineralization leads to fractures and deformities. Mineralization is impaired due to a deficiency of hydroxyapatite, a compound primarily consisting of calcium and phosphorus. Treatment of these disorders depends on the underlying cause, but normally includes high doses of different vitamin D preparations and calcium supplements.

In addition to vitamin and mineral replacement therapy, several different approaches are employed for treatment of bone disorders such as osteoporosis and osteomalacia. As described in Chapter 7, the main components of bone homeostasis are cells (osteoblasts and osteoclasts), cytokines, minerals and hormones (parathyroid hormone, the vitamin D family and calcitonin). The drugs used in bone disorders affect these components as described below and summarized in Figure 15.1.

Oestrogens

Through the reproductive years of a woman's life, oestrogens inhibit osteoclast recruitment and oppose the bone-resorbing

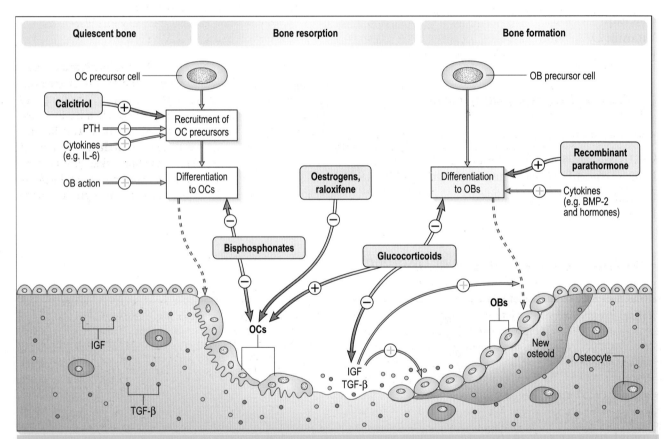

Figure 15.1.   The bone-remodelling cycle and the action of hormones, cytokines and drugs. In quiescent trabecular bone, cytokines such as insulin-like growth factor (IGF) and transforming growth factor-β (TGF-β), shown as dots, are embedded in the bone matrix. During bone resorption, osteoclast (OC) precursor cells, recruited by cytokines and hormones, are activated by osteoblasts (OB) to form mobile multinuclear osteoclasts, which then move along the bone surface resorbing bone and releasing the embedded cytokines. During bone formation, the released cytokines recruit osteoblasts, which lay down osteoid and embed cytokines IGF and TGF-β in it. Some OBs also become embedded, forming terminal osteocytes. The osteoid then becomes mineralized and lining cells cover the area (not shown). Oestrogens cause apoptosis (programmed cell death) of osteoclasts. Note that pharmacological concentration of glucocorticoids has the effects specified above, but physiological concentrations are required for osteoblast differentiation. BMP-2, bone morphogenic protein-2; PTH, parathormone (endogenous); rPTH, recombinant PTH; IL-6, interleukin-6. (Reproduced with permission from Rang et al., 2003.)

action of parathyroid hormone (PTH). Oestrogens may also stimulate calcitonin secretion and inhibit release of some important cytokines. After the menopause ovarian function decreases, and endogenous oestrogen production falls accordingly, removing an important factor in maintenance of bone integrity. Many women therefore experience rapid bone loss with increased risk of fractures of hip, vertebrae, humerus or wrists. Bone loss and fracture rate can, however, be reduced with administration of exogenous oestrogen, so-called hormone replacement therapy (HRT). Oestrogen is very effective in prevention of osteoporosis if administered in the immediate postmenopausal period, and there is increasing evidence that it is beneficial also more than 10 years after the menopause.

Oestrogens can be administered orally, transdermally (patches) or topically (creams or pessaries for local effect in the vagina).

Other benefits from oestrogen therapy in menopausal women:

- relief from menopausal discomforts such as hot flushes and vaginal dryness and itching
- favourable effect on lipid profile ($\uparrow$HDL, $\downarrow$LDL).

Because of the favourable effect on lipid profile, it has been suggested that hormone replacement therapy may reduce the incidence of stroke and myocardial infarction. However, large clinical trials have failed to demonstrate any effects on the risk of coronary heart disease.

The most common side effects of oestrogen therapy include breast tenderness, peripheral oedema, headache, nausea and vomiting. In postmenopausal women oestrogen frequently causes menstruation-like bleedings. Cyclic administration may be effective in relieving these adverse effects. Studies have shown that women taking hormone replacement therapy have an increased risk of deep vein thrombosis and pulmonary embolism. Prolonged oestrogen exposure is associated with increased risk of hyperplasia of the endometrium and possible transformation to cancer. In long-term HRT a progestogen is therefore added to prevent endometrial cancer. Possibly, there is also an increased risk of breast cancer with long-term HRT, so breast awareness is particularly important in women receiving HRT.

Oestrogen receptor modulators

Because the side effects of HRT can limit long-term therapy, the so-called selective (o)estrogen receptor modulators (SERMs) have been developed. These agents have antagonist properties at most oestrogen receptors, but act as agonists at oestrogen receptors in bone. *Raloxifene*, which has been approved for prevention and treatment of postmenopausal osteoporosis, appears not to induce breast tenderness, endometrial hyperplasia, menstrual bleeding, or endometrial cancer. Increased risk of venous thromboembolism is, however, reported. SERMs offer no relief from vasomotor menopausal symptoms such as hot flushes.

Bisphosphonates

The bisphosphonates adsorb onto hydroxyapatite crystals at sites of active bone resorption, where they can remain for months or years, until the bone is resorbed. They reduce the turnover of bone through three distinct mechanisms (of which the first two are the most important):

- inhibition of osteoclast recruitment
- promotion of osteoclast apoptosis (cell suicide)
- indirect stimulation of osteoblast activity.

Etidronate and *alendronate* are the bisphosphonates most commonly prescribed. All bisphosphonates must be taken on an empty stomach, since absorption is impaired by food, and particularly by milk. Alendronate and risendronate also require the patient to stand or sit upright for at least 30 minutes after swallowing the tablets, to reduce the risk of oesophageal reactions. Gastrointestinal side effects such as nausea and abdominal pain are common to all bisphosphonates. Occasionally, these agents may also produce bone pain.

Clinical uses of bisphosphonates

- treatment of Paget's disease
- prevention and treatment of postmenopausal osteoporosis (together with, or as an alternative to, oestrogens)
- treatment of malignant hypercalcaemia
- etidronate is also licensed for treatment of corticosteroid-induced osteoporosis.

Calcitonin

Calcitonin is an endogenous hormone secreted by the thyroid gland. It exerts its physiological function, which is to lower serum calcium concentration when elevated, mainly by inhibiting osteoclast activity. Calcitonin can be administered intranasally or by injection. Natural porcine and synthetic human calcitonin preparations are available, but clinically synthetic salmon calcitonin (*salcatonin*) is used. Patients receiving calcitonin therapy, should also be administered calcium and vitamin D supplements.

Calcitonin has a good safety profile. Nausea and gastro-intestinal discomfort are the main adverse effects. In the initial phases of therapy patients may experience facial flushing or dermatitis, but these reactions usually decline with continued therapy. Subcutaneous administration is believed to have less risk of causing inflammation at the site of injection, than does intramuscular administration. Calcitonin is also reported to have an analgesic effect in women with osteoporotic vertebral fractures.

Clinical uses of calcitonin

- Reduction of plasma calcium levels in hypercalcaemia
- Pain relief and reduction of neurological complications in Paget's disease
- Prevention and treatment of postmenopausal and corticosteroid-induced osteoporosis.

PTH fragments

One of the physiological effects of parathyroid hormone (PTH) is bone resorption. Paradoxically, once-daily injections of PTH fragments have been shown to have the opposite effect. *Teriparatide*, which constitutes the active part of PTH, has recently been approved for treatment of osteoporosis. Data have indicated that teriparatide not only prevents bone loss, but can also stimulate bone formation.

Calcium

Along with phosphate, calcium is the main mineral in bone. Adequate calcium intake throughout life is essential for attaining normal bone mass. In corticosteroid-induced and postmenopausal osteoporosis, calcium supplements are important adjuncts to oestrogen, calcitonin and bisphosphonates. They are not likely to affect bone metabolism in women having sufficient calcium intake, but are beneficial in elderly people who often suffer from decreased calcium absorption due for example to vitamin D deficiency (see below).

The use of calcium supplements rarely leads to hypercalciuria or kidney stone, since homeostatic mechanisms decrease intestinal absorption when intake is excessive. Constipation is the main side effect from calcium supplements.

Vitamin D

Vitamin D enhances gastrointestinal absorption and decreases renal excretion of calcium. Vitamin D deficiency results in a hypocalcaemic state where one of the compensatory mechanisms activated is bone resorption. Elderly people often have an inadequate vitamin D status due to one or both of two reasons:

- Endogenous production of vitamin D_3 in the skin requires exposure to sunlight, which may be minimal, particularly in institutionalized patients.
- Dietary vitamin D intake is often decreased in the elderly.

In osteoporosis treatment, vitamin D is used to ensure sufficient calcium absorption. Clinically, *ergocalciferol* (vitamin D_2) is the main preparation used. Fish liver oils are rich in *cholecalciferol* (vitamin D_3), which is also available as an alternative to ergocalciferol in tablets and injections. Both these compounds need to be hydroxylated in the kidney to give the active form of vitamin D. *Alfacalcidol* and *calcitriol* are hydroxylated vitamin D derivatives, and do not require activation in the kidney. These agents should therefore be prescribed for vitamin D therapy in patients with severe renal impairment.

Recommended therapeutic dose for elderly patients is vitamin D 800 units per day with calcium 600–800 mg per day.

Concomitant use of calcium and vitamin D may allow a reduction in the calcium dose, since intestinal absorption should be increased. Excessive intake of vitamin D causes hypercalcaemia with symptoms like constipation, depression, weakness and fatigue. Precipitation of calcium stones in the kidney may result if the hypercalcaemia persists.

Drug-induced osteoporosis

Several drugs used in other conditions have the potential of precipitating osteoporosis. Unlike menopause-associated osteoporosis, this drug-induced form can occur at any age. Loop diuretics, as well as caffeine, are known to cause calciuria. Alcohol may inhibit calcium absorption from the gastrointestinal tract, and cigarette smoking appears to have an anti-oestrogenic effect. These are all risk factors, but the drugs that confer the highest increase in risk of developing osteoporosis are the ones discussed below.

The drugs with the highest potential of osteoporosis induction are:

- glucocorticoids
- gonadotrophin-releasing hormone (GnRH) agonists
- heparin.

Glucocorticoids

One of the troublesome side effects of glucocorticoid therapy is alteration of bone metabolism. The incidence of steroid-induced osteoporosis is not known, but it has been estimated that as much as half of patients receiving glucocorticoid therapy will be affected. Glucocorticoids are believed to disturb bone homeostasis through several mechanisms. Inhibition of osteoblast function, induction of hyperparathyroidism and interference with sex hormone production in the testes and ovaries are among the proposed mechanisms.

Strategies to reduce the risk of glucocorticoid-induced osteoporosis include:

- use the lowest effective dose
- local administration (inhaled or topical)
- vitamin D and calcium supplements
- hormone replacement therapy or oestrogen receptor modulators in postmenopausal women.

GnRH agonists

Analogues of gonadotrophin-releasing hormone (GnRH) are indicated for conditions such as infertility, endometriosis and breast and prostate cancer. Continuous administration of these agents results in a shutdown of the pathways from the hypothalamus, via the pituitary, to the gonads (the ovaries and testes). The secretion of sex hormones from the gonads is reduced as a result, and this interferes with bone homeostasis. Bone loss can be rapid, and some guidelines therefore recommend that GnRH agonists should not be administered for more than 6 months.

Heparin

Long-term use of the anticoagulant heparin has been reported to increase the risk of developing osteoporosis. Mechanisms involving increased activity of PTH and collagenase, as well as decreased production of the active vitamin D form, have been suggested. However, the actual number of patients identified with heparin-induced osteoporosis remains small. Recent studies of one of the high-risk groups, namely women receiving heparin during pregnancy, have concluded that the osteopenic effect is low. Data also indicate that the low-molecular-weight heparins have less effect on bone metabolism as compared to unfractionated heparin.

DRUGS USED IN RHEUMATIC DISEASES AND GOUT

Symptomatic, analgesic treatment of rheumatoid disorders is normally accomplished with anti-inflammatory agents, which can belong either to the corticosteroid class, or to the non-steroidal anti-inflammatory drugs (NSAIDs). Suppression of the rheumatic disease process itself, however, requires the use of one or more of the so-called disease-modifying antirheumatic drugs (DMARDs). Recently, a separate class of biological agents attacking the tumour necrosis factor have been added to the spectrum of drugs used in rheumatoid arthritis. The following section focuses on antirheumatic drug therapy and drugs used for the treatment of gout.

Non-steroidal anti-inflammatory drugs (NSAIDs)

NSAIDs are most frequently used without prescription for minor pains and aches. In gout and rheumatic diseases they are first-line agents for relief of pain and inflammation, but have no effect on the progressive joint destruction.

Pharmacological actions

The NSAIDs are an extensive class of drugs, with more than 50 different agents available on the market. *Aspirin, ibuprofen, naproxen* and *paracetamol* are some well-known examples. Common to most of them are a relatively high incidence of side effects and three major types of pharmacological actions:

- anti-inflammatory
- analgesic
- antipyretic (lowering raised temperature).

(Paracetamol differs from the other NSAIDs in having analgesic and antipyretic effects, but minimal anti-inflammatory activity.)

All these effects are related to the main mode of action for the NSAIDs, namely inhibition of the enzyme arachidonate cyclo-oxygenase (COX). This enzyme catalyses the conversion of arachidonic acid to prostaglandins and thromboxanes. There are several subtypes of the COX enzyme, of which COX-1 and COX-2 are the most important. COX-1 is highly expressed in the gastrointestinal tract, kidneys and platelets, where it is responsible for the production of protective and regulatory prostaglandins. COX-2, on the other hand, is found in low levels in healthy tissues. During inflammation, COX-2 is upregulated, giving rise to high levels of prostaglandin E_2, the major contributor to the local inflammatory reaction. Traditional NSAIDs inhibit both forms of the enzyme, COX-2 inhibition being responsible for the anti-inflammatory action. COX-1 inhibition is believed to mediate unwanted effects, such as gastrointestinal bleeding. In recent years, COX-2 selective agents, such as *celecoxib, rofecoxib* and *parecoxib*, have been approved for marketing. Although controversial, these agents are claimed to give fewer side effects than conventional NSAIDs, having equal anti-inflammatory activity.

Antipyretic effect

During inflammation, the pyrogen interleukin-1 (IL-1) is released from macrophages. IL-1 stimulates the production of prostaglandins, most importantly prostaglandin E_2, (PGE_2), that act on the temperature centre in the brain, resulting in elevation of the set-point for temperature. The antipyretic effect of NSAIDs is largely due to inhibition of prostaglandin generation in the hippocampus, the brain region where the temperature centre is located.

Analgesia

Prostaglandins are not mediators of pain themselves, but have a sensitizing effect on nociceptors, thus potentiating the pain-producing effect of bradykinin. In conditions associated with elevated prostaglandin levels, NSAIDs produce analgesia through inhibition of prostaglandin synthesis. Analgesic therapy is described in the 'Analgesics' section later in this chapter.

Anti-inflammatory effect

In areas of acute inflammation, local tissues and blood vessels generate high levels of PGE_2 and PGI_2, and mast cells release PGD_2. These are powerful vasodilators, which through a synergistic effect with other inflammatory vasodilators such as histamine and bradykinin, increase blood flow in areas of inflammation. The vasodilation facilitates the effects of histamine and bradykinin to increase permeability of post-capillary venules. Increased blood flow and permeability cause the redness and swelling characteristic of acute inflammation. In chronic inflammation; cells of the macrophage type also release PGE_2 and thromboxane A_2 (TXA_2).

By blocking the synthesis of prostaglandins and thromboxanes, NSAIDs directly reduce the vasodilating component of the inflammatory response. By reducing blood flow in the inflammatory area, NSAIDs also reduce the effects of histamine and bradykinin on vascular permeability, giving less oedema.

Common adverse effects

NSAIDs have a high incidence of unwanted effects, the gastrointestinal side effects dyspepsia, nausea and vomiting being the most frequent. Up to 75% of patients on chronic NSAIDs have mucosal damage and are consequently at risk of developing serious haemorrhage. Particularly high-risk individuals include the elderly and patients with a history of peptic ulcer disease or gastrointestinal bleeding, liver or renal disease, or on chronic corticosteroid therapy. The gastrointestinal adverse events are proposedly caused mainly by COX-1 inhibition, which blocks the synthesis of prostaglandins that normally inhibit acid secretion, protect the mucosa and modulate mucosal blood flow.

High risk factors for development of gastrointestinal complications following NSAID therapy:

- Age of 65 years and over
- Previous clinical history of gastroduodenal ulcer, gastrointestinal bleeding or gastroduodenal perforation
- Concomitant use of medications that are known to increase the likelihood of upper gastrointestinal adverse events, e.g. steroids and anticoagulants
- Presence of serious co-morbidity, such as cardiovascular disease, renal or hepatic impairment, diabetes and hypertension
- Requirement for the prolonged use of maximum recommended doses of standard NSAIDs

(Source: National Institute for Clinical Excellence, Technology Appraisal No. 27, July 2001)

Other common adverse effects of NSAIDs:

- Skin reactions: Mostly mild rashes, urticaria and photosensitivity reactions. Most common with *mefenamic acid* and *sulindac*.
- Renal effects: NSAIDs may precipitate reversible renal ischaemia and renal insufficiency in susceptible patients. *Sulindac* is reported to have less effect on renal prostaglandin synthesis than other NSAIDs.
- CNS effects: Dizziness and headache. Highest incidence with *indomethacin*.
- *Aspirin* may precipitate bronchospasm attacks in aspirin-sensitive asthmatics.

Strategies to reduce gastrointestinal toxicity of NSAIDs

- Concomitant food intake.
- *Misoprostol* (prostaglandin E_1 analogue). Inhibits gastric acid secretion and increases mucosal blood flow and secretion of mucus and bicarbonate.
- Proton-pump inhibitors (e.g. *omeprazole*). Block the terminal step in gastric acid secretion.
- Histamine H_2 receptor antagonists (e.g. *cimetidine*, *ranitidine*). Reduce or eliminate gastric acid secretion.

Corticosteroids

(Corticosteroids are dealt with in the section 'Drugs used in management of asthma'. The section below focuses only on their use in rheumatic disorders.)

In treatment of rheumatic diseases, corticosteroids are reserved for cases where other anti-inflammatory therapy has proven unsuccessful, and for some specific indications:

- *polymyalgia rheumatica* and *giant cell (temporal) arteritis* (always treated with corticosteroids)
- *polyarteritis nodosa* and *polymyositis* (usually treated with corticosteroids)

* *systemic lupus erythematosus* (sometimes treated with corticosteroids).

Three therapeutic strategies are employed for the use of corticosteroids in rheumatic diseases:

* low oral daily doses
* intra-articular injections
* intravenous pulses of high doses.

Low-dose oral corticosteroids can reduce swelling and tenderness in patients treated with NSAIDs or just started on DMARDs. However, the risk of toxic effects on bone, metabolism and several organ systems limits chronic use of corticosteroids.

Insoluble salts of *dexamethasone, hydrocortisone, methylprednisolone* or *triamcinolone* can be administered by intra-articular injection into some joints to relieve pain, increase mobility and reduce deformity. Injected directly into soft tissues, small doses of corticosteroids may also offer relief of inflammation in conditions like tennis elbow or compression neuropathies. Following injection, the joint should be rested for 1–2 days. Joint infections rarely occur, but multiple injections to the same joint may produce damage to the articular cartilage.

Intravenous pulses of high methylprednisolone doses may offer short-term effects in refractory rheumatoid arthritis. No long-term benefits or alteration of disease progression are seen with this treatment. Severe adverse effects such as seizures, cardiac arrhythmias and sudden death have been reported. The most common side effect, affecting more than half of patients treated, is dysgeusia (altered or reduced sense of taste).

Disease-modifying antirheumatic drugs (DMARDs)

This class of drugs is highly heterogeneous, the only common factors being that all agents have a slow onset of action, and that their mechanisms of action in rheumatoid diseases are rather unclear. Therapy is complicated by the slow onset of action, because patients may have to wait for several months to see whether the drug they are administered has any benefit. The DMARDs are second-line agents in the treatment of rheumatoid conditions. Although controversial, they are thought to affect the actual disease processes, unlike the NSAIDs, which only reduce symptoms. The DMARDs include sulfasalazine, antimalarials, gold compounds, penicillamine, immunosuppressants and leflunomide.

Sulfasalazine

Sulfasalazine is the most commonly used DMARD. Bacteria in the colon split sulfasalazine into the anti-inflammatory agent aminosalicylate and the antibiotic sulfapyridine. Both moieties are believed to contribute to the pharmacological effects, although the mechanism of action is unknown. Nausea, vomiting, headache, skin rash and liver effects are common side effects of sulfasalazine. Initially, neutropenia and thrombocytopenia may also occur, requiring periodical blood monitoring. Toxic epidermal necrolysis, a potentially life-threatening skin reaction, has been reported following sulfasalazine administration. Nevertheless, sulfasalazine has a better risk/benefit ratio than most DMARDs, and is favourable in that monitoring for its side effects can be based mostly on clinical presentation of the patient.

Antimalarials

The quinoline derivatives *chloroquine* and *hydroxychloroquine* are used mainly to treat and prevent malaria, but have also been shown to have antirheumatic effects. They act at least partly by accumulation and alkalinization inside lysosomes, thus interfering with the action of acid hydrolases within the phagocytic cells. Production of toxic oxygen metabolites, generation of IL-1 and several other components of the inflammation are also inhibited.

Although the results of studies comparing the effect of different DMARDs have generally been unfavourable to the antimalarials, their low toxicity makes these agents attractive therapeutic options. Unlike many DMARDs, these drugs are not associated with renal, hepatic or bone marrow toxicity in patients with rheumatoid arthritis (RA). However, skin rashes, headache and gastrointestinal side effects such as nausea, vomiting and abdominal pain may enforce discontinuation of therapy. Ocular adverse effects like retinopathy with colour vision changes occur, and all patients normally undergo ophthalmological examinations before and during treatment with the quinoline derivatives.

> Antimalarials may exacerbate psoriasis, and should not be used for psoriatric arthritis.

Trapping of chloroquine or hydroxychloroquine inside lysosomes leads to extensive accumulation of the drugs in tissues (particularly in lysosome-rich organs such as the liver). Consequently, the half-lives of drugs and metabolites are very long, explaining why it takes at least 3–4 months for the drugs to reach steady-state conditions. The onset of clinical antirheumatic effects may delay even longer.

Gold compounds

Gold salts reduce pain, joint swelling and progression of bone and joint damage. Their mechanism of action is not fully understood, but is believed to include inhibition of activity and release of lysosomal enzymes, decreased generation of toxic oxygen metabolites from phagocytes, reduced histamine release from basophils and mast cells, and inhibition of mitogen-induced lymphocyte proliferation. Gold salts can require 2–6 months before onset of clinical effects.

Two gold compounds are available: *sodium aurothiomalate*, which is administered by deep intramuscular injection, and *auranofin*, which is given orally. The gold complexes gradually accumulate in the tissues, not only in synovial cells in the joints, but also in the liver, the kidney, the adrenal cortex and in macrophages throughout the body. Half-life is 7 days initially, but increases as treatment continues. Therefore, gold therapy is initiated with dosing once a week, and maintained with dosing intervals of 2–4 weeks.

Aurothiomalate produces unwanted effects in one-third of patients treated, and severe reactions in up to 5% of patients. Adverse effects with auranofin are less frequent and severe. The most common side effects of gold salts are mouth ulcers, skin rashes (which can be irreversible), proteinuria and blood disorders. Peripheral neuropathy and hepatitis can occur. If therapy is discontinued when early symptoms appear, serious toxic effects are relatively rare.

Penicillamine

Penicillamine is a metal chelator, which prompted its use in Wilson's disease (hepatolenticular degeneration, in which copper accumulates in liver, kidneys, and brain) and heavy metal poisoning. However, in RA penicillamine is believed to act partly by interference with collagen maturation, and perhaps also by decreasing IL-1 synthesis and activity. In this context, its metal-chelating effects are only believed to account for unwanted disturbances of taste due to chelation of zinc. Effect studies have indicated that penicillamine is superior to chloroquine, gold compounds and antimalarials, and at least equal to sulfasalazine and methotrexate for RA therapy. About 75% of patients respond to penicillamine, but no effect is normally seen for the first 6–12 weeks, and the main response takes several months to develop.

Despite its potency, penicillamine is not a DMARD of choice. About 40% of patients treated experience adverse effects, among which bone marrow disorders like leukopenia and aplastic anaemia, and autoimmune reactions such as myasthenia gravis, polymyositis, systemic lupus erythematosus and Goodpasture's syndrome are the most serious. Proteinuria occurs in up to 30% of patients, but may resolve despite continuation of therapy. Anorexia, nausea, fever and taste disturbances are common initially, but normally disappear with continued treatment. Skin rashes, stomatitis and thrombocytopenia normally resolve after a dose reduction. To reduce side effects, penicillamine therapy is started at low dosage and increased slowly.

Immunosuppressant drugs

Methotrexate (MTX) is widely used in cancer therapy, but is also the DMARD of first choice because it is potent, has a more rapid onset of action than other DMARDs and is significantly less toxic. The cytostatic effects can be ascribed to MTX acting as a folic acid antagonist, thereby reducing the concentration of circulating purines and pyrimidines, essential components of DNA and RNA. Proliferation of immune cells and expression of cytokines may be affected through the same mechanism, offering an explanation for the suppressive effect on the rheumatic disease process. On the other hand, it has been proposed that the antirheumatic effects are independent of folic acid antagonism, since administration of folic acid to MTX-treated RA patients only reduces toxicity, and does not alter the efficacy.

Studies have shown that MTX is the only DMARD continued by more than 50% of patients for 5 years or more. Adverse events or lack of effect force about half to discontinue other DMARDs within 2 years. Clinical effect of MTX is often observed 2–3 weeks from initiation of therapy. Gastrointestinal side effects occur, but can be relieved with concomitant administration of folic acid. Elevation of liver enzymes, haemocytopenia and rarely pneumonitis are other adverse effects of MTX.

Other immunosuppressants such as *ciclosporin*, *azathioprine*, *cyclophosphamide* and *leflunomide* are more toxic, and are used only in patients who do not respond to other DMARDs.

> Use of *triple therapy*, with concomitant administration of *MTX*, *sulfasalazine* and *hydroxychloroquine*, is increasing.

Leflunomide

Leflunomide is a new DMARD that has been proved to slow down the disease progression in rheumatoid arthritis. Administered orally, leflunomide is converted to an active metabolite that blocks the synthesis of pyrimidines, which are necessary for the synthesis of new DNA. Some specific components of the immune system, the activated CD4+ T-cells, proliferate rapidly during initiation of rheumatoid arthritis. This proliferation is inhibited by the active leflunomide metabolite, since the T-cell is prevented from producing new DNA molecules prior to cell division.

Clinical trials have shown promising results for leflunomide in the treatment of rheumatoid arthritis. Both leflunomide monotherapy and combination therapy with MTX seem to reduce the rate of disease progression. In the clinical trials, gastrointestinal discomfort, skin rash, and reversible alopecia were the most common adverse events.

Biological antirheumatic agents

Cytokines are important factors in the pathogenesis of rheumatoid conditions, and a great deal of research has been aimed at finding agents that can interfere with the functions of these disease mediators. The tumour necrosis factor, TNF-α, is an inflammatory cytokine released primarily by synovial macrophages, and is critical to the release of pro-inflammatory and joint-destructive molecules in the synovium. *Etanercept* and *infliximab* are biological agents that bind to TNF-α, preventing its interaction with TNF receptors on the cell surface. Etanercept is given by subcutaneous injection, while infliximab is administered by intravenous infusion. Both agents have been approved for treatment of rheumatoid arthritis, as alternatives when DMARD therapy has proved inadequate. They may be given alone, or in combination with MTX.

Drugs used for treatment of gout

The characteristic periodic attacks of acute arthritis in gout are caused by deposition of uric acid crystals in the synovial tissue of joints. Uric acid is a product of purine metabolism, and the precipitation of crystals is due to overproduction of purines or decreased elimination of uric acid, or both. Drugs used in gout affect the disease by four different mechanisms:

- inhibition of uric acid synthesis (*allopurinol*)
- increased uric acid excretion (*uricosuric agents*)
- prevention of leucocyte migration into the joint (*colchicine*)
- anti-inflammatory and analgesic effects (*NSAIDs, corticosteroids*).

In acute attacks of gout, NSAIDs, colchicine and alternatively corticosteroids are used to relieve pain and inflammation. Allopurinol or uricosuric agents are used for long-term prophylactic treatment, where the goal is normalization of uric acid levels.

NSAIDs

First-line treatment of acute gout attacks is NSAIDs such as *diclofenac, indomethacin, ketoprofen, naproxen, piroxicam* and *sulindac*. The drugs are administered in high doses the first 1–3 days, then in lower doses as the pain has settled. If commenced early, the NSAIDs can even abort gout attacks. Salicylate NSAIDs, i.e. aspirin and its derivatives, are *not* indicated in gout, as these drugs compete with uric acid for secretion.

Colchicine

Colchicine inhibits migration of neutrophils into the joint by altering cell motility. If administered quickly after onset of symptoms, colchicine is believed to be as effective as the NSAIDs for relief of pain and inflammation. It is of particular value in patients with heart failure, because, unlike the NSAIDs, colchicine does not cause fluid retention. Resolution of pain, redness and swelling is normally achieved within 2–3 days after initiation of colchicine therapy. Pain relief is achieved after about 12 hours.

The use of colchicine is limited by a very narrow therapeutic window. The usual dosage regimen is an initial dose of 1 mg orally, followed by 0.5 mg every 2 hours until pain relief or the patient has received the maximum dose of 10 mg. This regimen is often interrupted because the patient develops gastrointestinal symptoms. Up to 80% of colchicine patients experience gastrointestinal adverse effects, such as severe nausea and vomiting, diarrhoea and abdominal pain. Dehydration may be a major complication of therapy. Large doses may precipitate gastrointestinal haemorrhage and renal and hepatic damage.

Corticosteroids

Intra-articular injection of corticosteroids is an alternative to NSAIDs and colchicine, and can provide quick pain relief when only one or two joints are involved. It is important that the diagnosis of acute gout is certain, since intra-articular steroids will aggravate infection if the attack is caused by septic arthritis.

Allopurinol

Long-term hypouricaemic therapy may be initiated in patients suffering from recurrent gout attacks. The drug of choice is *allopurinol*, which reduces the synthesis of uric acid by inhibiting the enzyme xanthine oxidase. Enzyme inhibition occurs through two distinct mechanisms. Firstly, allopurinol is structurally very similar to hypoxanthine, a precursor in the uric acid synthesis, and competes with hypoxanthine for binding to the enzyme. Secondly, allopurinol is converted to alloxanthine, which acts as a non-competitive inhibitor of the enzyme. The result is reduced concentration of insoluble uric acid in the tissues, plasma and urine, and thus reversal of the deposition of uric acid crystals in the tissues and kidney.

- Allopurinol therapy should not be initiated during an acute gout attack, as this may prolong the attack or precipitate a new one.
- NSAIDs or colchicine are commonly given for the first 3 months of allopurinol therapy to prevent precipitation of acute gout attacks.
- Acute attacks during allopurinol therapy should be treated with NSAIDs or colchicine, without altering the allopurinol regimen.

Unwanted effects of allopurinol are few. Hypersensitivity reactions occur, mainly pronounced as skin rashes. These may develop into serious reactions if therapy is continued, but subside upon early discontinuation.

> Allopurinol enhances the effect of the following drugs:
> - mercaptopurine and azathioprine (metabolized by xanthine oxidase)
> - cyclophosphamide
> - oral anticoagulants.

Uricosuric agents

Uricosuric agents increase excretion of uric acid by competitive inhibition of its active reabsorption at the renal tubule. *Sulfinpyrazone* can be used instead of allopurinol, or in conjunction with it in cases where allopurinol monotherapy is insufficient. *Probenecid* is another alternative. Uricosuric agents are ineffective in patients with poor renal function, and should be avoided in patients with urate nephropathy and those who overproduce uric acid. Initial doses should be low to reduce the risk of stone formation in the kidney and precipitation of acute gout attacks.

> Patients taking uricosuric agents should have a high fluid intake to reduce the risk of stone formation in the kidney.

> Alcohol, diuretics (especially thiazides) and low-dose aspirin can induce gout.

DRUGS USED IN NEUROMUSCULAR DISORDERS

This section describes the actions of drugs acting at the neuromuscular junction, or used for disorders of the neuromuscular system.

Treatment of myasthenia gravis

In myasthenia gravis the neuromuscular junction is attacked by an autoimmune response evoked against nicotinic acetylcholine receptors. To overcome the resulting transmission failure, patients are given drugs that aim either to directly enhance cholinergic transmission at the synapse, or to suppress the underlying immune reaction.

Inhibitors of acetylcholinesterase

First-line treatment of myasthenia gravis is inhibition of acetylcholinesterase (AChE), the enzyme responsible for breakdown of the neurotransmitter acetylcholine. AChE inhibitors render each acetylcholine molecule released into the synaptic cleft less likely to be hydrolysed, and hence more likely to interact with the remaining postsynaptic receptors (Fig. 15.2). *Pyridostigmine* is often preferable to *neostigmine*, because of a longer duration of action. Other examples of AChE inhibitors are *distigmine* and *edrophonium*. The latter is used mainly for diagnosis of myasthenia gravis, and to determine whether ongoing anticholinergic therapy is optimal.

AChE inhibitors cause parasympathomimetic side effects such as increased gastrointestinal motility, slowing of the heart frequency, and increased secretion of sweat, saliva, and gastric acid. These effects are due to increased stimulation of muscarinic acetylcholine receptors, and can be reduced by administration of the muscarinic antagonist *atropine*.

Improvement of function in myasthenia gravis patients can be dramatic. However, if the disease has progressed too far, the number of remaining receptors may be too low to produce an adequate potential at the postsynaptic membrane, and AChE inhibitors will have very little effect. AChE inhibitors are also used and misused for several other purposes, ranging from symptomatic treatment of Alzheimer's disease to crop protection (as insecticides) and warfare (as nerve gases).

Immunosuppression

Because of the immunological basis of the disease, myasthenia gravis patients may also benefit from immunosuppressant therapy. The drugs most commonly used are *corticosteroids* with a wide variety of dosage regimens. Addition of *azathioprine* may allow a reduction in the corticosteroid dose.

Muscle relaxants

Muscle relaxants are employed for relief of pathological muscle spasm and spasticity, and for muscle relaxation during surgery.

Skeletal muscle relaxants

Dantrolene is the drug of choice for treatment of chronic muscle spasm or spasticity, because it produces fewer central side effects than the other skeletal muscle relaxants. While the other muscle relaxants act through centrally mediated processes, dantrolene inhibits skeletal muscle contraction directly by preventing calcium release from the sarcoplasmic reticulum.

The centrally acting muscle relaxants reduce the background tone of the muscle through different mechanisms of

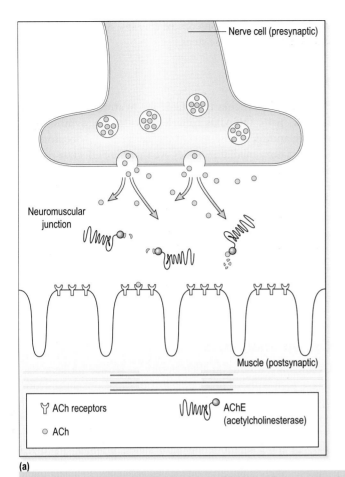

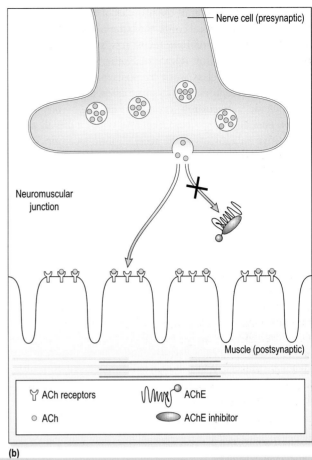

Figure 15.2.   Cholinergic synapse, AChE. (a) After release from the presynaptic cell, acetylcholine (ACh) is rapidly hydrolysed by acetylcholinesterase (AChE). A fraction of the released neurotransmitters reaches the postsynaptic receptors, and fulfils the signal transduction. (b) AChE inhibitors prevent the breakdown of ACh, allowing a larger fraction to reach the postsynaptic receptors. In myasthenia gravis, AChE inhibitors can increase stimulation of remaining ACh receptors.

action. These drugs do, however, to some extent also affect the ability of the muscles to carry out voluntary movements. Problems with postural control, for example, can often be inflicted with central muscle relaxation therapy. Other centrally mediated side effects, such as sedation, drowsiness and confusion, are also common with this class of drugs.

Baclofen is effective in treatment of spasticity caused by disorders such as multiple sclerosis or spinal cord injury. Cerebral spasticity caused by birth injury is, however, not treated with baclofen. It acts as an agonist at presynaptic GABA$_B$ receptors, thereby inhibiting activation of motor neurons in the spinal cord. In addition to the side effects mentioned above, baclofen produces motor incoordination, nausea and sometimes behavioural effects.

Benzodiazepines (BDZs) act on GABA$_A$ receptors, increasing their sensitivity to GABA. Independently of their sedative effect, BDZs reduce muscle tone, and can offer relief from a variety of muscle spasms. *Diazepam* is normally used, but other drugs in this class also display muscle-relaxant properties. BDZs occasionally produce hypotonia. Other side effects are the same as when these drugs are used for anxiolytic therapy.

Local muscle spasms can be treated with injection of botulinum toxin into the muscle.

Short-term symptomatic relief of muscle spasms can also be achieved with *carisoprodol* or *methocarbamol*. Carisoprodol is analgesic as well as muscle-relaxing, and is normally used for pain relief in the acute phase of lumbago and other painful conditions in the spine. Drowsiness is a common side effect, but normally resolves with dose reduction.

Neuromuscular blocking drugs

Neuromuscular blocking agents are not employed in neuromuscular disorders, but are used as adjuncts to anaesthesia.

They produce relaxation of the muscles of the abdomen, the diaphragm and the vocal cords, the latter allowing passage of a tracheal tube. *Botulinum toxin* acts presynaptically by inhibiting acetylcholine release. All other clinically important drugs in this class work by postsynaptic blockade of acetylcholine receptors, and, in some cases, also by ion channel blockade. *Atracurium, cisatracurium, gallamine, mivacurium, pancuronium, rocuronium* and *vecuronium* all act as competitive antagonists at the acetylcholine receptors of the motor endplate, and are referred to as non-depolarizing blocking agents. *Suxamethonium*, on the other hand, is an agonist at acetylcholine receptors, and is therefore referred to as a depolarizing blocking agent. Because it diffuses very slowly from the receptor, suxamethonium causes prolonged depolarization, and thus blockade of neurotransmission.

ANALGESICS

Severe pain states are treated with drugs acting on the central nervous system (CNS), mainly opioid analgesics. Pain from injury, surgery, trauma, arthritis and cancer can, however, often be relieved with non-steroidal anti-inflammatory drugs (NSAIDs), which act mainly through peripheral effects. The main classes of analgesic drugs are:

- NSAIDs
- opioid analgesics
- analgesic adjuncts.

The analgesic ladder

The three-step analgesic ladder offers a guideline for analgesic treatment (Fig. 15.3). However, patients presenting with severe pain may be taken directly to step 2, or even administered strong opioids (step 3) without climbing the first two steps. Especially in analgesic treatment of progressed cancer patients, recent recommendations turn to early onset and

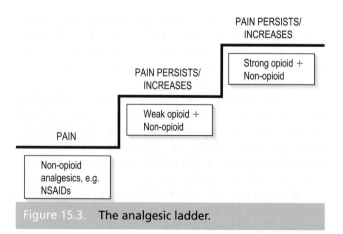

Figure 15.3.   The analgesic ladder.

rapid escalation of strong opioid therapy. Analgesic adjuncts may be used at all three steps.

NSAIDs

NSAIDs are particularly suitable for treatment of musculo-skeletal pain. NSAIDs interfere with the synthesis of prostaglandins, substances that sensitize nociceptors to inflammatory mediators. They are therefore effective in pain states associated with inflammation or tissue damage. Examples are muscular pain, arthritis, bursitis, toothache, dysmenorrhoea, postoperative pain and cancer metastases in bone. For short-term treatment, the agents of choice are *aspirin, paracetamol* and *ibuprofen*. More potent, longer-acting drugs like *naproxen, diclofenac* and *piroxicam* are used for chronic pain. NSAIDs are more thoroughly described in the section on drugs used in rheumatic diseases and gout, earlier in the chapter.

Opioid analgesics

Opioids are unique in their ability to reduce moderate to severe pain without producing loss of consciousness. Strong opioids, among which morphine is the standard drug, are used to treat severe acute, chronic, or terminal malignant pain. Weak opioids, such as codeine and buprenorphine, are used in mild to moderate pain states. Opioids are often abused because of their euphoric effects. Drug abuse is the subject of Chapter 16.2.

Receptors

Opioids are by definition agents producing morphine-like effects that are blocked by antagonists such as naloxone (used for reversal of opioid overdoses). They act on opioid receptors, and their main pharmacological actions are mediated by three receptor subtypes:

- μ (mu) receptors. Responsible for most of the analgesia produced by opioids. Also responsible for respiratory depression, euphoria, sedation and physical dependence.
- δ (delta) receptors. Contribute to analgesia, respiratory depression and gastrointestinal effects.
- κ (kappa) receptors. Produce analgesia at the spinal level. Responsible for dysphoria, but produce relatively few side effects.

Pharmacological effects

Besides analgesia, which is centrally mediated, opioid analgesics produce a range of other pharmacological effects on the CNS and on the gastrointestinal tract. The main side effects are respiratory depression and constipation. Tolerance to the analgesic effect is often a problem, requiring either an increase in dosage or substitution with another opioid.

Effects on the CNS:

- *Analgesia.* Opioids may produce analgesia at both spinal and brain level, the latter being reflected by a reduction in the affective component of pain.
- *Respiratory depression.* At therapeutic doses, opioids act on the respiratory centre in the brain to produce respiratory depression. This is the most common cause of death in acute opioid poisoning, whereas in chronic therapy, tolerance develops relatively rapidly.
- *Euphoria.* Drug addicts use opioids like *morphine* or *diamorphine* (heroin) to achieve euphoria. The euphoria does, however, depend strongly on which opioid drug is used, and on the circumstances. In chronic pain management, euphoria and addiction are rarely a problem, and opioids can instead be beneficial in reducing pain-related anxiety in addition to being analgesic.
- *Nausea and vomiting.* These side effects are very common, but normally transient. Antiemetics are co-administered during the initiation phase of opioid therapy.
- *Cough suppression.* Some opioids, such as *codeine* and *pholcodine*, produce this effect at subanalgesic doses, and are therefore employed as cough medicines.

Gastrointestinal effects:

- *Constipation.* Opioids reduce motility and secretions in many parts of the gastrointestinal system, frequently resulting in severe constipation. Stool softeners and laxatives are required in long-term opioid therapy.

Strong opioids

Morphine is the standard strong opioid analgesic. It has a duration of effect of about 4 hours (oral sustained release formulations with longer duration are available). Unlike the NSAIDs, morphine has no ceiling effect as the dose is increased.

Other strong opioids like *pethidine* and *dextromoramide* offer few advantages over morphine. *Methadone*, however, has proven beneficial in some patients who experience serious side effects with morphine. *Fentanyl* is administered transdermally through a self-adhesive patch, which is changed every 72 hours. Fentanyl is used for maintenance treatment of chronic cancer pain.

Weak opioids

Weak opioids, like *codeine* and *dextropropoxyphene*, are used for pain that is not responsive to non-opioid analgesics, although their therapeutic value is questionable. The main adverse effects are drowsiness and constipation, the latter limiting their use in long-term analgesic therapy. Dextropropoxyphene has a longer duration of action than codeine, and is somewhat less potent. Combined preparations of paracetamol and codeine or dextropropoxyphene are common. *Dihydrocodeine* has no clear advantages or disadvantages compared to codeine.

Patient-controlled analgesia (PCA)

Patients with for instance chronic malignant pain can control their own analgesia with PCA systems. Most PCA devices deliver a baseline infusion of an opioid drug, and when activated by the patient, the device delivers an additional bolus dose. A lockout period prevents overdosage and delivery of a second dose before the previous one has had an effect. Overall opioid consumption appears to be higher with PCA systems than with traditional administration, but without serious side effects.

Analgesic adjuncts

Antidepressants

Anxiety and depression often follow chronic pain, implying a role for antidepressant drugs in pain management. However, some of these drugs appear to be analgesic, independently of their psychotropic effects. The tricyclic antidepressant (TCA) drug *amitriptyline* is frequently used for chronic neuropathic pain states, including headache, facial pain, lower back pain, arthritis and denervation pain. TCAs inhibit reuptake and storage of noradrenaline and serotonin, which at least partially explains their ability to increase pain tolerance. Pain often precipitates sleep disturbances, and central serotonin enhancement may also contribute to reduce this problem.

Anticonvulsants

The antiepileptic agents *carbamazepine*, *phenytoin* and *valproate* suppress spontaneous neuronal firing by various actions on sodium channels and GABA systems, and are used to treat lancinating, burning pain, for instance following amputation or back surgery. The anticonvulsants frequently produce intolerable adverse effects, of which nausea, dizziness, slurred speech, ataxia, skin rashes and somnolence are the most common. Carbamazepine and phenytoin are furthermore potent inducers of hepatic enzymes, thus increasing the metabolism of several other drugs.

Other agents

The neuroleptic drug *methotrimeprazine* has an analgesic effect equivalent to morphine, without causing habituation or respiratory depression. It is effective in treatment of mild to moderate pain conditions, but sedative and anticholinergic side effects strongly limit its use.

Benzodiazepines (BDZs) such as *clonazepam* are used in the management of neuropathic and atypical facial pain, and *diazepam* may be used for skeletal muscle relaxation and anxiolysis in acute or spinal cord injury. However, BDZs produce habituation and withdrawal effects, and it has even been claimed that they can exacerbate pain.

Antihistamines such as *hydroxyzine* and *promethazine* may have some analgesic activity, and are sometimes used in acute pain, cancer pain or tension headache.

Clonidine and *guanethidine* are agonists at α_2-adrenergic receptors in the CNS, and act by presynaptic inhibition of noradrenaline release. These agents may be useful in spinal cord injury and neuropathic and sympathetically mediated pain.

Local anaesthetics

Lidocaine (*lignocaine*), *prilocaine* and *bupivacaine* can produce postoperative analgesia locally if applied directly to wounds or injected near a sensory nerve or plexus. When injected epidurally, local anaesthetics block the spinal nerves serving both superficial and deep tissues, thus also producing analgesia in deep internal organs. Epidural injections are effective in postoperative and labour pain, as well as in pain arising from several non-malignant and malignant dieases.

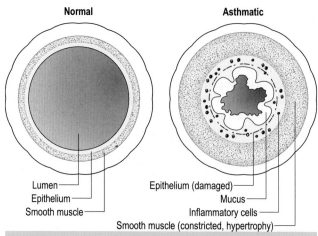

Figure 15.4.   Narrowing of airways in asthma.

DRUGS USED IN OBSTRUCTIVE PULMONARY DISEASES

Obstructive pulmonary diseases comprise asthma, chronic bronchitis and emphysema. The latter two conditions are included in the term chronic obstructive pulmonary disease (COPD). Pathologies of lung parenchyma are reversible but elements of bronchial hyperresponsiveness are regarded as irreversible. Asthma is characterized by narrowing of the airways as a result of bronchial hyperresponsiveness, excessive bronchial secretions, and airway inflammation (Fig. 15.4). The airway obstruction in asthma is usually reversible either spontaneously or with treatment. Drugs used in these disorders either act symptomatically by bronchodilation, or attack the actual underlying inflammatory process. To minimize side effects and ensure a rapid onset of action, the preferred route of administration is by inhalation.

Drugs used in management of asthma

Figure 15.5 outlines the treatment of chronic asthma in adults and schoolchildren.

Bronchodilators

There are three different classes of bronchodilating agents used in asthma, all with distinct mechanisms of action (Fig. 15.6). First-line agents are the adrenoceptor agonists. Theophylline or antimuscarinic bronchodilators are added at some later stage in therapy. The bronchodilators have little or no effect on inflammation, but are effective in reversing acute bronchoconstriction and preventing bronchospasm.

Adrenoceptor agonists

Adrenaline (epinephrine) and noradrenaline (norepinephrine) have a wide range of physiological actions, mediated through several subtypes of adrenoceptors (Fig. 15.7).

β_1-Stimulation produces increased cardiac rate and force, whereas the β_2 subtype is responsible for dilation or relaxation of smooth muscle in many organs, including the airways, the blood vessels, the bladder and the uterus. The bronchodilating effect of β-adrenergic agonists is due to direct stimulation of β_2-adrenoceptors.

The adrenoceptor agonists used for relief of asthmatic symptoms are termed β_2 selective, because they act preferentially on the β_2 subtype. However, all β_2-agonists also stimulate other adrenoceptor subtypes to some extent, and may cause adverse effects in organ systems away from the respiratory tract. Therefore, agents with high β_2-selectivity, such as *salbutamol* and *terbutaline*, have replaced the older, less selective agonists such as *orciprenaline* and *isoprenaline*.

Administration of β-agonists by inhalation is preferred because:

- the drug reaches its site of action more rapidly
- systemic absorption is lower, causing fewer side effects
- lower doses are allowed, since first-pass metabolism is avoided.

Orally administered drugs must cross the gastrointestinal membranes and the liver in order to reach the systemic circulation. The loss as the drugs pass through these sites during absorption is termed first-pass metabolism, and strongly regulates the amount of drug that reaches its site of action.

The β_2-agonists used in asthma are of two categories:

- short-acting agents such as *salbutamol* and *terbutaline* with an onset of effect within minutes and peak effect within 30 minutes

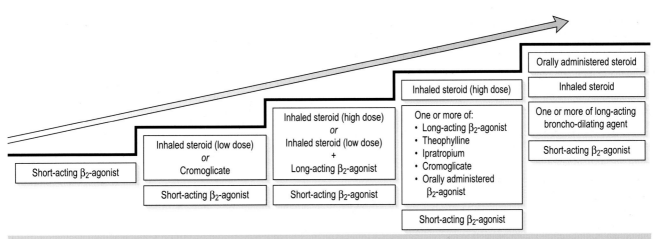

Figure 15.5. The five-step ladder: treatment of chronic asthma in adults and schoolchildren.

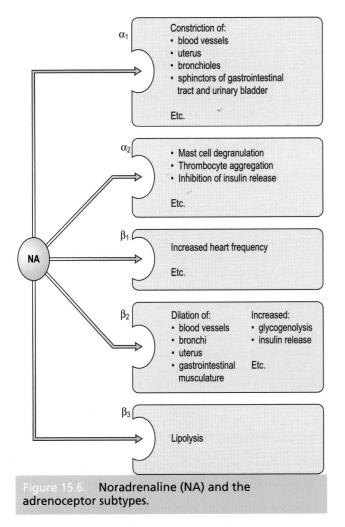

Figure 15.6. Noradrenaline (NA) and the adrenoceptor subtypes.

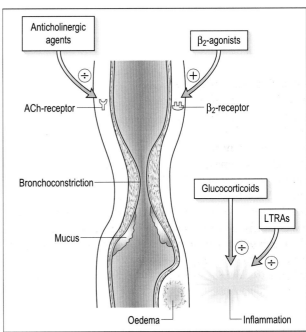

Figure 15.7. Schematic presentation of the mechanisms of action of β_2-agonists, muscarinic agonists and theophylline. LTRAs, leukotriene receptor antagonists.

The short-acting agonists are used to control symptoms on an 'as required' basis, and are included in all steps in the therapeutic ladder in Figure 15.5. They provide bronchodilation for 4–6 hours after administration. The long-acting agonists give bronchodilation for as much as 12–24 hours. These are not used 'as needed,' but are given twice daily as adjunctive therapy if asthma is poorly controlled by inhaled glucocorticoids (steps 3–5 in Fig. 15.5).

Acute adverse effects of oral and inhaled β_2-agonists are mainly due to stimulation of β_2-adrenoceptors in skeletal muscle and vascular smooth muscle, and include fine tremor

• long-acting agents such as *salmeterol*, which require 10–20 minutes to produce bronchodilation, and reach maximum effect 2–4 hours after administration.

(particularly in the hands) and headache (Fig. 15.6). As mentioned above, stimulation of β_1- and β_2-adrenoceptors in myocardial tissue results in tachycardia and palpitations, but these side effects are unlikely to pose a problem unless there is a pre-existing cardiovascular disease.

Anticholinergics

Inhaled *ipratropium* and *oxitropium* are not first-line agents, but may provide additional bronchodilation in patients not responding adequately to optimal doses of β_2-agonists and corticosteroids. They act by blocking muscarinic acetylcholine receptors in the bronchi, thus relaxing bronchoconstriction caused by excessive cholinergic stimulation (Fig. 15.7). Most mediators involved in asthmatic responses act only partially through cholinergic stimulation. Antimuscarinic agents are therefore less effective than β_2-agonists and theophylline, whose dilating effects are independent of the cause of bronchoconstriction.

The anticholinergic bronchodilators have a slower onset of action than β_2-agonists, but last longer. Administered by inhalation these agents are remarkably free of adverse effects because of minimal systemic absorption.

Ipratropium and oxitropium are particularly helpful in the elderly where asthma is often complicated by a degree of chronic obstructive pulmonary disease.

Theophylline

Theophylline is a relatively weak bronchodilator compared with inhaled β_2-agonists, but can provide additional benefit in cases where corticosteroid and β_2-agonist therapy is insufficient. Although theophylline has been used in both chronic and acute asthma for over 50 years, its mechanism of action is still largely unknown. The bronchodilating effects are, at least partially, believed to be due to inhibition of phosphodiesterase enzymes, which are important in intracellular signal transduction. Anti-inflammatory and immunomodulatory effects of theophylline have also been observed, but the clinical relevance of these is uncertain.

Theophylline therapy is complicated by some of its pharmacological properties:

- very narrow therapeutic window
- large inter-individual variations in theophylline metabolism
- metabolism vulnerable to many drug–drug interactions.

Theophylline has a very narrow therapeutic window, the toxic dose being only marginally higher than the therapeutic. Addition of theophylline to therapy therefore increases the risk of side effects.

Side-effects of theophylline

- At concentrations slightly above effective therapeutic level:
  - gastrointestinal symptoms (anorexia, nausea and vomiting)
  - CNS effects (nervousness and tremor)
  - generally mild and temporary.
- At higher concentrations:
  - Serious, potentially fatal, cardiovascular and CNS effects such as arrhythmia and seizures. In children, seizures can be precipitated even by theophylline concentrations at the upper limit of the therapeutic range.
- Minor toxicity symptoms may not precede more severe toxicity, so the potentially life-threatening effects can only be predicted reliably with plasma concentration measurements.

Several pharmacokinetic aspects further complicate theophylline therapy. Theophylline is metabolized in the liver, and there is considerable variation in its half-life between individuals. Liver disease, cardiac failure, viral infections and administration of drugs that inhibit hepatic enzymes (e.g. rifampicin) can lead to reduced theophylline metabolism, and hence a longer half-life and higher plasma concentrations. Heavy drinking and cigarette smoking as well as a large number of drugs (e.g. oral contraceptives, cimetidine and some antibiotics) induce the hepatic enzymes responsible for theophylline breakdown, and hence shorten its half-life.

Theophylline is normally given orally. Sustained-release preparations are used to avoid high plasma concentrations following administration. A single dose of sustained-release theophylline given at bedtime is useful in controlling nocturnal asthma and early morning wheezing.

Severe asthma attacks that do not respond to β_2-agonists can be treated with very slow intravenous injections of *aminophylline*, a theophylline preparation where ethylenediamine has been introduced to increase solubility.

Theophylline and caffeine are constituents of tea and coffee. Both are naturally occurring methylxanthines, and their chemical structures differ only by a single methyl (—CH_3) group.

Glucocorticoids

Corticosteroids

Steroid compounds secreted by the adrenal gland are called corticosteroids. The principal effects of the corticosteroids are either on carbohydrate and protein metabolism (glucocorticoid effects), or on water and electrolyte balance (mineralocorticoid effects). Naturally occurring corticosteroids display some degree of both types of effects.

Glucocorticoids (i.e. steroids with predominantly glucocorticoid effects) also possess anti-inflammatory and immunosuppressive activity, which make them therapeutically useful in a wide range of conditions. Mineralocorticoids are mainly used for replacement therapy, *fludrocortisone* being the most commonly used drug.

Glucocorticoids, particularly inhaled, are the cornerstone of asthma therapy. They are not bronchodilators, and have no role in treatment of the immediate asthmatic phase. Their potent anti-inflammatory actions, however, have made them first-line agents for management of chronic asthma.

Mechanisms of action

After entering a cell, corticosteroids bind to specific receptors in the cytoplasm and induce conformational changes in the receptors, exposing a DNA-binding domain. The steroid–receptor complexes then translocate to the cell nucleus and bind in pairs to the DNA. This interaction switches the transcription of some genes on, while transcription of others is blocked (Fig. 15.8). For example, one glucocorticoid–receptor complex blocks transcription of the genes encoding the COX-2 enzyme, inhibiting production of COX-2 and hence decreasing generation of prostanoids at the site of inflammation.

Pharmacological actions

Glucocorticoid therapy strongly suppresses the early, vascular events of inflammation (redness, pain, swelling), as well as the later phases, involving proliferation and repair processes. They affect all types of inflammatory reactions, regardless of the cause. In areas of acute inflammation glucocorticoids reduce influx and activity of leucocytes. In both chronic and acute inflammatory conditions they inhibit generation of inflammatory and immune mediators, such as complement factors of the blood, some immunoglobulins, and several cytokines and eicosanoids. The immunosuppressive effects of glucocorticoids are employed, for example, in autoimmune conditions (e.g. rheumatoid arthritis), or for prevention of graft rejection following transplantations.

Other pharmacological effects of glucocorticoids include:

- metabolic actions on carbohydrates (decreased uptake and utilization of glucose, increased glycogen breakdown), proteins (increased catabolism, decreased anabolism) and fat (redistribution)
- reduced release of endogenous glucocorticoids (negative feedback).

Clinical use in asthma

Systemic. Continuous therapy with oral glucocorticoids such as *prednisolone* is indicated only in chronic asthma that shows little or no response to other anti-asthmatic drugs. In order to reduce systemic side effects (see below), it is important that the lowest effective doses of oral glucocorticoids are given. High doses of inhaled glucocorticoids are administered concomitantly to minimize oral steroid requirements. Acute attacks of asthma are treated with short courses of oral glucocorticoids, starting with a high dose and reducing the dosage after a few days as the attack is under control. Severe acute attacks are treated with intravenous *hydrocortisone*, followed by oral prednisolone.

Inhaled. Anti-inflammatory therapy with inhaled glucocorticoids is recommended for all but the mildest asthmatics. *Beclometasone*, *budesonide* and *fluticasone* appear to be equally effective, all three producing substantial improvement in the inflammation and bronchial hyperresponsiveness characteristic of asthma. Alleviation of symptoms is normally achieved 3 to 7 days after initiation. The inhaled agents have a greatly reduced potential for systemic adverse effects compared to oral glucocorticoids.

Side effects

Large doses or continuous administration of systemic glucocorticoids are likely to produce unwanted effects. The most important are:

- osteoporosis (through effects on calcium and phosphate metabolism and on osteoblasts)
- increased susceptibility to infections (due to immunosuppression)
- Cushing's syndrome (with moon face, buffalo hump and abdominal obesity)
- tendency to hyperglycaemia

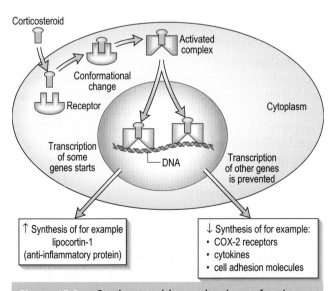

Figure 15.8.   Corticosteroids: mechanisms of action.

- posterior subcapsular cataracts
- muscle wasting and weakness.

Other side effects include acne, behavioural disturbances and growth suppression. Avascular necrosis of the head of the femur may occur as the blood supply to bone is affected. The patient's capacity to synthesize corticosteroids is suppressed by long-term steroid therapy, so sudden withdrawal of the drug may produce acute adrenal insufficiency.

Unwanted effects with inhaled steroids are uncommon, although oral fungal infections and voice problems can occur. Use of spacing devices decrease oropharyngeal deposition of the drug and reduce the severity of these side effects. Mouth rinsing with water following inhalation also reduces the risk of topical adverse effects. There is a risk of systemic effects such as adrenal suppression, growth suppression and osteoporosis with inhaled glucocorticoids, particularly with large doses. Again, use of spacers and mouth rinsing is helpful.

Cromoglicate and nedocromil

Cromoglicate and *nedocromil* have no bronchodilating effects, and are not indicated for treatment of acute asthma attacks. However, if given prophylactically they reduce the immediate phase of asthma as well as the late-phase inflammatory reactions. Some patients do not respond at all to cromoglicate or nedocromil therapy, but children generally respond better than adults.

Cromoglicate and nedocromil are effective in asthma induced by antigens, irritants or exercise, but β_2-agonists are generally preferred for prevention of exercise-induced attacks. Although indicated for the treatment of mild to moderate asthma, cromoglicate and nedocromil are considered alternatives in treatment of severe asthma. Inhaled corticosteroids are generally more effective, but long-term steroid therapy is associated with more side effects.

Adverse effects are infrequent and mostly limited to transient bronchospasm, cough and dry throat. Administration of an inhaled β_2-agonist quickly relieves the bronchospasm. Hypersensitivity reactions have been reported, but are rare. Because cromoglicate and nedocromil are administered by inhalation and are poorly absorbed into the bloodstream, they lack systemic effects and are often regarded as the safest anti-inflammatory therapy for children and during pregnancy.

The mechanism by which these drugs affect the asthmatic processes is uncertain. Cromoglicate has been shown to suppress neuronal reflexes triggered by stimulation of receptors for some irritant mediators involved in the asthmatic response. Interference with the release of neuropeptides and cytokines is also believed to contribute to the anti-asthmatic effects.

Leukotriene receptor antagonists

Along with the prostanoids, the leukotrienes are important inflammatory mediators derived from arachidonic acid. During inflammation eosinophils, mast cells, basophils and macrophages produce a certain type of leukotrienes, termed cysteinyl leukotrienes, which have been shown to contribute to the bronchial hyperresponsivity in asthmatics. It is believed that the cysteinyl leukotrienes are among the main mediators of both the early and late phases of asthma.

Leukotriene receptor antagonists (LTRAs), such as *montelukast* and *zafirlukast*, block the receptors for cysteinyl leukotrienes in the airways, and reduce bronchoconstriction and inflammatory parameters such as mucus secretion and leukotriene-induced formation of eosinophils in the blood and the respiratory system. Studies have indicated that the LTRAs possess an anti-inflammatory activity that is complementary to that presented by glucocorticoids. The LTRAs have been approved for treatment of mild or moderate asthma in patients not adequately controlled with an inhaled corticosteroid and a short-acting β_2-agonist.

Drug therapy of chronic obstructive pulmonary disease

Chronic obstructive pulmonary disease (COPD) is an incurable condition. However, management options such as physiotherapy, artificial ventilation and drug therapy can lengthen survival and improve quality of life for the patients. Therapeutic approaches to COPD have historically mirrored the treatment of asthma, but the benefits of glucocorticoid therapy generally seem to be far less in COPD patients, than in asthmatics.

Bronchodilators

Airway obstruction in COPD is considered to be irreversible, but bronchodilators do reverse airflow limitation in a significant proportion of patients. They may offer relief from symptoms such as wheeze and cough, and can increase exercise tolerance.

Anticholinergics

Increased muscle tone due to parasympathetic (vagal) stimulation is the major reversible component in COPD. The muscarinic antagonists ipratropium and oxitropium reverse the vagal tone, and have proved to be effective bronchodilators particularly in the elderly. Anticholinergic therapy in COPD may require higher doses than in treatment of asthma.

Adrenoceptor agonists

Inhaled short-acting β_2-agonists can produce additional bronchodilation when added to anticholinergic therapy, but can also have some benefit on their own. Anticholinergics have largely replaced adrenoceptor agonists as first-line agents for COPD, but the β_2-selective agents are still frequently used to control dyspnoea and to improve exercise tolerance.

Theophylline

Addition of theophylline to regimens of inhaled anticholinergics or β_2-agonists may give additive bronchodilation. However, theophylline is a weak bronchodilator and its use in COPD is mostly for patients who cannot use inhaled therapy, or whose disease does not respond to maximal doses of other bronchodilators. As with asthmatics, nocturnal cough and wheeze in COPD may be relieved with a single night-time dose of a sustained-release theophylline preparation.

Glucocorticoids

A therapeutic trial of an oral glucocorticoid or a high-dose inhaled glucocorticoid is recommended for patients uncontrolled on maximal bronchodilator therapy. Although there is little evidence suggesting a benefit of long-term steroid treatment for COPD, glucocorticoid treatment is often continued in patients responding to the steroid trial. The inhaled route is preferred in order to minimize systemic side effects.

> Long-term oxygen therapy prolongs survival in COPD patients.

REFERENCES AND FURTHER READING

General pharmacology and pharmacotherapy

Herfindal ET, Gourley DR (2000) Textbook of Therapeutics: Drug and Disease Management, 7th edn. Philadelphia: Lippincott Williams & Wilkins.

Rang HP, Dale MM, Ritter JM, Moore P (2003) Pharmacology, 5th edn. Edinburgh: Churchill Livingstone.

Walker R, Edwards C (2002) Clinical Pharmacy and Therapeutics. Edinburgh: Churchill Livingstone.

Bone disorders

Hulley S, Grady D, Bush T, et al. (1998) Randomized trial of estrogen plus progestin for secondary prevention of coronary heart disease in postmenopausal women. JAMA 280(7): 605–613.

Neer RM, Arnaud CD, Zanchetta JR, et al. (2001). Effect of parathyroid hormone (1–34) on fractures and bone mineral density in postmenopausal women with osteoporosis. N Engl J Med 344(19): 1434–1441.

Ruiz-Irastorza G, Khamashta MA, Hughes GR (2002) Heparin and osteoporosis during pregnancy: 2002 update. Lupus 11(10): 680–682.

Seeman E (2001) Raloxifene. J Bone Miner Metab 19(2): 65–75.

Rheumatic diseases and gout

Bombardier C, Laine L, Reicin A, et al. (2000) Comparison of upper gastrointestinal toxicity of rofecoxib and naproxen in patients with rheumatoid arthritis. VIGOR Study Group. N Engl J Med 343(21): 1520–1528.

Bondeson J (1997) The mechanism of action of disease-modifying antirheumatic drugs: a review with emphasis on macrophage signal transduction and the induction of proinflammatory cytokines. Gen Pharmacol 29(2): 127–150.

El Desoky ES (2001) Pharmacotherapy of rheumatoid arthritis: An overview. Curr Ther Res 62(2): 92–112.

Madhok R, Kerr H, Capell HA (2000) Recent advances: Rheumatology. BMJ 321: 882–885.

Pincus T, Marcum SB, Callahan LF (1992) Longterm drug therapy for rheumatoid arthritis in seven rheumatology private practices: II. Second-line drugs and prednisone. J Rheumatol 19: 1885–1894.

Rose BD, Post TW, Narins RG (1999) Chapter 6E: Prostaglandins and the Kidney. In UpToDate© in Nephrology (CD-ROM) 7(1): 1–7.

Schnitzer TJ (2001) Osteoarthritis management: The role of cyclooxygenase-2-selective inhibitors. Clin Ther 23(3): 313–326.

Silverstein FE, Faich G, Goldstein JL, et al. (2000) Gastrointestinal toxicity with celecoxib vs nonsteroidal anti-inflammatory drugs for osteoarthritis and rheumatoid arthritis: the CLASS study: A randomized controlled trial. JAMA 284(10): 1247–1255.

Simon LS, Yocum D (2000) New and future drug therapies for rheumatoid arthritis. Rheumatology 39(suppl 1): 36–42.

Neuromuscular disorders

Richman DP, Agius MA (2003) Treatment of autoimmune myasthenia gravis. Neurology 61(12): 1652–1661.

Analgesia

Lehmann KA (1999) Patient-controlled analgesia: An efficient therapeutic tool in the postoperative setting. Eur Surg Res 31(2): 112–121.

McQuay H (1999) Opioids in pain management. Lancet 353: 2229–2232.

Asthma and chronical obstructive pulmonary disease

Balzano G, Fuschillo S, Gaudiosi C (2002) Leukotriene receptor antagonists in the treatment of asthma: an update. Allergy 57(suppl 72): 16–19.

Barnes J (1999) Therapeutic strategies for allergic diseases. Nature 402(suppl): B31–B37.

Singh JM, Palda VA, Stanbrook MB, Chapman KR (2002) Corticosteroid therapy for patients with acute exacerbations of chronic obstructive pulmonary disease. Arch Intern Med 162: 2527–2536.

Summary of product characteristics

http://www.emea.eu.int/

Substance Abuse: Drug Toxicity and Overdose

Derek G. Waller

Most therapeutic drugs are developed for their ability to interfere with human homeostatic mechanisms in order to produce a beneficial response; only antimicrobial agents and parasiticides have the theoretical possibility of a therapeutic response without some direct action on human metabolic or physiological processes. Several therapeutic agents, for example atropine (belladonna), tubocurarine (curare), ergot alkaloids (causing St Anthony's fire), digoxin (digitalis) and dicoumarol (causing haemorrhagic disease in cattle) have actions that were first recognized as a result of either accidental or intentional poisonings. It is hardly surprising, therefore, that all drugs are capable of producing adverse effects.

The relationship between a drug and a poison was recognized five centuries ago when Paracelsus stated: 'all things are toxic and it is only the dose which makes a thing a poison'. Many of the medicines prescribed today were first used as plant extracts, for example digitalis glycosides and opium extracts. It was the identification and isolation of the active chemical entities in such plant extracts that allowed the dose and purity of the active ingredient to be controlled sufficiently to optimize the ratio between risk and benefit. The current vogue for 'natural, herbal remedies' may be considered to represent a backward step as far as the control of safety and efficacy of drugs is concerned.

Drug toxicity can develop during the normal therapeutic use of a drug or as a result of an acute overdose. In some cases, toxicity occurs in most treated patients because of the nature of the drug, for example cytotoxic agents used for cancer chemotherapy. Significant toxicity is rare with the majority of widely prescribed drugs when used at recommended dosages. There is considerable interpatient variability in the development of adverse reactions, and toxicity may be reduced by taking into account variables that are known to increase vulnerability prior to drug administration, such as age, concurrent disease or body weight, when selecting both the drug and the dosage. Usually a reduction in dosage or a change of drug during chronic treatment will reduce the severity of adverse effects (but see 'Immunological toxicity' below).

Toxicity following an acute overdose usually produces predictable adverse reactions, which may be life-threatening and/or prejudice long-term health. Rapid treatment is then required and this may be aimed at preventing further drug absorption, increasing drug elimination/inactivation and managing the adverse effects produced.

Part 1 of Chapter 16 is, therefore, divided into two main sections: drug toxicity, which discusses mechanisms for adverse effects produced both during normal drug therapy and after an overdose, and drug overdose, which is concerned with the management of the consequences of overdose.

DRUG TOXICITY

This section provides a framework for classifying adverse effects, rather than an exhaustive catalogue of drugs and their toxicities. The toxic effects of drugs are more numerous than their beneficial properties. Prescribers should be alert to both predicted and unexpected reactions to medicines and should consider the risk–benefit ratio for the particular patient and the suitability of alternative drugs and/or treatments. Patients should also be informed of the risk–benefit balance inherent in their treatment. Prescription information leaflets included with the dispensed medicine represent a useful way of providing such advice.

It should be appreciated that all drugs are associated with some risk of toxicity, although both the severity and incidence differ widely between drugs. The acceptability of a risk of toxicity is inversely related to the severity of the disease being treated; for example, serious idiosyncratic reactions with incidences of 1 in 10 000 have led to the withdrawal of some non-steroidal anti-inflammatory drugs (NSAIDs), whereas cancer chemotherapeutic agents may result in serious toxicity in nearly all patients. In addition 'one man's cure is another man's poison' because the beneficial effects of a drug in one situation (e.g. the antidiarrhoeal effect of opioids) may be an adverse effect in other circumstances (e.g. constipation, when used for pain relief). Therefore, even classification of the nature of effect into beneficial or adverse may depend on the condition being treated.

A useful indication of the safety margin available to the physician (and patient) is given by the therapeutic index (TI):

$$Therapeutic\ index = \frac{Dose\ resulting\ in\ toxicity}{Dose\ giving\ therapeutic\ response}$$

Drugs such as diazepam have a TI of about 50 and it is difficult for even the most inept doctor to poison patients with diazepam. In contrast, digoxin has a TI of only about 2 and for such drugs, toxicity may be precipitated by relatively small changes in dosage regimen, bioavailability or the clearance of the drug from the body. The TI relates to serious adverse effects and does not indicate the potential for minor unwanted effects, which can inconvenience the patient enough for them to stop treatment.

Types of drug toxicity

Toxicity is frequently divided into two main types:

- type A: these effects are dose related and largely predictable
- type B: these effects are not dose related but are idiosyncratic and unpredictable.

Our understanding of the mechanisms involved in toxicity has increased greatly in recent years, and this provides a useful framework for students to integrate future knowledge:

- pharmacological: type A
- biochemical: type A and some type B
- immunological: type B
- unknown: mostly type B?

Pharmacological toxicity

The toxic reaction is an extension of the known pharmacological properties of the drug at its site(s) of action (Table 16.1.1). There are numerous examples in this book where the adverse effects listed are a direct consequence of excessive therapeutic action (response 1 in Fig. 16.1.1).

Table 16.1.1.   Drugs with adverse effects that are related to their primary therapeutic properties

Drug	Adverse effect
Warfarin	Haemorrhage
Insulin	Hypoglycaemia
β-Adrenoceptor antagonists (beta-blockers)	Heart block when used as an antiarrhythmic
Loop diuretics	Hypokalaemia
General anaesthetics	Medullary depression
Acetylcholinesterase inhibitors	Muscle weakness

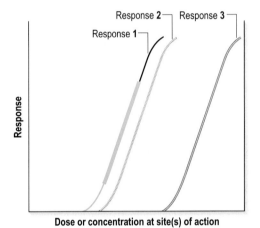

Dose or concentration at site(s) of action

Response 1
— low doses give a subtherapeutic response

— median doses give the desired therapeutic response

— high doses give an excessive or toxic response

Response 2
···· is a toxic effect (not related to the therapeutic effect)

Response 3
═══ is a toxic effect which normally is seen only in massive overdose or in subjects who are particularly susceptible

Figure 16.1.1.   Dose–response relationships in relation to toxicity.

The change in response with increase in dose from subtherapeutic to therapeutic to toxic has given rise to the concept of a 'therapeutic window' within which most patients should show a beneficial response with minimal risk of adverse effects (response 1 in Fig. 16.1.1). This concept is particularly valuable in the interpretation of measurements of drug concentrations in plasma to monitor compliance and to assess likely response (Table 16.1.2).

In many other cases, the toxic reaction may be unrelated to the primary therapeutic effect (Table 16.1.3) and may be caused by a secondary or alternative effect that is not the primary aim of the treatment given (response 2 in Fig. 16.1.1). This toxicity would usually be present to a limited extent in patients receiving therapeutic doses (e.g. response 2 in Fig. 16.1.1).

The separation of therapeutic and toxic dose–response curves is a measure of the TI. If these are very close (e.g. response 2 in Fig. 16.1.1) then there is little safety margin and most patients will exhibit some degree of toxicity, for example myelosuppression with cytotoxic anticancer drugs.

A high TI (response 3 in Fig. 16.1.1) results from a form of toxicity that would not be seen with normal therapeutic doses, for example heart failure caused by myocardial depression in patients with normal left ventricular function taking beta-blockers. However, some patients may be uniquely sensitive to the toxic effect because of their genetics or their physical condition; for example, beta-blockers may precipitate heart failure in patients with pre-existing impaired left ventricular function.

Pharmacological toxicity is the most common cause of adverse effects. Such toxicity can be minimized by an assessment of the risk–benefit balance for the individual patient. This should take into account factors that may influence both pharmacokinetics and sensitivity, including age, physiological status (e.g. renal function), concurrent medication, disease processes, environmental aspects (e.g. smoking), etc.

Because of the predictable nature of pharmacological toxicity, it is possible to co-prescribe drugs that will minimize toxic effects. Examples include anti-emetics given with cancer chemotherapy, vitamin B_6 given with isoniazid, and leucovorin (folinic acid) given after methotrexate.

Biochemical toxicity

This toxicity or tissue damage is caused by an interaction of the drug, or an active metabolite, with cell components, especially macromolecules. A generalized scheme is given in Figure 16.1.2. For most approved drugs, this form of toxicity is characterized during both preclinical studies in animals and early clinical trials, for example by monitoring changes in serum enzyme levels.

In some situations, an understanding of the mechanism of toxicity has allowed the development of appropriate treatments. An example is the key observation that the thiol (-SH) group of the tripeptide glutathione provides a cytoprotective

Table 16.1.2.   Therapeutic windows based on plasma concentrations

Drug	Therapeutic concentration range[a]		Toxic response
	Minimum	Maximum[b]	
Aspirin (analgesia) (μg/ml)	20	300	Tinnitus, metabolic acidosis
Carbamazepine (μg/ml)	4	10	Drowsiness, visual disturbances
Digitoxin (ng/ml)	15	30	Bradycardia, nausea
Digoxin (ng/ml)	0.8	3	Bradycardia, nausea
Gentamicin (μg/ml)	2	12	Ototoxicity, renal toxicity
Kanamycin (μg/ml)	10	40	Ototoxicity, renal toxicity
Phenytoin (μg/ml)	10	20	Nystagmus, lethargy
Theophylline (μg/ml)	10	20	Tremor, nervousness

[a] The values given represent average values only, patients will vary in their inherent sensitivity and response to particular concentrations. The concept of a therapeutic window also applies to situations where the response can be measured directly (e.g. blood clotting control with warfarin and hypoglycaemia with oral hypogycaemics).

[b] The maximum concentration may be based on toxicity related to the primary therapeutic response (e.g. carbamazepine) or an unrelated effect (e.g. gentamicin).

Table 16.1.3.   Drugs with adverse effects unrelated to their primary therapeutic use

Drug	Adverse effect
Opioid analgesic	Respiratory depression when used for analgesia
Beta-blocker	Reduction in heart rate when used for hypertension
Anticonvulsant	Sedation, when used for epilepsy

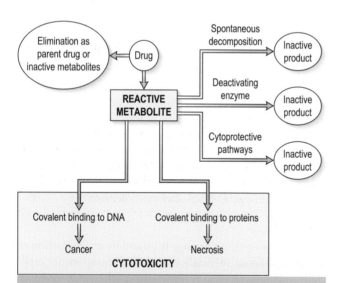

Figure 16.1.2.   Metabolism and toxicity. The extent of cytotoxicity depends on (i) the balance between the activation process and alternative pathways of elimination of the parent drug, and (ii) the balance between inactivation of the reactive metabolite and the production of biochemically adverse effects. Therapeutics interventions are aimed at either increasing elimination of the parent drug or enhancing cytoprotective pathways.

mechanism for preventing cell damage caused by highly reactive chemical species, such as certain drug metabolites (see below). The nature of the cell damage caused depends on the stability of the reactive chemical (metabolite); extremely unstable metabolites may bind covalently to and inactivate the enzyme that forms them; more stable species may diffuse to a distant site, for example DNA, and initiate changes, such as cancer. Some examples of biochemical toxicity and their treatment are given below.

Paracetamol

Paracetamol-induced hepatotoxicity represents the results of an imbalance between inactivation of paracetamol via conjugation with glucuronic acid and sulphate and activation via oxidation by cytochrome P450 to an unstable metabolite that binds covalently to proteins and causes cell necrosis. Low doses are safe because they are eliminated by conjugation with little oxidation. However, in overdose the conjugation reactions are saturated and there is increased cytochrome P450-mediated oxidation to an unstable quinone-imine metabolite (Fig. 16.1.3). Early after an overdose, much of the toxic metabolite is inactivated by a cytoprotective pathway involving glutathione, but as the available glutathione becomes depleted there is increased covalent binding and cell death. This mechanism explains the site of toxicity (centrilobular necrosis in the liver because of the large amounts of cytochrome P450 present) and the increased toxicity seen in patients treated with inducers of cytochrome P450 (especially alcohol-related induction of CYP2E1). An understanding of the mechanism of toxicity of paracetamol led to the development of treatment with acetylcysteine, which enhances the cytoprotective processes by providing an additional source of thiol groups for conjugation of the active metabolite and protection of thiol groups in proteins (see below).

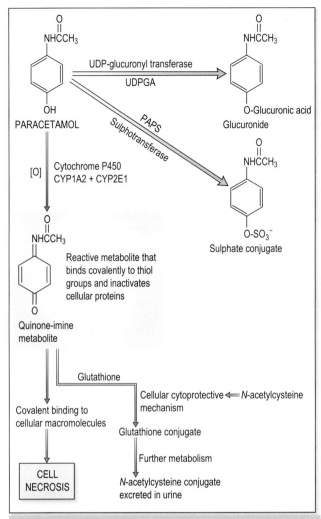

Figure 16.1.3.   Pathways of paracetamol metabolism. In overdose the concentrations of 3′-phosphoadenosine 5′-phosphosulphate (PAPS) (for sulphation) and glutathione (for cytoprotection) are depleted and extensive macromolecular binding leads to hepatocellular necrosis. UDPGA, uridine diphosphate glucuronic acid.

The sulphur-containing amino acid methionine can also prevent paracetamol-induced hepatotoxicity and a combination of paracetamol plus methionine (co-methiamol) is available. Such a formulation may prove to be of particular value to high-risk groups such as children (because of the greater risk of accidental overdose) and alcoholics (because of the possibility of induction of CYP2E1 and depressed glutathione levels).

Cyclophosphamide

Cyclophosphamide is an anticancer drug that is converted to highly toxic metabolites which are eliminated in the urine and cause haemorrhagic cystitis. This can be prevented by prior treatment with mesna (mercaptoethane sulphonic acid), which possesses both a thiol group for cytoprotection and a highly polar sulphonic acid group, which results in high renal excretion and delivery of this cytoprotective molecule to the bladder epithelium. Because of its polarity, mesna is absorbed from the gut slowly and incompletely but is eliminated rapidly. It is, therefore, given intravenously prior to cyclophosphamide and to cover the period of maximum excretion of toxic metabolites. It is not yet known if mesna will also protect the urinary bladder from the delayed consequence of cyclophosphamide, that is from bladder cancer that arises about 10–20 years after initial treatment.

Isoniazid

Isoniazid, which is used for the treatment of tuberculosis, causes hepatitis in about 0.5% of patients. This is believed to occur through increased formation of a reactive metabolite, *N*-acetylhydrazine, which is formed by acetylation followed by oxidative metabolism. Fast acetylators form more *N*-acetylhydrazine than do slow acetylators but, unexpectedly, they are not more sensitive to isoniazid toxicity. The biochemical basis for the susceptibility of some patients to the hepatotoxic metabolite is not known; it is possibly related to the balance between further activation of *N*-acetylhydrazine (by cytochrome P450-mediated oxidation) and detoxication of *N*-acetylhydrazine, which is by further acetylation. Consequently, fast acetylators may produce more active metabolite and also inactivate it more rapidly.

Chloroform

Chloroform is no longer used clinically because of hepatotoxicity, which is mediated by the generation of reactive free radicals during its metabolism.

Spironolactone

Spironolactone is oxidized by cytochrome P450. The metabolite formed in the testes binds to and destroys testicular cytochrome P450 and this causes a decrease in the metabolism of progesterone to testosterone (which is also catalysed by a cytochrome P450). This effect, combined with an antiandrogenic action at receptor sites, results in gynaecomastia and decreased libido.

Aromatic amines and nitrites

Aromatic amines, such as the antileprosy drug dapsone and some antimalarials, may cause both haemolysis and methaemoglobinaemia through the generation of toxic metabolites. The active metabolite is formed in the liver and released into the circulation. In the presence of oxygen, the active metabolite oxidizes haemoglobin (Fe^{2+}) to methaemoglobin (Fe^{3+}) and is oxidized itself (Fig. 16.1.4). Because of the large amounts of haemoglobin in the blood, compared with the amount of drug given, this would be inconsequential, except that the

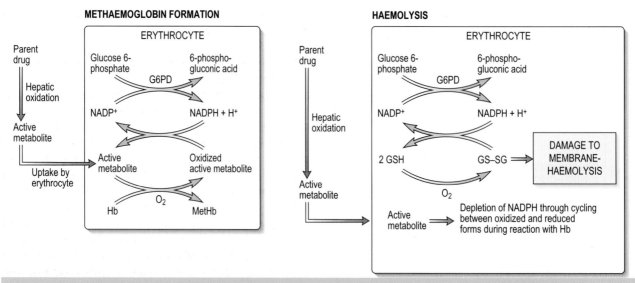

Figure 16.1.4.   Mechanisms of methaemoglobinaemia and haemolysis. Hb, haemoglobin; G6PD, glucose 6-phosphate dehydrogenase; GS-SG, glutathione dimer (oxidized form); GSH, glutathione (reduced form); NADP, nicotinamide-dinucleotide phosphate. High concentrations of reduced glutathione are necessary for maintaining cell membrane integrity; a build-up of oxidized glutathione is associated with haemolysis. The active metabolite may also react with glutathione directly to lower GSH concentrations.

oxidized active metabolite can be recycled back to the active metabolite by reduction with NADPH (reduced nicotinamide adenine dinucleotide phosphate) in the erythrocyte. Consequently, one molecule of the metabolite is able to oxidize many molecules of haemoglobin. The recycling depends on the presence of NADPH, which is formed during the metabolism of glucose 6-phosphate via glucose 6-phosphate dehydrogenase (G6PD) (Fig. 16.1.4). Haemolysis arises from accumulation of oxidized glutathione (GS–SG in Fig. 16.1.4) in the erythrocyte; oxidized glutathione accumulates because recycling of the drug metabolite linked to the formation of methaemoglobin causes depletion of NADPH, which is the cofactor essential for the reduction of oxidized glutathione.

The amounts of G6PD, and hence of NADPH, are determined genetically and the incidence of G6PD deficiency is high in Afro-Caribbeans and very high in Mediterranean races, such as the Kurds. Such subjects have limited NADPH reserves and, therefore, have a decreased ability to reduce either the oxidized drug metabolite or the oxidized glutathione (Fig. 16.1.4). Because they have insufficient NADPH to drive the interconversion of the oxidized active metabolite and the active metabolite, they are less susceptible to drug-induced methaemoglobinaemia. However, the deficiency in NADPH means that this can be depleted rapidly and the oxidized glutathione cannot be reduced; therefore they are very susceptible to haemolysis. Given the geographical distribution of G6PD deficiency, it is ironic that the amino groups associated with this form of toxicity are found in drugs used to treat tropical infections.

Immunological toxicity

Immunological toxicity is frequently referred to as 'drug allergy' and is the form of toxicity with which patients may be most familiar, for example penicillin allergy. Immunological mechanisms are implicated in a number of common adverse effects, such as rashes and fever, but may also be involved in organ-directed toxicity. Although the term allergy may not be strictly correct for all forms of immunologically mediated toxicity, it is probably better than hypersensitivity, which has also been used to describe an elevated sensitivity to any mechanism or effect.

Low-molecular-weight compounds (<1100 Da) are not able to elicit an allergic response unless the compound, or a metabolite, forms a stable or covalent bond with a macromolecule. The process has been recognized for many years and is summarized in Figure 16.1.5.

Immunologically mediated toxicity shows a wide range of characteristics:

- toxicity is unrelated to pharmacological toxicity but has been implicated in some forms of biochemical toxicity following the formation of a reactive, covalently binding metabolite
- toxicity is unrelated to dose: once the antibody has been produced even very small amounts of antigen can trigger a reaction
- there is normally a lag of at least 3 days between initial exposure and the development of symptoms; however, the first dose of a subsequent treatment may give an immediate reaction

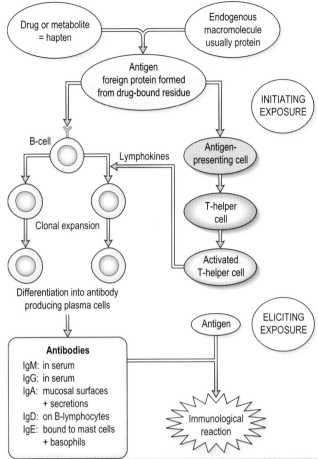

Figure 16.1.5.   Mechanisms of drug allergy. The initial exposure produces an antigen, which results in the production of antibodies via a B-cell clonal expansion and differentiations; this is stimulated by activated T-helper cells. The eliciting exposure occurs later (usually at least 3 days later, during which time therapy may or may not be continuing); antigen–antibody interaction exposes a complement-binding site, which triggers the reaction. The nature of the immunological reaction depends on the nature of the antibody and/or localization of the antigen. Immunosuppressant drugs such as cyclophosphamide, methotrexate and azathioprine act primarily to block the clonal expansion stage; ciclosporin is highly selective and prevents helper T-cell activation without myelosuppression.

- cross-reactivity is possible between compounds that share the same antigen-determinant or antibody-recognition moiety, such as the penicilloyl group of penicillins
- the incidence varies between different drugs, for example from about 1 in 10 000 for phenylbutazone-induced agranulocytosis to 1 in 20 for ampicillin-related skin rashes
- the response is idiosyncratic but genetically controlled; individual responsiveness cannot be predicted, but individuals who have a history of atopic disease are more likely to develop a drug allergy.

The effects produced may be subdivided into the classical four types of allergic reaction:

- Type I: immediate or anaphylactic reactions. These are mediated via IgE antibodies attached to the surface of basophils and mast cells; the release of numerous mediators, for example histamine, 5-hydroxytryptamine (5HT) and leukotrienes, produces effects that include urticaria, bronchial constriction, hypotension, oedema and shock. A skin-prick challenge test usually produces an acute inflammatory response. Examples of drugs having this type of effect are penicillins and peptide drugs such as crisantaspase.
- Type II: cytotoxic reactions. The antigen is formed by the drug binding to a cell membrane; subsequent interaction of this antigen with circulating IgG, IgM or IgA antibodies activates complement and initiates cell lysis. Loss of the carrier cell can result in thrombocytopenia (e.g. digitoxin, cephalosporins, quinine), neutropenia (e.g. phenylbutazone, metronidazole), and haemolytic anaemia (e.g. penicillins, rifampicin (rifampin) and possibly methyldopa).
- Type III: immune-complex reactions. The antigen–antibody interaction occurs in serum and the complex formed is deposited on endothelial cells, basement membranes, etc. to initiate a more localized inflammatory reaction, for example arteritis and nephritis. Examples include serum sickness (urticaria, angio-oedema, fever) with penicillins, lupus erythematosus-like syndrome with hydralazine and procainamide (especially in slow acetylators) and possibly NSAID-related nephropathy.
- Type IV: cell-mediated reactions. Reaction to the eliciting exposure is delayed. The reactions occur mostly in skin through the formation of an antigen between the drug (hapten) and skin proteins. This is followed by an infiltration of sensitized T-lymphocytes, which recognize the antigen and release lymphokines to produce local inflammation, oedema and irritation, for example contact dermatitis.

In addition to true immunologically mediated toxicity, as described above, there are examples of so-called 'allergic' reactions, such as aspirin hypersensitivity, which show many of the characteristics given above (e.g. rashes, induction of asthma in susceptible patients, cross-reactivity with other aromatic acids such as benzoates) but for which a true immunological basis has not been demonstrated.

It has been estimated that 'drug allergy' accounts for about 10% of adverse drug reactions but that severe reactions are very rare. For example, only about 5 patients in 10 000 develop an anaphylactic reaction to penicillins, but about one-half of these are sufficiently serious to warrant hospital treatment, which is directed to alleviating the effects on the airways and heart, and preventing further mediator release. However, given the large numbers of patients receiving drugs such as penicillins, 'drug allergy' is an important source of iatrogenic morbidity.

SELF-POISONING AND DRUG OVERDOSE

Self-poisoning can be either accidental or deliberate. Approximately a quarter of a million episodes are believed to occur each year, although less than 40% of these reach hospital. Deaths from self-poisoning still average about 2000 each year in England and Wales. Accidental poisoning is common in children under 5 years of age, at which age it often involves household products as well as medicines. A second peak of self-poisoning occurs in the teens and early twenties, when it is more frequent in girls. The incidence then progressively falls with increasing age. Most deliberate self-poisoning represents 'parasuicide' or attention-seeking behaviour. True suicide attempts comprise a minority of events, occurring most frequently in patients over 45 years. However, it is important to recognize that the severity of poisoning bears little relationship to suicidal intent. About 30% of the deaths from deliberate overdose are in patients over 65 years of age: self-poisoning at this age occurs most often in response to depression or specific life events such as bereavement.

The drugs most frequently used for self-poisoning are benzodiazepines, analgesics and antidepressants. Alcohol is often taken together with these drugs. It is important to attempt to identify the cause of the poisoning since it may influence treatment. However, it should be remembered that information from the patient about which drug was taken, how much and the time of overdosing is frequently unreliable.

Management principles

The management of drug overdose has a number of principal aims (Fig. 16.1.6).

Managing adverse effects

Immediate measures

There are certain immediate measures required when someone presents with a possible drug overdose or poisoning:

- remove person from contact with poison if appropriate, for example gases, corrosives
- assess vital signs: pulse, respiration and pupil size; inspect the person for injury
- ensure a clear airway; if breathing but unconscious, place in the coma position
- obtain a clear history if possible
- preserve any evidence, for example bottles, written notes, etc.

Supportive measures

Examples of drugs producing specific unwanted effects in overdose are shown in Table 16.1.4. There are a number of effects produced by drug overdose that will require supportive measures (Fig. 16.1.7).

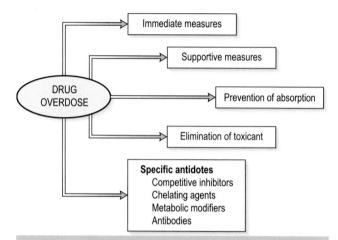

Figure 16.1.6.   Principles underlying the management of drug overdose.

Cardiac or respiratory arrest.   These may result from a toxic effect of the drug on the heart, depression of the respiratory centre or from metabolic disturbance. Assisted ventilation, ranging from mouth-to-mouth or Ambu-bag inflation to use of a ventilator may be required. In some circumstances, recovery is possible even after prolonged resuscitation.

Hypotension.   A low blood pressure is common in severe poisoning with central nervous system (CNS) depressants. It should be treated if accompanied by poor tissue perfusion or low urine output. Depression of the vasomotor centre can cause arterial dilation and peripheral venous pooling, producing a low central venous pressure. This should be raised to $10–15\,cmH_2O$ (measured from the midaxillary line) by intravenous infusion of a colloid solution, such as dextran polymers. If hypotension occurs with a normal or raised central venous pressure, this suggests myocardial depression. Positive inotropic drugs such as the β_1-adrenoceptor agonist dobutamine should then be used.

Arrhythmias.   Disturbances of cardiac rhythm should only be treated if they are severe. Ventricular arrhythmias causing hypotension often require intervention, but caution should be exercised if there is a long Q–T interval on the ECG, since the tachycardia often fails to respond to standard anti-arrhythmic drugs. It is essential to correct metabolic derangements that predispose to arrhythmias, for example hypothermia, hypoxia, hypercapnia, hypo- or hyperkalaemia and acidosis.

Convulsions.   These may be caused by a treatable underlying change such as hypoxia, hypoglycaemia or hypocalcaemia, or they may be a direct toxic effect of the drug on neuronal function. Lorazepam or diazepam intravenously (or rectal diazepam if the intravenous route is unavailable) is the treatment of choice. Artificial ventilation with neuromuscular blockade is used if the fits cannot be controlled.

Table 16.1.4.   Complications of acute poisonings

Complications	Cause	Examples of poisons
Cardiac arrest	Direct cardiotoxicity	Many
	Hypoxia	Many
	Electrolyte/metabolic disturbance	Many
Central nervous system depression		Many
Convulsions	Direct neurotoxicity	Tricyclic antidepressants, theophylline
	Hypoxia	Many
Hypotension	Myocardial depression	Beta-blockers, tricyclic antidepressants, dextropropoxyphene
	Peripheral vasodilation	Many
Arrhythmia	Direct cardiotoxicity	Beta-blockers, tricyclic antidepressants, verapamil, digoxin
	Hypoxia	Many
	Electrolyte/metabolic disturbance	Many
Renal failure	Hypotension	Many
	Rhabdomyolysis	Narcotic drugs, hypnotics, ethanol, carbon monoxide
	Direct nephrotoxicity	Paracetamol, heavy metals
Hepatic failure	Direct hepatotoxicity	Paracetamol, carbon tetrachloride
Respiratory depression	Direct neurotoxicity	Sedatives, hypnotics, narcotics

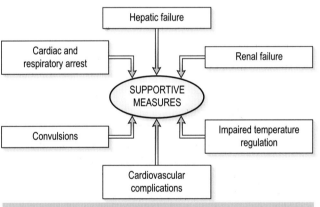

Figure 16.1.7.   Main effects of overdose requiring supportive measures.

Renal failure.   Kidney damage is usually a consequence of prolonged hypotension. Other causes include a direct nephrotoxic effect of the drug and renal damage produced by the products of toxic muscle necrosis (rhabdomyolysis).

Hepatic failure.   This usually results from the direct toxic effects of specific agents, such as paracetamol.

Impaired temperature regulation.   Hypothermia is common, caused by depression of metabolic rate with reduced heat production and by increased heat loss from cutaneous vasodilatation. It is common with phenothiazines or barbiturates, but is seen with any prolonged coma. Rewarming, preferably by wrapping in a 'space blanket', reduces the risk of serious ventricular arrhythmias. By contrast, CNS stimulants such as ecstasy can produce hyperthermia, as does aspirin by uncoupling cellular oxidative phosphorylation.

Reducing toxicity

The amount of poison that is available to cause the adverse effects can be reduced by:

- minimizing further absorption
- maximizing elimination
- negating effects with antidotes, etc.

Prevention of absorption of poisons

There are three principal methods of preventing further absorption of the drug:

Emesis.   Vomiting can be induced in a conscious person who has not ingested a corrosive agent. Stimulation of the pharynx can be tried in children but is often ineffective. Ipecacuanha is sometimes advocated to induce vomiting. It is a plant extract, containing emetine and cephaeline, that irritates the stomach and stimulates the medullary vomiting centre. Most people vomit within 30 min and prolonged vomiting can occur. There are doubts as to its effectiveness in removing drug from the stomach and the unwanted effects of ipecacuanha (nausea, drowsiness and lethargy) may mask symptoms of the overdose; in consequence the routine use of emetics is no longer recommended.

Gastric aspiration and lavage.   This should not be considered in unconscious or drowsy persons without protection of the airway by an endotracheal tube to prevent aspiration of gastric contents into the lungs. It should never

Table 16.1.5.   Drug adsorption onto activated charcoal

Drug/compounds not adsorbed	Drugs/compounds adsorbed
Acids	Aspirin
Alkalis	Carbamazepine
Cyanide	Dapsone
DDT (insecticide)	Digoxin
Ethanol	Ecstacy
Ethyleneglycol (antifreeze)	Paraquat (herbicide)
Ferrous salts	Phenobarbital
Lead	Quinine
Lithium	Sustained-release preparations
Mercury	Theophylline
Methanol	Tricyclic antidepressants
Organic solvents	

be used after ingestion of corrosives or petroleum products. A large-bore orogastric tube is used to aspirate gastric contents initially and then to lavage with doses of water at body temperature. Its effectiveness is unproven. Gastric lavage is normally only used for up to 1 h after ingestion of a significant amount of drug. There may be benefit for up to 4 h after aspirin and/or in unconscious persons and for up to 4–6 h after a life-threatening overdose of tricyclic antidepressants, but activated charcoal is now preferred.

Activated charcoal.   This formulation has a large adsorbent area and is given as a suspension in water. Activated charcoal adsorbs, or binds, the drug and retains it in the gastrointestinal lumen; not all drugs are adsorbed onto charcoal (Table 16.1.5). About 10 g of charcoal is required to every 1 g of poison, which makes it impractical for poisons that are usually ingested in large quantities, for example paracetamol. An initial dose of 50 g charcoal for adults can prevent drug absorption if given within 1 h of drug ingestion (later after poisoning with modified release preparations, or drugs with anticholinergic properties that delay gastric emptying). Repeated administration of 50 g every 4 h over 24–36 h achieves further adsorption of drug in the small intestine. Drug is continuously being transferred in both directions across the gut wall, with the concentration gradient normally favouring net absorption. If drug in the bowel is adsorbed onto the charcoal, this lowers the free concentration and can result in net transfer into the gut and enhanced elimination of the compound from the body. This is useful for overdose with barbiturates, carbamazepine, dapsone, quinine and theophylline. Charcoal should not be given to drowsy or comatose persons, because of the risk of aspiration into the lungs. Constipation is the major unwanted effect of charcoal; charcoal should not be given in the absence of bowel sounds because of the risk of obstruction.

Elimination of poisons
There are three principal methods of enhancing elimination of the drug: activated charcoal (see above), renal elimination and haemodialysis/haemoperfusion.

Renal elimination.   Forced diuresis with intravenous infusion of large quantities of fluid has been advocated in the past for drugs that are mostly eliminated unchanged by the kidney or if renally excreted metabolites are toxic. A major potential disadvantage of forced diuresis is serious disturbance of fluid or electrolyte balance, and therefore it is not recommended. Altering urine pH can be effective in increasing the renal elimination of drugs that are weak electrolytes. This is achieved by increasing the ionization of the drug, which reduces reabsorption from the renal tubule by lowering its lipid solubility. Only a modest increase in urinary flow rate is required. Weak acids, such as salicylates, are more readily excreted in alkaline urine (alkaline diuresis) while the converse is true for weak bases (acid diuresis). Alkalinization of the urine can be achieved with sodium bicarbonate and acidification with ammonium chloride.

Haemodialysis or haemoperfusion.   These are reserved for the most severely poisoned patients, and large amounts of drug must be retained in the plasma (a low apparent volume of distribution) for the techniques to be successful. Haemodialysis relies on diffusion of the drug across a semipermeable membrane from blood to the dialysis fluid, and is used for salicylates, phenobarbital, methanol, ethylene glycol and lithium. Haemoperfusion involves adsorption of drug from blood as it passes down a column containing activated charcoal or a resin; it is used for short- or medium-acting barbiturates, chloral hydrate, meprobamate and theophylline.

Specific antidotes
Antidotes are only available for a minority of drugs commonly involved in poisonings. Some important examples are given below.

Competitive inhibitors
- Atropine acts at muscarinic receptors to block the parasympathetic effects of organophosphorus insecticides. It is given by intravenous or intramuscular injection.
- Naloxone acts at opioid receptors to reverse the effects of narcotic analgesics. Its short half-life, compared to those of most opioids, means that repeated injections or an infusion are usually needed.
- Flumazenil is an antagonist at benzodiazepine receptors. It is rarely needed for the treatment of intentional overdose, because fatalities are uncommon with this class of drug and flumazenil can cause convulsions in benzodiazepine-dependent persons. It is of value in reversing the effects of benzodiazepines when toxicity occurs in those with chronic liver disease.

Chelating agents.   Chelating agents act by forming a complex with the drug or chemical, which reduces the free (active) drug concentration:

- desferrioxamine for ferrous ions; by intravenous infusion
- dicobalt edetate for cyanide; by intravenous injection
- dimercaprol for antimony, arsenic, bismuth, gold and mercury; it is used with sodium calcium edetate for lead; by intramuscular injection
- penicillamine for lead; by regular oral dosing
- sodium calcium edetate for lead; by intravenous infusion
- sodium nitrite, together with sodium thiosulphate, for cyanide; both by intravenous injection.

Compounds that affect drug metabolism

- Ethanol is used in the treatment of methanol poisoning, because it acts as a competitive substrate for alcohol dehydrogenase, preventing formation of the toxic metabolites formaldehyde and formic acid.
- *N*-Acetylcysteine provides a substrate for conjugation of the cytotoxic metabolite of paracetamol when the natural conjugating ligand, glutathione, is depleted.

Antibodies.   Digoxin can be neutralized in severe poisoning by specific antibody fragments. The antibodies are raised in sheep and cleaved to remove the antigenic crystalline (Fc) portion of the molecule while retaining the specific antigen-binding fragment (Fab).

Some specific common poisonings

Paracetamol

Paracetamol overdose can be fatal, with about 200 deaths occurring each year in England and Wales. Metabolism of paracetamol takes place in the liver, mainly producing non-toxic conjugates (Fig. 16.1.3). A small amount is oxidized by the cytochrome P450 system to a reactive intermediate, N-acetyl-*p*-benzoquinone imine (NAPBQI), that is inactivated by conjugation with the thiol group on glutathione. When hepatic glutathione is depleted (which occurs readily in overdose) oxidative stress, coupled with NAPBQI-mediated denaturation of protein, produce hepatic necrosis. Similar processes in the kidney can cause renal tubular necrosis.

In the first 24 h, there are few symptoms apart from nausea, vomiting, abdominal pain and sweating; these usually settle. Liver damage begins within 24 h after a large overdose, producing right upper quadrant pain and tenderness. Jaundice is apparent by 36–48 h and liver damage is maximal by 3–4 days. Severe liver failure, requiring transplantation for survival, can ensue. The most sensitive measures of liver damage are the prothrombin time, or the international normalized ratio (INR), and the plasma unconjugated bilirubin. Renal failure is seen in about a quarter of patients with severe liver damage.

Activated charcoal in large doses is recommended within 1 h of a potentially serious paracetamol overdose. Since antidotes

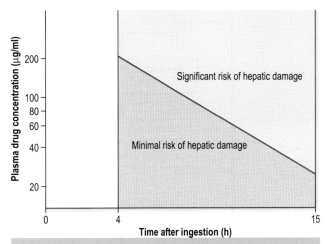

Figure 16.1.8.   Relationship between plasma paracetamol concentration and the risk of liver damage.

are most effective when given early, blood should be analysed for paracetamol if there is any suspicion of poisoning. Antidotes used in paracetamol poisoning replace glutathione as a thiol donor in the liver; glutathione cannot enter liver cells from the blood and so a substitute is given.

Methionine can be given orally as an initial measure, but not with or after activated charcoal, because methionine can compete with paracetamol for adsorption. Methionine should not be used if there is vomiting, or started more than 10–12 h after ingestion of paracetamol, since its efficacy in late poisoning is unknown. More than 4 h after the overdose, treatment with intravenous acetylcysteine is preferred for potentially serious poisoning, and should be started prior to the analysis of a plasma paracetamol concentration. A graph is available (Fig. 16.1.8) to indicate the risk of liver damage for a given plasma paracetamol concentration related to the time after ingestion. The plasma concentration before 4 h is unreliable because absorption and distribution are still occurring. High plasma concentrations after 15 h must be inferred by extrapolation of the graph. Treatment is only necessary if potentially toxic paracetamol concentrations are detected. It is important to realize that toxicity can occur at much lower plasma paracetamol concentrations under certain circumstances:

- concurrent use of drugs such as alcohol or phenytoin that induce liver cytochrome P450 and hence increase the formation of the reactive metabolite
- pre-existing liver disease
- malnourished/anorexic persons
- infection with human immunodeficiency virus (HIV).

All such individuals should be treated if plasma paracetamol concentrations are only one-half of those shown in Figure 16.1.8.

Treatment used to be confined to the first 15 h after overdose, but recent evidence suggests that liver damage can be

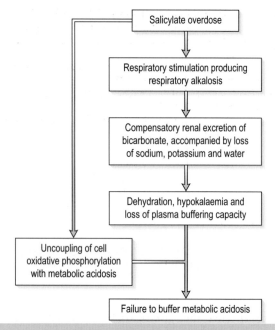

Figure 16.1.9. **The metabolic consequences of salicylate overdose.**

reduced even when the antidote is delayed for up to 20–30 h. It may be useful even later after ingestion to reduce the severity of established liver damage.

Salicylates

Although salicylate poisoning is becoming less common, there are still about 150 deaths each year in England and Wales. Aspirin is hydrolysed rapidly to salicylic acid after absorption but further metabolism, by conjugation, is rate-limited. Symptoms of toxicity are nausea, vomiting, abdominal pain, tinnitus, deafness, hyperventilation and sweating. Agitation frequently occurs in adults, but children become comatose. The chain of metabolic events produced by aspirin is shown in Figure 16.1.9.

Activated charcoal is recommended for reducing absorption if given early. Correction of fluid, electrolyte and acid–base balance is fundamental to successful management; a fluid deficit of 3–4 litres is not unusual in severe poisoning. Forced alkaline diuresis is no longer advocated to enhance salicylate elimination; simple alkalinization of the urine with 1.26% sodium bicarbonate to raise the pH above 7.5 is effective and safer. In severe poisoning, especially if there is severe metabolic acidosis, haemodialysis is the treatment of choice.

Tricyclic antidepressants

Approximately 400 deaths per year occur in England and Wales from overdose with tricyclic antidepressants. Antimuscarinic effects delay gastric emptying and oral activated charcoal is used routinely for up to 4 h after the overdose. Drowsiness

and confusion are followed by convulsions and coma in more severe poisoning. Cardiac depression can produce hypotension. Serious arrhythmias such as ventricular tachycardia can occur, and ECG monitoring is recommended for at least 24 h. Arrhythmias frequently respond to correction of acidosis or hypoxia. If this is not successful, phenytoin or direct current shock can be used. Antiarrhythmic drugs that depress cardiac contractility should be avoided.

Opioid analgesics

The triad of signs characteristic of opioid overdose are respiratory depression, pinpoint pupils and impaired consciousness. They can be reversed rapidly by naloxone, which is a competitive antagonist at opioid μ-receptors. After the response to an initial intravenous bolus dose of naloxone, it is often necessary to give repeated boluses or a continuous infusion because the half-life of naloxone is very short compared with those of most opioids. In poisoning with buprenorphine, the effect of naloxone is often incomplete, and assisted ventilation may also be needed. In poisoning with co-proxamol (dextropropoxyphene with paracetamol), especially if taken with alcohol, acute cardiovascular collapse can occur within 30 min of ingestion. Acute poisoning with organophosphorus insecticides can produce signs that are similar to those with opioids, but naloxone will have no effect.

Ecstasy

Ecstasy (methylenedioxymethamphetamine; MDMA) toxicity is characterized by tachycardia, hyperreflexia, hyperpyrexia and initial hypertension followed by hypotension. In severe cases, delirium, convulsions, coma and cardiac dysrhythmias may occur. MDMA is metabolized by CYP2D6, and genetic differences in this enzyme may result in wide interindividual differences in susceptibility to the toxic effects of MDMA. Some patients may present with hyponatraemia, possibly as a result of drinking excessive water as a precaution against dehydration. Treatments include activated charcoal, but only for up to 2 h post-ingestion since MDMA is absorbed rapidly, and diazepam for agitation or convulsions.

ACKNOWLEDGEMENT

Chapters 16.1 and 16.2 first published in: Waller DG, Renwick AG, Hillier K (2001) Medical Pharmacology and Therapeutics. Edinburgh: WB Saunders. Reproduced with permission.

REFERENCES AND FURTHER READING

Bateman DN (1994) NSAIDs: time to re-evaluate gut toxicity. Lancet 343: 1051–1052.
Buckley NA, Dawson AH, Whyte IM, Henry DA (1994) Greater toxicity in overdose of dothiepin than of other tricyclic antidepressants. Lancet 343: 159–162.

Buckley NA, Dawson AH, Whyte IM, O'Connell DL (1995) Relative toxicity of benzodiazepines in overdose. BMJ 310: 219–221.

Edwards JG (1995) Suicide and antidepressants. Controversies on prevention, provocation, and self poisoning continue. BMJ 310: 205–206.

Henry JA, Alexander CA, Sener EK (1995) Relative mortality from overdose of antidepressants. BMJ 310: 221–224.

Jick SS, Dean AD, Jick H (1995) Antidepressants and suicide. BMJ 310: 215–218.

Lee WM (1995) Drug-induced hepatotoxicity. N Engl J Med 333: 1118–1127.

Park BK, Kitteringham NR, Pirmohamed M, Tucker GT (1996) Relevance of induction of human drug-metabolising enzymes: pharmacological and toxicological implications. Br J Clin Pharmacol 41: 477–491.

Roujeau JC, Stern RS (1994) Severe adverse cutaneous reactions to drugs. N Engl J Med 331: 1272–1285.

Vale JA, Proudfoot AT (1995) Paracetamol (acetaminophen) poisoning. Lancet 346: 547–552.

Waring RH, Emery P (1995) The genetic origin of responses to drugs. Br Med Bull 51: 449–461.

Substance Abuse: Drug Abuse and Dependence

Derek G. Waller

Drug abuse is defined as self-administration of any drug in a manner that differs from the approved use in that culture. A number of therapeutic drugs are abused because of their effects on the nervous system. Examples in Western society include hypnotics, anxiolytics and opioid analgesics. This chapter also covers other drugs that are encountered in clinical practice primarily because of their abuse, such as ecstasy or cannabis, or because of their potential to cause dependence, such as nicotine and ethanol. The effects of many drugs of abuse are often complicated by the impurity and multiple constituents of samples of the abused drug.

Most drugs with potential for abuse also produce dependence. This is a syndrome that exists when an individual continues compulsively to take a drug because of the pleasurable effect it produces, often despite adverse social consequences or medical harm that it might produce. Dependence produces varying degrees of need for the drug, from mild desire to a craving.

Dependence may be psychological, caused by the unpleasant psychological reaction (dysphoria) that occurs on drug withdrawal, or physical, when there are abnormalities of behaviour and autonomic symptoms on withdrawal. Physical dependence causes symptoms on drug withdrawal that can be provoked by the use of a specific antagonist to the drug. Habituation to the use of a drug (shown by adverse psychological reactions on stopping use) is a far more powerful stimulus to drug-seeking behaviour than physical withdrawal symptoms.

THE BIOLOGICAL BASIS OF DEPENDENCE

Dependence is related to dopaminergic activity in the mesolimbic system of the brain. This system is involved in regulation of mood and affect, but also in motivation and reward processes (producing responses varying from slight mood elevation to intense pleasure or euphoria in response to food intake, sexual activity etc.). The mesolimbic system is activated by impulses arising in the ventral tegmental area of the brain. These impulses are relayed through the medial forebrain bundle, via the nucleus accumbens, to the prefrontal cortex. Stimulation of postsynaptic dopamine D_2 receptors (possibly the D_4 subtype), acting via G_i (inhibitory G proteins) to reduce the generation of the intracellular second messenger cAMP in the nucleus accumbens, is central to much drug-seeking behaviour.

Most drugs of abuse directly or indirectly release dopamine in the nucleus accumbens, and drug withdrawal leads to reduced dopaminergic function in the same area. Other changes in the mesolimbic system, including reduced 5-hydroxytryptamine (5HT, serotonin), gamma-aminobutyric acid (GABA) and noradrenaline, and increased glutamate, opioid and acetylcholine-mediated neurotransmission, also have a role in the genesis of dependence.

Neuroadaptive changes that occur with repeated use of an addictive drug lead to sensitization of the mesolimbic system to further drug administration. In the nucleus accumbens, the acute effect of dependence-inducing drugs such as morphine is to inhibit adenylate cyclase and reduce intracellular generation of the second messenger cAMP. With chronic use, inhibitory autoreceptor upregulation in the ventral tegmental area reduces dopamine release in the nucleus accumbens. In the nucleus accumbens there is loss of D_2 receptor-mediated inhibition and a compensatory increase in adenylate cyclase activity. This produces supersensitivity of D_1 excitatory receptors, and thus tolerance to further doses of the drug. Larger doses are then necessary to maintain normal function in the mesolimbic system, let alone achieve a pleasurable response.

The increase in adenylate cyclase activity in the nucleus accumbens reduces the motivational response to normal rewards. This is probably critical to producing drug dependence, since the drug becomes essential to maintain a 'normal' level of pleasure. Drug cessation decreases dopamine release in the nucleus accumbens and precipitates the psychological withdrawal reaction. Drug craving may also be related to neural input to the mesolimbic pathway from the amygdala, that are involved in emotion and conditioned responses. By contrast, physical dependence on a drug is unrelated to activity in the mesolimbic system and arises from excessive noradrenergic output from the locus ceruleus, a structure in the base of the brain that is involved in arousal and vigilance.

DRUGS OF ABUSE

Central nervous system stimulants

Several drugs that have central stimulant properties are abused and produce dependence. Those more commonly encountered are considered here.

Cocaine

Cocaine is usually taken as the hydrochloride salt. 'Crack' cocaine is the free base form named after the crackling sound produced when it is smoked.

Mechanism of action and effects

The psychomotor effects of cocaine are due to inhibition of neuronal presynaptic catecholamine reuptake into nerve terminals. This in turn may activate opioid systems in the brain, with upregulation of μ-receptors. Cocaine binds strongly to the catecholamine reuptake transporters, particularly inhibiting dopamine and to a lesser extent noradrenaline reuptake. Reduced serotonin reuptake may contribute to wakefulness. Changes in various pituitary neuroendocrine functions occur with more prolonged use; in particular, release of corticotrophin and luteinizing hormone (LH) is enhanced.

Tolerance to the psychomotor effects of cocaine is limited. One of the metabolites of cocaine, norcocaine, has direct vasoconstrictor activity.

Effects of cocaine include:

- intense euphoria
- alertness and wakefulness
- increased confidence and strength
- heightened sexual feelings
- indifference to concerns and cares
- severe psychological, but not physical, dependence through the reinforcing effect of the rapid onset, yet brief duration of action; this develops particularly rapidly with 'crack' cocaine
- despondency and despair rapidly follow withdrawal; after chronic use, withdrawal can produce a dysphoric mood with fatigue, vivid dreams, insomnia or excessive sleeping, increased appetite and either psychomotor retardation or agitation
- toxic psychosis, with delusions of great stamina, occurs with chronic use
- in overdose, excessive catecholamine concentrations produce convulsions, hypertension, cardiac rhythm disturbances and hyperthermia (due to excessive muscle activity and reduced heat loss); if severe, death can occur from respiratory depression and circulatory collapse. The cardiovascular toxicity can be treated with combined α- and β-adrenoceptor blockade, and seizures by intravenous diazepam
- cocaine snuff produces necrosis of the nasal septum through its vasoconstrictor action
- exposure in utero leads to impaired brain development and other teratogenic effects.

Pharmacokinetics

Cocaine, as the hydrochloride salt, is used orally, intranasally or by intravenous injection; the latter route gives an intense and rapid onset of effect. 'Crack' cocaine is prepared by mixing with sodium bicarbonate or ammonia and water, then heating to remove the hydrochloride. In this free base form it is smoked, which produces an effect similar to intravenous use. Cocaine is metabolized by plasma esterases and its half-life is very short.

Management of cocaine dependence

There are no recognized drug treatments for cocaine dependence. Prolonged behavioural treatments remain the main approach. Tricyclic antidepressants (especially desipramine) are sometimes advocated for the severe depression that can occur on withdrawal.

Amphetamine and derivatives

Amphetamine, methamphetamine ('speed', 'uppers') and 3,4-methylenedioxymethamphetamine (MDMA, 'ecstasy') are all drugs of abuse.

Mechanism of action and effects

Amphetamine and related drugs have indirect sympathomimetic effects, releasing cytosolic monoamines from CNS neurons. This action (principally as a consequence of dopamine release) produces CNS stimulation, which is most marked in the reticular formation but occurs in many other areas of the brain. The D-isomer (dexamphetamine) is twice as potent as the L-isomer of amphetamine in its central stimulant activity. Effects include the following:

- Euphoria, similar to that experienced with cocaine. This is particularly intense after intravenous use.
- Reduced fatigue and increased alertness for repetitive tasks.
- Anorexia.
- Psychotic behaviour during repeated use over a few days or with acute intoxication, causing hallucinations, paranoia and aggressive behaviour and repetitive actions. Acute intoxication can cause convulsions and death.
- Peripheral sympathomimetic effects can lead to hypertension and cardiac arrhythmias.
- Tolerance develops rapidly to some of the central effects of amphetamine, such as anorexia, presumably through central monoamine depletion. Tolerance to the euphoric effects and motor stimulation is slower.
- Withdrawal leads to prolonged sleep followed by fatigue, depression, anxiety, craving and increased appetite.

MDMA (ecstasy) produces euphoria similar to that of amphetamine but with less stimulant effect. Disturbance of thermoregulatory homeostasis occurs, leading to a syndrome resembling heat stroke with hyperthermia and dehydration, usually after exertion in hot environments. Stimulation of antidiuretic hormone release can cause thirst and water intoxication, a consequence of water retention and hyponatraemia. The toxic effects of MDMA include cardiac arrhythmias, convulsions, muscle damage and severe metabolic acidosis, which may be fatal. The long-term toxicity is unknown.

Pharmacokinetics

Although amphetamine is sometimes used intravenously or via nasal inhalation, absorption from the gut is rapid and complete. Amphetamine readily crosses the blood–brain barrier. About half is excreted unchanged in the urine, and the rest is metabolized in the liver. The half-life of amphetamine varies according to urine flow and pH; if the urine is acid then greater ionization increases excretion to produce a short half-life. By contrast, if urine pH is high, then the half-life is long because of renal tubular reabsorption of the drug. Metabolites of amphetamine are believed to contribute to the psychotic effects seen with long-term use.

Ecstasy is usually taken orally. It undergoes hepatic metabolism via CYP2D6, and polymorphism of this enzyme may explain some of the serious intoxication that occurs with the drug. The half-life is short.

Nicotine and tobacco

Mechanism of action

Over 300 chemical compounds are present in tobacco smoke. However, the actions of nicotine are central to the pharmacological effects of smoking. Nicotine has dose-related peripheral actions. At low doses, stimulation of aortic and carotid chemoreceptors enhances sympathetic nervous system activity. At higher doses, there is direct stimulation of the nicotinic N_1 receptors on autonomic ganglia. At even higher doses, nicotine acts as a ganglion-blocking agent. Initial stimulation of autonomic nervous tissue is therefore followed by depression. Effects on the CNS are mediated by presynaptic nicotinic receptors structurally distinct from those in the periphery. Stimulation of CNS nicotinic receptors increases neuronal permeability to sodium and potassium, and enhances release of neurotransmitters such as dopamine and glutamate. These receptors are found in the mesocortical and mesolimbic dopaminergic systems, in projections from the ventral forebrain to the cortex that mediate arousal, and in hippocampal projections where stimulation enhances learning and short-term memory. Tolerance to the CNS effects of nicotine is rapid.

Effects of nicotine and tobacco

Tobacco components including nicotine have effects on a number of organ systems.

Respiratory effects. The lungs are the first area to be in contact with the chemical components of tobacco smoke and are also exposed to particles and gases. Tars and other irritants, rather than nicotine, are responsible for the chronic damage to the lungs.

- An increase in blood carboxyhaemoglobin concentration (from carbon monoxide in tobacco smoke) decreases oxygen-carrying capacity. This may be important in ischaemic heart disease, increasing the chance of provoking angina.
- Increased mucus secretion, with reduction of activity of bronchial cilia and consequent decreased clearance of lung secretions, leads to chronic bronchitis.
- Progressive destruction of the supporting tissue in the bronchioles produces emphysema and chronic obstructive lung disease. Smoking is now the major cause of this condition.
- The risk of lung cancer is increased to about 20 times that of a non-smoker. Inhalation of tobacco smoke is a major contributory factor and explains the greater risk in cigarette smokers. Giving up smoking reduces the risk progressively over about 10 years of abstinence. The constituent of tobacco smoke responsible for altering DNA structure and initiating the cancer process remains controversial, but the relationship between smoking and lung cancer has been confirmed by numerous epidemiological studies. Compared with non-smokers, passive smokers also have a 20–25% increased risk of lung cancer.

Cardiovascular effects

- Stimulation of the autonomic nervous system and sensory receptors in the heart increases heart rate, blood pressure and cardiac output.
- The risk of cardiovascular disease is increased by smoking cigarettes, but not by pipe and cigar smoking, and it occurs at a younger age. The overall risk of death from coronary artery disease is doubled in smokers compared with non-smokers, but the magnitude of the effect is related to the number of cigarettes smoked. Peripheral vascular disease and stroke are also increased. Even passive smokers have an excess risk of vascular disease of 25%. The major reason for the excess of events is accelerated formation of atheromatous plaques, although contributory effects include increased plasma fatty acids and enhanced platelet aggregability. The risk of vascular disease falls over the first 3–5 years after stopping smoking to a level close to that of non-smokers.

Psychological effects. The psychological effects of smoking are substantial, as indicated by the difficulties experienced by those 'giving up smoking'.

- Decreased appetite, with weight gain on stopping smoking.
- Emotional dependence on nicotine and the physical act of smoking is powerful. Physical withdrawal is less marked but includes restlessness, irritability, anxiety, depression, difficulty concentrating, sleep disturbance and increased appetite.

Other effects. Nicotine and smoking have a number of other effects:

- Peptic ulceration is twice as common in smokers.
- Smoking in pregnancy, especially during the second half, has several effects. The most important is an increased risk of a low-birthweight child, and increased perinatal mortality. The vasoconstrictor effects of nicotine are responsible. Physical and mental development is slowed until at least age 7 years in children born to mothers who smoked during pregnancy.
- Smoking induces several hepatic cytochrome P450 isoenzymes, and increases the clearance of drugs such as theophylline and imipramine.

Pharmacokinetics of nicotine

Nicotine is absorbed from the mouth in its un-ionized form, which is found in the less acidic environment of cigar and pipe tobacco smoke. Acid cigarette smoke ionizes nicotine, which can then only be absorbed in significant amounts from the larger surface area of the lung. About 10% of the nicotine from a cigarette is absorbed, but at a faster rate than from cigars or a pipe, giving a higher, but less prolonged, peak plasma concentration. Nicotine can also be absorbed transdermally. It is metabolized in the liver and has a short half-life. The major metabolite, cotinine, has a longer half-life than nicotine and its plasma concentration can be used as a monitor of smoking behaviour.

Dependence on and withdrawal from nicotine

Withdrawal is often difficult to achieve unless motivation is high. Patients should be supported by counselling about health gains and advice on overcoming problems, such as weight gain. Behavioural therapy as an aid to quitting has a success rate of 20% at 1 year. Pharmacotherapy is often used to reduce the intensity of withdrawal symptoms.

Nicotine replacement therapy. Smokers adjust their smoking habit to maintain plasma nicotine concentrations just above a threshold that averts withdrawal symptoms. The plasma concentration falls rapidly within 1–2 hours of the last cigarette, and rather more slowly after smoking a cigar or pipe. The resultant craving for nicotine can be reduced by nicotine replacement. This can be delivered from transdermal patches, by chewing gum or via an inhaler (with most absorption occurring in the mouth) or via a nasal spray. The delivery method determines the speed at which plasma nicotine concentration rises; this is most rapid after nasal spray. The individual can choose the most appropriate vehicle for their needs and preferences. Established cardiovascular disease is a caution for, but not a contraindication to, nicotine replacement therapy. Behavioural therapy enhances the success rate achieved by nicotine replacement therapy. Use of nicotine replacement therapy doubles the chance of achieving abstinence.

Bupropion. This is an atypical antidepressant; unlike other antidepressants its use is associated with smoking cessation rates equal to, or slightly greater than, nicotine replacement therapy. Used with nicotine replacement therapy, bupropion produces a modest increase in the chance of stopping. It is a weak inhibitor of neuronal reuptake of noradrenaline and dopamine, and probably works by enhancing mesolimbic dopaminergic activity. It is used in a modified-release formulation and has a long half-life. Elimination is by hepatic metabolism to active metabolites. Treatment is usually started 1 week before a 'quit date'. Unwanted effects include anxiety, headache, insomnia and dry mouth. There is an increased risk of epileptic seizures, and bupropion should be avoided if there is a history of fits.

Psychotomimetic agents

Hallucinogens

Lysergic acid diethylamide (LSD), psilocybin ('magic mushrooms'), mescaline (from peyote cactus) and the synthetic drug dimethyltryptamine (DMT) are adrenergic hallucinogenics that have structural similarities to monoamine neurotransmitters. They share several properties, including cross-tolerance.

Mechanism of action and effects

The actions of hallucinogens on the brain are probably related to postsynaptic $5HT_2$ receptor stimulation in the cerebral cortex and locus ceruleus, a region of the midbrain that receives sensory signals. LSD also produces presynaptic $5HT_{1A}$ receptor blockade in the dorsal raphe neurons, inhibiting firing of neuronal projections to the forebrain. Tolerance to LSD occurs rapidly, and appears to be related to downregulation of these receptors. The actions of LSD, psilocybin and mescaline are similar. LSD is the most potent hallucinogen.

- Visual hallucinations are frequent, especially with high doses, and auditory acuity is accentuated. There may be an overlap of sensory impressions so that music is 'seen' or colours 'heard', which can produce severe anxiety. Time appears to pass slowly. Emotions are altered, with either elation or depression, and rapid mood swings can occur. The overall experience can produce a 'good' or a 'bad' trip, and can vary in the same individual on different occasions.
- Serious psychotic reactions can occasionally occur, and long-term psychotic disorders can be precipitated. The other unpleasant persistent effect in some individuals is 'flashback', seeing bright flashes, or haloes or trails attached to moving objects.
- Physical consequences of CNS stimulation include dizziness, weakness, drowsiness and paraesthesiae.
- Excessive sympathetic nervous system stimulation with large doses produces nausea, salivation, lacrimation, dizziness, mydriasis, tremor, hyperthermia, tachycardia and hypertension.
- Tolerance can occur within 5 days.
- Emotional dependence is frequent but physical dependence is not seen.

Pharmacokinetics

Oral absorption of these drugs is good. Physical effects begin after about 20 minutes, but psychoactive effects are delayed for 2–4 hours and then last up to 12 hours. DMT has a rapid onset of hallucinogenic action in 15–30 minutes, but the duration is only 1–2 hours. Elimination is by hepatic metabolism, and the half-lives are short.

Cannabis

Cannabis can be smoked as marijuana, which consists of dried leaves or flowers of the *Cannabis sativa* (hemp) plant, or as resin extracted from the leaves of the plant and then dried, known as hashish. Solvent extraction of the resin produces cannabis oil, which can be added to tobacco. The hallucinogenic effects of cannabis are much less marked than those of the adrenergic hallucinogens.

Mechanism of action and effects

The constituent compounds (cannabinoids) interact with specific CB_1 receptors in the brain. These receptors, coupled to G_i proteins that reduce intracellular cAMP production, and inhibit cell membrane calcium and potassium channels, have a natural ligand called anandamide (an arachidonic acid derivative). The receptors are found in greatest density in areas of the brain involved in cognition and pain recognition (cerebral cortex), memory (hippocampus), reward (mesolimbic system), and motor coordination (substantia nigra and cerebellum).

- The psychomotor effects result largely from the cannabinoid tetrahydrocannabinol (THC) and one of its metabolites 11-hydroxy-THC, which produce euphoria, heightened intensity of sensations, and relaxation. Occasionally panic reactions, hallucinations and depersonalization occur. Psychotic reactions are rare except in predisposed individuals. Recent memory is markedly impaired and complex mental tests are less well executed, although the user may perceive that their performance is enhanced. Motor incoordination may affect driving ability.
- Effects on the cardiovascular system include tachycardia and increased systolic blood pressure with a postural fall.
- The tars inhaled during chronic use predispose to heart disease, chronic bronchitis and lung cancer.
- THC has an anti-emetic action.
- Tolerance to the psychomotor effects of cannabis occurs with regular use, but it is not addictive.

Pharmacokinetics
Metabolism of THC is extensive, with some active metabolites being produced. The high lipid solubility of THC means that absorption from the lung or gut is high, with a large volume of distribution and a correspondingly long half-life. The psychomotor effects, however, only last 2–3 hours after inhalation.

Dissociative anaesthetics
Phencyclidine (PCP) and ketamine differ from adrenergic hallucinogens in their mode of action. Both drugs were developed as anaesthetics, but PCP was wthdrawn because of adverse effects.

Mechanism of action and effects
Both drugs block the excitatory effects of glutamate, an excitatory neurotransmitter, at NMDA (N-methyl-D-aspartate) receptors. These receptors are abundant in the cortex, basal ganglia and sensory pathways of the CNS. PCP also releases dopamine from nerve terminals in a similar manner to amphetamine. The term dissociative anaesthetic refers to the feelings of detachment (dissociation) from the environment and self produced by the drugs. These are not true hallucinations.

- Acute effects include euphoria, decreased inhibition, a feeling of immense power, analgesia and altered perception of time and space and depersonalization. Ketamine creates a 'mellow, colourful wonderworld'.
- Catatonic rigidity can occur, followed by ataxia and slurring of speech.
- Adverse experiences include confusion, restlesness, disorientation and impaired judgement. Irritability, paranoia,

depression and anxiety are also common. Psychotic reactions are precipitated in susceptible people.
- Ketamine can produce near death experiences.
- Persistent abuse of PCP leads to memory loss, speech and thought difficulties, and depression that persist for months after the last use.
- Tolerance is unusual, but psychological dependance occurs.

Pharmacokinetics
PCP is rapidly absorbed from the gut, nose or lungs after smoking. Effects are seen within minutes of ingestion and usually last 4–6 hours. It is a weak base that is excreted in the urine. It is also excreted into the stomach, and reabsorbed by the small intestine. The half-life is very long at 2–3 days. Ketamine is used intravenously. It is metabolized in the liver and has a short half-life.

CNS depressants
Benzodiazepines
Examples include diazepam and temazepam.

Mechanism of action and effects
Benzodiazepines bind to specific regulatory sites that are closely linked to the $GABA_A$ receptor. When a benzodiazepine binds to its receptor, it induces a conformational change that enhances affinity of the receptor for the inhibitory neurotransmitter GABA. GABA promotes influx of Cl^- into the cell, leading to membrane hyperpolarization and decreased cell excitability. Benzodiazepines act only in the presence of GABA to enhance GABA-mediated opening of the ion channel; they have no direct action on the channel (Fig. 16.2.1). The consequent increased inhibitory neurotransmission produces the following effects:

- sedation, because of reduced sensory input to the reticular activating system
- sleep induction at high concentrations of drug
- anxiolysis as a consequence of actions on the limbic system and hypothalamus
- anticonvulsant activity.

Benzodiazepines have several undesirable effects:

- drowsiness, which may cause problems with driving or operating machinery
- confusional states (more common in the elderly)
- impaired memory
- incoordination or ataxia
- potentiation of the sedative effects by other CNS depressant drugs, for example alcohol
- tolerance and dependence.

Tolerance.   Tolerance to the effects of benzodiazepines is common. Hypnotic effects are lost quite early but the rebound insomnia on withdrawal can perpetuate benzodiazepine use.

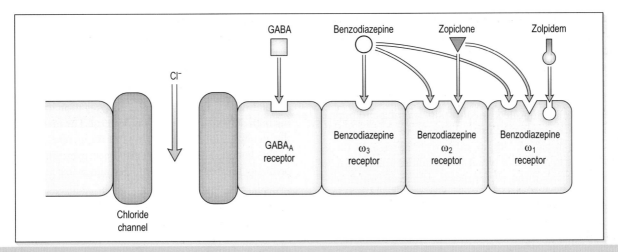

Figure 16.2.1.   Subtypes of benzodiazepine receptors (ω_{1-3}) modulate the activity of the gamma-aminobutyric acid (GABA) type A receptor, which facilitates the opening of Cl^- channels. Compounds such as zolpidem are thought to act selectively on the ω_1 subtype of the benzodiazepine receptor and this may explain why it lacks anticonvulsant and muscle relaxant activity. Barbiturates have similar effects on the Cl^- channel but act by modulating the channel rather than the benzodiazepine receptor.

Dependence.   Dependence with physical and psychological withdrawal symptoms is frequent during long-term use. The risk is highest in individuals with personality disorders or a previous history of dependence on alcohol or drugs, and more likely to occur if high doses of benzodiazepine are used. Restricting their use to a maximum of 4 weeks will minimize the risk of dependence. With long-acting drugs, withdrawal symptoms may be delayed by up to 3 weeks. Anxiety is the most frequent symptom and can take up to a month to resolve. Insomnia, depression or abnormalities of perception such as altered sensitivity to noise, light or touch also occur. More severe reactions include toxic psychosis or convulsions. Gradual withdrawal of a benzodiazepine over 4 to 8 weeks is desirable after long-term use although complete withdrawal may take up to a year. Lorazepam is a potent benzodiazepine with a relatively short action that proves particularly difficult to stop because of the intensity of withdrawal symptoms, which arise a few hours after withdrawal. Substitution by the longer-acting drug diazepam may be helpful before withdrawal is attempted. There are no proven treatments for reducing symptoms associated with withdrawal, but beta-blockers and sedative tricyclic antidepressants such as amitriptyline have been used.

Pharmacokinetics

Most benzodiazepines are well absorbed from the gut. Many, including diazepam, are subsequently metabolized in the liver to active compounds that contribute to a prolonged duration of action through relatively slow elimination from the body. Metabolism of some benzodiazepines, for example temazepam, produces inactive derivatives. Hypnotic benzodiazepines, such as temazepam, are rapidly absorbed and

Table 16.2.1.   Possible mechanisms of action of alcohol

Inhibition of monoamine oxidase B in neurons
Inhibition of Na^+/K^+-ATPase in neuronal membranes
Increased neuronal adenylate cyclase activity
Decreased intracellular phosphatidylinositol system activity, leading to reduced Ca^{2+} availability
Enhanced opioid δ-receptor activation

their lipid solubility ensures ready penetration into the brain. This produces a fast onset of sedation, then sleep. A brief duration of action is desirable to avoid hangover sedation in the morning; this can be achieved if the drug is inactivated in the liver (e.g. temazepam). Repeated dosing, particularly with long-acting compounds such as diazepam, increases the risk of accumulation with a prolonged sedative effect.

Diazepam and some other benzodiazepines can be given by intravenous injection for rapid onset of effect. Diazepam is available in solution for rectal administration.

Flumazenil is a selective antagonist at benzodiazepine receptors, and can be used to reverse the effects of acute overdosage.

Alcohol (ethyl alcohol, ethanol)

Mechanism of action and effects

Alcohol has multiple actions on the CNS. Non-specific actions such as increased fluidity of neuronal cell membranes (cf. general anaesthetics) may be important by reducing Ca^{2+} flux across the cell membrane, but several other actions have been described (Table 16.2.1). Overall, alcohol facilitates central inhibitory neurotransmission, particularly enhancing the effects of gamma-aminobutyric acid (GABA), and is therefore a general CNS depressant. There is an initial depression of inhibitory neurons, particularly in the mesolimbic system, which produces a sense of relaxation, but this is followed by progressive depression of all CNS functions. Mental processes that are modifed by education, training and previous experience are affected first, while relatively 'mechanical' tasks are less impaired. Despite subjective impressions, there is no increase in mental or physical capabilities unless anxiety had previously reduced performance. All effects are closely related to blood alcohol concentration (Table 16.2.2). In chronic alcoholics, tolerance to many of the psychological effects of alcohol is seen. Alcohol intake is usually measured in units (Table 16.2.3).

Table 16.2.2. The effects of alcohol at various plasma concentrations

Plasma concentration (mg/100 ml)	Effects
30	Mild euphoria owing to suppression of inhibitory pathways in the cortex; the individual is more talkative, emotionally labile with loss of self-control; the risk of accidental injury is increased
80	The legal limit for driving in the UK; the risk of serious injury in a road accident is more than doubled
100–200	Speech becomes slurred and motor coordination is impaired
>300	Often produces loss of consciousness
>400	Frequently fatal as a result of respiratory and vasomotor centre depression

Table 16.2.3. Alcohol content of alcoholic drinks

1 unit alcohol is about 10 g and is found in:

½ pint of beer, lager, cider
1½ pints low-alcohol beer, lager, cider
⅓ pint strong beer, lager, cider
⅕ pint extra strong beer, lager, cider
1 glass of wine (8 units per 75 cl bottle)
1 small measure of sherry (13 units per bottle)
1 standard measure of spirits (30 units per bottle)
⅔ bottle of 'alcopop'

Other effects of alcohol

Alcohol has a range of effects.

Cardiovascular effects

- A modest alcohol intake may have protective effects on the circulation, by inhibiting platelet aggregation and increasing high density lipoprotein cholesterol. The form in which the alcohol is taken is probably not important. The extent of this beneficial effect may have been overestimated; it is probably greatest at 1 unit per day and is lost when intake exceeds 3–4 units per day.
- Higher intake of alcohol has pressor effects that raise blood pressure, possibly through increased vascular sensitivity to catecholamines. This increases the risk of coronary artery disease and stroke.
- Cardiac arrhythmias can be provoked by high alcohol intake, particularly atrial fibrillation. This can occur after an alcoholic binge ('holiday heart') or following more chronic abuse.
- Alcoholic cardiomyopathy is a dilated cardiomyopathy that is only partially reversible with abstinence, and can lead to heart failure. An average intake of 10 units alcohol daily for 8–10 years can produce this condition.

Liver

- Hypoglycaemia occurs as a consequence of the metabolism of alcohol in the liver. The metabolic process generates excess protons, which encourages the conversion of glucose via pyruvate to lactate and predisposes to lactic acidosis. Alcoholics often have a low-carbohydrate diet, which compounds the hypoglycaemia. Hypoglycaemia tends to occur several hours after heavy alcohol intake and can contribute to convulsions on alcohol withdrawal.
- The lactic acidosis created by alcohol metabolism in the liver impairs the renal excretion of uric acid, which predisposes to gout.
- Lactic acidosis also facilitates synthesis of saturated fatty acids, which accumulate in the liver, leading to a fatty liver, possibly with altered liver function. Plasma triglycerides are also increased.
- Alcoholic hepatitis is usually a consequence of short-term heavy alcohol abuse. It can be fatal.
- Cirrhosis occurs with prolonged alcohol abuse, but individual susceptibility varies widely. On average, consumption of more than 8 units per day for at least 10 years is required for cirrhosis to occur in men. About two-thirds of this amount creates the same risk for women. Established cirrhosis reduces the first-pass metabolism and clearance of drugs eliminated by the liver.
- Chronic intake of alcohol induces several hepatic drug-metabolizing enzymes from the cytochrome P450 family, which decreases the effectiveness of some therapeutic drugs, for example warfarin, phenytoin and carbamazepine.

Other gastrointestinal consequences
- Erosive gastritis can occur as a result of stimulation of gastric secretions.
- Pancreatitis is probably caused by raised triglycerides or by pancreatic duct obstruction by proteinaceous secretions induced by alcohol.

Sexual function
- Sexual desire is often increased by alcohol, but the ability to sustain penile erection is reduced, possibly because of the vasodilator actions of alcohol.
- Direct damage to the Leydig cells of the testis reduces the circulating testosterone, leading to reduced libido, infertility and a loss of the male distribution of body hair. Altered steroid metabolism in the liver leads to an increase in circulating oestrone in males, which causes gynaecomastia.

Neuropsychiatric effects
- A combination of alcohol toxicity with vitamin B_6 and thiamine deficiency in the diet of alcoholics predisposes to peripheral neuropathy and dementia. Specific mid-brain damage can result and produces the syndromes of Wernicke's encephalopathy and Korsakoff's psychosis.
- Alcohol has anticonvulsant properties and withdrawal predisposes to convulsions, even in individuals without a history of epilepsy.
- Alcohol can disturb sleep patterns, with decreased REM (rapid eye movement) sleep and increased stage 4 sleep during intoxication. Withdrawal increases REM sleep with associated nightmares.
- Dose-related memory impairment can be caused by suppressed hippocampal function.
- Subdural haematoma is more common after head injury in heavy drinkers, perhaps as a consequence of cerebral atrophy.

- Depression or anxiety states are more common in heavy drinkers.

Carcinogenesis and teratogenesis
- Cancer of the mouth, oesophagus and liver are more common with heavy alcohol use. Colon and breast cancer may also be increased.
- The fetal alcohol syndrome is believed to be caused by the effects of alcohol on neuronal adhesion molecules that regulate neuronal migration. Heavy maternal drinking during pregnancy leads to impaired learning and memory in the child. Genetic factors may be involved in the susceptibility of the fetus to these problems.

Pharmacokinetics

Although ethanol is absorbed from the stomach, the majority is absorbed from the small intestine, due to its larger surface area. High concentrations of alcohol (above 20%) and large volumes inhibit gastric emptying and delay absorption, as do foods high in fat or carbohydrate. Peak blood alcohol concentrations, therefore, depend on the dose and strength of the alcohol and on whether or not it was taken with food. Once absorbed, alcohol undergoes substantial first-pass metabolism in the liver. Distribution of alcohol is fairly uniform and the ready passage across the blood–brain barrier and high cerebral blood flow ensure rapid access to the CNS. The effects on the brain are more marked when the concentration is rising, indicating a degree of acute tolerance.

Metabolism occurs mainly in the liver (Fig. 16.2.2), more than 90% being oxidized, while the rest is removed unchanged in expired air in close proportion to the blood concentration (the basis of the alcohol breath test) or the urine. Alcohol metabolism shows saturation kinetics due to the limited supply of nicotine adenine nucleotide (NAD^+) cofactor for the

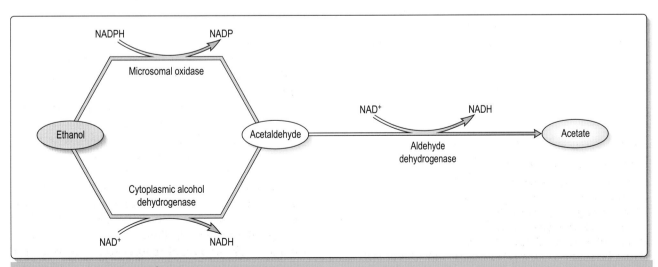

Figure 16.2.2. The metabolism of alcohol. Alcohol dehydrogenase is responsible for 80–90% of the metabolism of ethanol.

oxidative process. The maximum rate of alcohol metabolism averages 8 g per hour. The extent of first-pass metabolism of alcohol is related to the speed of absorption; thus with slower absorption, such as when alcohol is taken with food, less alcohol will reach the systemic circulation. The initial metabolic reaction is mediated by alcohol dehydrogenase, producing acetaldehyde. This is further metabolized by aldehyde dehydrogenase to acetic acid (Fig. 16.2.2). Accumulation of acetaldehyde in the circulation is responsible for many of the unpleasant effects of a hangover.

Small amounts of alcohol are metabolized via the microsomal ethanol oxidizing system (CYP2E1), the activity of which is increased by enzyme inducers such as alcohol itself (which does not affect the activity of alcohol dehydrogenase).

Some drugs, such as metronidazole and chlorpropamide, inhibit aldehyde dehydrogenase, leading to acetaldehyde accumulation if alcohol is taken with them. Typical 'hangover' effects of flushing, sweating, headache and nausea then occur after small amounts of alcohol. Genetic deficiencies in alcohol and aldehyde dehydrogenases occur particularly among Asians, leading to low levels of alcohol or aldehyde metabolism.

Alcohol abuse and dependence

There are no reliable estimates of the number of people in the UK with alcohol-related problems although it has been suggested that 1–2% of the population are affected. The distribution curve for alcohol consumption is continuous but skewed at the upper end; the risk of alcohol-related problems rises with the average alcohol intake. Up to 30% of hospital admissions are for alcohol-related problems, although the contribution of heavy drinking is often unrecognized. Screening for alcohol abuse can be carried out by obtaining a complete history of alcohol intake and, if necessary, using the CAGE questions (Table 16.2.4). Abnormal measurements of both the mean corpuscular volume (MCV) of red cells (which is raised with increasing alcohol intake because of an effect of alcohol on the cell membrane) and the liver enzyme γ-glutamyl transpeptidase (γGT) will identify about 75% of people with an alcohol problem.

Psychological dependence on alcohol is common but physical dependence also occurs. Withdrawal symptoms occur 6–24 hours after the last drink in dependent persons. If mild, these are related to autonomic hyperactivity and include

anxiety, agitation, tremor, sweating, anorexia, nausea and retching. Convulsions can occur through neuronal excitation. Insomnia, tachycardia and hypertension are common with more severe withdrawal reactions. The most severe form of withdrawal is *delirium tremens*, with confusion, paranoia, visual and tactile hallucinations. Delirium tremens can cause death from respiratory and cardiovascular collapse.

If an individual is drinking excessively, controlled drinking may be an option. However, if there is alcohol dependence or alcohol-related problems, then abstinence is usually preferable.

Controlled detoxification is usually undertaken with a sedative agent, such as a benzodiazepine, to attenuate withdrawal symptoms. Chlordiazepoxide is usually used, decreasing the dose over 7–10 days. Clomethiazole is sometimes used, but carries a greater risk of dependence. Clonidine (a presynaptic α2-adrenoceptor agonist at the vasomotor centre in the brain) can be useful, by reducing the excessive sympathetic stimulation that accompanies withdrawal. Beta-blockers may be helpful for the same reason. Multivitamin preparations containing an adequate amount of thiamine should be given for 1 month to prevent Wernicke's encephalopathy. Relapse is common after withdrawal from alcohol.

Two drugs are licensed in the UK to assist in the management of chronic alcoholism. Disulfiram, an inhibitor of acetaldehyde dehydrogenase, causes unpleasant hangover symptoms after small amounts of alcohol. Given alone, or with psychosocial rehabilitation, it can help to maintain abstinence. Acamprosate inhibits the excitatory amino acid glutamate by antagonism at the NMDA receptor, although several other contributory effects have been suggested. It has few unwanted effects, is non-addictive and can be used to reduce craving for alcohol.

Opioid analgesics

Examples include morphine, diamorphine (heroin), buprenorphine, pethidine, codeine, pentazocine and fentanyl.

Opioid is a term used for both naturally occurring and synthetic molecules that produce their effects by combining with opioid receptors. Use of the term opiate analgesics (specifically drugs derived from the juice of the opium poppy, *Papaver somniferum*) or narcotic analgesics (which literally means a 'stupor-inducing pain killer') is no longer preferred.

Mechanism of action

The brain produces several neuropeptides known as opioid peptides, which act as neurotransmitters via specific opioid receptors. Among these are the pentapeptide enkephalins: these contain the amino acid sequence Tyr-Gly-Gly-Phe linked to either leucine or methionine and are called leu- and met-enkephalin. A third compound is dynorphin, but the most potent is β-endorphin ('endogenous morphine'), a 31

Table 16.2.4. The CAGE questionnaire for alcoholism

Have you ever felt you could **C**ut down on your drinking?
Have people **A**nnoyed you by criticizing your drinking?
Have you ever felt bad or **G**uilty about your drinking?
Have you ever had a drink first thing in the morning to steady your nerves or get rid of a hangover (**E**ye-opener)?

A score of yes to one question or more should lead to further evaluation of the patient for alcoholism.

amino acid peptide with met-enkephalin at its carboxyl end. Opioid peptides are formed from larger precursor peptides.

There is a distinctive regional distribution of opioid peptides in the CNS with high concentrations in the limbic system and spinal cord, a distribution similar to that for opioid receptors. These regions also contain high concentrations of a neutral endopeptidase (enkephalinase), which rapidly hydrolyses the pentapeptides into fragments.

Morphine and related analgesics produce their effects by acting at specific opioid receptors in the CNS. Three major classes of opioid receptor have been identified that mediate distinct effects (Table 16.2.5). Opioid receptors are coupled to inhibitory G-proteins; stimulation reduces the intracellular generation of cAMP by adenylate cyclase. The G-proteins are also directly coupled to K^+ channels. When these channels in the pain pathways are opened, neurons become hyperpolarized. The resultant inhibition of voltage-gated Ca^{2+} channels in the presynaptic neurons reduces neurotransmitter release. In the periaqueductal grey matter of the brain, opioids enhance descending inhibitory serotonergic neuronal activity to the substantia gelatinosa of the dorsal horn. This is achieved by suppression of activity in inhibitory interneurons. At the spinal level, analgesia results from inhibition of the release of the pain pathway mediator, substance P, from dorsal horn afferent neurons. This is due to presynaptic inhibition of neurotransmitter release in the afferent nociceptive fibres. Opioids also reduce the sensitivity of peripheral nociceptive neurons to pain stimuli, particularly in inflamed tissues.

The various endogenous opioid peptides show preferential receptor-binding affinities, for example, β-endorphin binds equally to μ- δ- and κ-receptors, dynorphin binds mainly to k-receptors and the enkephalins bind mainly to δ-receptors. Opioid drugs also show receptor selectivity and can have agonist, partial agonist or antagonist properties.

- Pure agonists: these act principally at the μ-receptors and include morphine, diamorphine, pethidine (meperidine), methadone, codeine and dextropropoxyphene. Apart from methadone, they also have weak agonist activity at δ- and κ-receptors.
- Mixed agonist–antagonist: pentazocine has agonist effects at the κ-receptor (and to a lesser extent the δ-receptor) and is a weak μ-receptor antagonist.
- Mixed partial agonist–antagonist: buprenorphine is a potent partial agonist at the μ-receptor and has antagonist activity at κ-receptors.
- Opioids with additional properties; for example meptazinol is a μ-receptor agonist with muscarinic receptor agonist activity, while tramadol is a μ-receptor agonist that also inhibits neuronal noradrenaline and 5-hydroxytryptamine (5HT) reuptake. Enhanced amine-mediated neurotransmission potentiates descending inhibitory pain pathways.

Effects and unwanted effects

Analgesia. The paleospinothalamic pathway and limbic system are rich in opioid receptors; therefore, the analgesia produced by morphine is most effective for chronic visceral pain. In addition to its antinociceptive effect, morphine alters the perception of pain making it less unpleasant. Opioids have no anti-inflammatory effect and morphine can even release the inflammatory mediator histamine locally at the site of an injection. Analgesia produced by morphine is often associated with an elevated sense of well-being (euphoria, mediated by μ-receptors) whereas opioid administration to a pain-free subject can produce the opposite effect (dysphoria, mediated by κ-receptors). Pure μ-receptor agonists are the most powerful opioid analgesics. However, some pure μ-receptor agonists have a low affinity for the receptor (e.g. dextropropoxyphene) or unwanted effects prevent the use of high doses (e.g. codeine). The ceiling effect of partial agonists is lower. If a person receiving high doses of a potent pure μ-receptor antagonist is given a μ-receptor partial agonist (e.g. buprenorphine) or a μ-receptor antagonist (e.g. pentazocine) then some of the pure agonist molecules will be displaced from receptor sites by the less effective molecules, and in dependent individuals withdrawal symptoms can be produced (see below).

Respiratory depression. The sensitivity of the respiratory centre to stimulation by carbon dioxide is reduced by morphine, which decreases respiratory drive. Respiratory paralysis is a common cause of death in opioid overdose. Meptazinol and tramadol are claimed to cause less respiratory depression than other opioids.

Suppression of the cough centre. Opioids possess an antitussive action although the mechanism is unclear. Compounds such as codeine and dextromethorphan are highly effective for cough suppression despite having relatively weak analgesic effects.

Table 16.2.5. Effects of opioid receptors

Mu (μ)
  Analgesia (supraspinal $μ_1$, spinal $μ_2$)
  Respiratory ($μ_2$)
  Euphoria
  Miosis
  Physical dependence
  Sedation
Kappa (κ)
  Analgesia (spinal)
  Sedation
  Miosis
  Dysphoria
Delta (δ)
  Analgesia (spinal)
  Respiratory depression

CNS excitation

Vomiting. Opioids stimulate the chemoreceptor trigger zone. Emesis is more common in ambulatory individuals, but tolerance can occur.

Miosis. Stimulation of the third nerve nucleus results in pupillary constriction. Pinpoint pupils, together with coma and slow respiration, are signs of opioid overdose.

Peripheral effects

Gastrointestinal tract. There is a general increase in resting tone of the gut wall and sphincters, but a decrease in propulsive activity. Thus opioid administration is associated with constipation. Pethidine has less activity in the gastro-intestinal tract than equi-analgesic doses of morphine. The effects of morphine on the gut are largely a result of hyper-polarization of cells in the myenteric plexus, but there is some additional central action.

Cardiovascular and respiratory systems. Opioids have limited effects on the circulation and lungs; hypotension and bronchoconstriction can occur with morphine, possibly because of histamine release.

Other systems. Opioids have minor effects on other systems; for example, there is an increase in tone of the bladder wall and sphincter, which can lead to urinary retention. Changes in the release of some pituitary hormones may be mediated via inter-ference with the actions of opioid peptide hormones.

Tolerance and dependence

Tolerance results from changes in the functioning of opioid receptors during continuous opioid administration. In response to the inhibitory effects of morphine on intracellular cAMP generation, there is increased synthesis of stimulatory G-proteins and adenylate cyclase in an attempt to restore homeostasis. Therefore, more drug is necessary to produce the same effect.

Tolerance is associated with increased firing of neurons in the noradrenergic pathways of the locus ceruleus, which is rich in inhibitory opioid receptors. Dependence may be in part caused by effects on opioid neurons radiating from this region to the ventral tegmental area. The dopaminergic pathway projecting from the ventral tegmental area to the nucleus accumbens is believed to be involved in the euphoria of opioid administration.

Tolerance occurs rapidly during chronic opioid administration, despite constant plasma drug concentrations. Tolerance develops to analgesia, euphoria, respiratory depression and emesis but much less to the constipatory effects or miosis. A high degree of cross-tolerance is shown by many opioids; consequently, individuals who develop tolerance to one opioid will usually be tolerant to another. However, not all opioids show cross-tolerance. The non-uniform nature of tolerance and cross-tolerance may be a result of the multi-plicity of opioid receptors.

Dependence manifests itself as a withdrawal syndrome, which can be precipitated when individuals who are abusing the drug have their intake stopped or are given an opioid antagonist or partial agonist. The withdrawal effects during the first 12 hours, such as nervousness, sweating and craving, are largely psychological since they can be alleviated by the administration of a placebo. Following this period the effects of physiological dependence manifest themselves, for example dilated pupils, anorexia, weakness, depression, insomnia, gastrointestinal and skeletal muscle cramps, increased respiratory rate, pyrexia, piloerection with goose-pimples and diarrhoea. The time course for the development and loss of these symptoms varies among the opioids. In the case of morphine, the maximum withdrawal effects occur quickly (about 1–2 days) and subside rapidly (about 5–10 days) but the intensity of the symptoms may be intolerable.

By contrast, withdrawal from methadone is a slow process because of its very long half-life, but the effects are far less intense (peak effect at almost 1 week and symptoms persist for about 3 weeks). Therefore, morphine- or heroin-dependent subjects are often transferred from their drug of abuse to methadone prior to withdrawal. Methadone also promotes tolerance, and therefore produces less euphoria than morphine or heroin. After a period of chronic treatment with methadone, the methadone dosage is gradually reduced and the person undergoes a more tolerable withdrawal.

More recently, buprenorphine has been used as an alternative to methadone, due to the low severity of withdrawal symptoms. It can be given for a 6-day rapid detoxification, but long-term maintenance has shown promise for reducing relapse. Buprenorphine blocks the 'high' from illicit opioid use. Combined with high intensity psychosocial group therapy treatment, up to 75% success rate has been reported after 1 year.

Rapid in-hospital tapering of opioids over 2 weeks has an 80% success rate; as an outpatient, slow tapering over 6 months is more successful, but still only leads to a 40% withdrawal rate. Detoxification from opioids can also be helped by the presynaptic α_2-adrenoceptor agonists clonidine or lofexidine (a clonidine analogue with fewer unwanted effects). This inhibits the excessive sympathetic nervous system activity associated with opioid withdrawal. Lacrimation, rhinorrhoea, muscle pain, joint pain and gastrointestinal symptoms are all reduced by clonidine or lofexidine. By contrast, lethargy, insomnia and restlessness persist despite treatment.

Pharmacokinetics of individual agents

Opioids can be given by intravenous or intramuscular injection, by subcutaneous infusion, or orally. Morphine can also be given as a suppository, while buprenorphine is formulated for buccal absorption. Other opioids such as fentanyl or tramadol can be delivered transdermally. Some opioids (e.g. morphine, pethidine, pentazocine) show a low and variable absorption from the gut. Diamorphine is a prodrug that is rapidly hydrolysed in the circulation to morphine. Opioids undergo hepatic metabolism, although some are also excreted renally. Most opioids have short or intermediate half-lives. Fentanyl has a short half-life, but its effects persist for several hours after removing the transdermal patch owing to build-up of a subcutaneous drug reservoir.

ANDROGENS AND ANABOLIC STEROIDS

Androgens

Naturally occurring androgens are 19-carbon steroids synthesized in the adrenal cortex and gonads. They have characteristic actions on the reproductive tract and other tissues as well as an anabolic effect on metabolism. A number of synthetic androgenic steroids have been developed. When the predominant action of these molecules is anabolic rather than on reproductive tissues the substance is described as an 'anabolic steroid'. Although there are a few medical uses for such compounds, they have achieved notoriety because of their abuse by athletes to enhance muscle development.

Testosterone is the most powerful and major androgen secreted by the Leydig cells of the testis in response to the gonadotrophin luteinizing hormone. The adrenal cortex, stimulated by ACTH, releases a greater proportion of dehydroepiandrosterone and androstenedione (Fig. 16.2.3).

Testosterone

Actions of testosterone

The actions of testosterone are in part due to its metabolite dihydrotestosterone. The latter is produced in the prostate, skin and reproductive tissues by the action of the enzyme 5α-reductase. Dihydrotestosterone has a higher affinity for the androgen receptor than testosterone. Actions include:

- Sexual differentiation in the fetus.
- Sexual development of the male testis, penis, epididymis, seminal vesicles and prostate at puberty, and maintenance of these tissues in the adult.
- Spermatogenesis in the adult.
- Stimulation and maintenance of sexual function and behaviour.
- Metabolic actions. Testosterone is a powerful anabolic agent producing a positive nitrogen balance with an increase in the bulk of tissues such as muscle and bone. In the skin sebum production is increased, which can provoke acne. Growth of axillary, pubic, facial and chest hair is stimulated. In the liver, testosterone increases the synthesis of several proteins including clotting factors, but decreases high-density lipoprotein (HDL) synthesis. Testosterone also induces several liver enzymes including steroid hydroxylases.
- Haematological actions. Testosterone stimulates production of erythropoietin by the kidneys leading to a higher haemoglobin concentration in men than women.

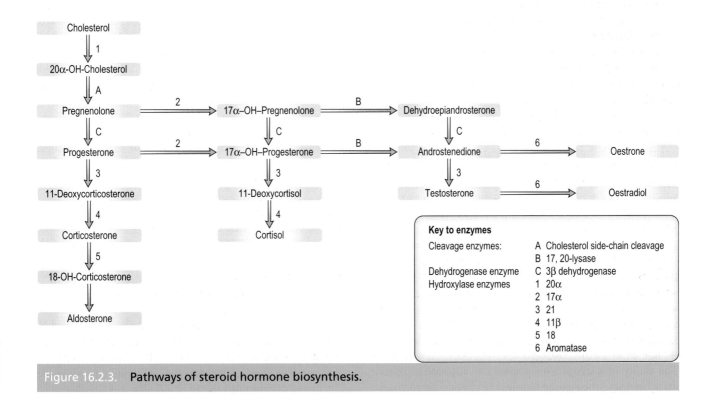

Figure 16.2.3. Pathways of steroid hormone biosynthesis.

Pharmacokinetics

Oral preparations. Testosterone is well absorbed from the gut but is almost completely degraded by first-pass metabolism in the gut wall and liver. Esterification to form $17-\beta$ hydroxyl derivatives creates a hydrophobic compound. Of these, testosterone undecanoate is absorbed via lacteals into the lymphatic system, thus avoiding hepatic metabolism. It can, therefore, be given orally.

Testosterone esters for depot injection. The most popular form of replacement therapy for hypogonadal men is a regular intramuscular injection of a testosterone ester in oily solution. Testosterone is absorbed gradually after ester hydrolysis at the site of injection. Examples include testosterone enanthate and testosterone propionate.

Transdermal delivery. A patch containing testosterone can be used to treat hypogonadism. It is usually applied to the back, abdomen, upper arm or thigh, rotating the site daily to avoid skin irritation.

Subcutaneous implant. A pellet of crystalline testosterone provides a reservoir for gradual absorption of testosterone into the systemic circulation for up to 4 months. A minor surgical procedure is necessary, and therefore this method of delivery is rarely used.

Circulating androgens are bound largely to a specific transport protein, sex hormone binding globulin (SHBG), which has a greater affinity for androgens than for oestrogen.

Unwanted effects

- Conversion to oestrogens by aromatase results in gynaecomastia in some patients (Fig. 16.2.3).
- Suppression of gonadotrophin release with diminished testis size and reduced spermatogenesis.
- Increased risk of prostate cancer.
- Cholestatic jaundice.

Anabolic steroids

Examples include nandrolone and stanozolol.

Anabolic steroids are most frequently encountered as drugs of abuse to improve athletic performance. In medical practice there are few indications for these compounds with little evidence for efficacy. Stanozolol is given orally and nandrolone as an ester by intramuscular injections in a depot formulation.

Unwanted effects

- Androgenic effects may be troublesome in women.
- Stanozolol can cause cholestatic jaundice and liver tumours after long-term use.

Abuse of anabolic steroids

The ability of androgens to promote an increase in muscle mass has led to their abuse to improve physical performance by athletes, weightlifters and bodybuilders. Often several different androgens are used for prolonged periods, perhaps with a brief 'drug-free' period. Abused compounds include testosterone, nandrolone, stanozolol and others licensed only for veterinary use. The consequences of abuse include:

- weight gain from muscle hypertrophy and fluid retention
- acne in adolescent and young men
- decreased testicular size and reduced sperm count
- hepatotoxicity with cholestasis, hepatitis or occasionally hepatocellular tumours
- atherogenic changes in the plasma lipids with a rise in plasma LDL cholesterol and a fall in HDL cholesterol; this may predispose to premature vascular disease
- psychological disturbance including changes in libido, increased aggression and psychotic symptoms.

REFERENCES AND FURTHER READING

Ashworth M, Gerada C (1997) Addiction and dependence – II: alcohol. BMJ 315: 358–360.

Bagatell CJ, Bremner WJ (1996) Androgens in men – uses and abuses. N Engl J Med 334: 707–714.

Balfour D, Benowitz N, Fagerström K, et al. (2000) Diagnosis and treatment of nicotine dependence with emphasis on nicotine replacement therapy. Eur Heart J 21: 438–445.

Barlecchi CE, MacKenzie TD, Schrier RW (1994) The human cost of tobacco. N Engl J Med 330: 907–912, 975–980.

Cherny NI (1996) Opioid analgesics. Drugs 51: 713–737.

Davis RM (1997) Passive smoking: history repeats itself. BMJ 315: 961–962.

Garbutt JC, West SL, Carey TS, et al. (1999) Pharmacological treatment of alcohol dependence. JAMA 281: 1318–1325.

Gerada C, Ashworth M (1997) Addiction and dependence. I: Illicit drugs. BMJ 315: 297–299.

Gonzalez G, Oliveto A, Kosten TR (2002) Treatment of heroin (diamorphine) addiction. Drugs 62: 1331–1343.

Hall W, Solowij N (1998) Adverse effects of cannabis. Lancet 352: 1611–1616.

Hall W, Zador D (1997) The alcohol withdrawal syndrome. Lancet 349: 1897–1900.

Leshner AI (1996) Molecular mechanism of cocaine addiction. N Engl J Med 335: 128–129.

Mendelson JH, Mello NK (1996) Management of cocaine abuse and dependence. N Engl J Med 334: 965–972.

O'Connor PG, Schottenfeld RS (1996) Patients with alcohol problems. N Engl J Med 338: 592–602.

Raw M, McNeill A, West R (1999) Smoking cessation: evidence based recommendations for the health care system. BMJ 318: 182–185.

Rigotti A (2002) treatment of tobacco use and dependence. N Engl J Med 346: 506–512.

Schaffer A, Naranjo CA (1998) Recommended drug treatment strategies for the alcoholic patient. Drugs 56: 571–585.

Sutherland G (2002) Current approach to the management of smoking cessation. Drugs 62 (Suppl 2): 53–61.

Swift RM (1999) Drug therapy for alcohol dependence. N Engl J Med 340: 1482–1490.

Ward J, Hall W, Mattick RP (1999) Role of maintenance treatment in opioid dependence. Lancet 353: 221–226.

Index

Note: Abbreviations used are: BMD = bone mineral density; CNS = central nervous system; COPD = chronic obstructive pulmonary disease; ECF = extracellular fluid; NSAIDs = non-steroidal anti-inflammatory drugs.

Page numbers in **bold** refer to figures, those in *italics* to tables.